# Recent Progress in Veterinary Science

# Recent Progress in Veterinary Science

Editor: Peter Jones

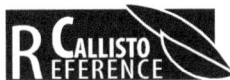

R CALLISTO REFERENCE

www.callistoreference.com

**Callisto Reference,**
118-35 Queens Blvd., Suite 400,
Forest Hills, NY 11375, USA

Visit us on the World Wide Web at:
www.callistoreference.com

ISBN: 978-1-64116-145-9 (Hardback)

**Cataloging-in-Publication Data**

Recent progress in veterinary science / edited by Peter Jones.
    p. cm.
Includes bibliographical references and index.
ISBN 978-1-64116-145-9
1. Veterinary medicine. 2. Animals--Diseases. 3. Animal health. I. Jones, Peter.
SF745 .R43 2019
636.089--dc23

# Table of Contents

# Preface

I am honored to present to you this unique book which encompasses the most up-to-date data in the field. I was extremely pleased to get this opportunity of editing the work of experts from across the globe. I have also written papers in this field and researched the various aspects revolving around the progress of the discipline. I have tried to unify my knowledge along with that of stalwarts from every corner of the world, to produce a text which not only benefits the readers but also facilitates the growth of the field.

Veterinary science is concerned with the prevention, diagnosis and treatment of animal diseases. Pets, livestock, lab animals, zoo animals and wild animals are all studied in veterinary science. It is also engaged in developing measures for animal welfare. Research in veterinary science explores interventions for the prevention and treatment of different diseases. It also includes research at human-animal interfaces such as zoonotic diseases, food safety, wildlife and ecosystem health. This book covers in detail some existing theories and innovative concepts revolving around veterinary science. Different approaches, evaluations, methodologies and advanced studies have been included herein. The topics covered in this book offer the readers new insights in this field.

Finally, I would like to thank all the contributing authors for their valuable time and contributions. This book would not have been possible without their efforts. I would also like to thank my friends and family for their constant support.

**Editor**

# Characterization of *Brucella abortus* mutant strain Δ22915, a potential vaccine candidate

Yanqing Bao[1], Mingxing Tian[1], Peng Li[1], Jiameng Liu[1], Chan Ding[1] and Shengqing Yu[1,2]*

## Abstract

*Brucellosis*, caused by *Brucella* spp., is an important zoonosis worldwide. Vaccination is an effective strategy for protection against *Brucella* infection in livestock in developing countries and in wildlife in developed countries. However, current vaccine strains including S19 and RB51 are pathogenic to humans and pregnant animals, limiting their use. In this study, we constructed the *Brucella abortus* (*B. abortus*) S2308 mutant strain Δ22915, in which the putative lytic transglycosylase gene *BAB_RS22915* was deleted. The biological properties of mutant strain Δ22915 were characterized and protection of mice against virulent S2308 challenge was evaluated. The mutant strain Δ22915 showed reduced survival within RAW264.7 cells and survival in vivo in mice. In addition, the mutant strain Δ22915 failed to escape fusion with lysosomes within host cells, and caused no observable pathological damage. RNA-seq analysis indicated that four genes associated with amino acid/nucleotide transport and metabolism were significantly upregulated in mutant strain Δ22915. Furthermore, inoculation of Δ22915 at $10^5$ colony forming units induced effective host immune responses and long-term protection of BALB/c mice. Therefore, mutant strain Δ22915 could be used as a novel vaccine candidate in the future to protect animals against *B. abortus* infection.

## Introduction

Brucellosis is a zoonotic disease epidemic in Asia, South and Central America, and sub-Saharan Africa [1]. It is caused by the genus *Brucella*, which infects millions of livestock and more than half a million people annually [2, 3]. Infection leads to reduction of animal productivity and debilitating disease in humans and causes economic losses and public health threats. Currently, vaccination of healthy animals is an effective strategy for protecting livestock from *Brucella* infection in developing countries and protecting wildlife in developed countries [4]. Vaccine strains such as S19, RB51 and Rev.1 have been extensively applied over the past decades with promising effects. These results stress the value of live attenuated vaccines. However, residue pathogenicity to humans and pregnant animals, and potential virulence reversion risks require the development of safer and better vaccines [5, 6].

Site-directed, unmarked deletion is an effective method for identifying virulence genes and constructing attenuated strains as *Brucella* vaccines. For example, acid shock protein 24 (*asp24*), ATP-binding/permease protein (*cydC*, a component of the cydDC operon), phosphoribosylamine-glycine ligase (*purD*), nitric oxide reductase activation protein (*norD*), high-affinity zinc uptake system (*zunA*), sigma factor (*rpoE1*, $\sigma^{E1}$) and teichoic acid ABC transporter ATP-binding protein (*BAB_RS18515*) are involved with *Brucella* virulence [7–13]. Deletion of these genes reduces *Brucella* virulence, but they maintain excellent immunogenicity to activate the host immune response. These mutants provide protection against wild-type, virulent *Brucella* challenge in mouse models [13–17], making them potential vaccine candidates.

In a previous study, we identified a series of genes associated with *B. abortus* S2308 virulence using miniTn5 transposon mutagenesis (unpublished data). One mutant with the gene *BAB_RS22915* interrupted by miniTn5 showed highly attenuated virulence in BALB/c mice. *BAB_RS22915* encodes a putative lytic transglycosylase

*Correspondence: yus@shvri.ac.cn
[1] Shanghai Veterinary Research Institute, Chinese Academy of Agricultural Sciences (CAAS), Shanghai, China
Full list of author information is available at the end of the article

that is a homolog of membrane-bound lytic transglycosylase B (MltB). MltB cleaves the $\beta$-(1→4)-glycosidic bond between the $N$-acetylmuramic acid and $N$-acetylglucosamine residues of bacterial heteropolymer peptidoglycan [18]. In addition to bacterial cell wall recycling [19] and antibiotic resistance [20], MltB is also involved in assembly of macromolecular transport systems such as the type IV secretion system in Gram-negative bacteria [21]. We expected that deletion of BAB_RS22915 would make the S2308 strain a good potential vaccine candidate; to investigate this, we generated the site-directed deletion mutant strain Δ22915. The virulence and protection capability of the mutant strain were evaluated. Our results demonstrated that the mutant strain Δ22915 was a highly attenuated strain and provided long-term, effective protection against wild-type, virulent strain S2308 challenge. These results suggested the mutant could be used as a novel vaccine candidate in the future.

## Materials and methods
### Ethics statement
This study was performed in strict accordance with the recommendations in the Guide for the Care and Use of Laboratory Animals of the Institutional Animal Care and Use Committee guidelines set by Shanghai Veterinary Research Institute, Chinese Academy of Agricultural Sciences (CAAS). BALB/c mice (SLAC, Experimental Animal Inc., Shanghai, China) were kept in cages and given water and food ad libitum under biosafety conditions. The protocol for animal experiments was approved by the Committee on the Ethics of Animal Experiments of Shanghai Veterinary Research Institute, CAAS (shvri-MO-0135).

### Bacterial strains, cell lines and plasmids
The virulent B. abortus S2308 strain was from American Type Culture Collection (ATCC, Manassas, VA, USA). Vaccine strain RB51 was kindly provided by Professor Qingming Wu from China Agriculture University, Beijing. Both strains were cultured in tryptic soy broth (TSB, Difco, Becton–Dickinson, Sparks, MD, USA) or tryptic soy agar (TSA) at 37 °C with 5% $CO_2$. B. abortus S2308 with nalidixic acid resistance was induced with nalidixic acid at 50 μg/mL and preserved in our laboratory. Escherichia coli DH5α competent cells (Tiangen, Beijing, China) were cultured in Luria–Bertani (LB) media at 37 °C. Murine macrophage RAW 264.7 cells were from ATCC and cultured in Dulbecco's modified Eagle medium (DMEM, Hyclone, GE Lifesciences, Logan, UT, USA) media with 10% fetal bovine serum (FBS, Gibco, ThermoScientific, Grand Island, NY, USA) at 37 °C with 5% $CO_2$. The suicide pSC plasmid with the sacB gene [22]

was preserved in our laboratory and used to construct a site-directed mutant strain.

### Construction of the mutant strain Δ22915
The Δ22915 strain was constructed as described previously [23]. Primers for construction were designed using the sequence of BAB_RS22915 in the B. abortus S2308 genome (GenBank Code: NC_007618.1). Fragments that flanked BAB_RS22915 were amplified in two independent PCR reactions using PrimeSTAR Max Mix (TaKaRa, Dalian, China) with primer pairs BAB_RS22915 UF/BAB_RS22915 UR, and BAB_RS22915 DF/BAB_RS22915 DR. Recovered PCR products were used for overlap PCR to produce joint sequences with primer pairs BAB_RS22915 UF/BAB_RS22915 DR. PCR products were purified, digested with XbaI and ligated into pSC. A recombinant plasmid with the correct sequence was designated pSC-Δ22915 and introduced into DH5α.

Allelic replacement was employed to delete BAB_RS22915 from the wild-type strain S2308. According to the method described previously [23], S2308 was cultured and collected by centrifugation at the exponential phase. After an ice bath for 15 min, S2308 was washed twice with ice-cold sterile water. Bacteria were resuspended in 10% (v/v) glycerin water and 3–5 μg recombinant pSC-Δ22915 plasmid was added on ice. After electroporation, transformed S2308 were immediately transferred to prewarmed TSB media and cultured overnight. Bacteria were cultured on TSA plates with ampicillin at 100 μg/mL. A single exchanged mutant was selected and inoculated into TSB without antibiotics and cultured on TSA containing 5% (w/v) sucrose to produce a second exchange mutant. At least ten colonies per plate were collected for identification with PCR or quantitative real-time PCR (qRT-PCR). Primer pair BAB_RS22915 FF/BAB_RS22915 FR, flanking the gene coding sequence, and primer pair BAB_RS22915 OF/BAB_RS22915 OR, partially overlapping the deleted sequence, were used to identify gene deletions. Colonies with length-reduced fragment from BAB_RS22915 FF/BAB_RS22915 FR pair and no fragment from BAB_RS22915 OF/BAB_RS22915 OR pair were selected as BAB_RS22915 deleted mutant. Primer pairs RT-22910 F/RT-22910 R, RT-22920 F/RT-22920 R and RT-22915 F/RT-22915 R were used for qRT-PCR to identify if BAB_RS22915 deletion had polar effects on flanking gene transcription. Deletion mutants were designated Δ22915. Primers and plasmids are listed in Table 1.

### Extraction and silver staining of Brucella lipopolysaccharide (LPS)
Mutant strain Δ22915 and wild-type strain S2308 were cultured in TSB and collected at the exponential phase

**Table 1  Strains, plasmids and primers used in this study**

| Primers or plasmids | Description | Source or reference |
|---|---|---|
| **Bacterial strains** | | |
| *B. abortus* S2308 | Wild type strain; smooth phenotype | ATCC |
| RB51 | Vaccine strain; rough phenotype | This study |
| Δ22915 | *BAB_RS22915* gene deletion mutant strain; smooth phenotype | This study |
| *Escherichia coli* (DH5α) | F⁻ φ80*lacZ*ΔM15Δ(*lacZYA-argF*)U169 *rec*A1 *end*A1 *hsd*R17(r$_k^-$, m$_k^+$) *pho*A *sup*E44 *thi*-1 *gyr*A96 *rel*A1 λ⁻ | Tiangen |
| **Plasmids** | | |
| pSC | Amp$^R$; pUC19 plasmid containing *SacB* gene | [22] |
| **Primers** | | |
| BAB_RS22915 UF | GC<u>TCTAGA</u>CGTATATTCATCATCCGCAG (*Xba*I underlined) | This study |
| BAB_RS22915 UR | TGAGTTGATCCTGCGTCAGACTGAGGCGATAATCTTCATG | This study |
| BAB_RS22915 DF | CATGAAGATTATCGCCTCAGTCTGACGCAGGATCAACTCA | This study |
| BAB_RS22915 DR | GC<u>TCTAGA</u>GACATTGGAGGTGATTGCC (*Xba*I underlined) | This study |
| BAB_RS22915 FF | GCCACCCAACTTAGCGTGAG | This study |
| BAB_RS22915 FR | AAGTGGCGGCACCAAGAG | This study |
| BAB_RS22915 OF | GATGGCAAGGTCGATCTG | This study |
| BAB_RS22915 OR | GCCTGTCGAGAAGTTCCTG | This study |
| RT-22910 F | AAAGCACCGTTTTGCTCATC | This study |
| RT-22910 R | GCCAGACGGTTCATGTAGTG | This study |
| RT-22920 F | CCTCATCTGGAAAGTGCTGC | This study |
| RT-22920 R | CGAGAAAGAGTCCAAGCGTG | This study |
| RT-22915 F | ATAATGCCGTCAACATGCCG | This study |
| RT-22915 R | GGAAATGAGGCGCTTGGAAA | This study |
| RT-GAPDH F | GACATTCAGGTCGTCGCCATCA | [23] |
| RT-GAPDH R | TCTTCCTTCCACGGCAGTTCGG | [23] |

$^R$ Antibiotic resistance.

with centrifugation. Bacterial LPS was extracted with LPS Extraction Kits (iNtRON, Seoul, Korea). Samples were loaded on 12.5% polyacrylamide gels for SDS-PAGE and silver staining to validate LPS integrity. After electrophoresis, gels were fixed with periodic acid solution (0.3 M periodic acid, 40% v/v ethanol, 5% v/v acetic acid) at room temperature for 20 min. After washing with ultrapure water three times, gels were stained with silver–ammonia solution (0.02 M NaOH, 1.3% v/v ammonia water, 0.67% w/v AgNO₃) at room temperature for 10 min. Gels were washed with ultrapure water to remove free Ag⁺ and incubated with coloring solution (0.005% w/v citric acid, 0.005% v/v formaldehyde) for 5–10 min. Reactions were halted with 10% (v/v) acetic acid solution and gels were imaged with an Odyssey Infrared Imaging System (LI-COR Biosciences, Lincoln, NE, USA).

### RNA extraction and quantitative real-time PCR

Strains Δ22915 and S2308 were cultured in TSB and collected at the exponential phase. Total RNA was extracted with TRIzol RNA isolation reagent (Ambion, Carlsbad, CA, USA). Genomic contamination was removed with Turbo DNA-free kits (Ambion). RNA was subjected to reverse transcription with PrimeScript RT reagent kits (TaKaRa) at 37 °C for 10 min, then 85 °C for 5 s for cDNA templates. GoTaq qPCR master mix (Promega, Fitchburg, WI, USA) was used for qRT-PCR, according to the manufacturer's instruction: 1 μL cDNA, 0.5 μL forward or backward primer (10 μM), 8 μL nuclease-free water and 10 μL 2× GoTaq qPCR master mix were added. Reactions were on a Mastercycler ep Realplex system (Eppendorf, Germany) at 95 °C for 2 min, 40 cycles at 95 °C for 15 s, 60 °C for 1 min and a melting curve. Genes were tested in triplicate and the GAPDH gene was the internal control. Primers were designed according to the wild-type strain S2308 genome (GenBank Code: NC_007618.1 and NC_007624.1) with National Center for Biotechnology Information (NCBI) Primer-BLAST [24]. Relative transcription levels were calculated with the $2^{-\Delta\Delta Ct}$ method.

### Growth assays

Bacterial growth was measured at optical density 600 nm (OD$_{600}$). Strains Δ22915 and S2308 were cultured in TSB for growth curves as described [22]. Freshly cultured bacteria were diluted to OD$_{600}$ 1.0, then 1 mL was inoculated into 100 mL TSB and cultured at 37 °C at 200 rpm. $OD_{600}$ absorbance of aliquots was measured every 4 h.

## Bacterial adherence, invasion and intracellular survival assays

Bacterial adherence, invasion and intracellular survival were tested using RAW 264.7 cells. Cells were seeded in 24-well plates (Corning, NY, USA) at $2 \times 10^5$ per well and cultured in DMEM media with 10% FBS at 37 °C with 5% $CO_2$. After 20 h, cells were washed twice with phosphate-buffered saline (PBS, Hyclone) and counted. Cells were infected with strain Δ22915 or S2308 at 100 multiplicity of infection (MOI). Plates were centrifuged at $400 \times g$ for 5 min followed by 37 °C for 1 h. Cells were washed twice with PBS to remove nonadherent bacteria.

For adherence assays, wells of infected cells were incubated with 200 μL 0.2% (v/v) Triton X-100 (Sigma-Aldrich, St Louis, MO, USA) water solution for 10 min at 37 °C and 100 μL cell suspension was used for tenfold serial dilutions in PBS. Dilutions (100 μL) were spread on TSA plates and cultured at 37 °C with 5% $CO_2$ for 72 h. For invasion assays, cells were treated with DMEM containing 100 μg/mL gentamicin for 1 h to kill extracellular bacteria after infection. Colony forming units (CFUs) were counted to determine adherent and invading bacteria. Invasion ratio was calculated as the number of invading bacteria versus the number of adherent bacteria.

For intracellular survival assays, after killing extracellular bacteria, cells were cultured in DMEM with 0.5% FBS and 50 μg/mL gentamicin. At 2, 8, 24 and 48 h postinfection (hpi), cells were washed and incubated with 200 μL 0.2% (v/v) Triton X-100 water solution for 10 min at 37 °C. Then, 100 μL of each dilution was collected to determine CFUs per well. Numbers of recovered bacteria at each time point were determined and compared with *B. abortus* S2308 to evaluate intracellular survival capacity of Δ22915.

## Immunofluorescence assays

RAW 264.7 cells were cultured on 15-mm glass diameter coverslips (Thermo Scientific, Waltham, MA, USA) in 24-well plates and infected with strain Δ22915 or S2308 at 100 MOI as described above. At 4 and 24 hpi, cells were washed twice with PBS and fixed overnight in 4% (w/v) paraformaldehyde at 4 °C. After three washes with PBS, cells were incubated with PBS containing 0.5% (v/v) Triton-X100 at room temperature for 10 min, followed by blocking with 5% (w/v) bovine serum albumin in PBS at 37 °C for 30 min. Cells were incubated with primary antibody diluted in 0.05% (v/v) Tween-20 PBS (PBST) for 45 min at 37 °C. After three washes with PBST, cells were incubated with secondary antibody for 45 min at 37 °C. After washing with PBST, coverslips were incubated

with 4,6-diamidino-2-phenylindole at 2 μg/mL at room temperature. Coverslips were mounted on glass slides with Eukitt quick-hardening mounting medium (Sigma-Aldrich) and observed under laser scanning confocal microscope (Nikon D-Eclipse C1, Tokyo, Japan) with 100× oil immersion objective. Projections were saved in TIFF format and imported into Adobe Photoshop CS4 (Adobe Systems Incorporated, San Jose, CA, USA) to be merged. About 80–150 bacteria were counted randomly per coverslip and the percentage of lysosome-associated membrane protein 1 (LAMP-1) co-localized *Brucella*-containing vacuoles (BCV) was determined. Assays were performed in triplicate.

Rabbit anti-*Brucella* polyclonal antibody (1:500 dilution) was used to track intracellular bacteria. Rat LAMP-1 monoclonal antibody (1:1000 dilution, Abcam, USA) was used to track lysosomes. Goat anti-rabbit Alexa Fluor 488 and goat anti-rat Alexa Fluor 555 (Molecular Probes, Life Technologies, Eugene, OR, USA) were secondary antibodies at 1:1000 dilution.

## In vivo survival experiments

To investigate bacterial survival in vivo, strain S2308, strain Δ22915 and vaccine strain RB51 were intraperitoneally (IP) inoculated into 4- to 6-week-old female BALB/c mice ($n = 6$ per group) at $1 \times 10^5$ CFU. Mice were euthanized at 2, 4, 6, 9 and 12 weeks post infection (wpi). Spleens were collected, weighed and homogenized in 5 mL 0.25% (v/v) Triton X-100 water solution and 100 μL aliquots were used for tenfold serial dilutions plated on TSA to determine bacterial CFUs. One mouse per group was euthanized and spleens and kidneys were collected and fixed in 4% (v/v) formaldehyde for histopathological examination. Peripheral blood samples of mice infected with Δ22915 or S2308 were collected. Levels of TNF-α and IL-12p40 in sera were detected with enzyme linked-immunosorbent assay (ELISA) (Yaoyun, Shanghai, China) to evaluate inflammation.

## Construction of *Brucella*-specific transcriptome library

A *Brucella* transcriptome library was constructed for strand-specific RNA deep sequencing at Beijing Genomics Institute. Strains Δ22915 and S2308 were cultured in TSB media and total RNA was extracted with RiboPure Bacteria Kits (Ambion) and ribosomal RNA removed with TruSeq RNA Sample Prep Kits v2 (Illumina, San Diego, CA, USA). After RNA was fragmented, first-strand cDNA was synthesized with First Strand Master Mix and Super Script II (Invitrogen, Carlsbad, CA, USA) with a program of 25 °C for 10 min, 42 °C for 50 min and 70 °C for 15 min. Product was purified with Agencourt RNAClean XP Beads (Beckman Coulter, Fullerton, CA, USA), then Second Master Mix (Invitrogen) and dATP, dGTP, dCTP, dUTP mix was added to synthesize second-strand cDNA. After end repair and A-tailing, purified product was treated with uracil-$N$-glycosylase. Then, the cDNA fragments were enriched with several rounds of PCR using Phusion High-Fidelity DNA polymerase (New England Biolabs, Beverly, MA, USA) and universal PCR primers.

The fragment distribution of the library was checked with an Agilent 2100 bioanalyzer instrument (Agilent Technologies, Santa Clara, CA, USA) and quantity checked by quantitative PCR. The qualified library was amplified to generate the cluster on the flowcell (TruSeq PE Cluster Kit V3-cBot-HS, Illumina). The amplified flowcell was used for pair-end sequencing on a HiSeq 2000 System (TruSeq SBS KIT-HS V3, Illumina) with read lengths of 90 bp. Acquired reads were mapped to the *B. abortus* S2308 genome (GenBank Accession: NC_007618.1 and NC_007624.1) and annotated gene sets obtained from NCBI Gene [25] using HISAT [26] and Bowtie [27] tools.

Reads that matched annotated genes were analyzed for expression differences between Δ22915 and S2308. Expression levels were determined using RSEM [28] software and calculated with a fragments per kilobase of transcript per million mapped reads (FPKM) algorithm [29]. Genes with FPKM >2.0-fold between the two strains were considered differentially expressed and validated with qRT-PCR using the protocol described above and primers in Additional file 1.

### Animal immunization assays

Female BALB/c mice ($n = 5$ per group) at 4–6 weeks were IP inoculated with Δ22915 or RB51 at $1 \times 10^5$ CFU. Mice IP-inoculated with PBS were the blank controls. At 12 and 16 weeks post-vaccination (wpv), mice were challenged with $1 \times 10^4$ CFU *B. abortus* S2308 that was nalidixic acid resistant. One week after challenge, mice were euthanized and spleens collected. As described above, spleens were homogenized in 5 mL 0.25% (v/v) Triton X-100 water solution. Each 100 μL of aliquot was serially tenfold diluted and spread on TSA with 30 μg/mL nalidixic acid to determine bacterial loads. Anti-*Brucella* ELISA titers in serum were detected at 2, 4, 6, 9 and 12 wpv as described previously [13], using heat-killed and sonicated *B. abortus* S2308 as coating antigen. The highest dilution with $OD_{450}$ absorbance that was at least twice the mean value of the negative sample readings was used as the ELISA titer.

### Statistical analysis

CFU data from adherence, invasion and intracellular survival assays, in vivo persistence assay, and animal protection assay, as well as anti-*Brucella* ELISA titers from serum were converted to logarithmic numbers. Data were imported into GraphPad Prism 6 (Graph Pad Software, San Diego, CA, USA) for analysis. Statistical significance was determined using an unpaired or two-tailed Student's $t$ test. For group analysis, two-way ANOVA followed by Holm–Sidak's multiple tests was used. $P$ values less than 0.05 were considered statistically significant.

## Results

### Mutant strain Δ22915 was constructed without phenotype changes

A 1036-bp fragment was deleted from the *BAB_RS22915* coding gene sequence with a suicide plasmid (Figure 1A). qRT-PCR confirmed that *BAB_RS22915* gene expression was inactivated and did not influence flanking gene transcription (Figure 1B).

*Brucella* is reported to have a tendency to lose the O-antigen of LPS during mutant construction [30, 31]; this is a critical virulence factor for intracellular survival [32]. To identify if mutant strain Δ22915 had this spontaneous mutation, LPS purification and silver staining were performed. No LPS pattern changes were seen between strain Δ22915 and the wild-type strain S2308 (Figure 1C). Strain Δ22915 had a similar growth rate before 36 h when cultured in TSB, but a higher growth rate thereafter, compared with wild-type strain S2308 (Figure 1D), based on $OD_{600}$. Bacterial CFU were $5 \times 10^9$ CFU/mL for both strains at $OD_{600} = 1.0$.

### Strain Δ22915 showed reduced intracellular survival and failure to escape from lysosome fusion in RAW 264.7 cells

To evaluate if the *BAB_RS22915* gene was involved in *Brucella* invasion and intracellular survival, RAW 264.7 cells were infected with Δ22915 or S2308 at 100 MOI. Strain Δ22915 adhered to and invaded RAW264.7 cells as effectively as S2308. No significant difference was seen in adherence and invasion capacity between the mutant and wild-type strains (data not shown). However, the mutant strain showed reduced intracellular survival after 8 hpi; it was significantly reduced by more than tenfold at 24 hpi and thereafter, compared to S2308 (Figure 2A).

To determine if the intracellular survival defect of the mutant was associated with the capacity of BCVs to mature or its capacity for intracellular trafficking, we determined the number of LAMP-1 positive BCV at 4 and 24 hpi. Strain Δ22915 failed to exclude LAMP-1 at 24 hpi, which might be the reason for the decreased intracellular survival (Figures 2B and C). Stress resistance assays showed no difference in resistance to low pH or $H_2O_2$ between Δ22915 and S2308 (data not shown).

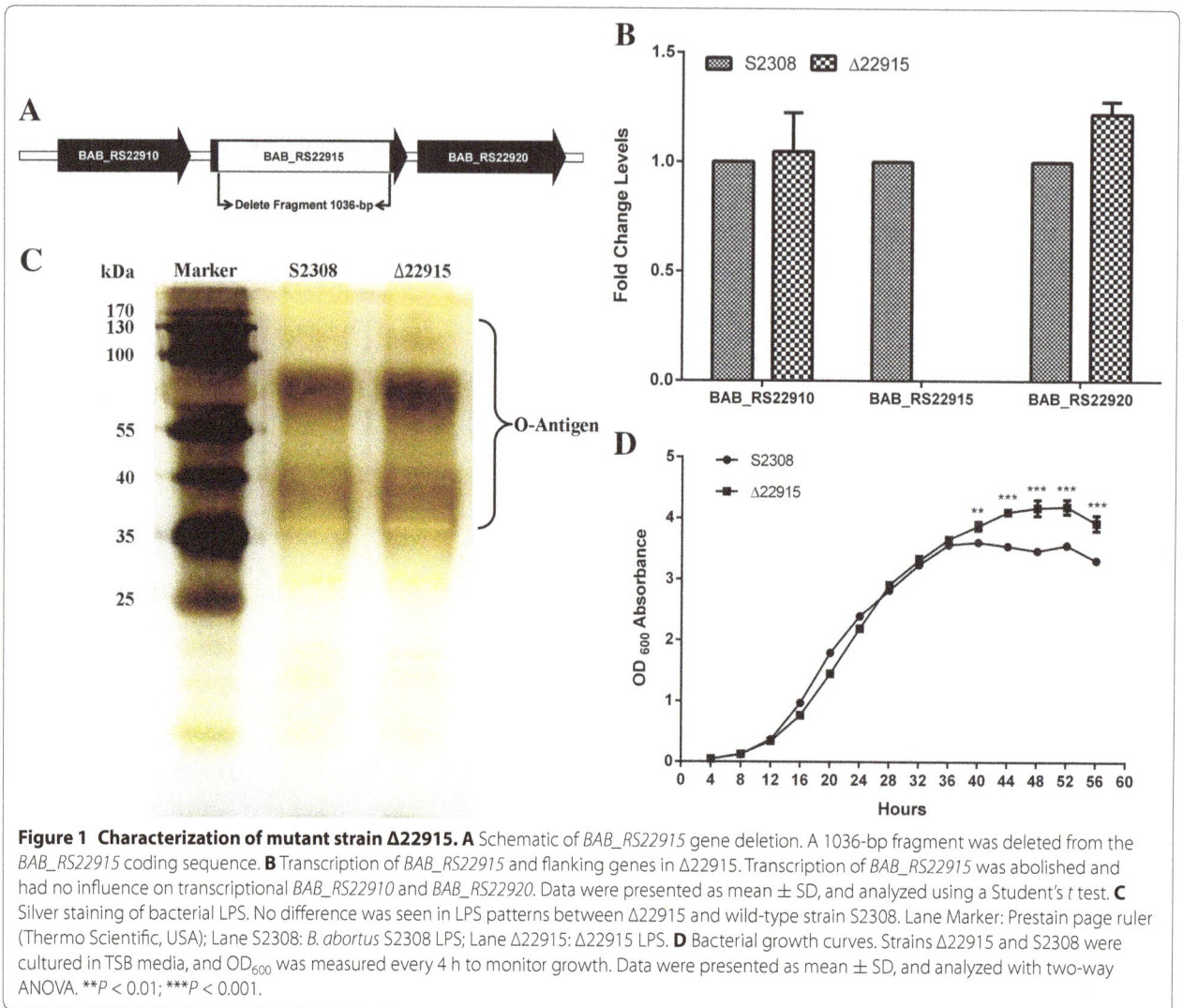

**Figure 1 Characterization of mutant strain Δ22915. A** Schematic of *BAB_RS22915* gene deletion. A 1036-bp fragment was deleted from the *BAB_RS22915* coding sequence. **B** Transcription of *BAB_RS22915* and flanking genes in Δ22915. Transcription of *BAB_RS22915* was abolished and had no influence on transcriptional *BAB_RS22910* and *BAB_RS22920*. Data were presented as mean ± SD, and analyzed using a Student's *t* test. **C** Silver staining of bacterial LPS. No difference was seen in LPS patterns between Δ22915 and wild-type strain S2308. Lane Marker: Prestain page ruler (Thermo Scientific, USA); Lane S2308: *B. abortus* S2308 LPS; Lane Δ22915: Δ22915 LPS. **D** Bacterial growth curves. Strains Δ22915 and S2308 were cultured in TSB media, and OD_{600} was measured every 4 h to monitor growth. Data were presented as mean ± SD, and analyzed with two-way ANOVA. **$P < 0.01$; ***$P < 0.001$.

## Strain Δ22915 is highly attenuated and induces no histopathological changes in mice

To evaluate the virulence of mutant strain Δ22915, bacteria were IP inoculated into female BALB/c mice at $1.0 \times 10^5$ CFU. Wild-type strain S2308 and vaccine strain RB51 were inoculated by the same route and dose as controls. Bacterial loads in spleens of Δ22915-infected mice were significantly reduced by around 1000-fold compared to S2308 infected mice at all time points investigated (Figure 3A). Splenomegaly was assessed by weighing spleens from infected mice. Spleen weight in wild-type-infected mice reached a peak at 4 wpi, then gradually decreased in the following weeks. Splenomegaly and spleen weight increases were not found in mice infected with Δ22915, which showed no significant differences from normal, uninfected spleens (Figure 3B). This result indicated the attenuated virulence of mutant strain Δ22915 in vivo.

Histopathological examination at 12 wpi showed that strain Δ22915 caused no observable pathological lesions (Figure 4A). In spleen of Δ22915-infected mouse, the boundary of red and white pulps was clear (indicated by arrows), and no reticular tissue proliferation or inflammatory cell infiltration was observed. On the other hand, wild-type strain S2308 caused extensive proliferation of reticular tissue and necrosis of mature lymphocytes in spleens, seen as an unclear boundary of red and white pulps. In kidney of Δ22915-infected mouse, the structure of renal tubules was intact. However, severe basophil infiltration, epithelial cell necrosis and atrophy was observed in renal tubules in S2308-infected mouse kidney. No observable lesions were found in organs of uninfected mice.

The production of proinflammatory cytokines TNF-α and IL-12p40 in peripheral blood was determined (Figures 4B and C). Strain Δ22915 induced significant less

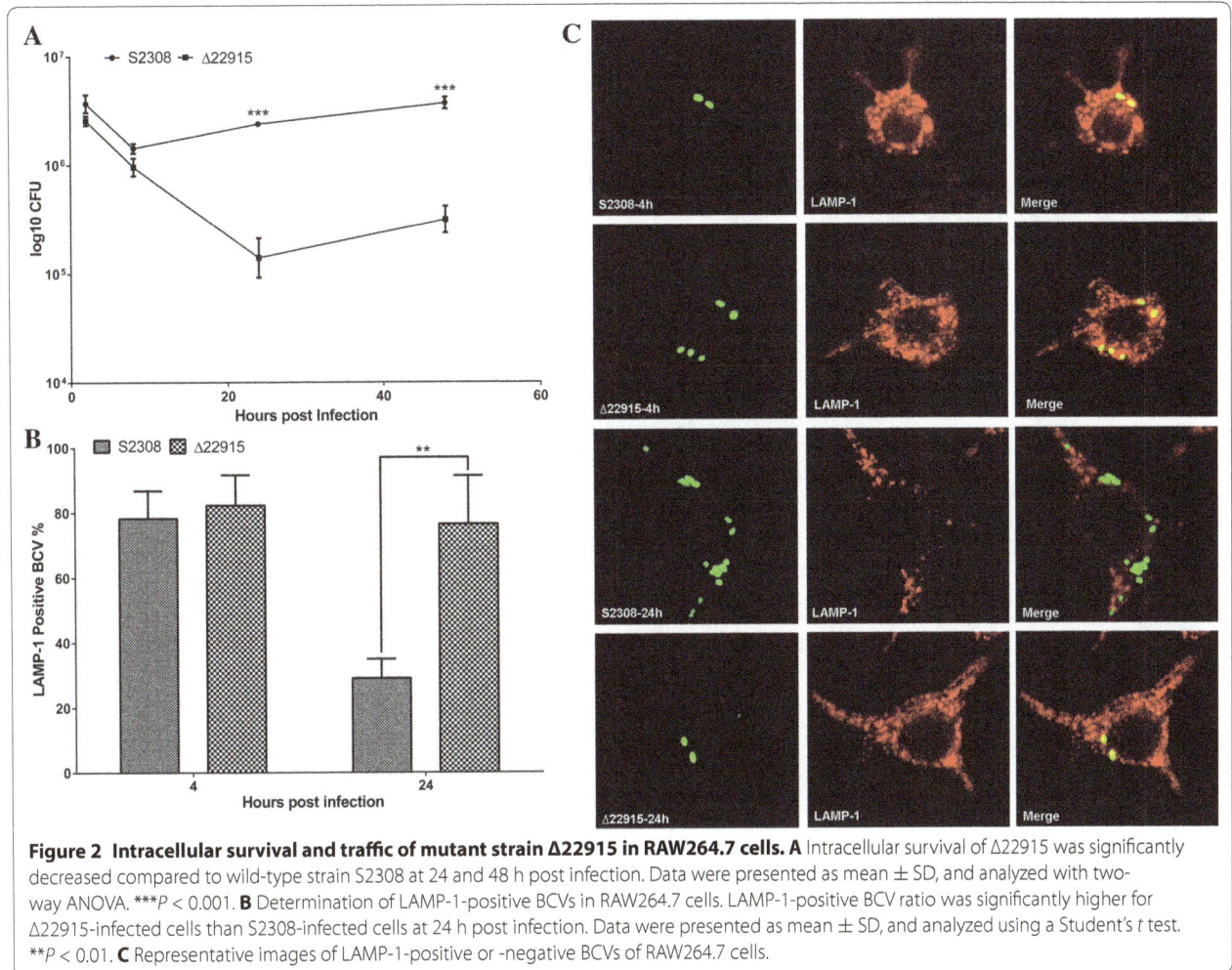

**Figure 2 Intracellular survival and traffic of mutant strain Δ22915 in RAW264.7 cells. A** Intracellular survival of Δ22915 was significantly decreased compared to wild-type strain S2308 at 24 and 48 h post infection. Data were presented as mean ± SD, and analyzed with two-way ANOVA. ***$P < 0.001$. **B** Determination of LAMP-1-positive BCVs in RAW264.7 cells. LAMP-1-positive BCV ratio was significantly higher for Δ22915-infected cells than S2308-infected cells at 24 h post infection. Data were presented as mean ± SD, and analyzed using a Student's $t$ test. **$P < 0.01$. **C** Representative images of LAMP-1-positive or -negative BCVs of RAW264.7 cells.

cytokines at all time points investigated, compared to strain S2308. However, the cytokine levels induced by strain Δ22915 were much higher than those in the normal, noninfected mice ($P < 0.001$). These results demonstrated that the virulence of the mutant strain Δ22915 was attenuated, facilitating its application as a novel vaccine candidate.

**Transcriptomic analysis**

The transcriptome of the mutant strain Δ22915 was compared with that of the wild-type strain S2308 using strand-specific RNA-Seq analysis. In total, 14 399 044 reads were acquired. The average mapping ratio was 97.38% for the reference genome and 78.94% for the reference genes. Analysis of the gene-matched reads revealed that 16 genes had a high probability of being dis-transcript by more than twofold in the mutant strain compared to the wild-type strain. qRT-PCR indicated that the transcription of six genes was upregulated, and four of them were upregulated more than tenfold (Table 2). EggNOG 4.5

[33] analysis showed that four genes were categorized as "amino acid/nucleotide transport and metabolism" and the other two had no designated functions. The product of the *BAB_RS17405* gene was involved with "nucleotide transport and metabolism" (Figure 5A). *BAB_RS17430* encoded a NADPH-dependent glutamate synthase (Figure 5B). *BAB_RS24460* and *BAB_RS30485* encoded two substrate-binding proteins of two amino acid ABC transporters (Figures 5C and D). *BAB_RS27765* encoded a hypothetical protein without known function (Figure 5E). *BAB_RS31735* encoded a putative amidohydrolase without known function (Figure 5F). These results indicated that the expression of amino acids/nucleotides transport and metabolism related protein was enhanced in the mutant strain Δ22915.

**Strain Δ22915 induces immune responses and protects against S2308 challenge**

After vaccination with the mutant strain Δ22915, *Brucella* antibodies in sera were measured using ELISA at

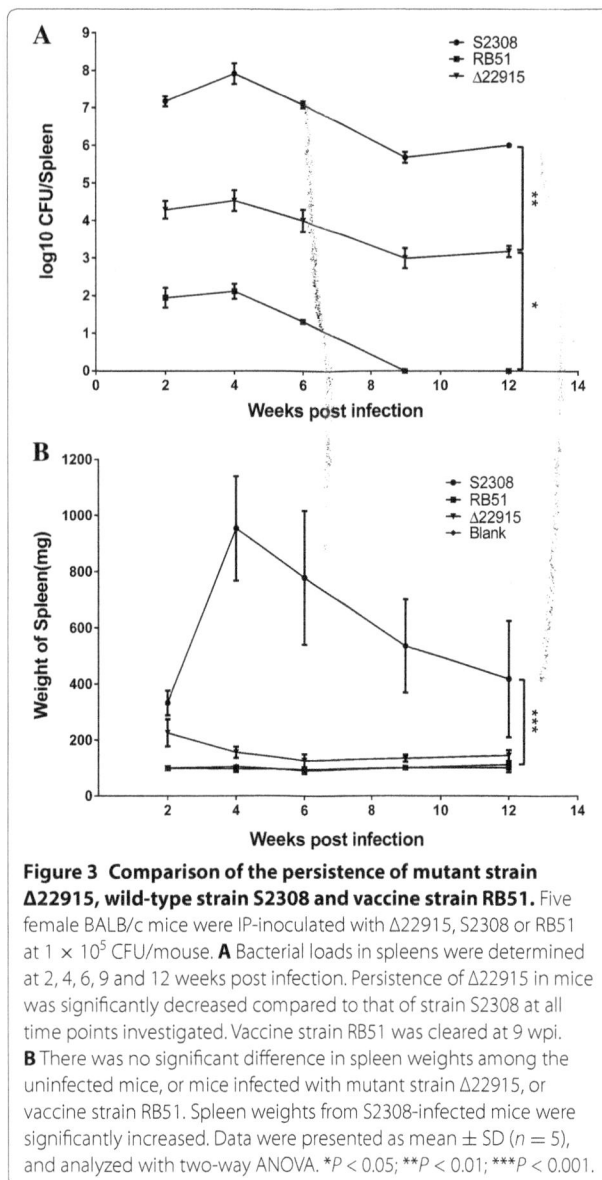

**Figure 3  Comparison of the persistence of mutant strain Δ22915, wild-type strain S2308 and vaccine strain RB51.** Five female BALB/c mice were IP-inoculated with Δ22915, S2308 or RB51 at $1 \times 10^5$ CFU/mouse. **A** Bacterial loads in spleens were determined at 2, 4, 6, 9 and 12 weeks post infection. Persistence of Δ22915 in mice was significantly decreased compared to that of strain S2308 at all time points investigated. Vaccine strain RB51 was cleared at 9 wpi. **B** There was no significant difference in spleen weights among the uninfected mice, or mice infected with mutant strain Δ22915, or vaccine strain RB51. Spleen weights from S2308-infected mice were significantly increased. Data were presented as mean ± SD ($n = 5$), and analyzed with two-way ANOVA. *$P < 0.05$; **$P < 0.01$; ***$P < 0.001$.

2, 4, 6, 9 and 12 wpv. Antibody was induced as early as 2 wpv, and reached a peak at 12 wpv (Figure 6A). Strain Δ22915 induced higher antibody titers than the vaccine strain RB51, suggesting that Δ22915 effectively activated host humoral immunity.

Protection of mice against challenge by wild-type strain S2308 was investigated. Mice vaccinated with strain Δ22915 were challenged with nalidixic-acid resistant S2308 at $1.0 \times 10^4$ CFU at 12 and 16 wpv. Mice vaccinated with strain RB51 and nonvaccinated mice were used as positive and negative protection controls, respectively. Spleens were collected at 1 week after challenge to determine bacterial loads. Strain Δ22915 provided better protection against S2308 challenge than vaccine strain RB51 (Figures 6B and C). No CFU was seen for S2308

in the Δ22915 vaccinated mice. More than 570 CFU/spleen were seen for S2308 counted in RB51-vaccinated mice. Bacterial loads in the nonvaccinated mice were 5290 CFU/spleen. This result showed that the mutant strain Δ22915 provided BALB/c mice with better protection against S2308 than RB51.

## Discussion

We successfully constructed the *B. abortus* mutant strain Δ22915 by deleting a 1036-bp fragment from the *BAB_RS22915* gene. Strain Δ22915 showed similar LPS phenotypes and adherence and invasion capacities compared to the wild-type strain S2308, but attenuated virulence, determined by in vivo and in vitro survival. We demonstrated that the decreased intracellular survival of strain Δ22915 was associated with the altered capacity to exclude lysosomes, an important step before *Brucella* reaches a replicative niche in endoplasmic reticulum [34]. This result suggested that the altered intracellular traffic contributed to decreased survival in RAW 264.7 cells.

MltB is a member of the lytic transglycosylase (LT) family that is involved in recycling bacterial cell walls to produce 1,6-anhydromuropeptides for bacterial growth [35]. However, inactivation of LTs does not inhibit bacterial growth in medium [36]. This finding indicates involvement of other pathways or gene upregulation to compensate for bacterial cell growth [37]. Thus, we investigated the gene expression in the whole genome using transcriptomic analysis, which indicated 16 genes were changed for their expression. qRT-PCR confirmed that four genes were upregulated by more than 10-fold; these were categorized into "amino acid/nucleotide transport and metabolism". Transcription of *BAB_RS24460* was upregulated 39-fold in the mutant strain Δ22915; this is the substrate-binding component of the branched-chain amino acid ABC transporter, responsible for the uptake of leucine, isoleucine and valine [38]; uptake mediated by this transporter contributes to bacterial growth [39], intracellular survival [40], and symbiosis between host and bacteria [41]. The *BAB_RS30485* gene, also known as the *PotD* gene, is the substrate-binding component of the polyamine ABC transporter that preferentially takes up spermidine [42]. *BAB_RS17430* encodes the α subunit of the NADPH dependent glutamate synthase that catalyzes the reductive transfer of the amide group of L-glutamine to C-2 of 2-oxoglutarate to produce L-glutamate [43]. This reaction is involved in nitrogen assimilation of *α-proteobacteria* to produce glutamine [44]. *BAB_RS17405* encodes a dihydropyrimidinase that is responsible for the second step of pyrimidine reductive catabolism to produce *N*-carbamoyl-b-alanine and *N*-carbamoyl-b-aminoisobutyric acid, respectively, from dihydrouracil and dihydrothymine [45]. To some

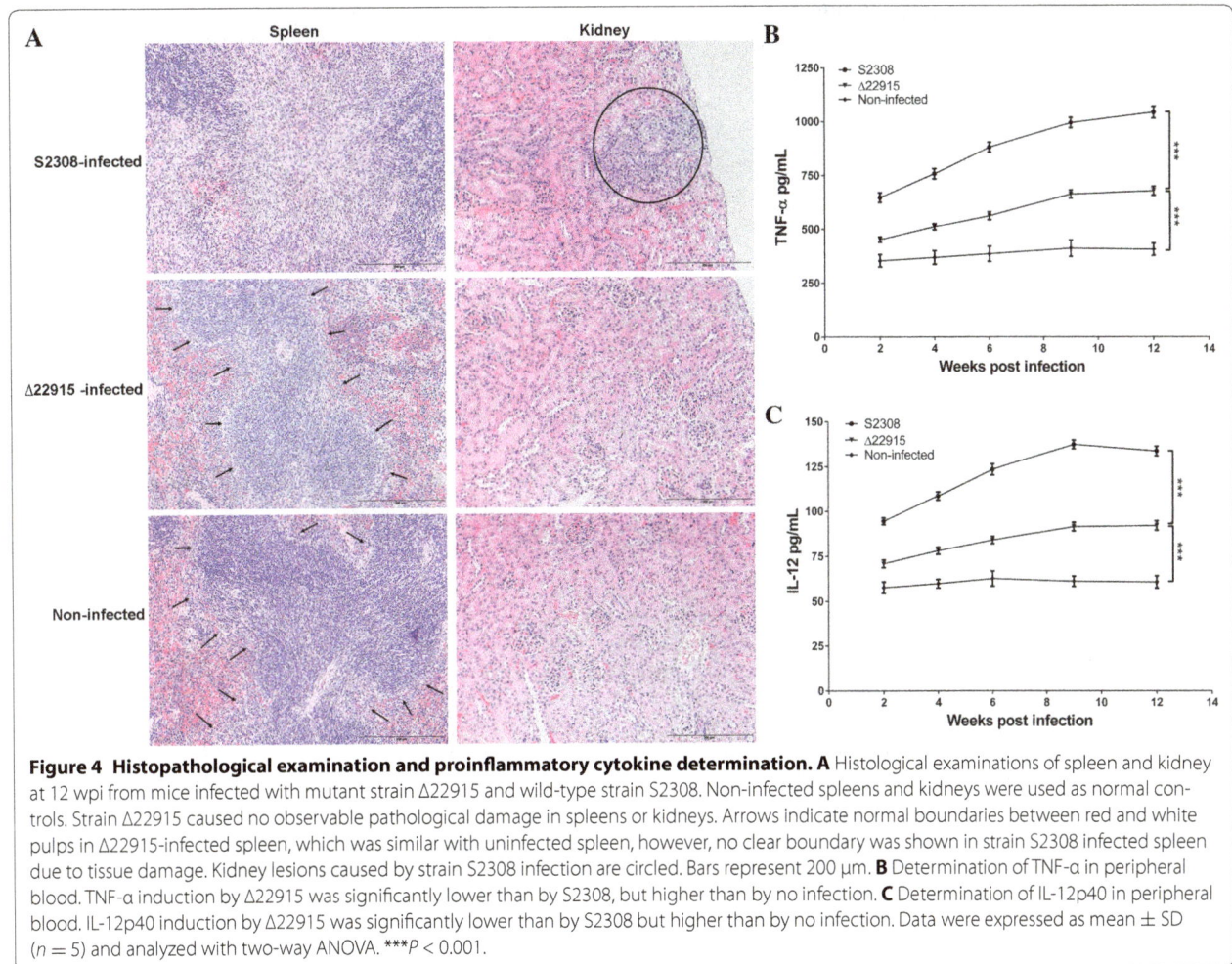

**Figure 4 Histopathological examination and proinflammatory cytokine determination. A** Histological examinations of spleen and kidney at 12 wpi from mice infected with mutant strain Δ22915 and wild-type strain S2308. Non-infected spleens and kidneys were used as normal controls. Strain Δ22915 caused no observable pathological damage in spleens or kidneys. Arrows indicate normal boundaries between red and white pulps in Δ22915-infected spleen, which was similar with uninfected spleen, however, no clear boundary was shown in strain S2308 infected spleen due to tissue damage. Kidney lesions caused by strain S2308 infection are circled. Bars represent 200 μm. **B** Determination of TNF-α in peripheral blood. TNF-α induction by Δ22915 was significantly lower than by S2308, but higher than by no infection. **C** Determination of IL-12p40 in peripheral blood. IL-12p40 induction by Δ22915 was significantly lower than by S2308 but higher than by no infection. Data were expressed as mean ± SD ($n = 5$) and analyzed with two-way ANOVA. ***$P < 0.001$.

bacteria, it functions as an important source of nitrogen [46]. We found that upregulated genes are mainly responsible for bacterial metabolism. Therefore, they might have contributed to the enhanced growth rate of strain Δ22915 in stationary stage cultures in TSB media. The upregulated genes might be related to the decreased intracellular survival of the mutant strain Δ22915. Bacterial ABC transporters and metabolism-related proteins are reported to provide animals with protection as vaccine candidates [47–49]. We assume the upregulation of these genes may enhance the antigenicity of Δ22915 to activate the immune response of macrophages, resulting in its decreased intracellular survival.

In vivo experiments indicated that strain Δ22915 persisted in mice for longer than 12 weeks, but caused no observable pathological damage. In addition, the mutant strain Δ22915 induced fewer inflammatory responses than the wild-type strain. In previous research, live attenuated Brucella with multiple disregulated genes protected against the wild-type strain S2308

[50]. This result suggested that testing whether mutant strain Δ22915 could be applied as a vaccine would be a worthwhile study. Vaccination with the mutant strain induced an effective immune response against the wild-type strain S2308. After vaccination with Δ22915, bacterial loads decreased until after 4 wpv, with specific antibody titers increasing to a peak at 12 wpv. The smooth type of the mutant strain Δ22915 induced higher levels of antibody than RB51, due to the dominant antigenicity of the O-antigen [51]. The adaptive cellular response is mainly responsible for the immunity against Brucella, but antibody against O-antigen or serum from smooth Brucella-infected animals participates in defense against challenge by wild-type Brucella [52]. In challenge assays, coinciding with the humoral response, strain Δ22915 provided longer and better protection than RB51 at 12 and 16 wpv. Unlike virB mutant Brucella [53], challenge by S2308 did not rescue the survival of Δ22915 (data not shown), confirming its safety as a vaccine candidate.

**Table 2  Real-time PCR verification of differentially expressed genes in mutant strain Δ22915**

| Gene locus[a] | Description of genes | Function[b] | Fold changes ($2^{-\Delta\Delta Ct}$) ±SD |
|---|---|---|---|
| BAB_RS24460 | Extracellular ligand-binding receptor | Amino acid transport and metabolism | 39.08 ± 4.25 |
| BAB_RS17405 | Dihydropyrimidinase | Nucleotide transport and metabolism | 20.50 ± 2.27 |
| BAB_RS30485 | Extracellular solute-binding protein family 1 | Amino acid transport and metabolism | 15.35 ± 1.80 |
| BAB_RS17430 | Oxidoreductase | Amino acid transport and metabolism | 12.67 ± 1.25 |
| BAB_RS31735 | Amidohydrolase | Function unknown | 3.63 ± 0.27 |
| BAB_RS27765 | Fumarylacetoacetate (Faa) hydrolase | Function unknown | 2.80 ± 0.22 |
| BAB_RS30280 | Quinone oxidoreductase | Energy production and conversion | 1.82 ± 0.20 |
| BAB_RS30270 | Abc transporter permease protein | Amino acid transport and metabolism | 1.70 ± 0.24 |
| BAB_RS26970 | Flagellar basal-body rod protein | Cell motility | 1.62 ± 0.31 |
| BAB_RS18915 | Gene transfer agent | Function unknown | 1.55 ± 0.22 |
| BAB_RS30285 | Transcriptional regulator, GntR family | Transcription | 1.52 ± 0.26 |
| BAB_RS30275 | Extracellular ligand-binding receptor | Amino acid transport and metabolism | 1.37 ± 0.14 |
| BAB_RS28745 | Abc transporter permease protein | Amino acid transport and metabolism | 1.37 ± 0.35 |
| BAB_RS 28215 | Transposase | Replication, recombination and repair | 1.25 ± 0.23 |
| BAB_RS27910 | Transcriptional regulator | Transcription | 0.81 ± 0.19 |
| BAB_RS22920 | Auxin efflux carrier | Function unknown | 0.76 ± 0.11 |

Genes with over twofold changes levels and high probability were further validated with qRT-PCR.

[a] Based on *B. abortus* S2308 genome (GenBank Code: NC_007618.1 and NC_007624.1).

[b] The functional categories of protein were predicted by searching through EggNOG database [33] with BLASTP.

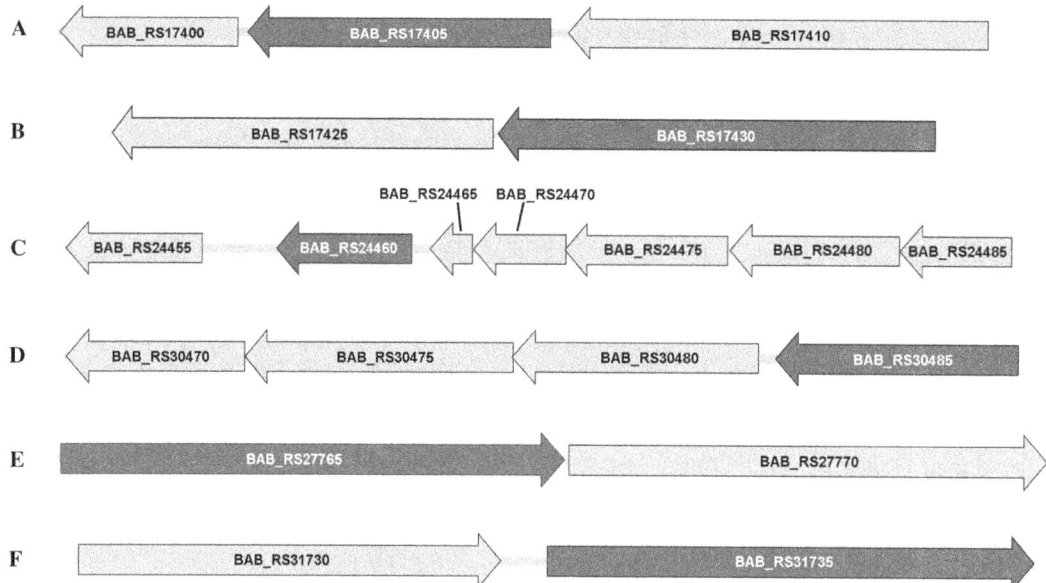

**Figure 5  Genetic organization of upregulated gene locus. A** *BAB_RS17405* encodes a dihydropyrimidinase on chromosome I of *B. abortus* S2308. It is flanked by a zinc-dependent allantoate amidohydrolase (*BAB_RS17410*) and a dihydrorhizobitoxine desaturase (*BAB_RS17400*). **B** *BAB_RS17430* encodes the α-subunit of NADPH dependent glutamate synthase on chromosome I of *B. abortus* S2308, downstream of β-subunit B of NADPH dependent glutamate synthase (*BAB_RS17425*). **C** *BAB_RS24460* encodes a substrate-binding protein on chromosome I of *B. abortus* S2308. It is flanked by genes for two hypothetical proteins without complete coding sequences (*BAB_RS24465* and *24470*), an ATP-binding protein with ATPase enzymatic activity (*BAB_RS24475*), two permease proteins (*BAB_RS24480* and *24485*) and another substrate-binding protein (*BAB_RS24455*). **D** *BAB_RS30485* encodes a substrate binding protein which is located on chromosome II of *B. abortus* S2308. It is flanked by two permease proteins (*BAB_RS30470* and *30475*) and another ATP-binding protein (*BAB_RS30480*). Both ABC transporters are predicted to be involved in amino acid transport and metabolism. **E** *BAB_RS27765* encodes a putative fumarylacetoacetate (Faa) hydrolase without known function. It is on chromosome II of *B. abortus* S2308, upstream of a gene for galactose 1-dehydrogenase (*BAB_RS27770*). **F** *BAB_RS31735* encodes a putative amidohydrolase without known function. It is on chromosome II of *B. abortus* S2308, downstream of a gamma-glutamyl-gamma-aminobutyraldehyde dehydrogenase (*BAB_RS31730*) gene. Arrows indicate direction of CDS. Except *BAB_RS27765* and *31735*, all other CDSs are on the complementary strand of the *B. abortus* S2308 genome. Tags of upregulated genes are indicated by a darker color.

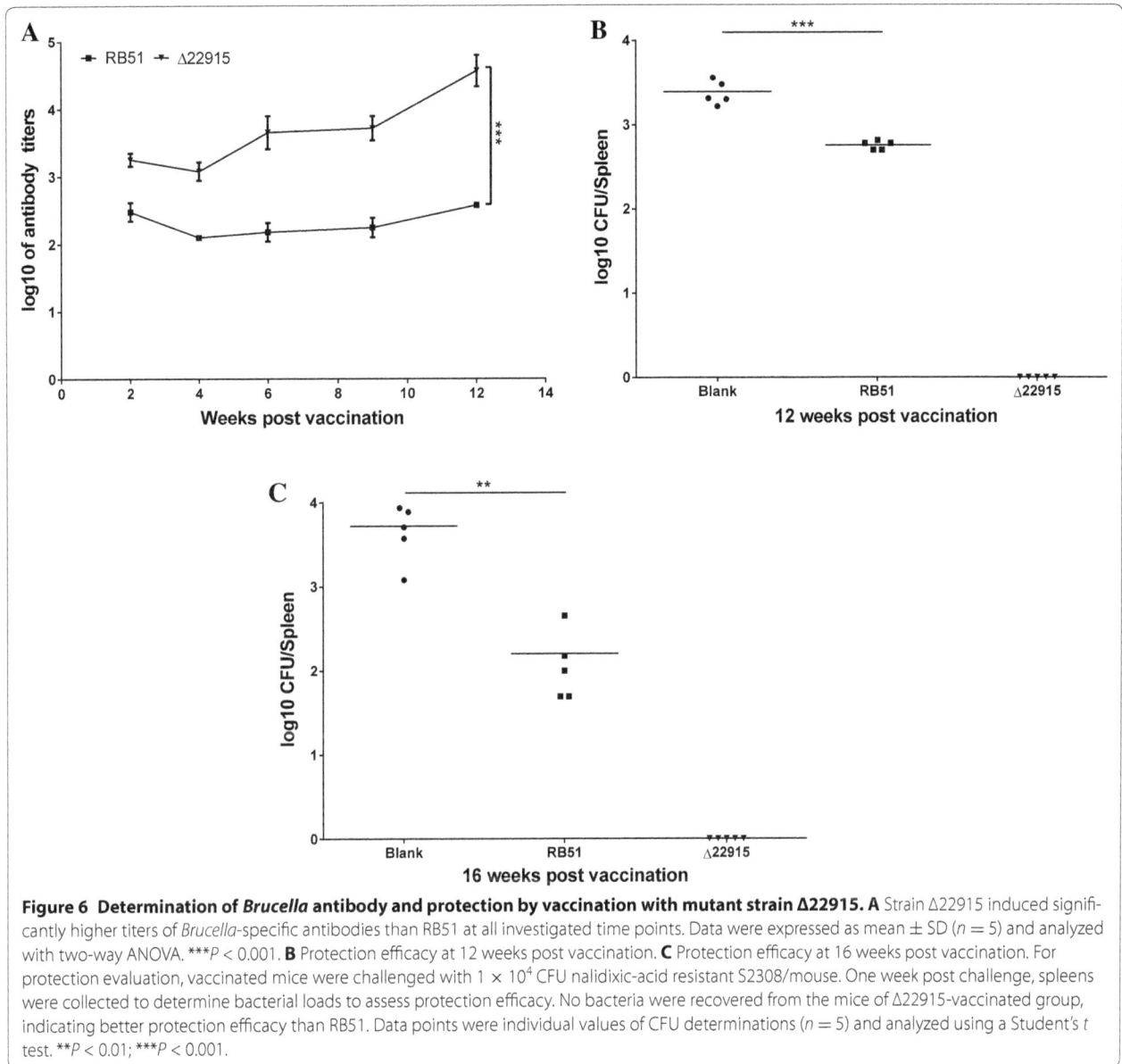

**Figure 6 Determination of *Brucella* antibody and protection by vaccination with mutant strain Δ22915. A** Strain Δ22915 induced significantly higher titers of *Brucella*-specific antibodies than RB51 at all investigated time points. Data were expressed as mean ± SD ($n = 5$) and analyzed with two-way ANOVA. ***$P < 0.001$. **B** Protection efficacy at 12 weeks post vaccination. **C** Protection efficacy at 16 weeks post vaccination. For protection evaluation, vaccinated mice were challenged with $1 \times 10^4$ CFU nalidixic-acid resistant S2308/mouse. One week post challenge, spleens were collected to determine bacterial loads to assess protection efficacy. No bacteria were recovered from the mice of Δ22915-vaccinated group, indicating better protection efficacy than RB51. Data points were individual values of CFU determinations ($n = 5$) and analyzed using a Student's *t* test. ***$P < 0.01$; ***$P < 0.001$.

In conclusion, using a suicide plasmid, we constructed a smooth-phenotype mutant strain Δ22915 with a deletion of the *BAB_RS22915* gene. In addition to altered intracellular traffic and attenuated survival, multiple genes involved in amino acid/nucleotide transport and metabolism were upregulated in the mutant strain. These genes may be associated with the attenuation of intracellular survival and require further research on their mechanism. Virulence of the mutant strain Δ22915 was significantly attenuated in BALB/c mice and provided better protection against *B. abortus* S2308 than RB51. This finding facilitated potential use of mutant strain Δ22915 as a novel vaccine candidate in the future.

**Competing interests**
The authors declare that they have no competing interests.

**Authors' contributions**
YB and MT performed the experiments, analyzed the data and prepared the manuscript. PL, JL, and CD contributed reagents, materials and analysis tools. SY designed the study and revised the manuscript. All authors read and approved the final manuscript.

**Acknowledgements**
This work was supported by the Scientific and Technical Innovation Project of the Chinese Academy of Agricultural Science (SHVRI-ASTIP-2014-8), the First-class General Financial Grant from the China Postdoctoral Science Foundation (2015M570184), the Shanghai Sailing Program (16YF1414600) and the National Basic Fund for Research Institutes, which is supported by the Chinese Academy of Agricultural Sciences (2016JB06).

## Author details

[1] Shanghai Veterinary Research Institute, Chinese Academy of Agricultural Sciences (CAAS), Shanghai, China. [2] Jiangsu Co-innovation Center for Prevention and Control of Important Animal Infectious Diseases and Zoonoses, Yangzhou, China.

## References

1. Pandey A, Cabello A, Akoolo L, Rice-Ficht A, Arenas-Gamboa A, McMurray D, Ficht TA, de Figueiredo P (2016) The case for live attenuated vaccines against the neglected zoonotic diseases brucellosis and bovine tuberculosis. PLoS Negl Trop Dis 10:e0004572

2. Pappas G, Papadimitriou P, Christou L, Akritidis N (2006) Future trends in human brucellosis treatment. Expert Opin Investig Drugs 15:1141–1149

3. Pappas G (2010) The changing Brucella ecology: novel reservoirs, new threats. Int J Antimicrob Agents 36(Suppl 1):S8–11

4. Olsen SC, Stoffregen WS (2005) Essential role of vaccines in brucellosis control and eradication programs for livestock. Expert Rev Vaccines 4:915–928

5. Fluegel Dougherty AM, Cornish TE, O'Toole D, Boerger-Fields AM, Henderson OL, Mills KW (2013) Abortion and premature birth in cattle following vaccination with Brucella abortus strain RB51. J Vet Diagn Invest 25:630–635

6. Ollé-Goig JE, Canela-Soler J (1987) An outbreak of Brucella melitensis infection by airborne transmission among laboratory workers. Am J Public Health 77:335–338

7. Lin J, Ficht TA (1995) Protein synthesis in Brucella abortus induced during macrophage infection. Infect Immun 63:1409–1414

8. Truong QL, Cho Y, Barate AK, Kim S, Hahn TW (2014) Characterization and protective property of Brucella abortus cydC and looP mutants. Clin Vaccine Immunol 21:1573–1580

9. Truong QL, Cho Y, Barate AK, Kim S, Watarai M, Hahn TW (2015) Mutation of purD and purF genes further attenuates Brucella abortus strain RB51. Microb Pathog 79:1–7

10. Loisel-Meyer S, Jimenez de Bagues MP, Basseres E, Dornand J, Kohler S, Liautard JP, Jubier-Maurin V (2006) Requirement of norD for Brucella suis virulence in a murine model of in vitro and in vivo infection. Infect Immun 74:1973–1976

11. Kim S, Watanabe K, Shirahata T, Watarai M (2004) Zinc uptake system (znuA locus) of Brucella abortus is essential for intracellular survival and virulence in mice. J Vet Med Sci 66:1059–1063

12. Kim HS, Caswell CC, Foreman R, Roop RM 2nd, Crosson S (2013) The Brucella abortus general stress response system regulates chronic mammalian infection and is controlled by phosphorylation and proteolysis. J Biol Chem 288:13906–13916

13. Zhang M, Han X, Liu H, Tian M, Ding C, Song J, Sun X, Liu Z, Yu S (2013) Inactivation of the ABC transporter ATPase gene in Brucella abortus strain 2308 attenuated the virulence of the bacteria. Vet Microbiol 164:322–329

14. Kahl-McDonagh MM, Ficht TA (2006) Evaluation of protection afforded by Brucella abortus and Brucella melitensis unmarked deletion mutants exhibiting different rates of clearance in BALB/c mice. Infect Immun 74:4048–4057

15. Yang X, Clapp B, Thornburg T, Hoffman C, Pascual DW (2016) Vaccination with a DnorD DznuA Brucella abortus mutant confers potent protection against virulent challenge. Vaccine 34:5290–5297

16. Willett JW, Herrou J, Czyz DM, Cheng JX, Crosson S (2016) Brucella abortus DrpoE1 confers protective immunity against wild type challenge in a mouse model of brucellosis. Vaccine 34:5073–5081

17. Truong QL, Cho Y, Park S, Kim K, Hahn TW (2016) Brucella abortus DcydCDcydD and DcydCDpurD double-mutants are highly attenuated and confer long-term protective immunity against virulent Brucella abortus. Vaccine 34:237–244

18. Reid CW, Legaree BA, Clarke AJ (2007) Role of Ser216 in the mechanism of action of membrane-bound lytic transglycosylase B: further evidence for substrate-assisted catalysis. FEBS Lett 581:4988–4992

19. Suvorov M, Lee M, Hesek D, Boggess B, Mobashery S (2008) Lytic transglycosylase MltB of Escherichia coli and its role in recycling of peptidoglycan strands of bacterial cell wall. J Am Chem Soc 130:11878–11879

20. Lamers RP, Nguyen UT, Nguyen Y, Buensuceso RN, Burrows LL (2015) Loss of membrane-bound lytic transglycosylases increases outer membrane permeability and beta-lactam sensitivity in Pseudomonas aeruginosa. Microbiologyopen 4:879–895

21. Koraimann G (2003) Lytic transglycosylases in macromolecular transport systems of Gram-negative bacteria. Cell Mol Life Sci 60:2371–2388

22. Gao J, Tian M, Bao Y, Li P, Liu J, Ding C, Wang S, Li T, Yu S (2016) Pyruvate kinase is necessary for Brucella abortus full virulence in BALB/c mouse. Vet Res 47:87

23. Tian M, Qu J, Han X, Ding C, Wang S, Peng D, Yu S (2014) Mechanism of Asp24 upregulation in Brucella abortus rough mutant with a disrupted O-antigen export system and effect of Asp24 in bacterial intracellular survival. Infect Immun 82:2840–2850

24. Ye J, Coulouris G, Zaretskaya I, Cutcutache I, Rozen S, Madden TL (2012) Primer-BLAST: a tool to design target-specific primers for polymerase chain reaction. BMC Bioinform 13:134

25. National Center for Biotechnology Information Gene. http://www.ncbi. nlm.nih.gov/gene. Accessed 6 Sep 2016

26. Kim D, Langmead B, Salzberg SL (2015) HISAT: a fast spliced aligner with low memory requirements. Nat Methods 12:357–360

27. Langmead B, Trapnell C, Pop M, Salzberg SL (2009) Ultrafast and memory-efficient alignment of short DNA sequences to the human genome. Genome Biol 10:R25

28. Li B, Dewey CN (2011) RSEM: accurate transcript quantification from RNA-Seq data with or without a reference genome. BMC Bioinform 12:323

29. Mortazavi A, Williams BA, McCue K, Schaeffer L, Wold B (2008) Mapping and quantifying mammalian transcriptomes by RNA-Seq. Nat Methods 5:621–628

30. Braun W (1946) Dissociation in Brucella abortus; a demonstration of the role of inherent and environmental factors in bacterial variation. J Bacteriol 51:327–349

31. Pei J, Kahl-McDonagh M, Ficht TA (2014) Brucella dissociation is essential for macrophage egress and bacterial dissemination. Front Cell Infect Microbiol 4:23

32. Gonzalez D, Grillo MJ, De Miguel MJ, Ali T, Arce-Gorvel V, Delrue RM, Conde-Alvarez R, Munoz P, Lopez-Goni I, Iriarte M, Marin CM, Weintraub A, Widmalm G, Zygmunt M, Letesson JJ, Gorvel JP, Blasco JM, Moriyon I (2008) Brucellosis vaccines: assessment of Brucella melitensis lipopolysaccharide rough mutants defective in core and O-polysaccharide synthesis and export. PLoS One 3:e2760

33. Huerta-Cepas J, Szklarczyk D, Forslund K, Cook H, Heller D, Walter MC, Rattei T, Mende DR, Sunagawa S, Kuhn M, Jensen LJ, von Mering C, Bork P (2016) eggNOG 4.5: a hierarchical orthology framework with improved functional annotations for eukaryotic, prokaryotic and viral sequences. Nucleic Acids Res 44:D286–D293

34. von Bargen K, Gorvel JP, Salcedo SP (2012) Internal affairs: investigating the Brucella intracellular lifestyle. FEMS Microbiol Rev 36:533–562

35. Goodell EW (1985) Recycling of murein by Escherichia coli. J Bacteriol 163:305–310

36. Kraft AR, Prabhu J, Ursinus A, Holtje JV (1999) Interference with murein turnover has no effect on growth but reduces β-lactamase induction in Escherichia coli. J Bacteriol 181:7192–7198

37. Vollmer W, Holtje JV (2001) Morphogenesis of Escherichia coli. Curr Opin Microbiol 4:625–633

38. Trakhanov S, Vyas NK, Luecke H, Kristensen DM, Ma J, Quiocho FA (2005) Ligand-free and -bound structures of the binding protein (LivJ) of the Escherichia coli ABC leucine/isoleucine/valine transport system: trajectory and dynamics of the interdomain rotation and ligand specificity. Biochemistry 44:6597–6608

39. Nikodinovic-Runic J, Flanagan M, Hume AR, Cagney G, O'Connor KE (2009) Analysis of the Pseudomonas putida CA-3 proteome during growth on styrene under nitrogen-limiting and non-limiting conditions. Microbiology 155:3348–3361

40. Gesbert G, Ramond E, Tros F, Dairou J, Frapy E, Barel M, Charbit A (2015) Importance of branched-chain amino acid utilization in Francisella intracellular adaptation. Infect Immun 83:173–183

41. Prell J, White JP, Bourdes A, Bunnewell S, Bongaerts RJ, Poole PS (2009) Legumes regulate Rhizobium bacteroid development and persistence by the supply of branched-chain amino acids. Proc Natl Acad Sci U S A 106:12477–12482

42. Furuchi T, Kashiwagi K, Kobayashi H, Igarashi K (1991) Characteristics of the gene for a spermidine and putrescine transport system that maps at 15 min on the Escherichia coli chromosome. J Biol Chem 266:20928–20933

43. Vanoni MA, Curti B (1999) Glutamate synthase: a complex iron–sulfur flavoprotein. Cell Mol Life Sci 55:617–638

44. Ronneau S, Moussa S, Barbier T, Conde-Alvarez R, Zuniga-Ripa A, Moriyon I, Letesson JJ (2016) Brucella, nitrogen and virulence. Crit Rev Microbiol 42:507–525

45. Wallach DP, Grisolia S (1957) The purification and properties of hydropyrimidine hydrase. J Biol Chem 226:277–288

46. Kim S, West TP (1991) Pyrimidine catabolism in *Pseudomonas aeruginosa*. FEMS Microbiol Lett 61:175–179

47. Biswas S, Biswas I (2013) SmbFT, a putative ABC transporter complex, confers protection against the lantibiotic Smb in Streptococci. J Bacteriol 195:5592–5601

48. Riquelme-Neira R, Retamal-Diaz A, Acuna F, Riquelme P, Rivera A, Saez D, Onate A (2013) Protective effect of a DNA vaccine containing an open reading frame with homology to an ABC-type transporter present in the genomic island 3 of *Brucella abortus* in BALB/c mice. Vaccine 31:3663–3667

49. Nol P, Olsen SC, Rhyan JC, Sriranganathan N, McCollum MP, Hennager SG, Pavuk AA, Sprino PJ, Boyle SM, Berrier RJ, Salman MD (2016) Vaccination of elk (*Cervus canadensis*) with Brucella abortus strain RB51 overexpressing superoxide dismutase and glycosyltransferase genes does not induce adequate protection against experimental *Brucella abortus* challenge. Front Cell Infect Microbiol 6:10

50. Lei S, Zhong Z, Ke Y, Yang M, Xu X, Ren H, An C, Yuan J, Yu J, Xu J, Qiu Y, Shi Y, Wang Y, Peng G, Chen Z (2015) Deletion of the small RNA chaperone protein Hfq down regulates genes related to virulence and confers protection against wild-type *Brucella* challenge in mice. Front Microbiol 6:1570

51. Ganesh NV, Sadowska JM, Sarkar S, Howells L, McGiven J, Bundle DR (2014) Molecular recognition of *Brucella* A and M antigens dissected by synthetic oligosaccharide glycoconjugates leads to a disaccharide diagnostic for brucellosis. J Am Chem Soc 136:16260–16269

52. Montaraz JA, Winter AJ, Hunter DM, Sowa BA, Wu AM, Adams LG (1986) Protection against *Brucella abortus* in mice with O-polysaccharide-specific monoclonal antibodies. Infect Immun 51:961–963

53. Nijskens C, Copin R, De Bolle X, Letesson JJ (2008) Intracellular rescuing of a *B. melitensis* 16 M virB mutant by co-infection with a wild type strain. Microb Pathog 45:134–141

# 2

# The role of phospholipase C signaling in bovine herpesvirus 1 infection

Liqian Zhu[1,2,4*†], Chen Yuan[1,2†], Xiuyan Ding[1,2,3], Clinton Jones[4] and Guoqiang Zhu[1,2*]

## Abstract

Bovine herpesvirus 1 (BoHV-1) infection enhanced the generation of inflammatory mediator reactive oxidative species (ROS) and stimulated MAPK signaling that are highly possibly related to virus induced inflammation. In this study, for the first time we show that BoHV-1 infection manipulated phospholipase C (PLC) signaling, as demonstrated by the activation of PLCγ-1 at both early stages [at 0.5 h post-infection (hpi)] and late stages (4–12 hpi) during the virus infection of MDBK cells. Viral entry, and de novo protein expression and/or DNA replication were potentially responsible for the activation of PLCγ-1 signaling. PLC signaling inhibitors of both U73122 and edelfosine significantly inhibited BoHV-1 replication in both bovine kidney cells (MDBK) and rabbit skin cells (RS-1) in a dose-dependent manner by affecting the virus entry stage(s). In addition, the activation of Erk1/2 and p38MAPK signaling, and the enhanced generation of ROS by BoHV-1 infection were obviously ameliorated by chemical inhibition of PLC signaling, implying the requirement of PLC signaling in ROS production and these MAPK pathway activation. These results suggest that the activation of PLC signaling is a potential pathogenic mechanism for BoHV-1 infection.

## Introduction

Bovine Herpesvirus 1 (BoHV-1) is an enveloped virus belonging to *Alphaherpesvirinae* subfamily member [1]. Acute infection of cattle with BoHV-1 generally results in inflammatory disease within the upper respiratory tract, nasal cavity, and ocular cavity, which leads to erosion of the mucosal surface. BoHV-1 also suppresses host immune responses by diverse mechanisms which lead to secondary infections [2]. BoHV-1 together with other viruses, such as bovine viral diarrhea viruses (BVDV), bovine respiratory syncytial virus (BRSV), parainfluenza-3 virus (PI3V) and bovine coronaviruses, and bacteria including *Mannheimia haemolytica*, *Pasteurella multocida*, *Histophilus somni* and *Mycoplasma* spp are the etiologies of life-threatening pneumonia known as bovine respiratory disease complex (BRDC), the most important disease in cattle [2–4]. BoHV-1 infection stimulates inflammasome formation [5], which contributes to BRDC by enhancing the inflammatory response in the lung. A BoHV-1 entry receptor, poliovirus receptor related 1, has been identified to be a BRDC susceptibility gene for Holstein calves [6], confirming the critical role of BoHV-1 as a cofactor for BRDC. BoHV-1 infection and the virus induced BRDC inflict a great economic lost to the cattle industry, worldwide [3].

It is known that BoHV-1 infection induces overexpression of pro-inflammatory cytokines, such as IL-1β and TNF-α that contribute greatly to the inflammatory response [7, 8]. In addition, we recently identified that BoHV-1 infection increases the generation of inflammatory mediator, reactive oxidative species (ROS) [9], which is also a potential mechanism to promote inflammatory response. Over-produced ROS mediated inflammatory response by diverse mechanisms in varied virus infections. In the context of Influenza virus or Dengue virus infection, ROS promotes the production of pro-inflammatory cytokines IL-1β and TNF-α [10–12]. In HSV-1 infected murine microglial cells, ROS mediated the regulation of some inflammation pertinent signaling, such as p38MAPK and Erk1/2 pathways [13]. In contrast, the activation of p38MAPK and Erk1/2 signaling by BoHV-1 infection is not mediated by over-produced ROS [14],

*Correspondence: lzhu3596@163.com; lqzhu@yzu.edu.cn; yzgqzhu@yzu.edu.cn
†Liqian Zhu and Chen Yuan contributed equally to this work
[1] College of Veterinary Medicine, Yangzhou University, 48 Wenhui East Road, Yangzhou 225009, Jiangsu, China
Full list of author information is available at the end of the article

though BoHV-1 and HSV-1 are genetically closed [9]. How BoHV-1 infection contributes to ROS production and the activation of p38MAPK and Erk1/2 signaling has yet to be found.

Phospholipase C (PLC) plays important roles in the regulation of inflammatory response with diverse mechanisms in varied cells, e.g. PLC signaling has been suggested to be involved in macrophage mediated inflammatory response by regulating ROS generation, inflammatory cytokine transcription, cell adhesion, and monocyte to macrophage differentiation [15–18]. NaCl-induced NLRP3 inflammasome activation in retinal pigment epithelial cells is partially dependent on the activities of PLC signaling [19]. The PLC family contains six members (β, γ, δ, ε, η and ζ) that are further subdivided into 13 isoforms, which are functionally dependent on the activation of a series of downstream signalings, such as protein kinase C (PKC) and calcium signaling [20]. It has been reported that PLCγ-1 signaling is required by influenza virus for efficient replication in both T-cells and human airway epithelial A549 cells, and for the virus induced inflammatory response mediated by macrophages [18, 21, 22], which highlighted the importance of PLC signaling in virus pathogenicity. However, the involvement of PLC signaling in BoHV-1 infection is unknown.

In this study, for the first time we investigated the role of PLC signaling in BoHV-1 infection. We demonstrated that BoHV-1 infection activated PLC signaling for efficient viral replication, increasing ROS generation and activation of Erk1/2 and p38MAPK signaling. These data collectively suggested that BoHV-1 infection regulated the generation of ROS and stimulation of Erk1/2 and p38MAPK signaling partially depending on PLC signaling. Our data suggest that PLC signaling is important for BoHV-1 infection and virus-induced inflammation.

## Materials and methods
### Antibodies and reagents
Antibodies against phospho-p38MAPK (Thr180/Tyr182), p38MAPK, phospho-p44/42 MAPK (Erk1/2) (Thr202/Tyr204), Erk1/2, phospho-PLCγ-1(Ser1248), PLCγ-1 and GAPDH, as well as HRP labeled secondary antibodies including goat anti-mouse IgG and goat anti-rabbit IgG were purchased from Cell Signaling Technology (Beverly, MA, USA). Fluorescein isothiocyanate (FITC) labeled goat anti-bovine IgG was purchased from Beijing Biosynthesis Biotechnology Co., Ltd (Beijing, China). PLC signaling inhibitors U73122 and edelfosine, intracellular ROS indicator 2′,7′- dichlorodihydrofluorescein diacetate (H2DCFDA), herpesvirus inhibitors phosphonoacetic acid (PAA) and Acyclovir (ACY), as well 3-(4,5-dimethylthiazol-2-yl)-2,5-diphenyl tetrazolium bromide (MTT)

were purchased from Sigma-Aldrich (St. Louis, MO, USA).

### Cells and virus
MDBK cells and RS-1 cells were maintained in DMEM (Gibco BRL) supplemented with 10% horse serum and fetal bovine serum (HyClone Laboratories, Logan, UT, USA), respectively. BoHV-1 (Colorado1 stain) was propagated in MDBK cells. Aliquots of virus stocks were stored at −70 °C until use. The virus was titrated in MDBK cells with results expressed as $TCID_{50}$/mL calculated using the Reed-Muench formula.

To inactivate BoHV-1 virus with UV-irradiation, virus stock was dispersed into 100-mm tissue culture dishes, and directly placed under a UV lamp (20 W) for 30 min. Complete inactivation of the virus was confirmed by the fact that no plaque was produced in MDBK cells exposed to the UV treated virus for 48 h.

### Cytotoxicity assays with MTT method
Cell viability was assessed by the MTT assay. MDBK or RS-1 cells were seeded into 96-well plates at $1 \times 10^4$ cells/well within a volume of 200 µL per well. Eight replicates were mock treated with DMSO, U73122 or edelfosine at various concentrations of 5 and 10 µM for 24 h at 37 °C. Thirty microliters MTT solution (2 mg/mL in PBS) were added to each well. The cells were then incubated for 4 h at 37 °C. The medium was replaced with 150 µL of DMSO for each well to solubilize the formazan. The plates were shaken on a rotary platform for 10 min. Finally, the absorbance value was measured at a wavelength of 550 nm using a Wellscan (Labsystems, Santa Fe, NM, USA). The mean optical density of the control was assigned a value of 100%.

### Virus replication inhibition assay
Serum starved MDBK cell in 24-wells plates were pretreated with inhibitors at the designated concentration for 1 h at 37 °C, then infected with BoHV-1 (MOI of 1) for 1 h along with the treatment of corresponding inhibitors. After extensive washing with PBS, DMEM (400 µL) with or without inhibitors was added to each well. At 24 hpi, viral yields were titrated in MDBK cells. The results are expressed as $TCID_{50}$/mL calculated using the Reed-Muench formula.

To test whether these inhibitors affected the viral entry or post entry stages of BoHV-1 infection, serum starved MDBK cells were incubated in 24-well plates with BoHV-1 (MOI = 1) for 1 h at 4 °C to allow the viruses to adsorb to the cell membrane but not to penetrate the cells. The cells were then subjected to extensive washing with ice-cold PBS. To identify the effect of PLC signaling on the virus entry process, pre-warmed fresh medium with DMSO, 5 μM of U73122, or 5 μM of edelfosine were added, and the cell cultures were quickly shifted to 37 °C for 1 h to allow the viruses enter the cells. The cells were then treated with citrate buffer (40 mM citric acid, 10 mM KCl, 135 mM NaCl, pH 3.0) for 1 min to inactivate cell membrane bound but unpenetrated virions [23, 24]. Subsequently, fresh medium was replaced and continuously incubated for 24 h at 37 °C. In parallel, to identify the effect of PLC signaling on the BoHV-1 post entry process, the virus adsorbed MDBK cells were first shifted to 37 °C for 1 h to allow the virus enter the cells followed by treatment with citrate buffer for 1 min, then incubated for 24 h at 37 °C in the absence or presence of U73122 and edlefosine, respectively. The virus yield was determined in MDBK cells with results expressed as $TCID_{50}$/mL.

To test whether PLC signaling affects the virus binding to MDBK cells, serum starved MDBK cells were incubated in 6-well plates in the absence or presence of PLC inhibitors at a concentration of 5 μM for 1 h at 37 °C to block PLC signaling. Then the cells were incubated with virus stock at 4 °C for 1 h to allow the viruses absorb to the cell membrane, in the absence or presence of corresponding PLC inhibitors. Then the cells were washed with ice-cold PBS, and subjected to two rounds of frozen-thawings to release cell membrane attached viruses. After centrifugation, the viral titer was determined in MDBK cells, with data expressed as $TCID_{50}$/mL.

### Flow cytometry assay

To analyze whether UV-inactivated BoHV-1 could bind to MDBK cells, the cells in 6-well plates were detached by treatment with 2 mM EDTA. After extensive washing with ice-cold PBS, the cells were incubated with infectious BoHV-1 or UV-inactivated BoHV-1 for 1 h at 4 °C allowing the viral particles to attach to the cells. The cells were then fixed with 4% paraformaldehyde for 15 min at room temperature, and stained with bovine anti-BoHV-1 serum followed by FITC-conjugated anti-bovine IgG. The cells were washed twice with ice-cold PBS, and the cell membrane bound viral particles were analyzed on FACS.

### Cellular ROS assay

MDBK cells in 24-well plates were pretreated with solvent DMSO, U73122 (2.5 μM) or edelfosine (5 μM) for 1 h, then infected with BoHV-1 (MOI = 10) in the presence of a corresponding inhibitor for 1 h. The uninfected control was treated with cell lysates from uninfected MDBK cells. After washing with PBS for three times, fresh medium containing inhibitor was added. At 4 hpi, the cells were washed with PBS and exposed to ROS fluorescence indicator H2DCFDA (50 μM) for 30 min at 37 °C. The reaction mixture was then replaced with PBS,

and images were acquired under a fluorescence microscope, the fluorescence intensity of cellular ROS was quantified with software Image-pro Plus 6.

### Western blot analysis

To test the kinetic variation of PLCγ-1 signaling, monolayers of MDBK cells were serum starved overnight in 60-mm dishes, infected with BoHV-1(MOI = 10) for 0.5, 1, 2, 4, 8 and 12 h. Cell lysate was prepared using lysis buffer (1% Triton X-100, 50 mM sodium chloride, 1 mM EDTA, 1 mM EGTA, 20 mM sodium fluoride, 20 mM sodium pyrophosphate, 1 mM phenylmethylsulfonyl fluoride, 0.5 g/mL leupeptin, 1 mM benzamidine, and 1 mM sodium orthovanadate in 20 mM Tris–HCl, pH 8.0).

To test the effect of U73122 and edelfosine on the designated signaling, MDBK cells were serum starved overnight in 60-mm dishes, pretreated with U73122 or edelfosine at the indicated concentrations for 1 h, then mock-infected or infected with BoHV-1 at 37 °C for 0.5 h along with the treatment by the corresponding inhibitors. Cell lysates were then prepared with the lysis buffer as described above.

Cell lysate was separated on an 8 or 10% SDS–polyacrylamide gel and proteins were transferred to a polyvinylidene difluoride (PVDF) membrane (Bio-rad, CA, USA). After blocking with 5% nonfat milk in Tris-buffered saline (TBS) buffer containing 0.05% Tween 20 (TBST), the membrane was incubated with designated primary antibody (1:1000). After extensive washing with TBST, the HRP-conjugated secondary antibody (1:1500) in the blocking reagent was then added. After extensive washing with TBST, immune reactive bands were detected using the enhanced chemiluminescence (ECL) reaction substrate (Millipore, USA). The band intensity was analyzed with software image J.

### Results

#### PLC signaling inhibitors U73122 and edelfosine inhibited BoHV-1 infection in bovine kidney cells (MDBK cells) and rabbit skin cells (RS-1 cells)

To test whether PLC signaling is involved in BoHV-1 infection, the effect of chemical inhibition of PLC signaling on viral replication in MDBK cells was first investigated. Since the chemical inhibitors may have an off target effect, we used two PLC signaling specific inhibitors U73122 and edelfosine for this evaluation in parallel. As shown in Figures 1A and B, the treatment of MDBK cells with U73122 or edelfosine resulted in a reduction of the virus yield in a dose-dependent manner. With the treatment of 1 and 5 μM of both inhibitors, the virus yield reduced a titer of ~1 and 2-log in comparison with the control samples, respectively. Acyclovir (ACY) a known inhibitor for herpesvirus was

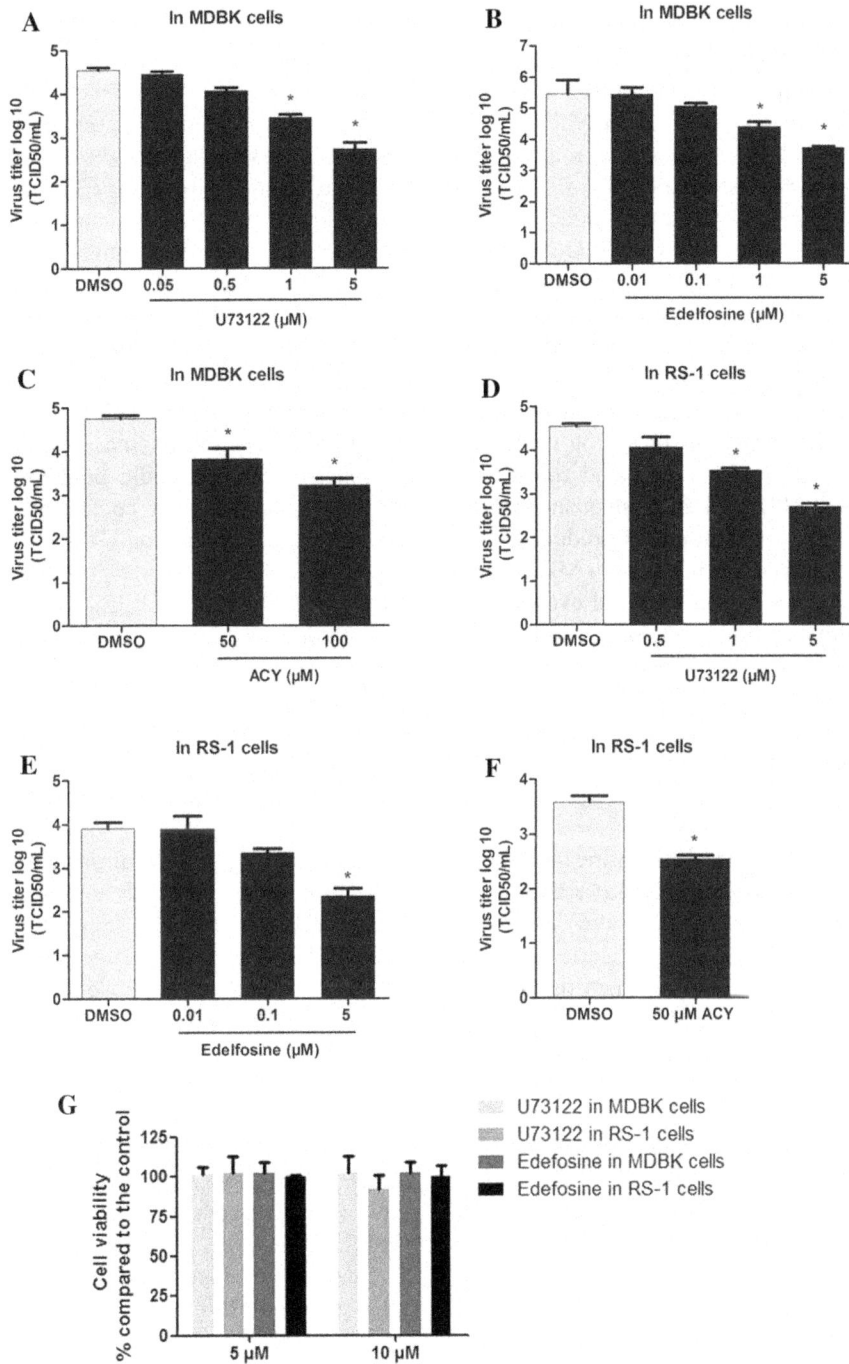

**Figure 1 Inhibitory effect of U73122 and edelfosine on BoHV-1 viral replication in vitro.** Inhibitory effect of U73122 (**A**), edelfosine (**B**) and ACY (**C**) on BoHV-1 replication in MDBK cells. Serum starved MDBK cells were pretreated with each inhibitor at indicated concentrations for 1 h, infected with BoHV-1(MOI = 1) for 24 h along with the treatment of corresponding inhibitor, respectively. The viral titer was determined with MDBK cells with the results expressed as $TCID_{50}$/mL. Inhibitory effect of U73122 (**D**), edelfosine (**E**) and ACY (**F**) on BoHV-1 replication in RS-1 cells. Serum starved RS-1 cells were pretreated with each inhibitor at the indicated concentrations for 1 h, infected with BoHV-1(MOI = 1) for 24 h along with the treatment of the corresponding inhibitor, respectively. The viral titer was determined with MDBK cells with results expressed as $TCID_{50}$/mL. (**G**) The cytotoxicity assay for both U73122 and edelfosine in either MDBK cells or RS-1 cells. MDBK cells or RS-1 cells were exposed DMSO, U73122 or edelfosine at the designated concentrations for 24 h. After incubation with MTT, the OD value was determined and compared to the control which was designated as 100%. Data represent three independent experiments. Significance was assessed with the student $t$ test (*$P < 0.05$).

introduced as a positive control. ACY at a concentration of 50 and 100 μM decreased the virus titer by ~0.9 and 1.5-log compared to the control, respectively (Figure 1C), validating the inhibitory effects of both U73122 and edelfosine on BoHV-1 replication in MDBK cells. These results suggest that PLC signaling is required for BoHV-1 infection in MDBK cells. Rabbit skin (RS-1) cells are also permissive for BoHV-1 productive infection [25]. To see whether the inhibitory effect of PLC inhibitors on BoHV-1 replication was bovine kidney cell specific, RS-1 cells were utilized for further evaluation. As can be seen in Figure 1D, E, both inhibitors at a concentration of 5 μM significantly reduced the virus yield in RS-1 cells. The known herpesvirus inhibitor ACY at a concentration of 50 μM decreased the virus titer of ~1-log compared to the control (Figure 1F), which validated the inhibitory effects of both U73122 and edelfosine on BoHV-1 replication in RS-1 cells. In addition, the reduced virus yield by both U73122 and edelfosine in both MDBK cells and RS-1 cells was not due to the chemical cytotoxicity, because both inhibitors at the tested concentrations did not show apparent cytotoxicity to neither MDBK cells nor RS-1 cells detected with the MTT assay (Figure 1G). Therefore, our data suggest that PLC signaling may affect BoHV-1 infection in a broad spectrum of cell types, in vitro.

### PLC signaling inhibitors U73122 and edelfosine inhibited BoHV-1 infection at the postbinding cell entry stages

Since PLC inhibitor of both U73122 and edelfosine could unanimously inhibit BoHV-1 replication in both MDBK and RS-1 cells, we further identified which stage(s) of the viral replication including virus binding, postbinding cell entry and post entry stages was affected in MDBK cells. As a result, both U73122 and edelfosine mainly affected the virus postbinding cell entry stages but not the post entry stages (Figures 2A and B). As virus attachment and cell entry are early events in the virus infection cycle, we further investigated the role of PLC signaling in virus attachment. As shown in Figure 2C, both U73122 and edelfosine treatment had no effect on BoHV-1 binding to the cell surface. These results suggest that PLC signaling may mainly contribute to the postbinding cell entry stages during BoHV-1 infection of MDBK cells.

### BoHV-1 infection activated PLCγ-1 signaling in MDBK cells

Since PLC signaling inhibitor apparently affected BoHV-1 replication in both MDBK and RS-1 cells, we further examined whether BoHV-1 infection affected PLC signaling by testing the kinetics of phosphorylated PLCγ-1(Ser1248) during virus infection of MDBK cells as previously described [18, 21]. In order to see the burst

effect of virus infection on the detected signaling, MDBK cells were infected with BoHV-1 (Colorado 1 strain) at a high MOI of 10. At 0.5, 1, 2, 4, 8 and 12 hpi, the cell lysate were prepared and subjected to western blot analysis. As shown in Figure 3A, the level of phospho-PLCγ-1(Ser1248) was first detected to increase at 0.5 hpi, then it decreased to the basal level from 1 to 2 hpi, and re-increased at 4 hpi, then remained at a high level until the end of the detected time point at 12 hpi.

Since the increased phosphorylation of PLCγ-1(Ser1248) could be detected at 0.5 hpi, we wondered whether this was related to viral entry. To address this question, the ability of UV-inactivated BoHV-1 virus to stimulate the phosphorylation of PLCγ-1(Ser1248) in MDBK cells was examined as previously described [21]. UV-inactivated virus could bind to the virus receptors and enter the cells, but could not express viral genes [26]. Here, the ability for UV-irradiated viral particles to bind to MDBK cells was confirmed with FACS assay (Figure 3C). As expected, UV-irradiated BoHV-1 could also increase the phosphorylation of PLCγ-1(Ser1248), compared to the control, though there is a minor reduced ability compared to the infectious viral particles (Figure 3B). This suggests that the virus entry would initially stimulate the phosphorylation of PLCγ-1(Ser1248) which corroborated the result that PLC signaling inhibitors affected the virus entry stage(s) (Figure 2A). We also supposed that de novo viral protein expression or DNA replication may potentially account for the enhanced phosphorylation of PLCγ-1(Ser1248) that occurred at 4, 8 and 12 hpi (Figure 3A). To test the hypothesis, MDBK cells were treated with phosphonoacetic acid (PAA), a specific inhibitor targeting the viral DNA polymerase [27], through virus infection. As a result, PAA treatment significantly inhibited the virus replication in MDBK cells (Figure 3E), and apparently reduced the phosphorylation of PLCγ-1(Ser1248) at 12 hpi but not at 0.5 hpi which was stimulated by BoHV-1 infection while PAA treatment only had a minor effect on viral induced phosphorylation of PLCγ-1(Ser1248) at 0.5 hpi (Figure 3E). Thus, de novo viral protein production and/or DNA replication seems to be correlated to the elevated levels of phosphorylated PLCγ-1(Ser1248).

### PLC signaling inhibitors U73122 and edelfosine inhibited Erk1/2 and p38MAPK signaling stimulated by BoHV-1 infection

As we know, the activated PLC signaling can stimulate calcium and PKC signaling [33]. In addition, multiple studies have demonstrated that Erk1/2 and p38MAPK signaling can be activated by PKC and increased intracellular calcium signaling [28, 29], suggesting that BoHV-1 may activate Erk1/2 and p38MAPK signaling through

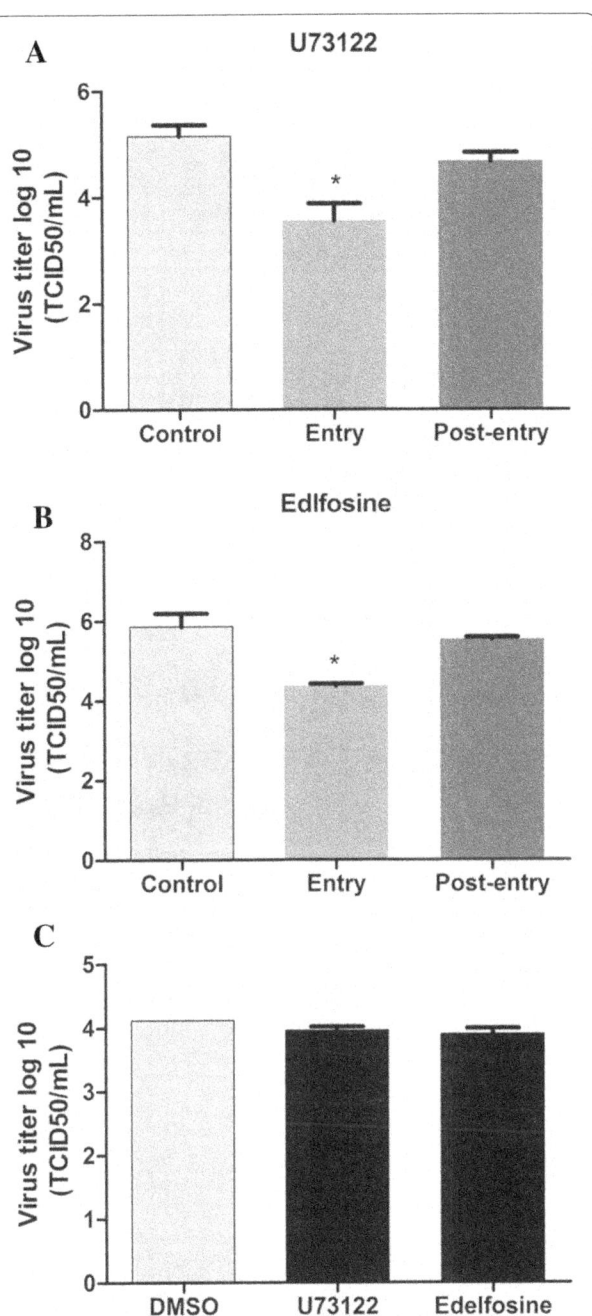

**Figure 2 Both U73122 and edelfosine affect virus entry.** Serum starved MDBK cells infected with BoHV-1 (MOI = 1) were treated with U73122 (**A**) and edelfosine (**B**) at a concentration of 5 µM, at the virus entry, or post-entry process, respectively. At 24 hpi the viral titer were determined in MDBK cells with results expressed as TCID50/mL. **C** Serum starved MDBK cells were incubated in the absence or presence of 5 µM of U73122 or 5 µM of edelfosine for 1 h at 37 °C. The virus in ice-cold DMEM containing fresh inhibitors was then allowed to adsorb to MDBK cells for 1 h at 4 °C. After freezing and thawing, the cell membrane bound viruses were titered in MDBK cells. Values represent three independent experiments. Significance was assessed with the student $t$ test (*$P < 0.05$).

PLC signaling. Therefore, the effects of U73122 and edelfosine on Erk1/2 and p38MAPK signaling in response to BoHV-1 infection were examined. As expected, both inhibitors decreased the levels of phosphorylated PLCγ-1(Ser1248) in a dose-dependent manner (Figures 4A and B; P-PLCγ-1 panel), validating the specific effect of these chemicals on PLC signaling. BoHV-1-induced activation of Erk1/2 and p38MAPK, was attenuated by U73122 and edelfosine in a dose-dependent manner (Figures 4A and B, P-Erk1/2 and P-p38MAPK panels). However, these inhibitor treatments did not have a dramatic effect on total steady state protein levels of PLCγ-1, Erk1/1 or p38MAPK following BoHV-1 infection (Figure 4C). Therefore, our results indicated that the activation of Erk1/2 and p38MAPK signaling by BoHV-1-infection was partially dependent on PLC signaling.

### PLC signaling inhibitors U73122 and edelfosine inhibited ROS generation stimulated by BoHV-1 infection

We recently reported that BoHV-1 infection promotes ROS production which depended on viral entry, and de novo protein expression and/or DNA replication [9]. Here, we additionally tested whether chemical inhibition of PLC signaling affected BoHV-1-induced ROS production. Our results indicate that the treatment of MDBK cells with PLC inhibitor of both U73122 (2.5 µM) and edelfosine (5 µM) led to decreased ROS production stimulated by BoHV-1 infection by 38.6 and 48.3%, respectively (Figure 5). It indicated that PLCγ-1 signaling may partially regulate ROS production in response to BoHV-1 infection.

### Discussion

In this study, for the first time we demonstrated that chemical inhibition of PLC signaling led to significant inhibition of BoHV-1 infection. Since chemical inhibitors may have off target effects, two specific inhibitors for PLC signaling U73122 and edelfosine were employed, in parallel, with both bovine kidney cells and rabbit skin cells. They unanimously show inhibitory effects on BoHV-1 infection in both cell cultures (Figure 1). Biphasic activation of PLCγ-1 signaling by BoHV-1 infection in MDBK cells corroborated the requirement of PLC signaling in the virus infection (Figure 3).

Since PLC signaling is potentially regulating intracellular calcium signaling, multiple evidence suggests that calcium signaling is important to mediate some virus entry processes, e.g., $Ca^{2+}$ is strictly required for the cell entry of Rubella virus [30], Ebola virus, Marburg virus, Lassa virus and Junin virus [31]. In this study, our findings suggest that PLC inhibitors of both U73122 and edelfosine could efficiently inhibit the virus postbinding cell entry process (Figure 2). It is possible that PLC signaling

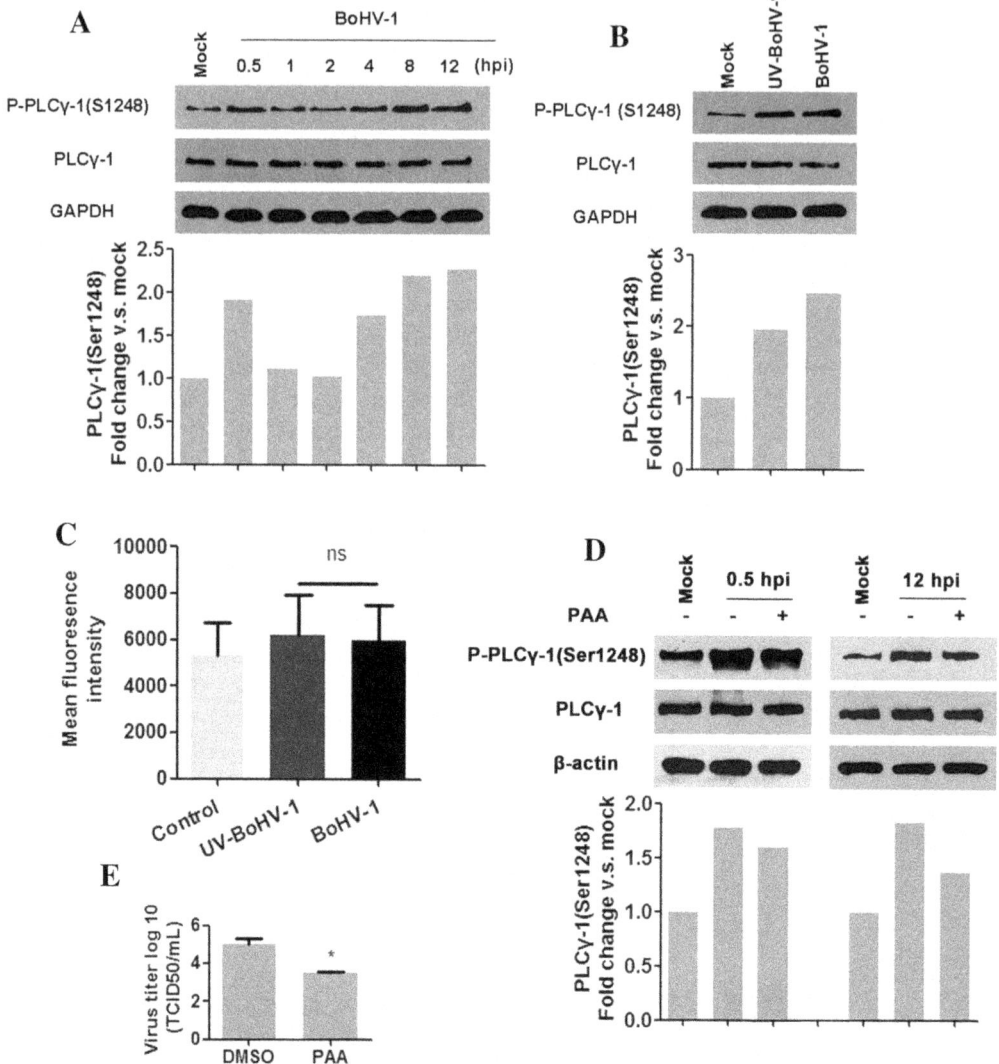

**Figure 3  BoHV-1 infection enhanced the phosphorylation of PLCγ-1 (S1248) in MDBK cells. (A)** Time course of PLCγ-1(Ser1248) phosphorylation following BoHV-1 infection. Serum starved MDBK cells were infected with BoHV-1 at an MOI of 10, and at indicated time points the cell lysates were prepared for western blotting. **(B)** MDBK cells were incubated with UV-irradiation inactivated virus or infectious virus at an MOI of 10 for 30 min, and then subjected to analysis of PLCγ-1(Ser1248) phosphorylation by western blotting. **(C)** The ability of UV-irradiation inactivated virus to bind to MDBK cells were analyzed with FACS. MDBK cells with or without viral particles attached were stained with bovine anti-BoHV-1 serum followed by FITC-conjugated anti-bovine IgG. The cell membrane bound viral particles were analyzed on FACS. The mean fluorescence intensity was analyzed. **(D)** Serum starved MDBK cells were infected with BoHV-1 at an MOI of 10 along with PAA treatment (100 μM). At 0.5 and 12 hpi the cell lysates for western blotting analysis were prepared, respectively. At 24 hpi the virus yield were determined in MDBK cells **(E)**. The band intensity was analyzed with software image J. Data are representative results of three independent experiments.

mediated BoHV-1 entry through the mobilization of calcium signaling, which needs further investigation.

We recently reported that BoHV-1 infection increased ROS production, which was required for efficient viral replication, and the oxidative stress contributes to mitochondrial dysfunction in MDBK cells [9]. However, the mechanism underlying the overproduction of ROS driven by BoHV-1 infection is still unknown. Here, we illustrated that inhibition of PLC signaling led to a significant decrease of ROS production induced by BoHV-1 infection (Figure 5), indicating that the virus induced ROS generation was partially regulated by PLC signaling.

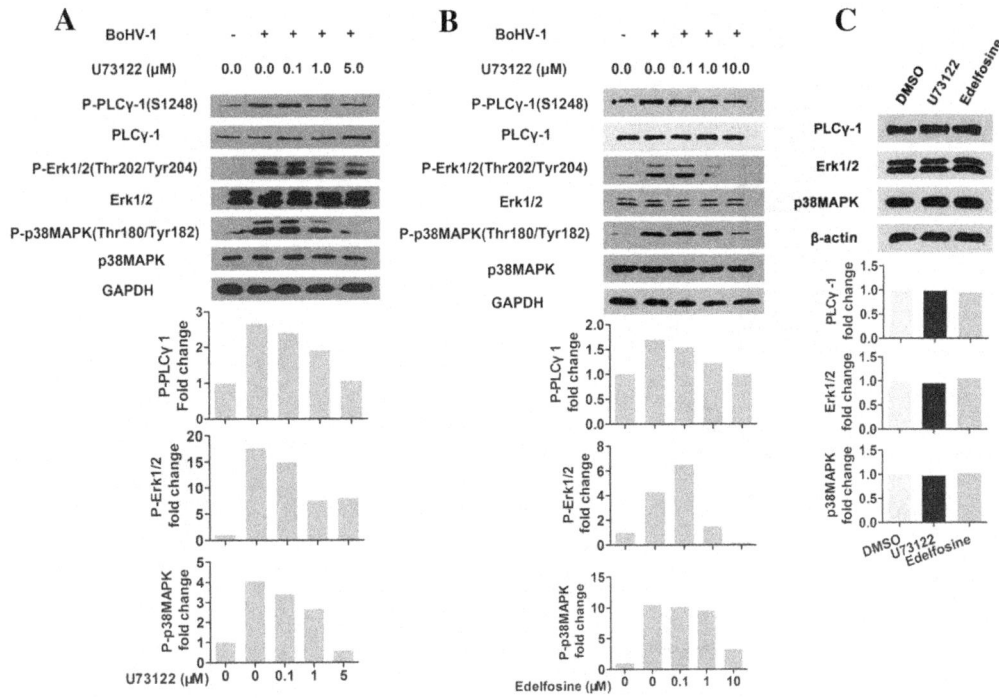

**Figure 4 Effect of U73122 and edelfosine on Erk1/2 and p38MAPK signaling in response to BoHV-1 infection.** Serum starved MDBK cells in 60-mm dishes were pretreated with U73122 (**A**) or edelfosine (**B**) at the indicated concentrations for 1 h, respectively, then infected with BoHV-1 (MOI = 10) in the presence of respective inhibitors for 0.5 h. (**C**) Serum starved MDBK cells in 60-mm dishes were exposed to DMSO, U73122 or edelfosine at the indicated concentrations for 1.5 h. Cell lysate was prepared and subjected to western blotting analysis. The band intensity was analyzed with software image J. The data are representatives of three independent experiments.

It is known that the NADPH (nicotinamide adenine dinucleotide phosphate) oxidases (NOXs) family including NOX1- to −5 and Duox1- to −2 are the main resource of ROS generation [32]. We previously identified that PLC signaling inhibitor U73122 inhibits ROS production partially through decreasing NOX2 expression in influenza virus PR8-infected human macrophage like cells (dU937 cells) [18]. However, antibodies suited for the detection of bovine NOXs are currently unavailable, and we could not identify whether NOXs expression is regulated by PLC signaling in the context of BoHV-1 infection. However, we know that BoHV-1 induced ROS production is partially regulated by PLC signaling.

Accordingly and in view of the extensive published evidence regarding the interaction between calcium signaling and MAPK pathways, as well as the mobilization of calcium signaling by PLC signaling [33], we further identified the effect of PLC signaling on Erk1/2 and

p38MAPK pathways. Here, we show that inhibition of PLC signaling attenuated the activation of Erk1/2 and p38MAPK signaling following BoHV-1 infection, but did not affect the steady state levels of both Erk1/2 and p38MAPK (Figure 3), indicating that PLC signaling partially mediates the activation of Erk1/2 and p38MAPK signaling stimulated by BoHV-1 infection. It is highly possible that BoHV-1 infection activates this MAPK signaling via the PLC/calcium signaling axis.

In summary, in this study we describe a so far unrecognized role of PLC signaling in BoHV-1 infection. For the first time we identified that PLC signaling is not only important for the BoHV-1 infection, but also important for the activation of Erk1/2 and p38MAPK signaling as well as excessive production of ROS induced by the virus infection. The activation of PLC signaling is a potential pathogenic mechanism for BoHV-1 infection. Therefore, pharmacological modulation of PLC signaling may provide

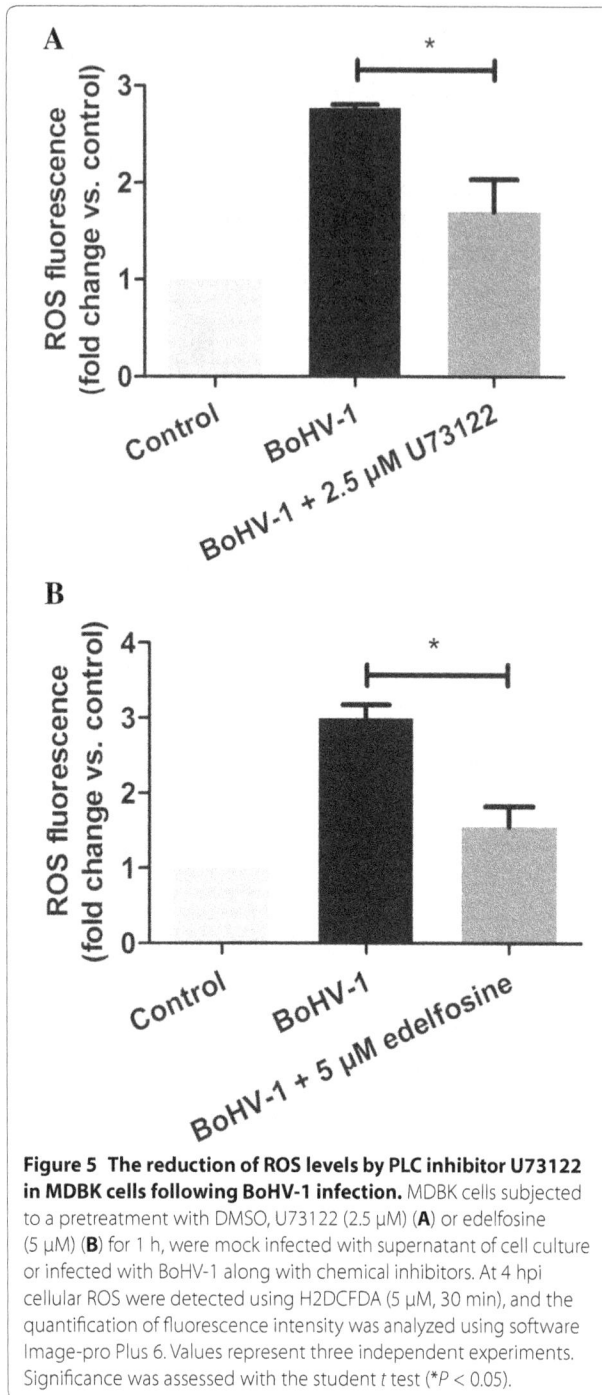

**Figure 5 The reduction of ROS levels by PLC inhibitor U73122 in MDBK cells following BoHV-1 infection.** MDBK cells subjected to a pretreatment with DMSO, U73122 (2.5 μM) (**A**) or edelfosine (5 μM) (**B**) for 1 h, were mock infected with supernatant of cell culture or infected with BoHV-1 along with chemical inhibitors. At 4 hpi cellular ROS were detected using H2DCFDA (5 μM, 30 min), and the quantification of fluorescence intensity was analyzed using software Image-pro Plus 6. Values represent three independent experiments. Significance was assessed with the student $t$ test (*$P < 0.05$).

a novel approach for fighting the virus through inhibition of both viral replication and inflammatory response.

**Competing interests**
The authors declare that they have no competing interests.

**Authors' contributions**
LZ participated in design of the study, analyzed the data and prepared the manuscript. CY carried out the experiments, XD cultured the cells. CJ revised

the manuscript, GZ coordinated the research. All authors read and approved the final manuscript.

**Acknowledgements**
We thank Dr. Leonard J Bello, University of Pennsylvania, USA for the kindly supplying BoHV-1 colorado1 stain and MDBK cells, Dr. Jumin Zhou, from Kunming Institute of Zoology, Chinese Academy of Sciences for kindly providing RS-1 cells. This research was supported by National Key Research and Development Program of China, Grant Nos. 2016YFD0500704, 2016YFD0500900, Chinese National Science Foundation, Grant No. 31472172, and partially supported by the Priority Academic Program Development of Jiangsu Higher Education Institutions (PAPD and TAPP).

**Author details**
[1] College of Veterinary Medicine, Yangzhou University, 48 Wenhui East Road, Yangzhou 225009, Jiangsu, China. [2] Jiangsu Co-innovation Center for Prevention and Control of Important Animal Infectious Diseases and Zoonoses, 48 Wenhui East Road, Yangzhou 225009, Jiangsu, China. [3] Test Center, Yangzhou University, 48 Wenhui East Road, Yangzhou 225009, Jiangsu, China. [4] Department of Veterinary Pathobiology, Oklahoma State University, Center for Veterinary Health Sciences, Stillwater, OK 74078, USA.

**References**
1.  Tikoo SK, Campos M, Babiuk LA (1995) Bovine herpesvirus 1 (BHV-1): biology, pathogenesis, and control. Adv Virus Res 45:191–223
2.  Jones C (2009) Regulation of innate immune responses by bovine herpesvirus 1 and infected cell protein 0 (bICP0). Viruses 1:255–275
3.  Jones C, Chowdhury S (2007) A review of the biology of bovine herpesvirus type 1 (BHV-1), its role as a cofactor in the bovine respiratory disease complex and development of improved vaccines. Anim Health Res Rev 8:187–205
4.  Fulton RW, d'Offay JM, Landis C, Miles DG, Smith RA, Saliki JT, Ridpath JF, Confer AW, Neill JD, Eberle R, Clement TJ, Chase CC, Burge LJ, Payton ME (2016) Detection and characterization of viruses as field and vaccine strains in feedlot cattle with bovine respiratory disease. Vaccine 34:3478–3492
5.  Wang J, Alexander J, Wiebe M, Jones C (2014) Bovine herpesvirus 1 productive infection stimulates inflammasome formation and caspase 1 activity. Virus Res 185:72–76
6.  Neibergs HL, Seabury CM, Wojtowicz AJ, Wang Z, Scraggs E, Kiser JN, Neupane M, Womack JE, Van Eenennaam A, Hagevoort GR, Lehenbauer TW, Aly S, Davis J, Taylor JF, Bovine Respiratory Disease Complex Coordinated Agricultural Project Research Team (2014) Susceptibility loci revealed for bovine respiratory disease complex in pre-weaned holstein calves. BMC Genom 15:1164
7.  Risalde MA, Molina V, Sánchez-Cordón PJ, Pedrera M, Panadero R, Romero-Palomo F, Gómez-Villamandos JC (2011) Response of proinflammatory and anti-inflammatory cytokines in calves with subclinical bovine viral diarrhea challenged with bovine herpesvirus-1. Vet Immunol Immunopathol 144:135–143
8.  Muylkens B, Thiry J, Kirten P, Schynts F, Thiry E (2007) Bovine herpesvirus 1 infection and infectious bovine rhinotracheitis. Vet Res 38:181–209
9.  Zhu L, Yuan C, Zhang D, Ma Y, Ding X, Zhu G (2016) BHV-1 induced oxidative stress contributes to mitochondrial dysfunction in MDBK cells. Vet Res 47:47
10. Ye S, Lowther S, Stambas J (2015) Inhibition of reactive oxygen species production ameliorates inflammation induced by influenza A viruses via upregulation of SOCS1 and SOCS3. J Virol 89:2672–2683
11. Amatore D, Sgarbanti R, Aquilano K, Baldelli S, Limongi D, Civitelli L, Nencioni L, Garaci E, Ciriolo MR, Palamara AT (2015) Influenza virus replication in lung epithelial cells depends on redox-sensitive pathways activated by NOX4-derived ROS. Cell Microbiol 17:131–145
12. Olagnier D, Peri S, Steel C, van Montfoort N, Chiang C, Beljanski V, Slifker M, He Z, Nichols CN, Lin R, Balachandran S, Hiscott J (2014) Cellular oxidative stress response controls the antiviral and apoptotic programs in dengue virus-infected dendritic cells. PLoS Pathog 10:e1004566

13. Hu S, Sheng WS, Schachtele SJ, Lokensgard JR (2011) Reactive oxygen species drive herpes simplex virus (HSV)-1-induced proinflammatory cytokine production by murine microglia. J Neuroinflamm 8:123

14. Zhu L, Yuan C, Huang L, Ding X, Wang J, Zhang D, Zhu G (2016) The activation of p38MAPK and JNK pathways in bovine herpesvirus 1 infected MDBK cells. Vet Res 47:91

15. Bae YS, Lee JH, Choi SH, Kim S, Almazan F, Witztum JL, Miller YI (2009) Macrophages generate reactive oxygen species in response to minimally oxidized low-density lipoprotein: toll-like receptor 4- and spleen tyrosine kinase-dependent activation of NADPH oxidase 2. Circ Res 104: 210–218 , 221 p following 218

16. Bae YS, Lee HY, Jung YS, Lee M, Suh PG (2017) Phospholipase Cγ in Toll-like receptor-mediated inflammation and innate immunity. Adv Biol Regul 63:92–97

17. Zhu L, Yuan C, Ma Y, Ding X, Zhu G, Zhu Q (2015) Anti-inflammatory activities of phospholipase C inhibitor U73122: inhibition of monocyte-to-macrophage transformation and LPS-induced pro-inflammatory cytokine expression. Int Immunopharmacol 29:622–627

18. Zhu L, Yuan C, Ding X, Xu S, Yang J, Liang Y, Zhu Q (2016) PLC-γ1 is involved in the inflammatory response induced by influenza A virus H1N1 infection. Virology 496:131–137

19. Prager P, Hollborn M, Steffen A, Wiedemann P, Kohen L, Bringmann A (2016) P2Y1 receptor signaling contributes to high salt-induced priming of the NLRP3 inflammasome in retinal pigment epithelial cells. PLoS One 11:e0165653

20. Vines CM (2012) Phospholipase C. Adv Exp Med Biol 740:235–254

21. Zhu L, Ly H, Liang Y (2014) PLC-γ1 signaling plays a subtype-specific role in postbinding cell entry of influenza A virus. J Virol 88:417–424

22. Fan K, Jia Y, Wang S, Li H, Wu D, Wang G, Chen JL (2012) Role of Itk signalling in the interaction between influenza A virus and T-cells. J Gen Virol 93:987–997

23. Chung CS, Huang CY, Chang W (2005) Vaccinia virus penetration requires cholesterol and results in specific viral envelope proteins associated with lipid rafts. J Virol 79:1623–1634

24. Zhu L, Ding X, Tao J, Wang J, Zhao X, Zhu G (2010) Critical role of cholesterol in bovine herpesvirus type 1 infection of MDBK cells. Vet Microbiol 144:51–57

25. Geiser V, Rose S, Jones C (2008) Bovine herpesvirus type 1 induces cell death by a cell-type-dependent fashion. Microb Pathog 44:459–466

26. Goodman AG, Smith JA, Balachandran S, Perwitasari O, Proll SC, Thomas MJ, Korth MJ, Barber GN, Schiff LA, Katze MG (2007) The cellular protein P58IPK regulates influenza virus mRNA translation and replication through a PKR-mediated mechanism. J Virol 81:2221–2230

27. Becker Y, Asher Y, Cohen Y, Weinberg-Zahlering E, Shlomai J (1977) Phosphonoacetic acid-resistant mutants of herpes simplex virus: effect of phosphonoacetic acid on virus replication and in vitro deoxyribonucleic acid synthesis in isolated nuclei. Antimicrob Agents Chemother 11:919–922

28. Li X, Yu H, Graves LM, Earp HS (1997) Protein kinase C and protein kinase A inhibit calcium-dependent but not stress-dependent c-Jun N-terminal kinase activation in rat liver epithelial cells. J Biol Chem 272:14996–15002

29. Heimfarth L, da Silva Ferreira F, Pierozan P, Loureiro SO, Mingori MR, Moreira JC, da Rocha JB, Pessoa-Pureur R (2016) Calcium signaling mechanisms disrupt the cytoskeleton of primary astrocytes and neurons exposed to diphenylditelluride. Biochim Biophys Acta 1860:2510–2520

30. Dube M, Rey FA, Kielian M (2014) Rubella virus: first calcium-requiring viral fusion protein. PLoS Pathog 10:e1004530

31. Han Z, Madara JJ, Herbert A, Prugar LI, Ruthel G, Lu J, Liu Y, Liu W, Liu X, Wrobel JE, Reitz AB, Dye JM, Harty RN, Freedman BD (2015) Calcium regulation of hemorrhagic fever virus budding: mechanistic implications for host-oriented therapeutic intervention. PLoS Pathog 11:e1005220

32. Bedard K, Krause KH (2007) The NOX family of ROS-generating NADPH oxidases: physiology and pathophysiology. Physiol Rev 87:245–313

33. White CD, Sacks DB (2010) Regulation of MAP kinase signaling by calcium. Methods Mol Biol 661:151–165

# 3

# Use of the mice passive protection test to evaluate the humoral response in goats vaccinated with Sterne 34F2 live spore vaccine

P. H. Phaswana[1], O. C. Ndumnego[1,3], S. M. Koehler[2,4], W. Beyer[2], J. E. Crafford[1] and H. van Heerden[1*]

## Abstract

The Sterne live spore vaccine (34F2) is the most widely used veterinary vaccine against anthrax in animals. Antibody responses to several antigens of *Bacillus anthracis* have been described with a large focus on those against protective antigen (PA). The focus of this study was to evaluate the protective humoral immune response induced by the live spore anthrax vaccine in goats. Boer goats vaccinated twice (week 0 and week 12) with the Sterne live spore vaccine and naive goats were used to monitor the anti-PA and toxin neutralizing antibodies at week 4 and week 17 (after the second vaccine dose) post vaccination. A/J mice were passively immunized with different dilutions of sera from immune and naive goats and then challenged with spores of *B. anthracis* strain 34F2 to determine the protective capacity of the goat sera. The goat anti-PA ELISA titres indicated significant sero-conversion at week 17 after the second doses of vaccine ($p = 0.009$). Mice receiving undiluted sera from goats given two doses of vaccine (twice immunized) showed the highest protection (86%) with only 20% of mice receiving 1:1000 diluted sera surviving lethal challenge. The in vitro toxin neutralization assay (TNA) titres correlated to protection of passively immunized A/J mice against lethal infection with the vaccine strain Sterne 34F2 spores using immune goat sera up to a 1:10 dilution ($r_s \geq 0.522$, $p = 0.046$). This study suggests that the passive mouse protection model could be potentially used to evaluate the protective immune response in livestock animals vaccinated with the current live vaccine and new vaccines.

## Introduction

Anthrax is a zoonotic disease caused by *Bacillus anthracis* that affects all mammals especially herbivorous mammals [1]. The main virulence factors are encoded by two plasmids, pXO1 and pXO2 [2]. The pXO1 encodes for the tripartite protein exotoxin (anthrax toxin) that consists of the cell-binding protective antigen (PA), and two enzymes known as lethal factor (LF) and edema factor (EF) [3]. The pXO2 encodes for the anti-phagocytic poly-D glutamic acid (PGA) capsule which protects the bacteria against phagocytosis [4].

Lethal toxin (LT) is formed by the binding of LF to PA while edema toxin (ET) formation occurs when EF binds to PA [2, 3]. The highly immunogenic PA therefore plays

a central role in the activation of both LT and ET and was shown to elicit a protective immune response against anthrax in both experimental animals and humans as reviewed by Little et al. [5]. Virulence of *B. anthracis* is also dependent on the presence of the anti-phagocytic capsule and the absence of either pXO1 or pXO2 will result in attenuation of the organism [6].

The current anthrax veterinary vaccine comprises of spores from the live, attenuated *B. anthracis* 34F2 strain developed in 1937 by Max Sterne and known as the Sterne live spore vaccine [7]. The vaccine is a stable uncapsulated mutant that produces all three toxin components of *B. anthracis* (PA, LF and EF) whilst still providing protective antigens [7, 8]. Humoral immunity develops 2–4 weeks after first vaccination and revaccination is recommended every 9–12 months (Anthrax vaccine leaflet, Onderstepoort Biological Products, South Africa, http://www.obpvaccines.co.za) [9]. In vivo

*Correspondence: henriette.vanheerden@up.ac.za
[1] Department of Veterinary Tropical Diseases, University of Pretoria, Onderstepoort 0110, South Africa
Full list of author information is available at the end of the article

assessment of the Sterne vaccine immunity mainly involved pathogenicity and efficacy testing during which guinea pigs were vaccinated with Sterne live spore vaccine and challenged with *B. anthracis* strain 17 JB (Pasteur II strain) [9]. The use of serological techniques for the detection of correlates of protection to anthrax vaccine was initiated with the search for efficacious human vaccines.

Until recently the few studies on the immune response induced by the Sterne live spore vaccine in ruminants were done by Turnbull et al. [10] and Shakya et al. [11]. Ndumnego and Kohler et al. [12] vaccinated Boer goats with one or two doses of Sterne 34F2 live spore vaccine and challenged them with fully virulent *B. anthracis* spores. All the goats receiving two vaccine doses survived virulent challenge whereas 60 and 80% of those vaccinated once survived. Sera collected post-challenge from these animals were used as the positive controls in this study. In this report, we evaluated the humoral immune response induced by the live spore anthrax vaccine in Boer goats using the anti-PA ELISA, an in vitro toxin neutralization assay (TNA) and a passive protection test in A/J-mice as first performed with large wild animals by Turnbull et al. [13].

## Materials and methods
### Sterne live spore vaccine
The Sterne live spore vaccine is produced by Onderstepoort Biological Products (OBP) in South Africa and consists of *B. anthracis* strain 34F2 (pXO1$^+$, pXO2$^-$) spores suspended in glycerine at a spore concentration of $6 \times 10^6$ per mL.

### Experimental animals
Healthy, age-matched female and emasculated male naive Boer goats were used for production of immune sera. These animals were sourced from livestock farms in Pretoria area (Gauteng Province, South Africa), confirmed to be PA-reactive antibody negative by ELISA and kept at the OBP experimental animal facility. The animals were fed pellets and hay with water ad libitum. They were dewormed following arrival and kept in a fenced, outdoor facility with concrete floors throughout the trial. All goats were kept together for the entire period of the experiment.

Six to eight weeks old female A/J mice were used in the passive protection test. A/J mice are deficient for the C5 complement component rendering them highly susceptible to the Sterne live spore vaccine strain [14]. These mice were obtained from Jackson Laboratories, USA, and maintained in pathogen-free conditions at the laboratory animal facility of the University of Pretoria Biomedical Research Centre (UPBRC) according to the South

African national standard for the care and use of animals for scientific purpose. All studies were approved by the animal ethics committee (AEC) of the University of Pretoria, South Africa (protocol approval number V083/13) and permission was granted (12/11/1/1) by the Department of Agriculture, Forestry and Fisheries, South Africa under the animals disease act (Act 35 Section 20, 1984).

### Vaccination regimen
The experimental group consisted of Boer goats ($n = 5$), immunized twice with the Sterne live spore vaccine ($6 \times 10^6$ per mL). One ml OBP Sterne vaccine was administered subcutaneously at week 0 and week 12 according to the manufacturer's instruction. A negative control group of Boer goats ($n = 3$) received only sterile saline (1 mL) instead of vaccine. The animals were bled before the initial vaccination (week 0) and at week 4 and week 17. Positive control sera ($n = 4$) were sourced from Boer goats which survived challenge with virulent anthrax spores after two vaccinations with the Sterne live spore vaccine in a previous study [12].

### Anti-PA antibody ELISA
Sera collected at weeks 0, 4 and 17 were analysed for PA-specific antibody using the ELISA as previously described by Hahn et al. [15] and Pombo et al. [16] with some modifications as described by Ndumnego et al. [17]. Endpoint titres of individual serum were defined as the reciprocal of the highest serum dilution giving an optical density of 0.1. Titres of < 50 were ascribed an arbitrary value of 0. Sera from immune goats ($n = 4$) that survived a virulent *B. anthracis* challenge and naive goats ($n = 3$) were used as positive and negative controls respectively.

### Toxin neutralization assay (TNA)
An in vitro toxin neutralization assay (TNA) was performed using a MTT [3-(4.5-dimethylthiazol-2-yl)–2.5-diphenyltetrazolium bromide] in a colorimetric cell viability assay with the J774A.1 macrophage cell line as previously described by Hering et al. [18] with slight modifications by Ndumnego et al. [17]. Briefly, serial diluted goat serum was incubated with PA and LF (List Biological Laboratories, USA) at concentrations of 500 and 400 ng/mL respectively before addition to overnight incubated macrophage cells. The following controls were added to each assay: a single dilution series of positive serum from a Sterne hyper-immunized goat which survived virulent challenge served as positive control [12], three wells (without cells) with medium and LT served as blanks, three wells (with cells) and LT served as toxin control and two wells with cells and culture media served as medium control. Cell viability was determined

by reading the optical density (OD) at 540 nm after the addition of the MTT tetrazolium dye. The neutralization titre of each serum was calculated by $NT_{50}$ = (sample OD − toxin control OD)/(medium control OD − toxin control OD) × 100 and expressed as the reciprocal of the highest serum dilution neutralizing 50% of the toxins.

### Passive transfer of serum and challenge in A/J mice

A/J mice ($n = 96$) were used in the passive protection tests as previously described by Turnbull et al. [13]. Briefly, serum from twice immunized individual goats ($n = 5$), collected on week 17, were used either undiluted or diluted in physiological saline (1:1000, 1:100, 1:50, 1:10, 1:5). Each of these dilutions were administered intraperitoneally (500 μL) to three A/J mice ($n = 3$ for each goat serum) for each dilution from individual goats ($n = 15$). Positive control mice ($n = 12$, three A/J mice for each goat serum) received undiluted sera from immune goats (n = 4) that survived a virulent B. anthracis challenge. Negative control mice ($n = 9$, three A/J mice for each goat serum) received undiluted sera from naïve goats ($n = 3$) as performed previously [13]. The mice were challenged after 24 h by subcutaneous inoculation with $1.92 \times 10^5$ spores [13] from Sterne 34F2 vaccine strain and monitored for survival over 14 days. Death due to anthrax was confirmed by re-isolation of B. anthracis from liver and spleen smear cultures on sheep blood agar. Survivors were euthanized by injecting a barbiturate overdose and confirmed free of Sterne spores following culture of liver and spleen.

### Statistics

We compared the immune response in Sterne vaccinated goats using ELISA and TNA with the passive protection test in mice. The relationship between individual ELISA, TNA antibody titres and time of survival was described using the Pearson's correlation coefficient. Differences in antibody titres (ELISA and TNA) between points of measurement were analysed using a two-tailed (paired) Student $t$ test. $p$ values of < 0.05 were considered statistically significant. The survival times for mice receiving different goat serum dilutions were analysed using the Kaplan–Meier method in SPSS Version 21 (IBM SPSS Statistics, USA). Log-rank test was used to compare the survival curves of test and control groups. The anti-PA and TNA linear plot was done using Sigma Plot (Systat software Inc, USA).

### Results
#### Anti-PA antibody ELISA and TNA

ELISA was performed to determine the serum IgG antibody levels against PA from individual sera collected at weeks 0, 4 and 17. Serum anti-PA antibody titres were very low in naïve animals, both the animals before the first vaccination and control animals injected with sterile saline. Titers in the latter group remained low until the end of the experiment. The anti-PA titres of each individual animal before vaccination (week 0), after first vaccination (week 4) and after second vaccination (week 17) are indicated in Figure 1. There was no significant difference in mean titres between week 0 and 4 ($p = 0.0913$) but there were significant differences between week 0 and 17 ($p = 0.009$) and between week 4 and 17 ($p = 0.019$). The goat anti-PA ELISA titres indicated significant sero-conversion at week 17 after the second doses of vaccine ($p = 0.009$).

An in vitro TNA was performed to assess toxin neutralizing antibodies in sera of vaccinated goats using murine J774A.1 macrophage cell line. Neutralizing antibody titres measured by the TNA assay varied among the individual animals. There were no detectable neutralizing titres in sera collected at week 0 (before vaccination). The TNA titres at week 4 were low and goat D6 and D20 did not give neutralization titres after the first vaccination. All five immune goat sera showed neutralizing activity at week 17 after the second vaccine dose (Figure 2). No significant differences were found between TNA titres at week 0 and 4 ($p = 0.218$), but there was significant difference in mean titres between week 0 and 17 ($p = 0.004$) and between week 4 and 17 ($p = 0.025$).

### Passive protection test

A total of 75 A/J mice were passively immunized with undiluted and diluted immune sera ranging from 1:1000, 1:100, 1:50, 1:10 and 1:5 collected at week 17 from individual goats immunized with Sterne live spore vaccine. The protective effect of the immune sera was assessed following challenge with B. anthracis 34F2 spores. The level of protection of the immune goat sera was dependent on the dilution used, while sera from the naïve goats failed to protect mice (Figure 3). All nine A/J mice that received negative (naive) goat sera died within 3 days of challenge, whereas all mice (12/12) that received serum from the positive controls (Sterne-immunized goats surviving lethal anthrax spores challenge) survived for 14 days (Figure 3).

Mice receiving immune goat sera at higher dilutions showed lower survival than those receiving sera at lower dilutions. Analysis of the survival curves showed no difference between the negative control and the 1:1000 diluted sera group ($p = 0.290$). However, survival curves from sera groups diluted 1:100 or less were significantly different from the negative control ($p \leq 0.004$). For the undiluted immune goat sera, 13 of the 15 (87%) mice survived the challenge and was no different from the positive control group ($p = 0.165$). Two mice injected with undiluted sera from vaccinated goats D6 and D20 only

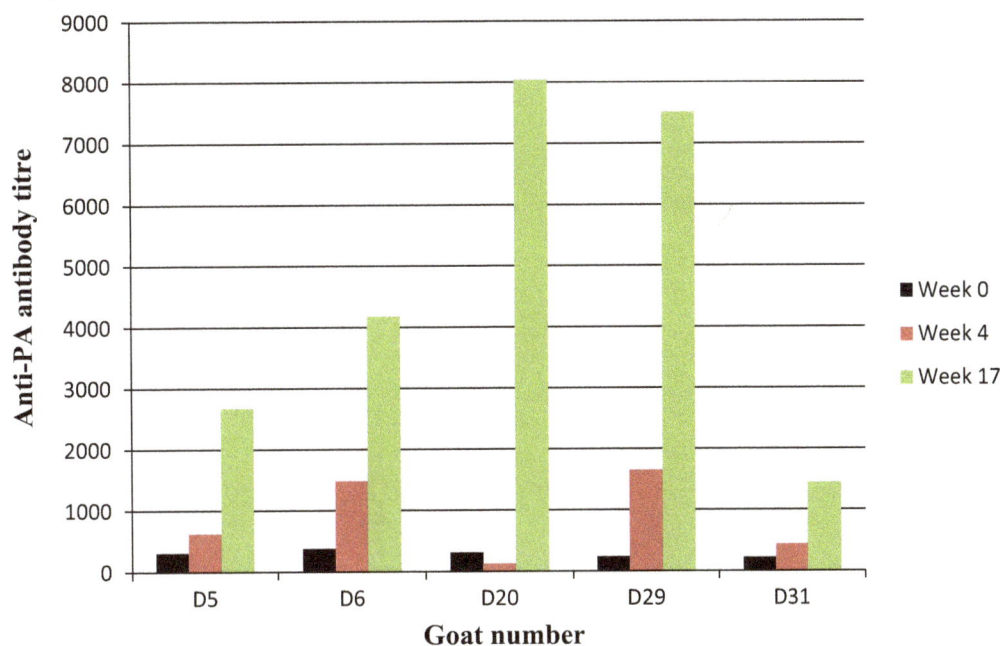

**Figure 1 Anti-protective antigen (PA) antibody titres as detected by ELISA following Sterne live spore vaccination of goats at week 0 and week 12.** Serum samples of individual goats (D5, D6, D20, D29 and D31) were collected and analysed before vaccination (week 0), 4 weeks after initial vaccination (week 4) and after the second vaccine dose (week 17). Mean anti-PA antibody titres detected by ELISA of positive control (Sterne live spore vaccinated goats) and negative control (naive goats) are indicated in Table 1.

died on day 12 (euthanized) and 14, respectively (Table 1). Both mice were confirmed positive for anthrax by isolation of *B. anthracis* from the spleen and liver. Mice that received undiluted immune serum had a mean survival of 13.9 days compared to the mice that received different dilutions for which survival ranged between 5 and 12 days depending on the dilution (Table 1). The 1:5, 1:10, 1:50, 1:100 and 1:1000 dilutions had 80, 47, 13, 13 and 20% survival rates respectively with most of the mice dying within the first 5 days (Figure 3; Table 1). There was no difference in survival times between 1:5 and the positive control groups ($p \geq 0.0829$). However, dilution of immune sera by 1:10 or more afforded significantly less protection to the mice when compared to the positive control ($p \leq 0.002$).

### Comparison of ELISA, TNA and passive protection test

The ELISA and TNA titres of sera from individual goats at week 17 (after second vaccine dose) showed no correlation ($r_s = 0.404$; $p < 0.135$). PA antibody measured in sera from individual vaccinated goats did not correlate with passive protection in A/J mice using either diluted or undiluted sera ($r_s \leq 0.487$; $p \geq 0.066$). Significant positive correlations between toxin neutralizing antibodies and protection of A/J mice were observed following passive transfer of immune goat sera diluted at 1:5 and 1:10 respectively (Table 2).

### Discussion

Results of this study demonstrate a potential protective capacity of the humoral response elicited in Sterne live spore vaccinated goats using the passive protection test in A/J mice. The passive mouse protection model can be effectively used to evaluate the immune response in livestock animals. A/J-mice were utilized because of their known susceptibility to toxigenic but non-encapsulated strains of *B. anthracis* such as Sterne or STI-1 [19], caused by a deficiency of C5 in the complement system [14]. A/J mice react in a dose-dependent manner unlike CBA/J and BALB/c mice to a challenge with those vaccine strains. Passively transferred goat immune sera protected A/J mice from lethal challenge with protection correlated to sera dilution levels. We observed that sera from twice immunized goats (goats vaccinated twice with Sterne live spore vaccine 12 weeks apart) with neutralizing antibody titres $\geq 200$ afforded robust protection against $1.92 \times 10^5$ *B. anthracis* Sterne strain spores challenge in the A/J mice model (Table 1). The number of goats ($n = 5$) as well as mice ($n = 3$ per assessed serum dilution) used in this study limited statistical power and results should be interpreted in this light. As the main focus was to investigate protection only the PA-ELISA IgG antibody titres in vaccinated and non-vaccinated goats were measured, but IgM antibody response can

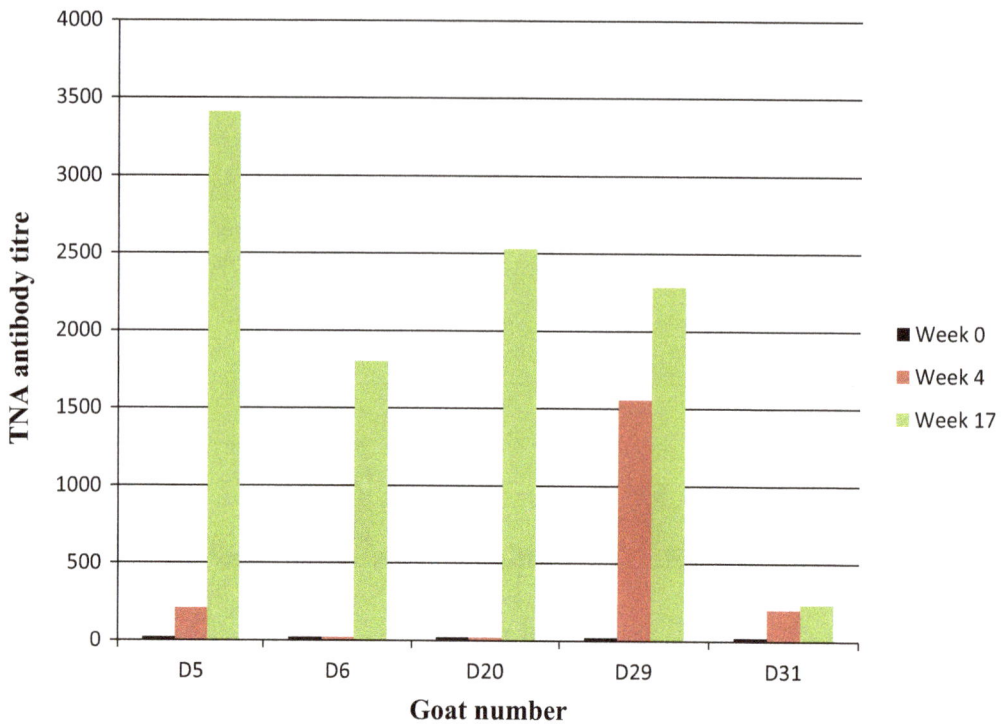

**Figure 2  Toxin neutralization antibody titres following Sterne live spore vaccination of goats at week 0 and week 12.** Serum samples of individual goats (D5, D6, D20, D29 and D31) were collected and analysed before vaccination (week 0), 4 weeks after initial vaccination (week 4) and after the second vaccine dose (week 17). Mean toxin neutralization antibody titres of positive control (Sterne live spore vaccinated goats) and negative control (naive goats) are indicated in Table 1.

be investigated in future. However, this study provides valuable insight in the potential use of immune assays and the passive protection test to measure presumptive protection conferred following vaccination with anthrax vaccines.

The *B. anthracis* TNA is a technique designed to measure the ability of toxin neutralizing antibody to protect certain susceptible cell lines from the lethal effects of anthrax toxin [20, 21]. TNA is not species dependent and has been developed for use with multiple species [18]. Here, the TNA titres directly correlated to survival in mice with 1:5 and 1:10 diluted immune goat sera in the passive protection test (Table 1). The inability to show correlation using undiluted sera was likely due to the almost uniform survival observed following challenge, with the two non-survivors protected for 12 and 14 days respectively (Table 1). We noticed that TNA titres of just over 200 can confer protection in the passive protection test performed in this study. Accordingly serum from goat D31 provided 100% (3/3) protection to A/J mice for undiluted sera (Table 1) despite a relatively low TNA antibody level but did not provide protection when diluted 1:10; 1:50 and 1:100. This is in line with data from guinea pig studies. Reuveny et al. [20] showed that TNA

titres as low as 220 will provide some level of protection. Toxin neutralization titres were absent to low, 4 weeks after the first vaccination but were evident at week 17. This supports the results published by Ndumnego et al. [12] who showed a strong increase in titres after a second vaccination of goats with the same vaccine (34F2).

Our study provides evidence that the mouse protection model can be effectively used to evaluate the immune response of target animals like livestock, thereby eliminating the ethical and logistical challenges associated with large animal trials. It also obviates the need of fully virulent *B. anthracis* strains for the challenge and consequent biosafety level specification. This test would be beneficial to assess presumptive protective capacities of new vaccine formulations against anthrax in animals prohibitive to be experimentally challenged (valuable livestock, endangered/critical wildlife populations). Moreover, it could be used to evaluate and monitor the presumptive protective capacity of vaccination procedures currently in veterinary use, e.g. to determine the herd immunity after a vaccination campaign. In order to unambiguously proof the significance of the correlation between the passive mouse protection test and TNA titres as an immunological correlate for protection in

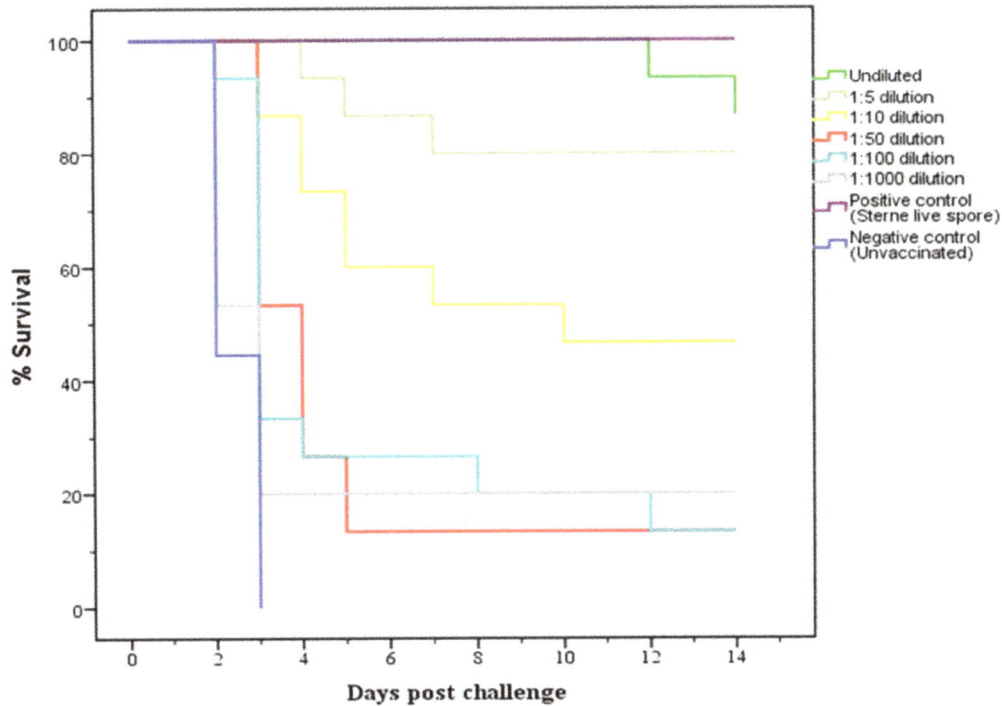

**Figure 3  Kaplan–Meier plots indicating the survival of A/J mice after passive transfer of naïve and immune goat sera at different dilutions.** For each group (undiluted and diluted), 500 µL of serum from each goat subject ($n = 5$) were inoculated into three A/J mice ($n = 15$ for each group). Positive control mice ($n = 12$, three A/J mice per goat) received undiluted sera from immune goats ($n = 4$) that survived a virulent *B. anthracis* challenge. Negative control mice ($n = 9$, three A/J mice per goat) received undiluted sera from naïve goats ($n = 3$). The mice were lethally challenged after 24 h with $1.92 \times 10^5$ spores per dose from the Sterne 34F2 vaccine strain.

**Table 1  Passive protection test results of A/J mice.**

| Goat serum | | | Survival (Time to death[b]) | | | | | |
|---|---|---|---|---|---|---|---|---|
| Animal | PA-ELISA (week 0) | TNA (week 0) | Undiluted sera | 1:5 | 1:10 | 1:50 | 1:100 | 1:1000 |
| D5[a] | 2680 (212) | 3410 (0) | 3/3 | 3/3 | 2/3 (11) | 0/3 (4, 4, 4) | 1/3 (3, 3) | 0/3 (2, 2, 2) |
| D6[a] | 4190 (380) | 1800 (0) | 2/3 (12) | 3/3 | 2/3 (5) | 0/3 (3, 3, 3) | 0/3 (2, 3, 3) | 1/3 (2, 3) |
| D20[a] | 8050 (310) | 2530 (0) | 2/3 (14) | 3/3 | 1/3 (4, 7) | 1/3 (3, 5) | 0/3 (3, 3, 12) | 0/3 (2, 2, 3) |
| D29[a] | 7510 (240) | 2280 (0) | 3/3 | 2/3 (5) | 2/3 (10) | 1/3 (3, 5) | 1/3 (3, 8) | 1/3 (3, 3) |
| D31[a] | 1450 (220) | 240 (0) | 3/3 | 1/3 (4, 7) | 0/3 (3, 3, 4) | 0/3 (3, 3, 4) | 0/3 (3, 3, 4) | 1/3 (2, 3) |
| Negative control[ac] | | | | | | | | |
| D13 | 590 (80) | 0 (0) | 0/3 (2, 2, 2) | | | | | |
| D39 | 100 (130) | 0 (0) | 0/3 (3, 2, 3) | | | | | |
| D77 | 120 (90) | 0 (0) | 0/3 (3, 3, 2) | | | | | |
| Positive control[d] | | | | | | | | |
| 8175 | 39 590 (212) | 5870 (0) | 3/3 | | | | | |
| 8182 | 17 000 (0) | 7300 (0) | 3/3 | | | | | |
| 8210 | 185 500 (173) | 17 380 (0) | 3/3 | | | | | |
| 8212 | 1 223 430 (405) | 35 720 (0) | 3/3 | | | | | |

[a]  Sera collected at 17 weeks

[b]  Time to death (in days) of non-surviving mice; Mice injected with undiluted and diluted hyper-immune goat sera and challenged with spores from the Sterne 34F2 vaccine strain 24 h later and immune sera were diluted from 1:5 to 1:1000

[c]  Sera collected from goats ($n = 3$) receiving sterile saline only; all mice died within 3 days of challenge with *B. anthracis* Sterne strain

[d]  Sera sourced from goats ($n = 4$) surviving virulent anthrax spores after two vaccinations with the Sterne live spore vaccine in a previous study [12]

**Table 2  Pearson correlation between toxin neutralizing titres (goat serum) and mouse survival.**

|                            | Undiluted sera | 1:5   | 1:10  | 1:50  | 1:100 | 1:1000 |
|----------------------------|----------------|-------|-------|-------|-------|--------|
| Pearson correlation ($r_s$) | 0.064          | 0.522 | 0.655 | 0.203 | 0.324 | −0.317 |
| Significance (2-tailed)    | 0.820          | 0.046 | 0.008 | 0.469 | 0.238 | 0.249  |

Toxin neutralization titres to survival in A/J mice following passive transfer of various dilutions of immune goat sera before challenge with spores from Sterne 34F2 vaccine strain. Correlation analysis was performed for each dilution using individual TNA titres and survival

various animal species more such data sets are needed. Then, one could imagine that in the future TNA titres could serve as the correlate for protection also for commercial vaccine production, making the animal challenge tests for vaccine batches obsolete.

Certainly, the final proof for the correlation of TNA titres and protection would need appropriate lethal challenge experiments with various animal species. As this approach is, correctly, considered unethical such data will have to be collected from further small scale experiments and, where possible, from epidemiological data of the veterinary field usage of commercial vaccines. For the latter it would be helpful to monitor by TNA the actual immune responses in various target animals.

## Abbreviations
*B. anthracis*: *Bacillus anthracis*; PA: protective antigen; ELISA: enzyme-linked immunosorbent assay; TNA: toxin neutralization assay; LF: lethal factor; EF: edema factor; LT: lethal toxin; ET: edema toxin; OBP: Onderstepoort Biological Products; LD: lethal dose; OD: optical density; MTT: 3-(4.5-dimethylthiazol-2-yl)-2.5-diphenyltetrazolium bromide.

## Competing interests
The authors declare that they have no competing interests.

## Authors' contributions
PHP did the experiments and wrote the manuscript. OCN was the responsible veterinarian for animal experiments, knowledge transfer of techniques to PHP used in this study, participated in the design of the study and drafting the manuscript. SMK assisted in passive protection experiment, knowledge transfer of techniques to OCN and participated in the design of the study. JC was the supervising veterinarian, participated in the design of the study. WB has been the principal investigator of the DFG project BE2157/4-1. He initiated the original vaccine studies and passive protection test. HvH participated in the design of the study, drafting the manuscript and providing funding. All authors participated in critical revision of manuscript. All authors read and approved the final manuscript.

## Acknowledgements
This work was supported financially by German Research Foundation (DFG); project BE2157/4-1 and Technology Innovation Agency (TIA, TAHC12-00041) in South Africa. We thank Ilse Janse van Rensburg at University of Pretoria Biomedical Research Centre for her help and expertise during passive protection test.

## Author details
[1] Department of Veterinary Tropical Diseases, University of Pretoria, Onderstepoort 0110, South Africa. [2] Department of Livestock Infectiology and Environmental Hygiene, Institute of Animal Science, University of Hohenheim, Emil-Wolff-Strasse 14, 70599 Stuttgart, Germany. [3] Present Address: Africa Health Research Institute, K-RITH Tower Building, Umbilo Road, Durban 4013, South Africa. [4] Present Address: Robert Koch Institute, Nordufer 20, 13353 Berlin, Germany.

## Funding
This work was supported financially by German Research Foundation (DFG); project BE2157/4-1 and Technology Innovation Agency (TIA, TAHC12-00041) in South Africa.

## References
1. Hambleton P, Carman JA, Melling J (1984) Anthrax: the disease in relation to vaccines. Vaccine 2:125–132
2. Farrar WE (1994) Anthrax: virulence and vaccines. Ann Intern Med 121:379–380
3. Pezard C, Berche P, Mock M (1991) Contribution of individual toxin components to virulence of *Bacillus anthracis*. Infect Immun 59:3472–3477
4. Makino S, Uchida I, Terakado N, Sasakawa C, Yoshikawa M (1989) Molecular characterization and protein analysis of the cap region, which is essential for encapsulation in *Bacillus anthracis*. J Bacteriol 171:722–730
5. Little SF, Ivins BE (1999) Molecular pathogenesis of *Bacillus anthracis* infection. Microbes Infect 1:131–139
6. Welkos SL (1991) Plasmid-associated virulence factors of non-toxigenic (pX01−) *Bacillus anthracis*. Microb Pathog 10:183–198
7. Sterne M (1939) The use of anthrax vaccines prepared from avirulent (uncapsulated) variants of *Bacillus anthracis*. Onderstepoort J Vet Sci Anim Ind 13:307–312
8. Turnbull PC, Broster MG, Carman JA, Manchee RJ, Melling J (1986) Development of antibodies to protective antigen and lethal factor components of anthrax toxin in humans and guinea pigs and their relevance to protective immunity. Infect Immun 52:356–363
9. OIE (2012) Anthrax. In: Manual of diagnostic tests and vaccines for terrestrial animals, 7th edn. http://www.oie.int/fileadmin/Home/eng/Health_standards/tahm/2.01.01_ANTHRAX.pdf
10. Turnbull PC, Doganay M, Lindeque PM, Aygen B, McLaughlin J (1992) Serology and anthrax in humans, livestock and Etosha National Park wildlife. Epidemiol Infect 108:299–313
11. Shakya KP, Hugh-Jones ME, Elzer PH (2007) Evaluation of immune response to orally administered Sterne strain 34F2 anthrax vaccine. Vaccine 25:5374–5377
12. Ndumnego OC, Köhler S, Crafford J, van Heerden H, Beyer W (2016) Comparative analysis of the immunologic response induced by the Sterne 34F2 live spore *Bacillus anthracis* vaccine in a ruminant model. Vet Immunol Immunopathol 178:14–21
13. Turnbull PC, Tindall BW, Coetzee JD, Conradie CM, Bull RL, Lindeque PM, Huebschle OJ (2004) Vaccine-induced protection against anthrax in cheetah (*Acinonyx jubatus*) and black rhinoceros (*Diceros bicornis*). Vaccine 22:3340–3347
14. Welkos SL, Keener TJ, Gibbs PH (1986) Differences in susceptibility of inbred mice to *Bacillus anthracis*. Infect Immun 51:795–800
15. Hahn UK, Alex M, Czerny CP, Böhm R, Beyer W (2004) Protection of mice against challenge with *Bacillus anthracis* STI spores after DNA vaccination. Int J Med Microbiol 294:35–44
16. Pombo M, Berthold I, Gingrich E, Jaramillo M, Leef M, Sirota L, Hsu H, Arciniega J (2004) Validation of an anti-PA-ELISA for the potency testing of anthrax vaccine in mice. Biologicals 32:157–163
17. Ndumnego OC, Crafford J, Beyer W, Van Heerden H (2013) Quantitative anti-PA IgG ELISA; assessment and comparability with the anthrax toxin neutralization assay in goats. BMC Vet Res 9:265
18. Hering D, Thompson W, Hewetson J, Little S, Norris S, Pace-Templeton J (2004) Validation of the anthrax lethal toxin neutralization assay. Biologicals 32:17–27
19. Beedham RJ, Turnbull PC, Williamson ED (2001) Passive transfer of protection against *Bacillus anthracis* infection in a murine model. Vaccine 19:4409–4416

# 4

# A longitudinal study of serological responses to *Coxiella burnetii* and shedding at kidding among intensively-managed goats supports early use of vaccines

Michael Muleme[1]*(ID), Angus Campbell[2], John Stenos[3], Joanne M. Devlin[1], Gemma Vincent[3], Alexander Cameron[1], Stephen Graves[3], Colin R. Wilks[1] and Simon Firestone[1]

## Abstract

Vaccination against *Coxiella burnetii*, the cause of Q fever, is reportedly the only feasible strategy of eradicating infection in ruminant herds. Preventive vaccination of seronegative goats is more effective in reducing shedding of *C. burnetii* than vaccinating seropositive goats. The age at which goats born on heavily-contaminated farms first seroconvert to *C. burnetii* has not yet been documented. In a 16-month birth cohort study, the age at which goats seroconverted against *C. burnetii* was investigated; 95 goats were bled every 2 weeks and tested for antibodies against *C. burnetii*. Risk factors for seroconversion were explored and goats shedding *C. burnetii* were identified by testing vaginal swabs taken at the goats' first kidding using a *com1* polymerase chain reaction assay. The first surge in the number of goats with IgM to *C. burnetii* was observed at week 9. Thus, a first vaccination not later than 8 weeks of age to control *C. burnetii* in highly contaminated environments is indicated. The odds of seroconversion were 2.0 times higher [95% confidence interval (CI) 1.2, 3.5] in kids born by does with serological evidence of recent infection (IgM seropositive) compared to kids born by IgM seronegative does, suggesting either In utero transmission or peri-parturient infection. The rate of seroconversion was 4.5 times higher (95% CI 2.1, 9.8) during than outside the kidding season, highlighting the risk posed by *C. burnetii* shed during kidding, even to goats outside the kidding herd. Shedding of *C. burnetii* at kidding was detected in 15 out of 41 goats infected before breeding.

## Introduction

*Coxiella burnetii* causes Q fever in humans, a disease that manifests with influenza-like symptoms including fever and pneumonia in approximately 30% of those acutely infected [1, 2]. Chronic Q fever is characterised by debilitating arthritis, myopathy and cardiac malfunction [1–6]. Recent reports of chronic Q fever among individuals that had never been diagnosed with acute disease draws attention to the need for increased detection and treatment of sub-clinical Q fever infections [1, 2, 7]. The impact of the disease is further highlighted by increasing reports of chronic Q fever in children and mortalities of up to 13% among chronic Q fever patients [7–11]. These potentially severe impacts of Q fever underscore the need to implement stringent prevention and control measures. It is therefore imperative to have evidence of how effective the different control measures are in the control of *C. burnetii* infections.

Many large Q fever outbreaks have been linked to farms with small ruminants and key control strategies have targeted reducing shedding of *C. burnetii* by the animals [12–15]. For example, a ban on breeding, culling of pregnant animals and vaccination of animals before breeding were used to control the large Q fever outbreak in the Netherlands [12–15]. Additionally, vaccination against *C. burnetii* in animals was shown to be more

*Correspondence: mmuleme@gmail.com;
michael.muleme@unimelb.edu.au
[1] Asia–Pacific Centre for Animal Health, Faculty of Veterinary and Agricultural Sciences, The University of Melbourne, Parkville, VIC 3010, Australia
Full list of author information is available at the end of the article

effective in reducing the shedding of the organism when carried-out in seronegative animals than in seropositive ones, underscoring the need to vaccinate animals before they are infected with *C. burnetii* [16–18].

The age at which most animals born on infected farms first seroconvert to *C. burnetii* has not been documented. Several previously published studies point to the possibility that goats get infected early in life. For example, during a human Q fever outbreak that was linked to a goat farm in France, 52% of 3–4-month-old kids were reported to have been seropositive to *C. burnetii*; and approximately 90% of these were reported to have been infected with *C. burnetii* before they started kidding [19]. Similarly, 33% (192/589) of kid goats in another study undertaken on a farm linked to a human Q fever outbreak, were reported to have been infected before they started kidding and shed *C. burnetii* at their first kidding despite being kept away from adult goats as soon as they were born [17]. These studies do not indicate when the goats first seroconverted to *C. burnetii* although some of the results point to a time before 4 months of age.

Based on modelling of *C. burnetii* transmission and control in Dutch dairy farms, Bontje et al. found that vaccination of goats was the only control measure that could eradicate *C. burnetii* infections from infected herds [20]. The models estimated that it would take 7 years to eradicate the disease from infected farms if goats were to be vaccinated 1 month before breeding annually for all the 7 years [21]. There is a possibility that eradication of *C. burnetii* on infected farms could be achieved in shorter timeframes if vaccination of goats against *C. burnetii* were implemented at the age when most animals had not seroconverted. The Dutch transmission models supported the value of preventive vaccination over vaccination of already infected animals [20, 21]. Similarly, experimental and field studies that were carried out to assess the effectiveness of phase 1 vaccines administered prior to breeding mostly reported that vaccination only reduced the level of shedding at the herd level but did not prevent infection. This may be due to most of the goats being infected by the time of vaccination [16, 18, 19, 22].

This study therefore aimed to establish the age at which goats born on an intensively-managed goat dairy associated with human cases of Q fever first seroconverted to *C. burnetii* to provide recommendations on the timing of vaccination against *C. burnetii*. Additional objectives included: describing and comparing the nature (time of occurrence, duration and titres) of antibody-mediated immune responses to *C. burnetii* of goats that first seroconverted before the target breeding age (28 weeks) to those of goats that seroconverted later, and identifying risk factors and estimating any production losses associated with goats seroconverting before the target breeding age.

## Materials and methods
### Study design
In this longitudinal cohort study, 95 goats were followed from birth for 16 months. The animals were kept under routine animal management conditions on a large intensive dairy goat enterprise in Victoria, Australia. The enterprise holds approximately 5000 milking goats which are synchronised to concentrate kidding at four times each year (at March, June, September and November), in herds on five farms. The enterprise also has a flock of 1100 paddock-grazed extensively-managed dairy sheep. The sheep flock is kept separately from the goat flock. Since 2013, the enterprise was associated with 18 confirmed human cases of Q fever and tested polymerase chain reaction (PCR) positive for *C. burnetii* on various clinical and environmental samples [23]. Approximately 250 goats kid on each of the farms in every one of four kidding seasons, at a kidding rate of approximately two kids per goat. Only female kids and males from high producing animals (elite males) are kept for raising and production.

In herds infected with caprine arthritis and encephalitis virus (CAEV), some kids are routinely "snatch-reared", i.e. removed from their does before they feed on colostrum to prevent transmission of CAEV. These were then bottle-fed pooled colostrum from a CAEV negative farm. The 95 goats (90 female and 5 elite males) in this study were on two of the farms ("GS" and "LC"), both of which were CAEV-positive herds that were previously shown to have a high prevalence of *C. burnetii* [24]. Therefore, the kids in this study were mostly snatch-reared and were bottle-fed colostrum (from the herd on a third farm, "FH", holding CAEV-negative, but *C. burnetii*- positive goats) within 8 h after birth. The colostrum is routinely heat-treated before it is fed to the goats. It is anticipated that heat-treatment would not lower the quality of immunoglobulins in the colostrum. The kid goats were then fed a milk replacer and weaned at approximately 10 weeks of age. At 28 weeks of age (target breeding age), the female goats that weighed $\geq$ 23 kg were mated using adult elite males (not the elite males followed in this study). The goats are routinely weighed at weaning and before breeding.

### Sample size
The minimum required sample size was estimated to be 40 kids to have 80% power of detecting a statistically significant difference between paired samplings (day 0–2 weeks sampling as well as 0–12 weeks) assuming seroconversion to *C. burnetii* would be very rare in kids between 0 and 2 weeks of age (< 1%) and that 20% of the kids would have seroconverted by 12 weeks of age; at a 5% chance of a type I error. Based on this sample size

calculation, with consideration of anticipated mortality, losses to follow-up and multivariable effects, 95 goats were recruited from two kidding seasons; 33 in March 2014 kidding season (cohort 1) and 62 in June 2014 kidding season (cohort 2). Goats in cohort 1 were recruited from farms GS and LC while goats from cohort 2 were recruited only from LC. All animal sampling was conducted with the approval of the University of Melbourne Animal Ethics Committee, Application Number 1413118.

### Examination of antibody-mediated immune responses to *C. burnetii* in goats from birth to 16 months of age

To investigate the age at which goats seroconvert to *C. burnetii* as well as to describe and compare antibody-mediated immune responses to *C. burnetii* among goats that seroconverted before and after the target breeding age, blood samples were taken from the recruited goats at birth (before feeding colostrum), then every 2 weeks for the first 7 months of life and then every 4 weeks until the end of the study, and tested for serum IgM and IgG antibodies against *C. burnetii* antigens using a previously validated indirect immunofluorescence assay (IFA) [24].

In this study, the IFA applied was on a dilution series commencing at 1:160. As described in detail elsewhere [24], at this cut-off there was minimal background fluorescence in negative control goat samples obtained from New Zealand, an OIE-declared *C. burnetii* free country. Appling a 1:160 cut-off, the IFA has also been shown to be highly sensitive for IgG (94.8%) and IgM antibodies (88.8%) [24]. The repeatability of the IFA was previously estimated to be 100% for IgG phase 1, 96.9% for IgG phase 2 and 78.1% for both IgM phase 2 and IgM phase 1 using samples re-tested after 3 months of storage at 4 °C [24]. The IFA slides were read by two experienced technicians with 94.4% agreement (Cohen's *Kappa* = 0.88) [24].

To quantify serum antibodies to *C. burnetii* two-fold serial dilutions of sera were prepared, from 1:160 (the previously validated cut-off value) to 1:1280, and tested for IgM and IgG antibodies against *C. burnetii* antigen using the IFA [24]. The testing of the twofold serial dilutions from 1:160 to 1:1280 was undertaken on sera from 54 of the 95 goats that were present throughout the first 12 months of the study. Among those excluded were animals that were lost to follow up, including those that died in the first 10 weeks of the study before immune responses were mounted. Repeat samples from each goat were also used to describe the duration of the immune response and the proportion of goats mounting secondary immune responses (immune responses that occur after the initial antibody response had declined). All samples were tested in duplicate for IgM and IgG against phase 1 and 2 *C. burnetii*.

Colostrum antibodies were identified through the occurrence of high IgG phase 1 titres in kid goats that were previously seronegative but seroconverted after feeding colostrum, as IgG antibodies occur late in the course of infection and are not expected to occur within 2 weeks in goats that had been negative. After the decay of IgG phase 1 maternal antibodies, new *C. burnetii* infections were considered to have occurred when serum IgM followed by IgG antibodies against phase 2 antigens were identified in previously seronegative goats or a twofold rise in antibody titre was detected following seroconversion to IgG phase 2, as is routine practice in human and veterinary *C. burnetii* diagnostics [25, 26]. Antibodies against the phase 2 antigens of *C. burnetii* appear early in the course of infection while antibodies against phase 1 antigens appear much later in the course of infection [25, 26]. Incidence rates were estimated using an animal time at risk denominator calculated as the number of weeks from birth to the sampling time immediately before the first seroconversion (from negative to positive for both IgM and IgG or ≥ twofold rise in IgG titre against phase 2) or loss to follow-up of each animal. Half of the time between the last negative sample and the first positive sample or loss to follow up was added to the length of time an animal was considered at risk [27].

Pooled colostrum collected from the CAEV-negative farm, FH, was tested for *C. burnetii* IgG antibodies to phases 1 and 2 *C. burnetii* using the *IDEXX* commercial ELISA kit validated for detecting antibodies in milk whey at a 1:5 dilution [24, 28]. Undiluted whey from the pooled colostrum was also tested for IgG and IgM antibodies against phase 1 and 2 *C. burnetii* using the IFA protocol that had been validated for use with goat serum, to ascertain the type of antibodies the goats obtained from colostrum, as described previously [24, 28]. The colostrum was also tested for *C. burnetii* DNA using a DNA extraction protocol and PCR assay targeting the *com 1* gene of *C. burnetii* as previously described [24, 29].

### Identification of risk factors associated with seroconversion to *C. burnetii* before breeding

The probability of remaining seronegative at the different sampling points until the target breeding age was estimated using survival analysis. Initially, three parametric models (namely the Weibull, the Cox proportional hazard model and the Exponential model) were constructed to estimate the probability of goats remaining seronegative from birth to breeding. These were then analysed for goodness of fit based on the Akaike information criterion (AIC) [30]. As the Weibull model displayed the best fit to the data, the probability density function of the time to first seroconversion (change from negative to positive for both IgM and IgG or ≥ twofold rise in IgG titre against phase 2) ($t$) was derived from the Weibull distribution using the equation:

$$f(t) = \alpha \lambda t^{\alpha-1} e^{\lambda t^{\alpha}}$$

where $f(t)$ is the probability density function of seroconversion at the different time points $t$; $\lambda > 0$ is the probability of seroconversion or scale parameter and $\alpha > 0$ is the shape parameter. $\alpha$ is $1/\sigma$, $\sigma$ being a variance-like parameter on the log-time scale. From this the survival (i.e. proportion yet to seroconvert at each timepoint), $S(t)$, was derived as:

$$S(t) = e^{-\lambda t \alpha}$$

The influence of qualitative risk factors including farm, cohort, *C. burnetii* exposure status of the source does, failure of passive transfer and the quality of passive transfer, on seroconversion was tested using the Weibull survival model. The *C. burnetii* exposure status of the source does was obtained by testing serum samples from the source does for IgG and IgM antibodies against *C. burnetii* at the time of birth of the study kid-goats. The occurrence of passive transfer was inferenced through the detection of IgG phase 1 maternally-derived antibodies in the study goats at 2 weeks of age while the quality of passive transfer was assessed using the titre of maternally-derived IgG phase 1 and 2 antibodies detected the kid-goats at 2 weeks of age as well as the detection of IgG phase 1 maternally-derived antibodies in kid goat sera after 4 weeks of age. The risk factors were included in separate univariable Weibull models to assess their influence on the probability of goats remaining seronegative or seroconverting at various times before the target breeding age. The univariable Weibull models testing the influence of risk factors on the probability of seroconversion is described by the equation:

$$\lambda_i = e^{-(\mu + \beta x_j)/\sigma}$$

where the influence of risk factor $x_j$, for the $i^{th}$ goat is modelled through the seroconversion probability parameter $\lambda_j$ and $\alpha = 1/\sigma$.

Kaplan–Meier survival curves and univariable Weibull regression coefficients were then generated for different factors at cohort, farm (farm of birth), doe (IgG and IgM serological status) and individual kid level (level and duration of antibodies to *C. burnetii* derived from colostrum) and used to assess how the different risk factors influence seroconversion. Multivariable Weibull regression models were constructed (based on appropriate fit to the data) including all factors statistically significant in univariable analysis at $p < 0.2$. The coefficients of the Weibull model were converted to hazard ratios using the *ConvertWeibull* package in R version 3.1.3 [31, 32], and only variables associated with the relevant outcome at $p < 0.05$ were retained in final models. The residuals and predicted values of the variables in the final models were analyzed and scaled-schoenfied residual plots were prepared for the variables in the final models.

To ascertain whether exposure to kidding periods resulted in increased numbers of infected goats, the rate of occurrences of IgM or IgG responses against *C. burnetii* during and outside the kidding season was compared using the animal time at risk denominator and the number of IgM and IgG responses as the numerator in the "compare 2 rates" function in Open Epi, version 3.01. The number of IgG and IgM responses were counted whenever a change from negative to positive to either IgM or IgG occurred during testing at the screening dilution. Primary and secondary IgM or IgG responses were considered to have occurred during the kidding period if they were detected within or 15 d after the kidding months. The extra 15 d were included to cater for the time required for antibody-mediated immune responses to occur in case goats became infected towards the end of the kidding season. Antibody-mediated immune responses that could have resulted from infections due to *C. burnetii* shed at either early kidding or late-term abortions, occurring within 2 weeks prior to the start of the kidding season, would fall within the kidding months and thus catered for in the "within kidding" counts of seroconversion. Only antibody-mediated immune responses that occurred after weaning (week 10) were included in this analysis as they were considered to be immune responses arising from environmental exposure to *C. burnetii* and not infection as neonates during the kidding process.

The period between any two consecutive sampling points from week 10 to the end of the study were classified as occurring "within" or "outside" the kidding season based on whether or not they fell during the kidding month and 15 d later. Animal time at risk "within" and "outside" the kidding period was computed for each animal as the number of weeks between the two consecutive sampling points if its samples tested negative at both points; half of the length of time between two sampling points if antibody-specific immune responses occurred (from negative to positive at 1:160 screening dilution), seroreversion (from a positive to either IgM or IgG at the 1:160 screening dilution to negative) or loss to follow-up occurred. For periods with one sampling point falling within the kidding season and the other outside the kidding season, the animal time at risk was divided equally between the within and outside kidding categories.

### Estimating the effect of pre-breeding seroconversions on shedding of *C. burnetii* at kidding and on production parameters

To estimate the proportion of shedding arising from goats that seroconverted before the target breeding age, vaginal swabs were obtained within 24 h of the goats' first kidding and tested using the real genomics DNA extraction protocol (Real Biotech Company) and a PCR targeting the *com1* gene of *C. burnetii* [29]. The difference in the risk of delayed kidding (not kidding by 12 months of age), delayed joining (not bred at 7 months) and shedding of *C. burnetii* among goats that seroconverted before the target breeding age and those that seroconverted after the target breeding age was estimated using two-by-two contingency tables, and comparing relative risks with estimation of 95% confidence intervals and Fisher's exact test statistic in STATA.

The association between seroconversion before breeding and outcomes of weight at weaning, and weight change between weaning and breeding, were estimated using multivariable linear regression models, and adjusting for cohort and farm, using STATA 13.0. The model residuals and the weight variables used were also analysed for normality in STATA 13.0.

## Results

### Antibody-mediated immune responses to *C. burnetii* in goats from birth to 16 months

No antibodies *against C. burnetii* were detected before goats were fed colostrum (Figure 1). High IgG antibody titres to phase 1 and phase 2 *C. burnetii* were detected after feeding colostrum (Figure 1). IgG antibodies against phase 1 *C. burnetii* were used to differentiate maternally-derived antibodies from responses to *C. burnetii* exposure; IgG antibodies against phase 1 waned by week 7 (median duration of presumably-colostrum derived antibodies: 7 weeks; inter-quartile range: 4–7 weeks). Of the 80 goats sampled after they had been fed colostrum, 71 (89%) became seropositive for IgG to phase 1 antibodies (presumably maternally-derived). Furthermore, all these, except one, were also positive for IgG antibodies against phase 2 *C. burnetii*. Colostrum was tested and found to have IgG antibodies to phase 1 and 2 *C. burnetii* antigens using ELISA (optical density [OD] of 1.09 at 0.40 cut-off) and IFA (titres of 1024 IgG to phase 1, 1024 IgG phase 2) and contained negligible amounts of IgM against phase 2 (IFA titre = 40) and no IgM to phase 1 *C. burnetii*.

IgM seroconversion to phase 2 *C. burnetii* occurred as early as week 2 after birth; however, the first surge in the number of goats that seroconverted to phase 2 *C. burnetii* was observed at 9 weeks of age (Figure 2). Similarly, IgM titres to phase 2 *C. burnetii* rose as early as 2 weeks into the study, but the first peak was observed at 9 weeks of age as shown in Figure 1. This was followed by a rise in IgG titres to phase 2 *C. burnetii* and a rise in IgG titres to phase 1 *C. burnetii* at 24 and 40 weeks of age in cohort 2 and cohort 1, respectively (Figure 1).

From birth to 10 weeks, 40 out of the 80 goats (50%) present at the second sampling point showed IgM seroconversion to phase 2 *C. burnetii* while between week 10 and week 28, another 17 out of the 76 (22%) goats present at week 10 showed IgM seroconversion to phase 2. From birth to week 10, IgG seroconversion to phase 2 was detected in 2 out of the 80 goats (3%) and between week 10 and week 28, a total of 38 out of the 76 goats (50%) showed IgG seroconversion to phase 2. One goat had IgG antibodies against phase 2 without a detectable IgM response against phase 2.

Nine goats did not have detectable IgG antibodies to phase 1 after feeding colostrum. Of these, seven goats showed IgM seroconversion to phase 2 by week 28 (three at week 2, three at week 7 and one at week 25) and only one seroconverted after week 28. One of the nine goats that did not have IgG to phase 1 after feeding colostrum died at week 4 before seroconverting to *C. burnetii*.

A total of 19 out of the 95 goats died by week 5, before any seroconversion was observed. Of these, only three had the initial IgG to phase 1 and 2 observed after feeding colostrum while one goat did not have IgG antibodies to phase 1 after feeding colostrum. The rest of these goats (15) died before the second sampling, thus their serological status after feeding colostrum could not be assessed. Another six goats died between week 5 and week 10, all of which had detectable IgG to phase 1 after feeding colostrum. One of these showed IgM seroconversions to phase 2. An additional eight deaths occurred between week 10 and week 28, all except one had IgG antibodies against phase 1 after feeding colostrum and only three had seroconverted with IgM against phase 2.

The crude incidence rate was seven seroconversions (95% CI 5.7, 8.9) per 100 goat weeks at risk. Equivalent interpretations include seven seroconversions per 100 goats at risk for 1 week, or per 50 goats followed for 2 weeks. Whilst there was no statistically significant difference in the rates when compared across time periods (from birth to weaning, weaning to target breeding age and after the target breeding age), see Table 1, there was a trend suggesting gradually increasing risk over time.

Secondary IgM against phase 2 was detected in 42 out of the 70 goats (60%) present at the time of weaning. A total of 24 of these secondary IgM immune responses occurred before the target breeding age and the other 18 occurred after the target breeding age. Secondary IgG immune responses against phase 2 were detected in only 11 goats, four of these occurring before the target breeding age. Only seven goats had a secondary IgM response against phase 1 and only one goat had a secondary IgG response against phase 1.

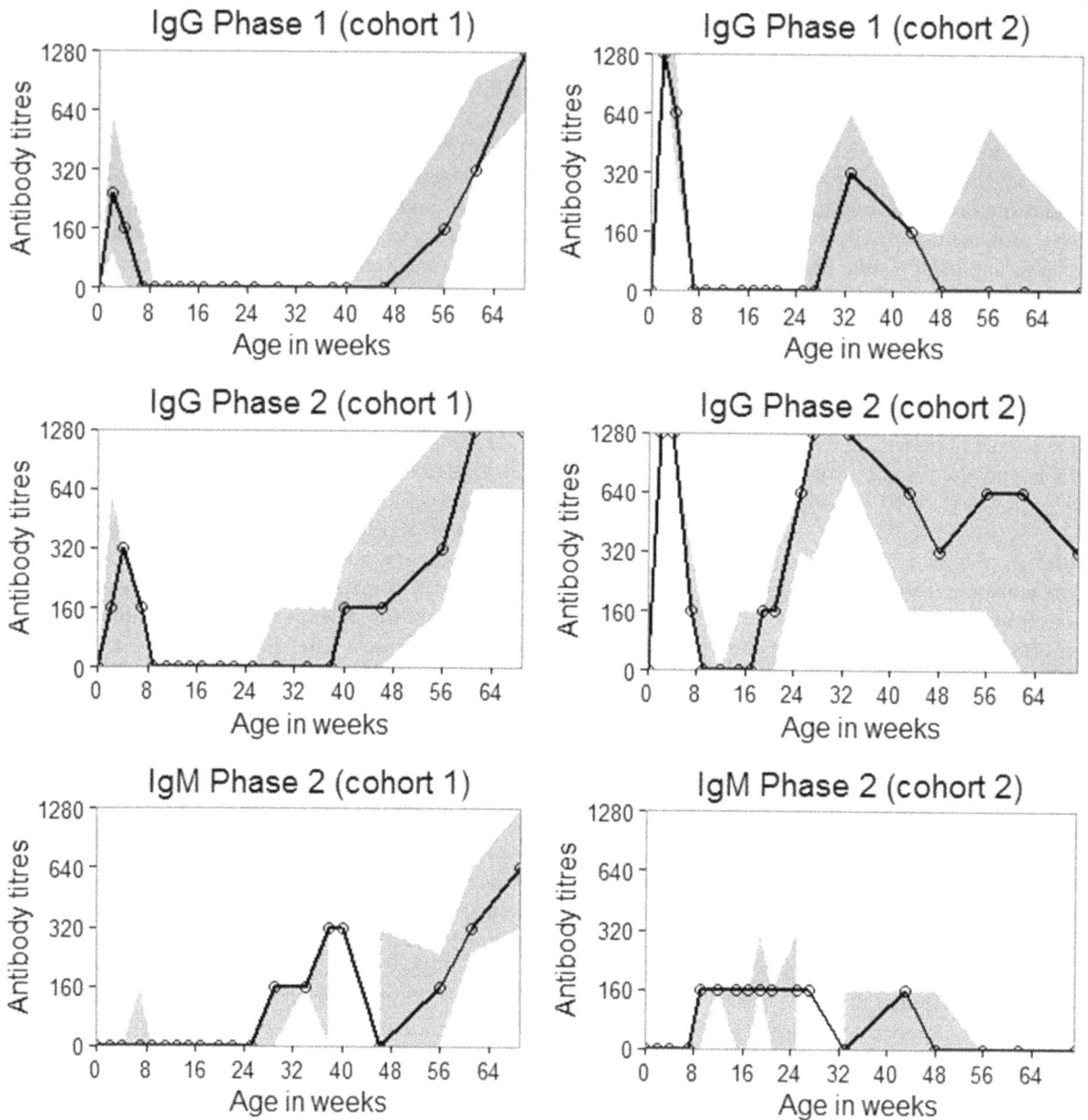

**Figure 1 Median and inter-quartile range of antibody titres against *C. burnetii* in intensively-managed goats**. High IgG titres against phase 1 and phase 2 were detected after feeding colostrum during the follow up of 95 kid-goats. IgG phase 1 antibodies against *C. burnetii* were used to differentiate maternally-derived antibodies from immune response to *C. burnetii* exposure; IgG antibodies against phase 1 waned by 7 weeks. IgM titres started to rise from 2 weeks of age and reached the first peak at 8 weeks of age. This was followed by a rise in IgG phase 2 titres. A rise in IgG phase 1 titres then followed at 24 weeks of age in cohort 2 and 40 weeks in cohort 1. The solid light grey band shows the inter-quartile range of titres while the solid black line shows the median titres.

The duration of IgG and IgM immune responses are described in Table 2. The duration of primary immune responses was significantly higher in cohort 2 than in cohort 1, except for IgM against phase 2 as shown in Figure 3. Overall, immune responses that occurred before the target breeding age were not statistically different from those that occurred after the target breeding age (Table 2).

### Risk factors associated with seroconversion to *C. burnetii* before breeding

The probability of goats remaining seronegative to *C. burnetii* for the first 28 weeks of life was 16.7% (95% CI 9.4, 29.4) (Additional file 1). The Weibull model had the best fit for these data with (AIC = 440.9) compared to the Cox proportional hazards model (AIC = 457.5) and the

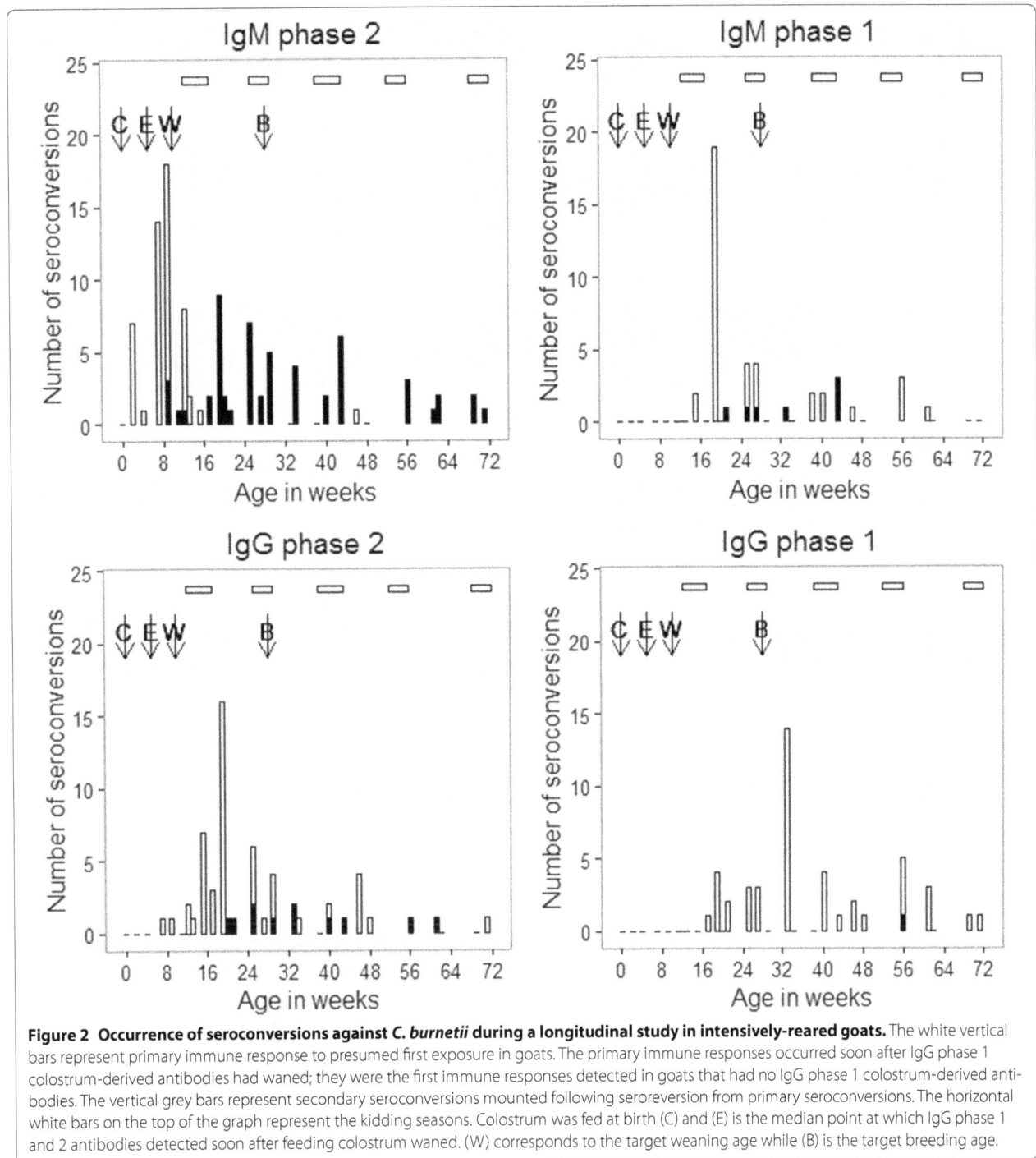

**Figure 2 Occurrence of seroconversions against *C. burnetii* during a longitudinal study in intensively-reared goats.** The white vertical bars represent primary immune response to presumed first exposure in goats. The primary immune responses occurred soon after IgG phase 1 colostrum-derived antibodies had waned; they were the first immune responses detected in goats that had no IgG phase 1 colostrum-derived antibodies. The vertical grey bars represent secondary seroconversions mounted following seroreversion from primary seroconversions. The horizontal white bars on the top of the graph represent the kidding seasons. Colostrum was fed at birth (C) and (E) is the median point at which IgG phase 1 and 2 antibodies detected soon after feeding colostrum waned. (W) corresponds to the target weaning age while (B) is the target breeding age.

Exponential model (AIC = 460.6). Being from farm GS, being a member of cohort 1, having colostrum-derived IgG phase 1 antibodies titres ≥ 320 and being born by an IgM seronegative doe were all associated with a higher probability of not seroconverting against *C. burnetii* before 28 weeks of age on univariate analysis as shown in Figure 4. Outputs of multivariable Weibull regression are presented

in Table 3, and for completeness, univariable results are presented in Additional file 2. The odds of seroconversion were 2.0 times higher [95% confidence interval (CI) 1.2, 3.5] in kids born by does with serological evidence of recent infection (IgM seropositive) compared to kids born by IgM seronegative does. Model residual analysis showed that the assumptions for the Weibull model were not violated.

**Table 1  The incidence rate of seroconversion to *C. burnetii* before and after the breeding age.**

| Time period (weeks) | Number at risk | Goat weeks at risk | Number of seroconversions | Incidence rate (per 100 goat weeks at risk) | Incidence rate ratio (95% CI) |
|---|---|---|---|---|---|
| 0–10 | 95 | 618.5 | 40 | 6.5 (4.6, 8.8) | 1.00 (reference) |
| 11–28 | 32 | 238.0 | 18 | 7.6 (4.5, 12.0) | 1.17 (0.67, 2.04) |
| 29–71 | 8 | 61.5 | 8 | 13.0 (5.6, 25.6) | 2.01 (0.94, 4.30) |
| Total | 135 | 918.0 | 64 | 7.0 (5.7, 8.9) | – |

10 weeks is the target weaning age, 28 weeks was the target breeding age in the intensively-managed goats on the study farm in Victoria, Australia, 2014–2015

*CI* confidence interval

**Table 2  Comparison of the duration of pre-breeding to post-breeding antibody responses to *C. burnetii* in goats.**

| Antibody type | Type of immune response | Time of occurrence | Duration of antibody responses in weeks | | | |
|---|---|---|---|---|---|---|
| | | | n (rev) | Mean | Median (range) | p value* |
| IgM phase 2 | Primary | Pre-breeding | 57 (55) | 10.9 | 5.5 (1.0, 51.0) | 0.570 |
| | | Post-breeding | 7 (7) | 5.9 | 6.0 (2.0, 12.0) | |
| | Secondary | Pre-breeding | 24 (24) | 10.4 | 9.0 (1.0, 34.0) | 0.523 |
| | | Post-breeding | 18 (18) | 8.4 | 4.0 (2.0, 33.0) | |
| IgG phase 2 | Primary | Pre-breeding | 40 (27) | 19.4 | 12.0 (1.0, 48.5) | 0.376 |
| | | Post-breeding | 14 (5) | 7.5 | 6.0 (2.5, 13.0) | |
| | Secondary | Pre-breeding | 4 (3) | 30.7 | 42.5 (3.0, 46.5) | 0.564 |
| | | Post-breeding | 7 (2) | 25.8 | 25.8 (17.0, 34.5) | |
| IgM phase 1 | Primary | Pre-breeding | 29 (29) | 5.1 | 4.0 (1.0, 12.0) | 0.197 |
| | | Post-breeding | 9 (7) | 2.9 | 3.0 (1.0, 6.0) | |
| | Secondary | Pre-breeding | 3 (3) | 1.3 | 1.0 (1.0, 2.0) | 0.127 |
| | | Post-breeding | 4 (4) | 2.9 | 3.5 (1.0, 3.5) | |
| IgG phase 1 | Primary | Pre-breeding | 40 (12) | 23.7 | 22.5 (5.0, 42.5) | 0.897 |
| | | Post-breeding | 14 (14) | 20.5 | 22.3 (5.0, 34.5) | |
| | Secondary | Pre-breeding | 0 (0) | – | – | – |
| | | Post-breeding | 1 (1) | 11.5 | – | |

Pre-breeding responses are those that started before the target breeding age while post-breeding responses are those that started after the target breeding age in intensively managed goats on the study farm in Victoria, Australia, 2014–2015

*rev.* number of antibody responses that seroreverted (moved from positive to negative) which were used in calculating the duration of serological positivity, *n* total number of antibody responses

*p* values derived using the Mann–Whitney U test comparing the duration of pre-breeding immune responses to the post-breeding immune responses

The rate of occurrence of IgG immune responses to *C. burnetii* was 4.5 times higher (95% CI 2.1, 9.8) within the kidding season than outside the kidding season among goats in cohort 2 (Additional file 4), whereas, the rate of occurrence of IgG immune responses was comparable within and outside the kidding season among goats in cohort 1.

### The effect of pre-breeding seroconversions on the shedding of *C. burnetii* and on production parameters

Overall, 18 out of 46 goats were detected as shedding *C. burnetii* by PCR at their first kidding. Shedding was detected in 15 out of the 41 goats that seroconverted before week 28, some of which remained seropositive until kidding (Additional file 5). Out of the five goats

that had not seroconverted by week 28, three goats had detectable *C. burnetii* DNA in vaginal swabs taken at their first kidding.

The proportion of goats that were joined on time was comparable in goats that seroconverted before 28 weeks (28/50 goats, 56.0%) and those that had not seroconverted by week 28 (6/8 goats, 75.0%). Similarly, the proportion of goats kidding on time was comparable in goats that seroconverted before week 28 (19/50 goats, 38.0%) and those that had not seroconverted by week 28 (5/8 goats, 62.5%).

The multivariable linear regression model showed no statistically significant difference in pre-breeding weight between goats that seroconverted early and those that seroconverted later (Table 4). At weaning, goats in cohort

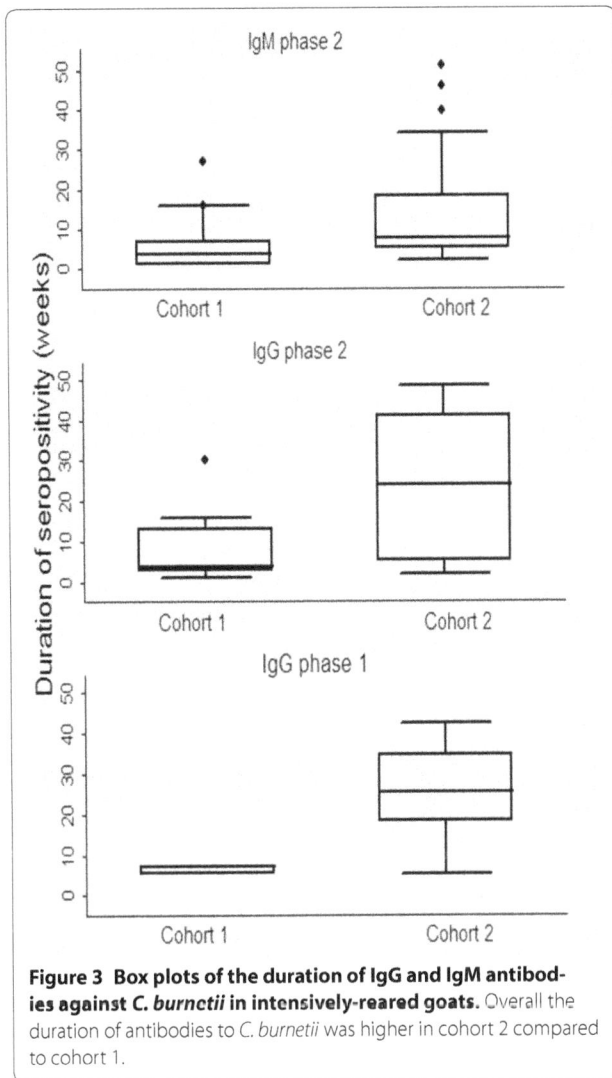

**Figure 3 Box plots of the duration of IgG and IgM antibodies against *C. burnctii* in intensively-reared goats.** Overall the duration of antibodies to *C. burnetii* was higher in cohort 2 compared to cohort 1.

2 weighed 4.8 kg less than goats in cohort 1 (95% CI 6.6, 3.1 kg less); and 30 out of the 49 goats (61%) with weaning weight records in cohort 2 had seroconverted to either IgG or IgM phase 2 by week 10 while only 5 out of the 13 of goats (39%) with weaning weight data in cohort 1 had seroconverted by week 10. Between the time of weaning and the target breeding age, goats in cohort 2 gained 5.3 kg more than goats in cohort 1 (95% CI 2.4, 8.1). Only 10 out of the 38 goats (26%) in cohort 2 seroconverted between weaning and the target breeding age compared to 6 out of the 12 goats (50%) in cohort 1. The distribution of the model residues and weight variables used in the model were within acceptable limits (skewedness ± 1).

## Discussion

To the best of our knowledge, this is the first birth cohort study to systematically investigate *C. burnetii* seroconversions in goats on infected farms over an extended period from birth. Furthermore, this study was undertaken in the absence of vaccination of goats or other control measures that would reduce the shedding of *C. burnetii* in infected goats. Therefore, the patterns of seroconversion or transmission described in this study can be considered representative of transmission of *C. burnetii* among young goats in a heavily contaminated intensive dairy herd.

Detection of antibodies in serum was considered the most effective way of detecting recent infection with *C. burnetii* in goats before breeding. Substantial quantities of *C. burnetii* are shed in milk, vaginal mucus and faeces around parturition due to massive replication of *C. burnetii* in the placenta [33–35]. However, shedding is only detectable over a very short timeframe and not before breeding [33–35]. Additionally, *C. burnetii* is present in low concentrations in blood, and for only a few days following infection, unlike antibodies which appear 1–3 weeks after infection and typically last for weeks to months depending on antibody class [26].

High proportions of goats had seroconverted to IgM and IgG against phase 2 *C. burnetii* by week 28 of the study which indicates that majority of the goats born on *C. burnetii* positive farms are infected early in life. Seroconversions were observed well before the goats were mated, which is contrary to the notion that trophoblasts are required for establishment of *C. burnetii* infection in ruminants. Infection of young non-pregnant goats with *C. burnetii* has been disputed in previous studies [17, 19, 36–39]. Although some studies suggest that *C. burnetii* requires trophoblasts for successful establishment of infection in ruminants [35, 36, 40, 41], we are not aware of any study that has investigated whether the absence of trophoblasts in young and male animals prevented the establishment of *C. burnetii* infection. Previous work has suggested that *C. burnetii* infections require trophoblasts to infect ruminants. This was hypothesised after observing primary replication and histopathological lesions only in trophoblasts following experimental infection of pregnant goats with *C. burnetii* [36]; that finding has been referenced in other studies [20]. However, it is possible that the organisms could have been present in other tissues in quantities undetectable by the methods used, as noted by the authors of the study [36].

Despite some studies suggesting that trophoblasts are required for establishing infection in ruminants, a number of studies investigating other aspects of *C. burnetii* on infected farms have reported a high proportion (> 50%) of seroconversions to *C. burnetii* in young ruminants before breeding [17, 19], which is similar to the level detected in our study. Another study reported a seroprevalence of 9.8% in 6-month-old goats that had been kept in a closed facility with no exposure to adult goats [39]. In

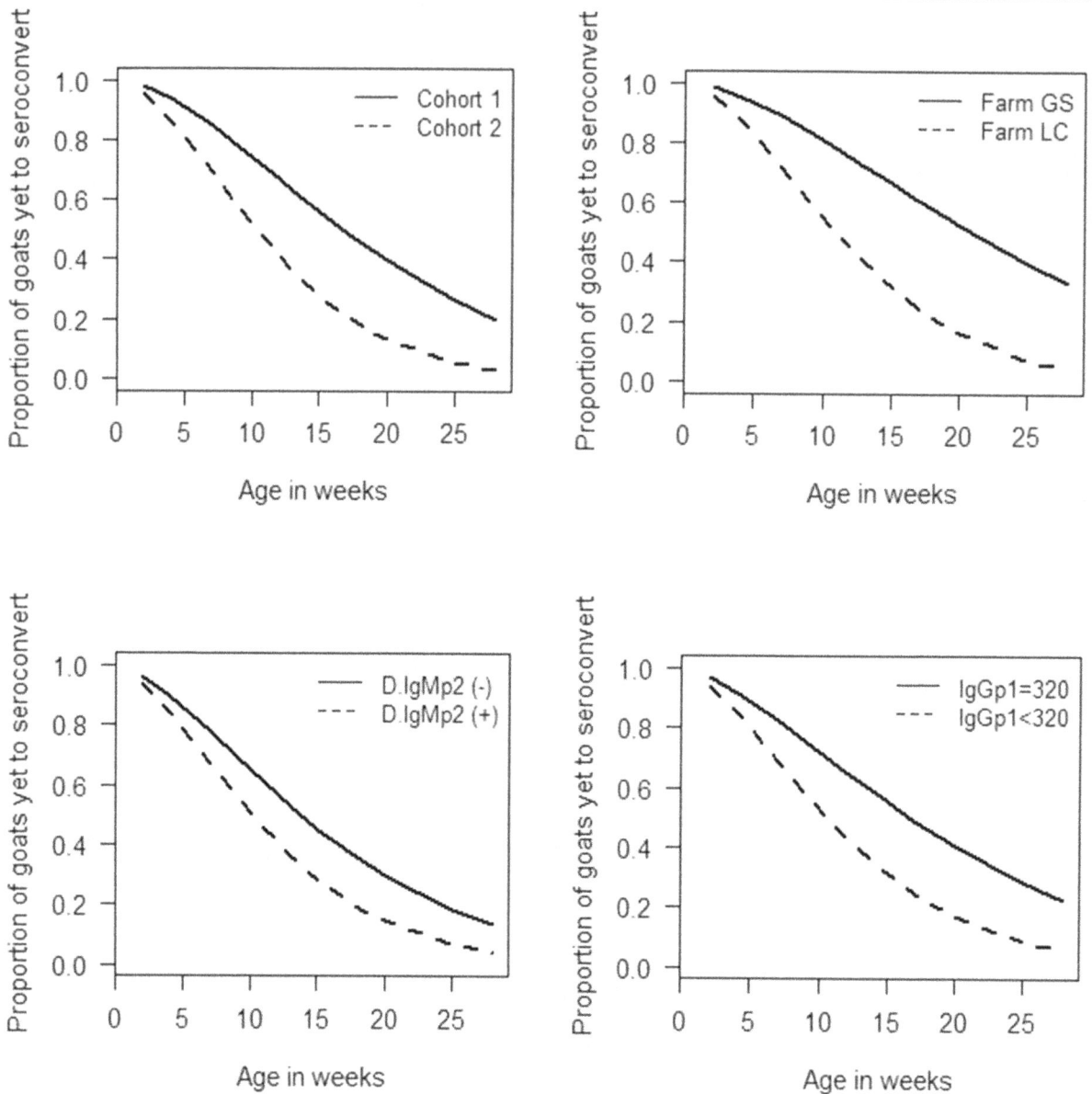

**Figure 4 Weibull survival curves comparing the pre-breeding probability of remaining seronegative to *C. burnetii* in goats.**
D.IgMp2 = IgM serological status of the source does with (D.IgMp2(−) representing negative does and (D.IgMp2(+) the positive ones. IgGp1 =colostrum derived antibody titres dichotomised at a cut-off of 320 (IgGp1). Goats in cohort 1, farm GS and those born by (D.IgMp2(−) as well as those with IgGp1 =320 had statistically significantly (*p* < 0.1) higher probabilities of remaining seronegative before breeding than goats from cohort 2, farm LC as well as those from D.IgMp2(+) and those with IgGp1 < 320 colostrum antibodies.

some instances, young animals were thought not to pose much risk in the transmission of *C. burnetii* thus excluding them from *C. burnetii* studies [16]. It is likely that the discrepancy in the proportion of young animals that seroconvert to *C. burnetii* among several studies [17, 19, 39] is highly dependent on the proportion of parent does shedding *C. burnetii* and the timing of the samplings relative to the progression of the outbreak. The proportion

of adult goats shedding *C. burnetii* is likely to increase over time in an uncontrolled outbreak thus increasing the dose of *C. burnetii* organisms each susceptible animal in the herd is exposed to; and henceforth increasing the number of animals infected with *C. burnetii*. It is not clear if the build-up in the proportion of goats shedding *C. burnetii* would be affected by development of immunity after repeated exposure to *C. burnetii* but one study

A longitudinal study of serological responses to Coxiella burnetii and shedding at kidding among...

41

**Table 3 Multivariable Weibull accelerated failure-time regression model assessing risk factors for seroconversion to *C. burnetii* before breeding.**

| Variable | Levels | n | Serocon. | Coef. | SE (Coef.) | p value | Survival rate ratio (95% CI) | Hazard ratio (95% CI) |
|---|---|---|---|---|---|---|---|---|
| Cohort | Cohort 2 | 62 | 42 | −0.60 | 0.11 | 0.001 | 0.55 (0.39, 0.78) | 2.73 (1.45, 5.16) |
|  | Cohort 1 | 33 | 16 | 0.00 (ref) |  |  | 1.00 | 1.00 |
| Doe IgM | Positive | 37 | 29 | −0.42 | 0.16 | 0.008 | 0.65 (0.48, 0.89) | 2.04 (1.19, 3.54) |
|  | Negative | 56 | 28 | 0.00 (ref) |  |  | 1.00 | 1.00 |
| Intercept | – | – | – | 3.89 | 0.35 | < 0.001 | – | – |

In intensively-reared goats in Victoria, Australia, 2014–2015. Interpretation: After adjusting for the effect of cohort, kids born by does that had positive IgM titres (Doe IgM = positive; indicating recent exposure) were 2.04 times more likely to seroconvert within the first 6 months of life compared to those born by IgM seronegative does. Log likelihood = −201.1. *Coef.* coefficient. Similarly, after adjusting for the effect of farm, kids born by does that had positive IgM titres were 2.23 times (95% CI 1.29, 3.86) more likely to seroconvert within the first 6 months of life compared to those born by IgM seronegative does; see Additional file 3

**Table 4 Multivariable linear regression analysis of the effect of seroconversions to *C. burnetii* on goat weights.**

| Model | Variable | Levels | n | Coef. | SE (coef.) | p value | 95% CI of Coef. |
|---|---|---|---|---|---|---|---|
| Effect of seroconversion on weight at weaning[a] | Cohort | Cohort 2 | 49 | −4.84 | 0.88 | < 0.001 | −6.61, −3.08 |
|  |  | Cohort 1 | 13 | 0.00 (ref) |  |  |  |
|  | Sex | Male | 4 | 3.64 | 1.46 | 0.016 | 0.71, 6.56 |
|  |  | Female | 58 | 0.00 (ref) |  |  |  |
|  | Time of first seroconversion | After 28 weeks | 10 | −0.33 | 1.00 | 0.740 | −1.03, 2.35 |
|  |  | 10–28 weeks | 17 | 0.66 | 0.84 | 0.435 | −2.36, 1.66 |
|  |  | 0–10 weeks | 35 | 0.00 (ref) |  |  |  |
|  | Intercept | – | – | 17.71 | 0.89 | < 0.001 | 15.93, 19.48 |
| Effect of seroconversion on weaning to breeding weight change[b] | Cohort | Cohort 2 | 38 | 5.27 | 1.41 | 0.001 | 2.43, 8.11 |
|  |  | Cohort 1 | 12 | 0.00 (ref) |  |  |  |
|  | Time of first seroconversion | After 28 weeks | 3 | 0.98 | 2.52 | 0.700 | −4.09, 6.04 |
|  |  | 10–28 weeks | 16 | −0.60 | 1.31 | 0.652 | −3.23, 2.04 |
|  |  | 0–10 weeks | 31 | 0.00 (ref) |  |  |  |
|  | Intercept | – | – | 7.67 | 1.40 | < 0.001 | 4.86, 10.49 |

Interpretation: [a] No statistically significant difference in weaning weight was observed between goats that seroconverted before breeding and those that seroconverted post-breeding after adjusting for cohort and sex. However, goats in cohort 2 had weighed 4.84 kg lower at weaning than goats in cohort 1

[b] Similarly, no statistically significant difference in weaning-breeding weight change was observed between goats that seroconverted before breeding and those that seroconverted post-breeding after adjusting for cohort. Surprisingly, goats in cohort 2 weighed 5.27 kg more than goats that had not seroconverted by breeding. Sex was not included in model[b] because all male animals were lost from the study by breeding time

reported that infected goats shed *C. burnetii* for at least two successive kiddings [34].

Furthermore, studies that detected *C. burnetii* organisms in spleens, liver, lungs, kidneys and hearts of young goats [18, 36, 37, 42] as well as interstitial non-suppurative pneumonia and granulomatous hepatitis lesions, similar to those observed in adult goats infected with *C. burnetii,* adds further evidence to the notion that goats can be infected early in life [42]. In most of these studies, it is apparent that diagnosis was made on a few tissues that were submitted, and the majority of the tissues were from kids that died perinatally as well as those that had been sacrificed after birth.

These studies provide useful clues to potential sites of replication and persistence of *C. burnetii* infection in non-pregnant young goats that could possibly result in shedding of low levels of the bacterium before breeding. However, the site of persistent *C. burnetii* infection in young ruminants is still unknown, unlike in adult goats where *C. burnetii* infection persists in the mammary glands and uterus resulting in continuous shedding of *C. burnetii* in milk long after kidding [43, 44]. The site of persistent infection in young animals needs to be investigated, notwithstanding the possibility that the organism may be present in low numbers below the detection limit of most diagnostic tools.

The initial rise in IgG phase 1 and IgG phase 2 following colostrum feeding is probably due to uptake of antibodies against *C. burnettii* in colostrum. This is further supported by the high concentrations of IgG specific for phase 1 and phase 2 as well as negligible quantities of IgM that were detected in colostrum. The IgG and IgM concentrations in colostrum reported by this study are in accordance with another study that reported colostrum IgG concentrations of 41.2 mg/mL and IgM concentrations of 1.9 mg/mL [45]. In the event of infection at birth or around the time of feeding colostrum, IgG antibodies to phase 1 against such infections would not be detectable within 2 weeks as IgG phase 1 antibodies appear much later in the course of infection [26, 36, 46, 47]. Thus, the extremely high IgG phase 1 and phase 2 antibody titres (Figure 2) observed in the serum of kids at 2 weeks were most likely derived from colostrum.

Early IgM responses were detected mostly in kids that did not receive sufficient colostrum. This suggests that antibodies and other immune components in colostrum are protective against *C. burnetii* infection. This further explains the surge in IgM and IgG immune responses after the IgG phase 1 colostrum antibodies (antibodies detected immediately after feeding colostrum) wane, around week 7 (median), and thus suggests that goats are at risk after the depletion of colostrum antibodies. These findings also suggest that, in this study, ingestion of colostrum was protective in goat kids.

Colostrum could also have been a source of *C. burnetii* infection although this appears not to have been the case in this study possibly due to heat treatment of colostrum before it is fed to the goats. In any case, it appears that infection resulting from ingestion of contaminated milk is not readily achieved and observations in humans ingesting contaminated milk failed to demonstrate resulting infection [48, 49]. It is therefore worthwhile to ensure that all goats are fed enough colostrum containing antibodies against *C. burnetii*, especially in instances where new-born goats are snatched from their mothers before they ingest colostrum. Perhaps, efforts could also be aimed towards increasing antibodies and immune components against *C. burnetii* in colostrum indirectly by giving a booster vaccination against *C. burnetii* to pregnant goats, as demonstrated in a vaccination trial of sows against porcine circovirus type 2 in pigs where the aim was to protect piglets from infection with this virus early in life [50]. Also, studies in which, pregnant animals were vaccinated using phase 1 *C. burnetii* vaccines have not reported any deleterious effects of the vaccine [22, 36].

In a dairy farm setting where new-born animals are restricted from receiving milk from their does, it seems reasonable to protect these animals as early as possible. However, considering the workload on intensive dairy farms during and immediately after kidding and the difficulty of ensuring that all kids receive adequate colostrum intake, we recommend vaccination be implemented not later than 8 weeks of age, i.e. preceding the majority of seroconversions in this study. We also recommend a booster dose to increase vaccine coverage, considering that antibodies derived from colostrum may still be present in some goats at 8 weeks of age and interfere with antibody production, even for inactivated vaccines like the Coxevac vaccine, (CEVA, France) used to vaccinate against *C. burnetii* in goats [51].

Cell-mediated immunity also plays an important role in protection against intra-cellular pathogens like *C. burnetii* and it is not affected by the presence of maternally derived antibodies, as demonstrated in a study that evaluated vaccination against Aujesky's disease in pigs [51–53]; early vaccination, even in the presence of maternal antibody, may still be protective. Some studies have however, shown that some components of the immune system, for example, the B cells derived from the intestinal lymphoid tissues are not produced until after 8 weeks of age in goats [54]. Ideally the best time to vaccinate the kids would be during the narrow window of opportunity that occurs between the decline of the colostrum-derived maternal antibodies and the synthesis of kid-endogenous antibody arising from their environmental exposure to *C. burnetii*. This is probably from 8 to 10 weeks of age.

The comparable duration of seropositivity and median antibody titres of goats that seroconverted prior to and after the target breeding age suggests similarity in exposure before and after breeding. The duration of seropositivity varied widely, which accords with what has been previously reported in another outbreak in the UK [39]. The finding that the IgG phase 2 and 1 responses last longer than the IgM phase 2 and 1 responses that precede them is consistent with what has been reported in human serology and in adult animal studies [26, 46]. However, the number of secondary IgM responses compared to IgG responses, described in Table 2, may have been confounded by the lower repeatability of the IFA for IgM (78.1%) compared to IgG antibodies (96.9%) as well as the lower sensitivity of the IFA for IgM (88.8%) compared to IgG antibodies (94.8%).

The difference in risk associated with the two cohorts from two different kidding times studied here suggests that differences in the level of *C. burnetii* shedding at each kidding season, and possibly different levels of exposure to *C. burnetii* at birth, or soon after, may influence timing of occurrence of seroconversions against *C. burnetii* infections. This could also indicate differences in colostrum quality and its administration. Similarly, the surge in IgM and IgG seroconversions that occurred prior to weaning could possibly be due to exposure to *C. burnetii* at birth. The difference in the risk of seroconversion at farm level points to variability in contamination or shedding patterns on the different farms on the property; animals on Farm GS were partly reared by less intensive small out-grower farms until 4 months of age, which may explain the lower risk of seroconversion compared to Farm LC.

The increased risk of seroconversion in kids born to IgM seropositive does suggests recent infections in these does and points to either in utero transmission of *C. burnetii* or periparturient transmission. In utero transmission of *C. burnetii* has not been confirmed but *C. burnetii* DNA has been detected in amniotic fluid as well as spleen and kidneys of live and aborted kids; histopathological lesions similar to those in infected adult goats have also been reported in new-born goats [18, 36, 38]. Another study has also shown goat embryos to be highly susceptible to *C. burnetii* infection in vitro [55]. However, there is a challenge in differentiating DNA present because of *C. burnetii* infection from that due to contamination from the heavily infected placentas. The majority of the reports of PCR positive results from tissues of aborted kids provided very little information on how the prevention of contamination of these tissues by DNA from the heavily infected placental tissues was achieved [18, 36, 37]. Perhaps, the demonstration of vertical transmission of *C. burnetii* using PCR needs to be complemented by other methods, such as immunohistochemistry, that detect *C. burnetii* within the cells in tissues of foetuses or newborn kid goats.

As expected, exposure to *C. burnetii* shed at subsequent kidding seasons could be playing a role in increasing the proportion of infected goats before the target breeding age. This was more evident in cohort 2, where the rate of occurrence of antibody mediated responses was 4.5 times higher within than outside the kidding season. The comparable rate of occurrence of immune responses within and outside the kidding season for cohort 1 could be a result of a proportion of these goats being reared on out-grower farms for the first 4 months of their lives. The occurrence antibody-mediated immune responses outside the kidding seasons points to other risks of exposure to *C. burnetii* in the environment; for example, contaminated straw, hay or pastures, as well as inhalation or ingestion of contaminated dust particles especially during dry and windy weather [56–58].

Although occurrence of IgM and IgG responses and not the conventional twofold rise in IgG against phase 2 or IgM followed by IgG were used in comparing outside and within kidding season exposure to *C. burnetii*, this seemed the most practical way of computing animal-time at risk given the shorter duration of IgM antibodies compared to IgG as shown in Table 2. Comparisons for within and outside kidding seasons were also restricted to either IgM and IgG to cater for the differences in duration of IgM and IgG seropositivity as well as the differences in repeatability and sensitivity of the IFA for IgM

and IgG antibodies. The detection of antibodies using the IFA may have been enhanced by repeated sampling and testing of samples in duplicate against IgG and IgM to phase 1 and 2 *C. burnetii* given that all IgG responses except one were preceded by IgM responses. The performance of the IFA may also have been enhanced by the quality of antigens used and the experience of the technicians in this instance, as these factors may influence the reproducibility of the test.

The shedding of *C. burnetii* by goats that seroconverted before breeding and remained seropositive through pregnancy underscores the role played by pre-breeding infections in the transmission of infection within the herd. Owing to mortality, we did not have a sufficiently large sample size at the end of the study to detect any statistically significant differences in *C. burnetii* shedding patterns between goats that seroconverted before breeding and those that seroconverted after breeding. Similarly, we were not able to detect any statistically significant reductions in weight gain at the individual animal level. These considerations are the focus of further ongoing studies. The high mortalities reaching up to 20% in the first months of follow-up were thought to result from a number of factors, including a poor-quality milk replacer and infectious causes like coccidiosis.

In summary, the first surge in the number of goats seroconverting with IgM antibodies to *C. burnetii* antigens was observed at 9 weeks of age, which underscores the need to vaccinate goats born on *C. burnetii* positive farms not later than 8 weeks of age. However, experimental studies are required to establish the effectiveness and feasibility of vaccinating goats at 8 weeks of age. It is expected that booster doses of vaccine will need to be administered to increase vaccine coverage. The shedding of *C. burnettii* by goats that remained seropositive after the initial seroconversion before the target breeding age provides more evidence supporting the notion that goats infected early in life can transmit *C. burnetii* to other goats and humans at their first kidding, underscoring the need to vaccinate young goats.

Post-weaning, the rate of seroconversion to *C. burnetii* was significantly higher within than outside the kidding seasons, this being more notable among goats in cohort 2, which were exposed to kidding season throughout the study period. Furthermore, goats from IgM seropositive does were two times more likely to seroconvert before the target breeding age, which points to either the occurrence of in utero transmission of *C. burnetii* or infection of goats during or shortly after birth.

Some of the goats that seroconverted before breeding shed *C. burnetii* at their first kidding, suggesting that goats infected early in life can be a risk for transmission of *C. burnetii* to susceptible animals in the herd.

No statistically significant reductions in weight gain at the individual animal level were observed among goats that seroconverted against *C. burnetii* before breeding.

## Additional files

**Additional file 1.** Kaplain-Meier survival curve showing the probability of intensively-reared kid goats remaining seronegative to *C. burnetii* before breeding, Victoria, Australia, 2015.

**Additional file 2.** Univariable assessment of the effect of risk factors on seroconversion against *C. burnetii* in goats.

**Additional file 3.** Multivariable Weibull accelerated failure time regression model assessing risk factors for seroconversion to *C. burnetii* before breeding in intensively-reared goats.

**Additional file 4.** Comparison of the rate of occurrence of antibody responses within and outside the kidding season in intensively managed goats.

**Additional file 5.** Median and inter-quartile range of antibody titres of goats in cohort 2 that shed *C. burnetii* at their first kidding during a Q fever outbreak farm.

**Competing interests**
The authors declare that they have no competing interests.

**Authors' contributions**
All authors participated in sample collection and analysis as well as in the writing of the manuscript. All authors read and approved the final manuscript.

**Acknowledgements**
We would like to acknowledge laboratory support from the Australian Rickettsial Reference Laboratory as well as support from staff at the affected farm and staff from the Mackinnon project.

**Funding**
No specific funding was provided for this work. All research was undertaken using resources at the institutions involved.

**Author details**
[1] Asia–Pacific Centre for Animal Health, Faculty of Veterinary and Agricultural Sciences, The University of Melbourne, Parkville, VIC 3010, Australia. [2] The Mackinnon Project, Faculty of Veterinary and Agricultural Sciences, The University of Melbourne, Werribee, VIC 3010, Australia. [3] Australian Rickettsial Reference Laboratory, Barwon Health, Geelong, VIC, Australia.

## References

1. Kampschreur LM, Hagenaars JC, Wielders CC, Elsman P, Lestrade PJ, Koning OH, Oosterheert JJ, Renders NH, Wever PC (2013) Screening for *Coxiella burnetii* seroprevalence in chronic Q fever high-risk groups reveals the magnitude of the Dutch Q fever outbreak. Epidemiol Infect 141:847–851
2. Schack M, Sachse S, Rödel J, Frangoulidis D, Pletz MW, Rohde GU, Straube E, Boden K (2014) *Coxiella burnetii* (Q fever) as a cause of community-acquired pneumonia during the warm season in Germany. Epidemiol Infect 142:1905–1910
3. Angelakis E, Edouard S, Lafranchi MA, Pham T, Lafforgue P, Raoult D (2014) Emergence of Q fever arthritis in France. J Clin Microbiol 52:1064–1067
4. Million M, Walter G, Thuny F, Habib G, Raoult D (2013) Evolution from acute Q fever to endocarditis is associated with underlying valvulopathy and age and can be prevented by prolonged antibiotic treatment. Clin Infect Dis 57:836–844
5. Levy PY, Carrieri P, Raoult D (1999) *Coxiella burnetii* pericarditis: report of 15 cases and review. Clin Infect Dis 29:393–397
6. Piquet P, Raoult D, Tranier P, Mercier C (1994) *Coxiella burnetii* infection of pseudoaneurysm of an aortic bypass graft with contiguous vertebral osteomyelitis. J Vasc Surg 19:165–168
7. Kampschreur LM, Delsing CE, Groenwold RHH, Wegdam-Blans MC, Bleeker-Rovers CP, de Jager-Leclercq MG, Hoepelman AI, van Kasteren ME, Buijs J, Renders NH et al (2014) Chronic Q fever in the Netherlands 5 years after the start of the Q fever epidemic: results from the Dutch chronic Q fever database. J Clin Microbiol 52:1637–1643
8. Briggs BJ, Raoult D, Hijazi ZM, Edouard S, Angelakis E, Logan LK (2016) *Coxiella burnetii* endocarditis in a child caused by a new genotype. Pediatr Infect Dis J 35:213–214
9. Francis JR, Robson J, Wong D, Walsh M, Astori I, Gill D, Nourse C (2016) Chronic recurrent multifocal Q fever osteomyelitis in children: an emerging clinical challenge. Pediatr Infect Dis J 35:972–976
10. Angelakis E, Mediannikov O, Socolovschi C, Mouffok N, Bassene H, Tall A, Niangaly H, Doumbo O, Znazen A, Sarih M (2014) *Coxiella burnetii*-positive PCR in febrile patients in rural and urban Africa. Int J Infect Dis 28:107–110
11. Chryssanthou E, Cuenca-Estrella M, Denning D (2006) Q fever in young children, Ghana. Mycopathologia 162:289–294
12. Delsing CE, Kullberg BJ (2008) Q fever in the Netherlands: a concise overview and implications of the largest ongoing outbreak. Neth J Med 66:365–367
13. Guigno D, Coupland B, Smith EG, Farrell ID, Desselberger U, Caul EO (1992) Primary humoral antibody response to *Coxiella burnetii*, the causative agent of Q fever. J Clin Microbiol 30:1958–1967
14. Smith DL, Ayres JG, Blair I, Burge PS, Carpenter MJ, Caul EO, Coupland B, Desselberger U, Evans M, Farrell ID et al (1993) A large Q fever outbreak in the West Midlands: clinical aspects. Respir Med 87:509–516
15. Lyytikäinen O, Ziese T, Schwartländer B, Matzdorff P, Kuhnhen C, Jäger C, Petersen L (1998) An outbreak of sheep-associated Q fever in a rural community in Germany. Eur J Epidemiol 14:193–199
16. Hogerwerf L, van den Brom R, Roest HI, Bouma A, Vellema P, Pieterse M, Dercksen D, Nielen M (2011) Reduction of *Coxiella burnetii* prevalence by vaccination of goats and sheep, the Netherlands. Emerg Infect Dis 17:379–386
17. de Cremoux R, Rousset E, Touratier A, Audusseau G, Nicollet P, Ribaud D, David V, Le Pape M (2012) *Coxiella burnetii* vaginal shedding and antibody responses in dairy goat herds in a context of clinical Q fever outbreaks. FEMS Immunol Med Microbiol 64:120–122
18. Arricau-Bouvery N, Souriau A, Bodier C, Dufour P, Rousset E, Rodolakis A (2005) Effect of vaccination with phase I and phase II *Coxiella burnetii* vaccines in pregnant goats. Vaccine 23:4392–4402
19. de Cremoux R, Rousset E, Touratier A, Audusseau G, Nicollet P, Ribaud D, David V, Le Pape M (2012) Assessment of vaccination by a phase I *Coxiella burnetii*-inactivated vaccine in goat herds in clinical Q fever situation. FEMS Immunol Med Microbiol 64:104–106
20. Bontje DM, Backer JA, Hogerwerf L, Roest HI, van Roermund HJ (2016) Analysis of Q fever in Dutch dairy goat herds and assessment of control measures by means of a transmission model. Prev Vet Med 123:71–89
21. van Asseldonk M, Bontje DM, Backer JA, Roermund HJ, Bergevoet RH (2015) Economic aspects of Q fever control in dairy goats. Prev Vet Med 121:115–122
22. Rousset E, Durand B, Champion JL, Prigent M, Dufour P, Forfait C, Marois M, Gasnier T, Duquesne V, Thiéry R, Aubert MF (2009) Efficiency of a phase 1 vaccine for the reduction of vaginal *Coxiella burnetii* shedding in a clinically affected goat herd. Clin Microbiol Infect 15:188–189
23. Bond KA, Vincent G, Wilks CR, Franklin L, Sutton B, Stenos J, Cowan R, Lim K, Athan E, Harris O et al (2015) One health approach to controlling a Q fever outbreak on an Australian goat farm. Epidemiol Infect 144:1129–1141
24. Muleme M, Stenos J, Vincent G, Wilks CR, Devlin JM, Campbell A, Cameron A, Stevenson MA, Graves S, Firestone SM (2017) Peripartum dynamics of

*Coxiella burnetii* infections in intensively managed dairy goats associated with a Q fever outbreak in Australia. Prev Vet Med 139(Pt A):58–66

25. Rousset E, Durand B, Berri M, Dufour P, Prigent M, Russo P, Delcroix T, Touratier A, Rodolakis A, Aubert M (2007) Comparative diagnostic potential of three serological tests for abortive Q fever in goat herds. Vet Microbiol 124:286–297

26. Roest HI, Post J, van Gelderen B, van Zijderveld FG, Rebel JM (2013) Q fever in pregnant goats: humoral and cellular immune responses. Vet Res 44:67

27. Thrusfield M (2013) Veterinary epidemiology. Elsevier, Amsterdam

28. Da Silva AS, Tonin AA, Camillo G, Weber A, Lopes LS, Cazarotto CJ, Balzan A, Bianchi AE, Stefani LM, Lopes STA, Vogel FF (2014) Ovine toxoplasmosis: indirect immunofluorescence for milk samples as a diagnostic tool. Small Rumin Res 120:181–184

29. Lockhart MG, Graves SR, Banazis MJ, Fenwick SG, Stenos J (2011) A comparison of methods for extracting DNA from *Coxiella burnetii* as measured by a duplex qPCR assay. Lett Appl Microbiol 52:514–520

30. Akaike H (1998) Information theory and an extension of the maximum likelihood principle. In: Selected papers of Hirotugu Akaike. Springer, Berlin. doi: 10.1007/978-1-4612-1694-0_15

31. Hubeaux S, Rufibach K (2014) SurvRegCensCov: Weibull regression for a right-censored endpoint with a censored covariate, arXiv preprint arXiv:1402.0432, https://arxiv.org/abs/1402.0432

32. R Core Team (2014) R: a language and environment for statistical computing. R Foundation for Statistical Computing. https://www.r-project.org/

33. Woldehiwet Z (2004) Q fever (*coxiellosis*): epidemiology and pathogenesis. Res Vet Sci 77:93–100

34. Berri M, Rousset E, Champion JL, Russo P, Rodolakis A (2007) Goats may experience reproductive failures and shed *Coxiella burnetii* at two successive parturitions after a Q fever infection. Res Vet Sci 83:47–52

35. Sánchez J, Souriau A, Buendía AJ, Arricau-Bouvery N, Martínez CM, Salinas J, Rodolakis A, Navarro JA (2006) Experimental *Coxiella burnetii* infection in pregnant goats: a histopathological and immunohistochemical study. J Comp Pathol 135:108–115

36. Roest HJ, van Gelderen B, Dinkla A, Frangoulidis D, van Zijderveld F, Rebel J, van Keulen L (2012) Q fever in pregnant goats: pathogenesis and excretion of *Coxiella burnetii*. PLoS One 7:e48949

37. Palmer NC, Kierstead M, Key DW, Williams JC, Peacock MG, Vellend H (1983) Placentitis and abortion in goats and sheep in Ontario caused by *Coxiella burnetii*. Can Vet J 24:60–61

38. Bouvery NA, Souriau A, Lechopier P, Rodolakis A (2003) Experimental *Coxiella burnetii* infection in pregnant goats: excretion routes. Vet Res 34:423–433

39. Reichel R, Mearns R, Brunton L, Jones R, Horigan M, Vipond R, Vincent G, Evans S (2012) Description of a *Coxiella burnetii* abortion outbreak in a dairy goat herd, and associated serology, PCR and genotyping results. Res Vet Sci 93:1217–1224

40. Ben Amara A, Ghigo E, Le Priol Y, Lépolard C, Salcedo SP, Lemichez E, Bretelle F, Capo C, Mege JL (2010) *Coxiella burnetii*, the agent of Q fever, replicates within trophoblasts and induces a unique transcriptional response. PLoS One 5:e15315

41. Waag DM, Thompson HA (2005) Pathogenesis of and immunity to *Coxiella burnetii*. In: Biological weapons defense, Springer, pp 185–207

42. Moore JD, Barr BC, Daft BM, O'Connor MT (1991) Pathology and diagnosis of *Coxiella burnetii* infection in a goat herd. Vet Pathol 28:81–84

43. Rodolakis A (2014) Zoonoses in goats: how to control them. Small Rumin Res 121:12–20

44. Rodolakis A, Berri M, Héchard C, Caudron C, Souriau A, Bodier CC, Blanchard B, Camuset P, Devillechaise P, Natorp JC et al (2007) Comparison of *Coxiella burnetii* shedding in milk of dairy bovine, caprine, and ovine herds. J Dairy Sci 90:5352–5360

45. Moreno-Indias I, Sánchez-Macías D, Castro N, Morales-delaNuez A, Hernández-Castellano LE, Capote J, Argüello A (2012) Chemical composition and immune status of dairy goat colostrum fractions during the first 10h after partum. Small Rumin Res 103:220–224

46. Peacock MG, Fiset P, Ormsbee R, Wisseman CL Jr (1979) Antibody response in man following a small intradermal inoculation with *Coxiella burnetii* phase I vaccine. Acta Virol 23:73–81

47. Powell OW, Stallman ND (1962) The incidence and significance of phase 1 complement-fixing antibody in Q fever. J Hyg 60:359–364

48. Krumbiegel ER, Wisniewski HJ (1970) Q fever in the Milwaukee area. II. Consumption of infected raw milk by human volunteers. Arch Environ Health 21:63–65

49. European Food Safety Association (2010) Q fever. EFSA J 8:1595–1709

50. Kurmann J, Sydler T, Brugnera E, Buergi E, Haessig M, Suter M, Sidler X (2011) Vaccination of dams increases antibody titer and improves growth parameters in finisher pigs subclinically infected with porcine circovirus type 2. Clin Vaccine Immunol 18:1644–1649

51. Niewiesk S (2014) Maternal antibodies: clinical significance, mechanism of interference with immune responses, and possible vaccination strategies. Front Immunol 5:446

52. Pomorska-Mól M, Markowska-Daniel I (2010) Interferon-γ secretion and proliferative responses of peripheral blood mononuclear cells after vaccination of pigs against Aujeszky's disease in the presence of maternal immunity. FEMS Immunol Med Microbiol 58:405–411

53. Toman R, Heinzen RA, Samuel JE, Mege JL (2012) Components of protective immunity, *Coxiella burnetii*: recent advances and new perspectives in research of the Q fever bacterium. Springer, Berlin, pp 91–104

54. Corpa JM, Pérez V, García Marín JF (2000) Differences in the immune responses in lambs and kids vaccinated against paratuberculosis, according to the age of vaccination. Vet Microbiol 77:475–485

55. Alsaleh A, Fieni F, Rodolakis A, Bruyas JF, Roux C, Larrat M, Chatagnon G, Pellerin JL (2013) Can *Coxiella burnetii* be transmitted by embryo transfer in goats? Theriogenology 80:571–575

56. Maurin M, Raoult D (1999) Q fever. Clin Microbiol Rev 12:518–553

57. Angelakis E, Raoult D (2010) Q fever. Vet Microbiol 140:297–309

58. Tigertt WD, Benenson AS, Gochenour WS (1961) Airborne Q fever. Bacteriol Rev 25:285–293

# 5

# Acquisition of resistance to avian leukosis virus subgroup B through mutations on *tvb* cysteine-rich domains in DF-1 chicken fibroblasts

Hong Jo Lee[1], Kyung Youn Lee[1], Young Hyun Park[1], Hee Jung Choi[1], Yongxiu Yao[2], Venugopal Nair[2] and Jae Yong Han[1,3]*

## Abstract

Avian leukosis virus (ALV) is a retrovirus that causes tumors in avian species, and its vertical and horizontal transmission in poultry flocks results in enormous economic losses. Despite the discovery of specific host receptors, there have been few reports on the modulation of viral susceptibility via genetic modification. We therefore engineered acquired resistance to ALV subgroup B using CRISPR/Cas9-mediated genome editing technology in DF-1 chicken fibroblasts. Using this method, we efficiently modified the tumor virus locus B (*tvb*) gene, encoding the TVB receptor, which is essential for ALV subgroup B entry into host cells. By expanding individual DF-1 clones, we established that artificially generated premature stop codons in the cysteine-rich domain (CRD) of TVB receptor confer resistance to ALV subgroup B. Furthermore, we found that a cysteine residue (C80) of CRD2 plays a crucial role in ALV subgroup B entry. These results suggest that CRISPR/Cas9-mediated genome editing can be used to efficiently modify avian cells and establish novel chicken cell lines with resistance to viral infection.

## Introduction

Avian leukosis virus (ALV) is a retrovirus that infects avian species, eventually causing tumors [1]. The ALV is a group VI virus of the family *Retroviridae*, and it can be divided into six subgroups, A–E and J, based on retroviral envelope glycoproteins that play a crucial role in host–virus interactions [2]. ALV-infected poultry display several symptoms, including lymphoblastic, erythroblastic and osteopetrotic tumors, and the virus can be transmitted both vertically and horizontally. The spread of ALV in poultry flocks therefore causes tremendous economic losses within the poultry industry [3].

Susceptibility and resistance to the virus depend largely on specific host receptors that interact with viral envelope proteins. Naturally occurring genetic mutations in the host receptors, or artificial expression of mutant receptors in host cells, can affect susceptibility to the virus. A four base pair (bp) insertion and 1 bp substitution in the tumor virus locus A (*tva*) gene confer resistance to ALV subgroup A [4], and mutations in the first intron of *tva* are also reported to reduce susceptibility to ALV subgroup A [5, 6]. Chickens with a 1 bp substitution in *tvb* creating an in-frame stop codon exhibit complete resistance to ALV subgroup B, and a single amino acid substitution (C125S) reduces susceptibility to ALV subgroups B, D and E [7, 8]. Resistance to ALV subgroup C is closely related to a 1 bp substitution in tumor virus locus C (*tvc*) that creates an in-frame stop codon [9]. Moreover, comparative studies suggest that variation in tryptophan 38 (W38) in the NHE1 gene explains the differences in susceptibility to ALV subgroup J among avian species [10, 11].

Despite the discovery of specific host receptors that are critical for ALV entry, there has been only one report on the acquisition of resistance to ALV subgroup C in

*Correspondence: jaehan@snu.ac.kr
[1] Department of Agricultural Biotechnology, College of Agriculture and Life Sciences, and Research Institute of Agriculture and Life Sciences, Seoul National University, Seoul 08826, South Korea
Full list of author information is available at the end of the article

avian species via genome editing of host receptor genes. This can be attributed partly to the lack of an efficient genome editing technology [9]. The recently developed clustered regularly interspaced short palindromic repeats (CRISPR)/CRISPR-associated (Cas9) system is a programmable genome editing technology [12] that has been widely adopted for use in many organisms, including mice, fish, pigs and cows [13–16]. Among avian species, CRISPR/Cas9 has also been used successfully for genome editing in chickens [17, 18].

We performed genome editing on the chicken host receptor gene *tvb*, which is related specifically to ALV subgroup B. Since chickens with premature stop codons in CRDs of TVB receptors exhibit resistance to ALV subgroup B, we sought to identify artificial mutations in CRDs of TVB receptors that cause similar effects [7]. We adopted the CRISPR/Cas9 system, an efficient programmable genome editing tool, for use in DF-1 chicken fibroblasts. We then evaluated the susceptibility of genetically modified hosts to ALV subgroup B using flow cytometry.

## Materials and methods

### Experimental animals and animal care
The care and experimental use of chickens were approved by the Institute of Laboratory Animal Resources, Seoul National University (SNU-150827-1). Chickens were maintained according to a standard management program at the University Animal Farm, Seoul National University, Korea. The procedures for animal management, reproduction and embryo manipulation adhered to the standard operating protocols of our laboratory.

### Construction of CRISPR/Cas9 expression vectors
We constructed all-in-one CRISPR/Cas9 vectors targeting *tvb*, with minor modifications. The CRISPR kit used for constructing multiplex CRISPR/Cas9 vectors was a gift from Takashi Yamamoto (Addgene Kit #1000000054) [19], and a neomycin resistance gene under the regulation of a thymidine kinase promoter was inserted into CRISPR/Cas9 vectors by *NotI* digestion and ligation (New England Biolabs, Ipswich, MA, USA). For the insertion of guide RNA sequences into CRISPR/Cas9 vectors, we synthesized sense and antisense oligonucleotides (Bionics, Seoul, Korea) and carried out annealing using the following thermocycling conditions: 30 s at 95 °C, 2 min at 72 °C, 2 min at 37 °C and 2 min at 25 °C. The oligonucleotides used are listed in Table 1.

### Culture of DF-1 chicken fibroblasts
DF-1 cells were maintained and subpassaged in Dulbecco's minimum essential medium (DMEM; Hyclone, Logan, UT, USA), supplemented with 10% fetal bovine

**Table 1  Primers used in this study**

| Primers | Sequence |
|---|---|
| TVB #1 F | 5'- CAC CGG CAG CTG AGC GCA TCG TGC G -3' |
| TVB #1 R | 5'- AAA CCG CAC GAT GCG CTC AGC TGC C -3' |
| TVB #2 F | 5'- CAC CGA ATG ACT TTC CCA AGT GCC T -3' |
| TVB #2 R | 5'- AAA CAG GCA CTT GGG AAA GTC ATT C -3' |
| TVB #1 seq F | 5'- AGC TGT CAG CTG GTG GAG TTC AC -3' |
| TVB #1 seq R | 5'- ATA GCG TCC AAT CTG GGT GAG CC -3' |
| TVB #2 seq F | 5'- TCT CCA CGT CTC GGC AGC AC -3' |
| TVB #1 seq R | 5'- CAG CTC TGC TCG GGC TCT CC -3' |

serum (FBS; Hyclone) and 1× antibiotic–antimycotic (ABAM; Thermo Fisher–Invitrogen, Carlsbad, CA, USA). DF-1 cells were cultured in an incubator at 37 °C in an atmosphere of 5% $CO_2$ at 60–70% relative humidity.

### Culture of White Leghorn (WL) chicken embryonic fibroblasts (CEFs)
All internal organs and limbs were removed from WL chicken embryos of 6-day-incubated fertilized eggs, and the remaining embryonic body was then dissociated using 0.05% (v/v) trypsin/ethylenediaminetetraacetic acid (Gibco, Grand Island, NY, USA) at 37 °C for 15 min. The limbs were used for genomic DNA extraction, and the dissociated cells were filtered through 70 mm nylon mesh filters and cultured in DMEM (Hyclone) containing 10% FBS (Hyclone) and 1% ABAM (Thermo Fisher–Invitrogen) in a 5% $CO_2$ atmosphere at 37 °C [20].

### Transfection and G418 selection of DF-1 cells
CRISPR/Cas9 vectors (3 µg) were mixed with Lipofectamine 2000 reagent (Thermo Fisher–Invitrogen) in Opti-MEM (Thermo Fisher–Invitrogen), and the mixture was applied to $5 \times 10^5$ DF-1 cells. Then, 6 h after transfection, transfection mixtures were replaced with DF-1 culture medium. Geneticin® Selective Antibiotic (G418; GIBCO Invitrogen, Grand Island, NY, USA) (300 µg/mL) was added to the culture medium 1 day after transfection. The complete selection period required up to 7 days.

### T7E1 assay
We adapted the T7E1 assay method from previous publications with minor modifications [21]. Genomic DNA was extracted from DF-1 cells after G418 selection. Genomic regions encompassing the CRISPR/Cas9 target sites were amplified using specific primer sets (Table 1). The amplicons were reannealed to form a heteroduplex DNA structure after denaturation. Subsequently, the heteroduplex amplicons were treated with 5 units T7E1 endonuclease (New England Biolabs) for

20 min at 37 °C and then analyzed by 1% agarose gel electrophoresis.

### Culture of single DF-1 cells and genomic DNA sequencing

After G418 selection, single DF-1 cells from the DF-1 cells treated with CRISPR vectors were seeded in individual wells of a 96-well plate with 100 μL culture medium. We checked the wells each day after seeding and, when the cells in each well were confluent, subpassaged the cells into a 48-well plate. These cells were then used for genomic DNA extraction. The genomic regions encompassing the CRISPR/Cas9 target sites in DF-1 and WL CEFs were amplified using specific primer sets (Table 1), and the PCR products were sequenced using the ABI Prism 3730 XL DNA Analyzer (Thermo Fisher–Applied Biosystems, Foster City, CA, USA). The sequences were analyzed against assembled genomes using BLAST (http://blast.ncbi.nlm.nih.gov).

### Virus production and infection

RCASBP-(B)-CN-EGFP was kindly provided by Dr. Yao and Dr. Nair (Pirbright Institute). CRISPR/Cas9 vectors (5 μg) were mixed with Lipofectamine 2000 reagent (Thermo Fisher–Invitrogen) in Opti-Mem (Thermo Fisher–Invitrogen), and the mixture was applied to $1 \times 10^6$ DF-1 cells. The mixture was replaced with DF-1 culture medium 6 h after transfection. One day after transfection we could detect green fluorescence in DF-1 cells, which indicated virus production. Cells were subpassaged, and the medium was changed 1 day after subpassaging. One day later, the medium containing virus was harvested and frozen at −70 °C until use. For viral infection, the medium containing virus was thawed at 37 °C and added to individual DF-1 and WL CEF clones. Four days post-infection, DF-1 and WL CEFs were observed using fluorescence microscopy (TU-80; Nikon, Tokyo, Japan) and analyzed using FACSCalibur (BD Biosciences, San Jose, CA, USA).

### Protein alignment and structure analysis

The protein sequences and bisulfide bond structures of human DR5 TRAIL receptor (NP_003833.4), mouse Tnfrsf10b (NP_064671.2), western clawed frog tnfrsf10b (NP_001004894.1), chicken TVB[S1] (NP_989446.2) and chicken TVB[S3] were analyzed using ClustalW.

### Statistical analysis

Statistical analysis system (SAS) software was used for analysis of ALV subgroup B susceptibility. Each treatment was compared using the least-squares method or Duncan's method, and the significance of the main effects was determined using analysis of variance in the SAS package. A *p* value < 0.05 was regarded as statistically significant.

## Results

### Virus production in DF-1 cells

To produce ALV subgroup B in chicken DF-1 cells, cells were transfected with the RCASBP-(B)-CN-EGFP vector. This vector contains a green fluorescent protein (GFP)-expressing cassette with ALV subgroup B *gag*, *env* and *pol* genes (Figure 1A). This allowed us to assess virus production in DF-1 cells based on GFP expression compared with wild type (WT) DF-1 cells (Figure 1B).

### Genome editing in tvb mediated by CRISPR/Cas9

To efficiently disrupt *tvb*, we designed two CRISPR/Cas9 vectors targeting two different sites within the gene. The TVB#1 vector (TVB#1) was designed to target the ATG sequence of *tvb*, which can inhibit gene translation. The TVB#2 vector (TVB#2) was designed to target exon 3 of *tvb*, which can cause frame shift mutations resulting in production of a stop codon in CRDs of TVB receptors [7] (Figure 2A). DF-1 cells transfected with TVB#1 and TVB#2 were successfully selected 7 days post-transfection using G418, and T7E1 analysis showed that the transfected cells had indel mutations in targeted loci (Figure 2B). The mutations were analyzed using the TA cloning method, and the mutation efficiencies of the two targeted loci were 70 and 45.5% in DF-1 cells transfected with TVB#1 and TVB#2, respectively (Figure 2C). The patterns of mutations were diverse in both experimental groups. In DF-1 cells transfected with TVB#1, we identified both deletions and insertions. In DF-1 cells transfected with TVB#2, only deletions mutations were identified (Figure 2C).

### Establishment of single DF-1 clones and genomic DNA analysis

To establish single *tvb*-mutated DF-1 clones, we picked single cells from DF-1 cells transfected with TVB#1 and TVB#2, respectively. The picked single cells became attached and actively proliferated (Additional file 1: A). We established several different clones from both TVB#1- and TVB#2- transfected DF-1 cells. Unfortunately, we obtained only clones with a 1 bp insertion before the ATG sequence from DF-1 cells transfected with TVB#1 (Additional file 2); therefore, we evaluated only the clones from DF-1 cells transfected with TVB#2. For 3–4 weeks, a total of 21 clones from DF-1 cells transfected with TVB#2 were established (Additional file 1: B), and the clones were then sequenced. Sequencing of the PCR products revealed a single clear peak in all samples, indicating that all DF-1 clones had diverse bi-allelic mutation patterns (Table 2; Additional file 3). Specifically, clone #17 had a 44 bp insertion in targeted loci, and clones #13, #16 and #28 had 15, 12 and 15 bp deletions, respectively, which could

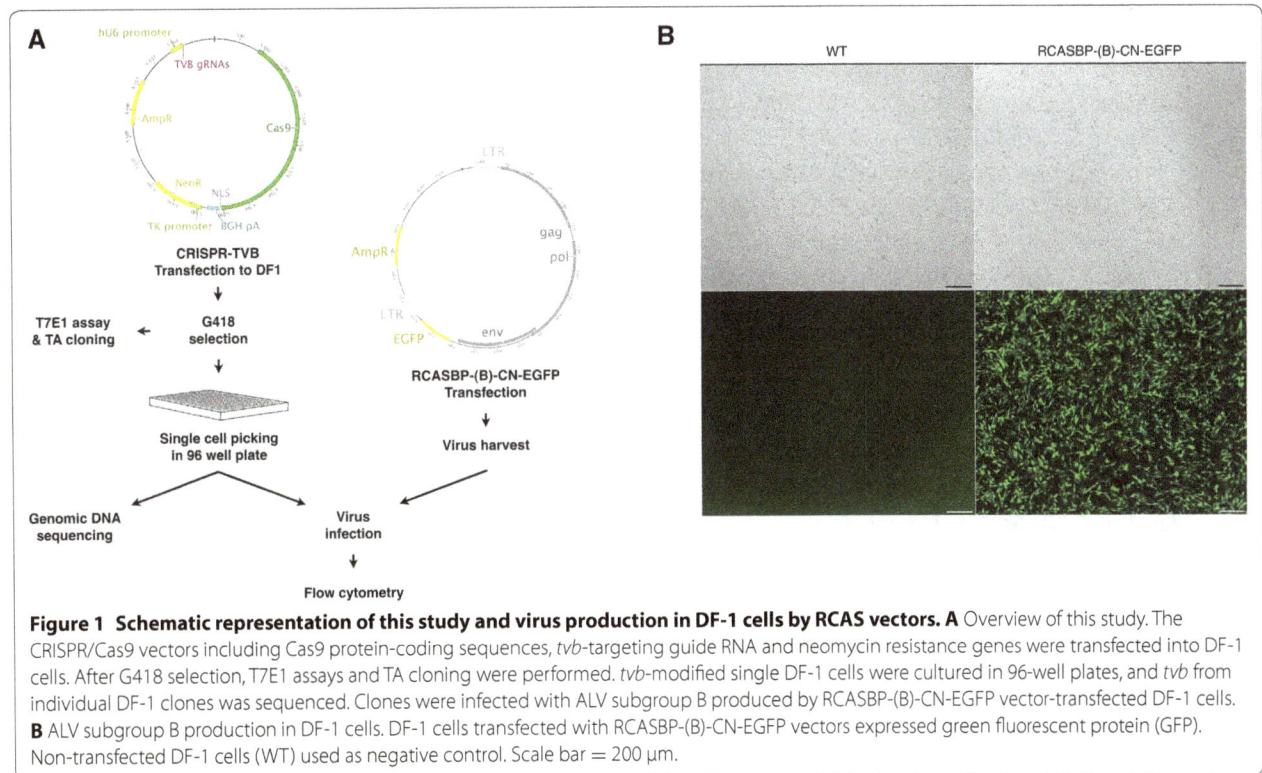

**Figure 1  Schematic representation of this study and virus production in DF-1 cells by RCAS vectors. A** Overview of this study. The CRISPR/Cas9 vectors including Cas9 protein-coding sequences, *tvb*-targeting guide RNA and neomycin resistance genes were transfected into DF-1 cells. After G418 selection, T7E1 assays and TA cloning were performed. *tvb*-modified single DF-1 cells were cultured in 96-well plates, and *tvb* from individual DF-1 clones was sequenced. Clones were infected with ALV subgroup B produced by RCASBP-(B)-CN-EGFP vector-transfected DF-1 cells. **B** ALV subgroup B production in DF-1 cells. DF-1 cells transfected with RCASBP-(B)-CN-EGFP vectors expressed green fluorescent protein (GFP). Non-transfected DF-1 cells (WT) used as negative control. Scale bar = 200 μm.

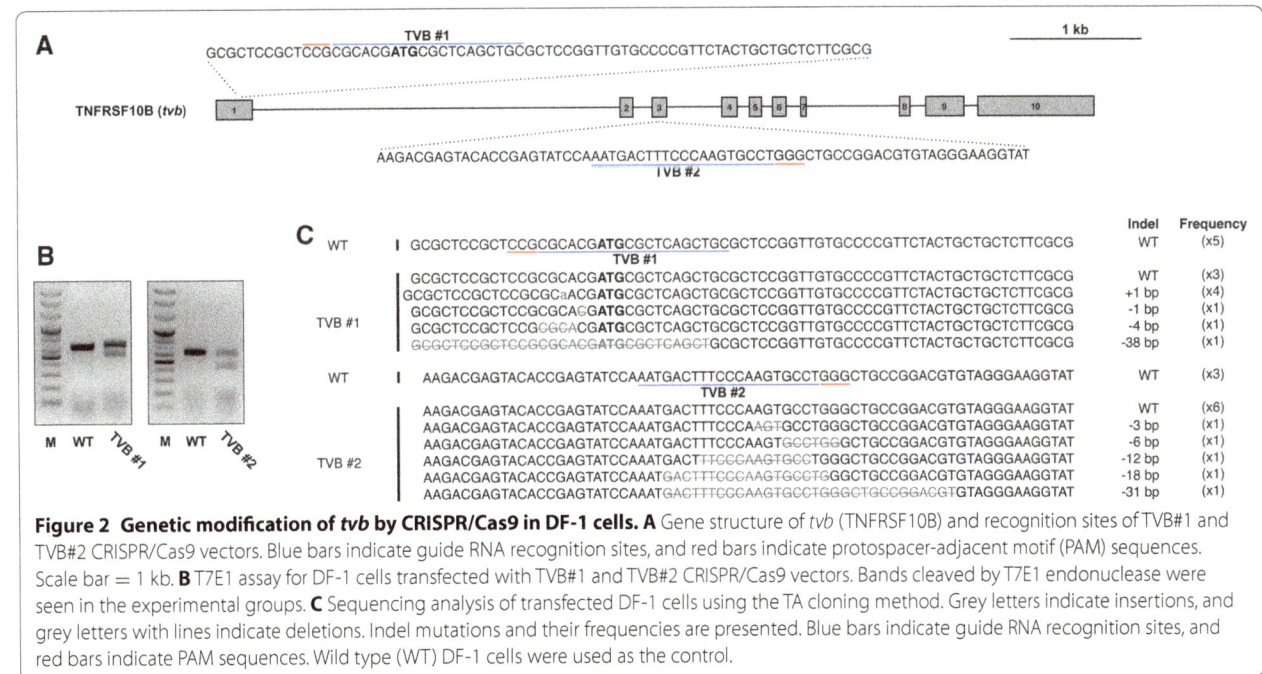

**Figure 2  Genetic modification of *tvb* by CRISPR/Cas9 in DF-1 cells. A** Gene structure of *tvb* (TNFRSF10B) and recognition sites of TVB#1 and TVB#2 CRISPR/Cas9 vectors. Blue bars indicate guide RNA recognition sites, and red bars indicate protospacer-adjacent motif (PAM) sequences. Scale bar = 1 kb. **B** T7E1 assay for DF-1 cells transfected with TVB#1 and TVB#2 CRISPR/Cas9 vectors. Bands cleaved by T7E1 endonuclease were seen in the experimental groups. **C** Sequencing analysis of transfected DF-1 cells using the TA cloning method. Grey letters indicate insertions, and grey letters with lines indicate deletions. Indel mutations and their frequencies are presented. Blue bars indicate guide RNA recognition sites, and red bars indicate PAM sequences. Wild type (WT) DF-1 cells were used as the control.

not induce frame shift mutations. Other clones (#2, #10, #14, #18, #19, #21, #23, #25 and #27) had deletions in targeted loci that caused frame shift mutations (Table 2).

**ALV subgroup B infection in single DF-1 clones and flow cytometry**

To verify the susceptibility of DF-1 clones to ALV subgroup B infection, clones from DF-1 cells transfected with

**Table 2 Sequencing results of *tvb*-modified DF-1 clones**

| ID | Sequence | Indel |
|---|---|---|
| WT | 5′-CAGTGCCTCCCAAGTAAGAAAGACGAGTACACCGAGTATCCA <u>AATGACTTTCCCAAGTGCCTGGG</u>CTGCCGGACGTGTAGGGAAGGTAT-3′ | WT |
| #1 | 5′-CAGTGCCTCCCAAGTAAGAAAGACGAGTACACCGAGTATCCA <u>AATGACTTTCCCAAGTGCCTGGG</u>CTGCCGGACGTGTAGGGAAGGTAT-3′ | WT |
| #2 | 5′-CAGTGCCTCCCAAGTAAGAAAGACGAGTACACCGAGTATCCA <u>AATGAC~~TTTCCCAAGTG~~CCTGGG</u>CTGCCGGACGTGTAGGGAAGGTAT-3′ | −11 bp |
| #3 | 5′-CAGTGCCTCCCAAGTAAGAAAGACGAGTACACCGAGTATCCA <u>AATGACTTTCCCAAGTGCCTGGG</u>CTGCCGGACGTGTAGGGAAGGTAT-3′ | WT |
| #7 | 5′-CAGTGCCTCCCAAGTAAGAAAGACGAGTACACCGAGTATCCA <u>AATGACTTTCCCAAGTGCCTGGG</u>CTGCCGGACGTGTAGGGAAGGTAT-3′ | WT |
| #9 | 5′-CAGTGCCTCCCAAGTAAGAAAGACGAGTACACCGAGTATCCA <u>AATGACTTTCCCAAGTGCCTGGG</u>CTGCCGGACGTGTAGGGAAGGTAT-3′ | WT |
| #10 | 5′-CAGTGCCTCCCAAGTAAGAAAGACGAGTACACCGAGTATCCA <u>AATGACTTTC~~CCAAGTGC~~CTGGG</u>CTGCCGGACGTGTAGGGAAGGTAT-3′ | −8 bp |
| #11 | 5′-CAGTGCCTCCCAAGTAAGAAAGACGAGTACACCGAGTATCCA <u>AATGACTTTCCCAAGTGCCTGGG</u>CTGCCGGACGTGTAGGGAAGGTAT-3′ | WT |
| #12 | 5′-CAGTGCCTCCCAAGTAAGAAAGACGAGTACACCGAGTATCCA <u>AATGACTTTCCCAAGTGCCTGGG</u>CTGCCGGACGTGTAGGGAAGGTAT-3′ | WT |
| #13 | 5′-CAGTGCCTCCCAAGTAAGAAAGACGAGTACACCGAGTATCCA <u>AATGACTTTCCCAAGTG~~CCTGGGCTGCCGGAC~~</u>GTGTAGGGAAGGTAT-3′ | −15 bp |
| #14 | 5′-CAGTGCCTCCCAAGTAAGAAAGACGAGTACACCGAGTATCCA <u>AATGACTTT~~CCCAAGTGC~~CTGGG</u>CTGCCGGACGTGTAGGGAAGGTAT-3′ | −8 bp |
| #16 | 5′-CAGTGCCTCCCAAGTAAGAAAGACGAGTACACCGAGTATCCA <u>AATGA~~CTTTCCCAAGTGC~~CTGGG</u>CTGCCGGACGTGTAGGGAAGGTAT-3′ | −12 bp |
| #17 | 5′-CAGTGCCTCCCAAGTAAGAAAGACGAGTACACCGAGTATCCA <u>AATGACTTTCCCAAGTG</u>agctgagcaaggacacctacgacgacga<u>CCTGG</u>acaacct <u>G</u>CTGgc<u>CCG</u>gatcggc<u>GACGTGTAGGGAAGGTAT</u>-3′ | +44 bp |
| #18 | 5′-CAGTGCCTCCCAAGTAAGAAAGACGAGTACACCGAGTATCCA <u>AATGACTTT~~CCCAAGTGC~~CTGGG</u>CTGCCGGACGTGTAGGGAAGGTAT-3′ | −8 bp |
| #19 | 5′-CAGTGCCTCCCAAGTAAGAAAGACGAGTACACCGAGTATCCA <u>AAT~~GACTTTCCCAAGTGCCTGGGCTGCCG~~</u>GACGTGTAGGGAAGGTAT-3′ | −26 bp |
| #20 | 5′-CAGTGCCTCCCAAGTAAGAAAGACGAGTACACCGAGTATCCA <u>AATGACTTTCCCAAGTGCCTGGG</u>CTGCCGGACGTGTAGGGAAGGTAT-3′ | WT |
| #21 | 5′-CAGTGCCTCCCAAGTAAGAAAGACGAGTACACCGAGTATCCA <u>AATGACTTTC~~CCAAGTG~~CCTGGG</u>CTGCCGGACGTGTAGGGAAGGTAT-3′ | −7 bp |
| #23 | 5′-CAGTGCCTCCCAAGTAAGAAAGACGAGTACACCGAGTATCCA <u>AATGACTTTC~~CCAAGTGC~~CTGGG</u>CTGCCGGACGTGTAGGGAAGGTAT-3′ | −7 bp |
| #24 | 5′-CAGTGCCTCCCAAGTAAGAAAGACGAGTACACCGAGTATCCA <u>AATGACTTTCCCAAGTGCCTGGG</u>CTGCCGGACGTGTAGGGAAGGTAT-3′ | WT |
| #25 | 5′-CAGTGCCTCCCAAGTAAGAAAGACGAGTACACCGAGTATCCA <u>AATGACTTTC~~CCAAGTGC~~CTGGG</u>CTGCCGGACGTGTAGGGAAGGTAT-3′ | −7 bp |
| #27 | 5′-CAGTGCCTCCCAAGTAAGAAAGACGAGTACACCGAGTATCCA <u>AATGACTTTCC~~CAAGTGCCTGGGCTGCC~~GGAC</u>GTGTAGGGAAGGTAT-3′ | −17 bp |
| #28 | 5′-CAGTGCCTCCCAAGTAAGAAAGACGAGTACACCGAGTATCCA <u>AATGACTTTCCCAAGTG~~CCTGGGCTGCCGGAC~~</u>GTGTAGGGAAGGTAT-3′ | −15 bp |

Underlining indicates the TVB#2 guide RNA recognition site and protospacer-adjacent motif (PAM) sequences

Strikethrough lines indicate deleted nucleotides and lowercase letters indicate inserted nucleotides

TVB#2 were infected with ALV subgroup B. Strong GFP expression was detected in nine different clones (#1, #3, #7, #9, #11, #12, #16, #20 and #24) compared with WT DF-1 cells at 4 days post-infection. We also found markedly lower levels of GFP expression in clones #2, #10, #14, #17, #18, #19, #21, #23, #25 and #27 and moderate levels of GFP expression in clones #13 and #28 (Figure 3A). The results of flow cytometric analysis showed that the proportions of GFP-expressing cells in DF-1 clones #1, #3, #7, #9, #11, #12, #16, #20 and #24 were 82.6, 93.8, 96.1,

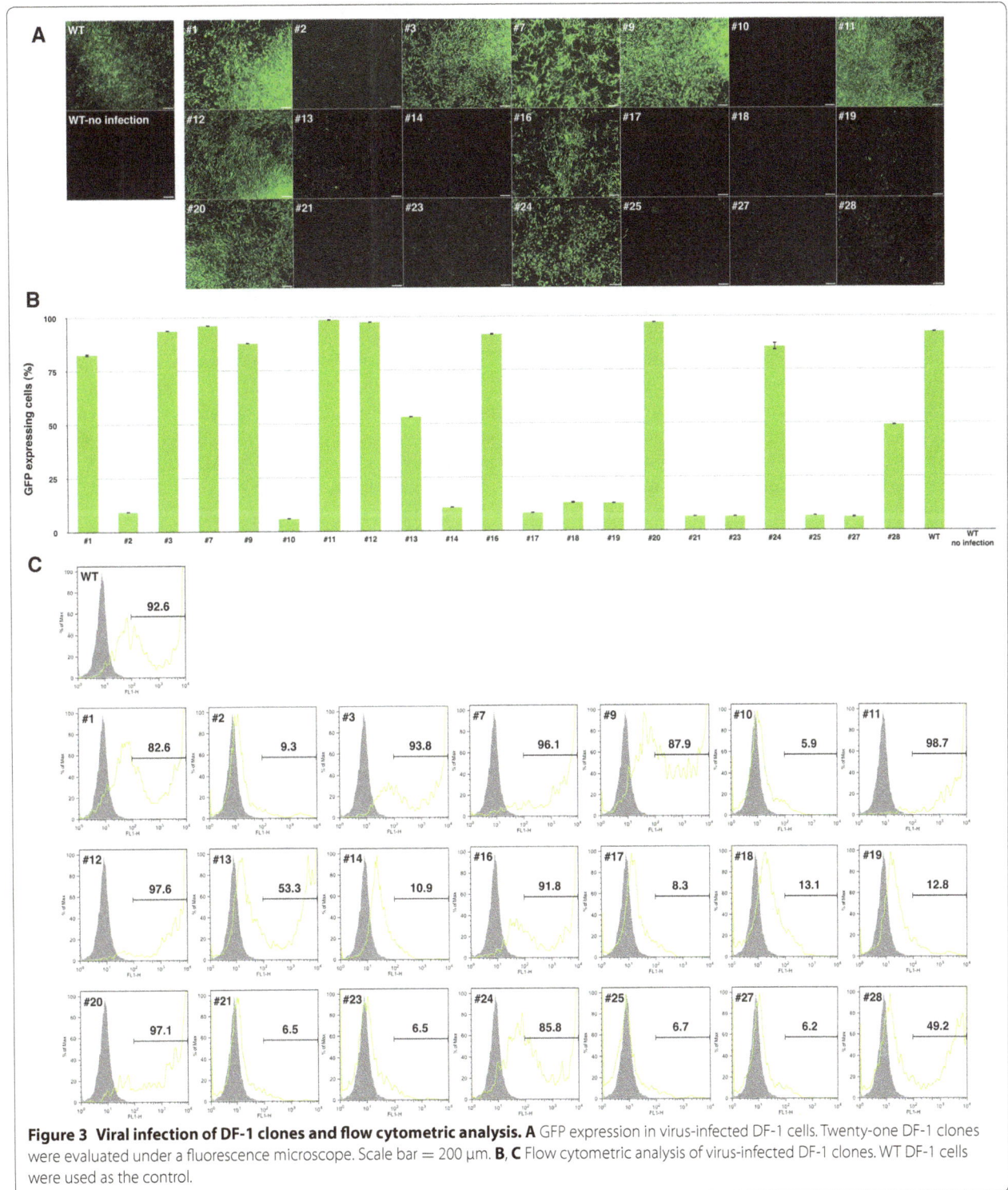

**Figure 3  Viral infection of DF-1 clones and flow cytometric analysis. A** GFP expression in virus-infected DF-1 cells. Twenty-one DF-1 clones were evaluated under a fluorescence microscope. Scale bar = 200 μm. **B**, **C** Flow cytometric analysis of virus-infected DF-1 clones. WT DF-1 cells were used as the control.

87.9, 98.7, 97.6, 91.8, 97.1 and 85.8%, respectively. The proportions of GFP-expressing cells in clones #2, #10, #14, #17, #18, #19, #21, #23, #25 and #27, which exhibited low levels of GFP expression, were 9.3, 5.9, 10.9, 8.3, 13.1, 12.8, 6.5, 6.5, 6.7 and 6.2%, respectively. The proportions of GFP-expressing cells in clones #13 and #28, which exhibited moderate levels of GFP expression, were 53.3 and 49.2%, respectively (Figures 3B and C).

### Amino acid sequence analysis

To identify the reason for the significantly reduced ALV group B susceptibility in *tvb*-mutated DF-1 clones, we analyzed their amino acid sequences. First, we compared the sequence of tumor necrosis factor receptor superfamily member 10B (TNFRSF10B) among humans, mice, frogs and chickens (TVB$^{S1}$ and TVB$^{S3}$). Sequence alignment analysis revealed highly conserved amino acid sequences in CRDs located in the extracellular receptor domain and cytoplasmic death domain (DD), which mediates the apoptosis signaling pathway. In particular, we located highly conserved cysteine residues in CRDs that formed bisulfide bonds (Figure 4A).

Next, we deduced the amino acid sequences of *tvb*-mutated DF-1 clones. Amino acid sequence analysis showed that clones #10, #14 and #18 shared the same amino acid sequences, as did clones #21, #23 and #25. Clones had mutations that generated an in-frame stop codon resulting in the production of a truncated protein similar to that of the WT *tvb$^r$*. Clones #13 and #28,

which expressed moderate levels of GFP, possessed the same mutations, including five amino acid deletions and one amino acid substitution from the 77th to 82nd amino acid positions of the TVB receptor. Clone #16, which expressed high levels of GFP, had four amino acids deletions from the 76th to 79th amino acid positions of the TVB receptor (Figure 4B). The mutations of nucleotides and deduced amino acids, and results of virus challenge in *tvb*-modified DF-1 clones were summarized in Table 3.

### Discussion

The acquisition of complete disease resistance is the ultimate goal of the agricultural industry and human society. However, despite the development of vaccines and improvements in quarantine facilities, complete disease control is elusive owing to economic costs and the rapid evolution of viruses. To overcome these limitations, targeted DNA modification using CRISPR/Cas9 technology has been used against a variety of viruses [22–27]. This system specifically targets and modifies the structure of viral genomes or host viral receptor genes and may therefore be used for efficient viral disease prevention without off-target events [28]. Therefore, in the present study, we used the CRISPR/Cas9-mediated genome editing method to confer resistance to ALV subgroup B in DF-1 chicken fibroblasts.

To evaluate the feasibility of CRISPR/Cas9-mediated genome editing for engineering resistance to ALV subgroup B, we first designed two CRISPR/Cas9 vectors

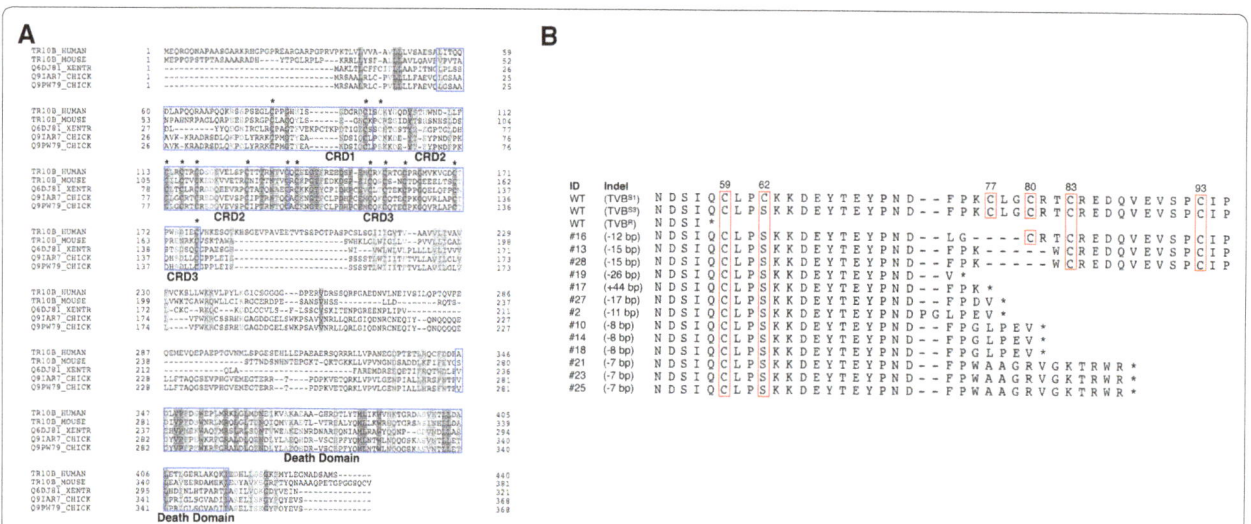

**Figure 4 Analysis of deduced amino acid sequences of *tvb*-modified DF-1 clones. A** Sequence alignment of human DR5 TRAIL receptor (NP_003833.4), mouse Tnfrsf10b (NP_064671.2), western clawed frog tnfrsf10b (NP_001004894.1) and chicken TVB$^{S1}$ (NP_989446.2). Blue boxes indicate cysteine-rich domains (CRDs) and death domains (DDs); shaded boxes indicated similarities among amino acid sequences. Asterisks indicate conserved cysteine residues. **B** Sequence alignment of deduced amino acids in *tvb*-modified DF-1 clones. Red boxes indicate conserved cysteine residues, and numbers indicate the order of the amino acids in TVB proteins. Asterisks indicate stop codons. WT with *tvb$^{s1}$*, *tvb$^{s3}$* and *tvb$^r$* genotypes were used as the control.

**Table 3 Mutations of nucleotides and deduced amino acids, and results of virus challenge in *tvb*-modified DF-1 clones**

| ID | Indel | Amino acid mutation | GFP expression (%) |
|----|-------|---------------------|---------------------|
| WT | WT | No mutation | Strong (92.6) |
| #16 | −12 bp | 4 amino acid deletion (76th to 79th positions) | Strong (91.8) |
| #13 | −15 bp | 5 amino acid deletion (77th to 80th positions) | Moderate (53.3) |
| #28 | −15 bp | 5 amino acid deletion (77th to 80th positions) | Moderate (49.2) |
| #19 | −26 bp | Premature stop codon | Low (12.8) |
| #17 | +44 bp | Premature stop codon | Low (8.3) |
| #27 | −17 bp | Premature stop codon | Low (6.2) |
| #2 | −11 bp | Premature stop codon | Low (9.3) |
| #10 | −8 bp | Premature stop codon | Low (5.9) |
| #14 | −8 bp | Premature stop codon | Low (10.9) |
| #18 | −8 bp | Premature stop codon | Low (13.1) |
| #21 | −7 bp | Premature stop codon | Low (6.5) |
| #23 | −7 bp | Premature stop codon | Low (6.5) |
| #25 | −7 bp | Premature stop codon | Low (6.7) |

specifically targeting two *tvb* loci for genetic mutations (Figure 2A). Chickens that have a naturally occurring single bp mutation in *tvb* are reported to be resistant to infection by ALV subgroups B, D and E, and this is thought to be because of the creation of a premature stop codon in the CRD1 domain [7]. To artificially generate a premature stop codon in *tvb* in DF-1 cells, we targeted the 3' region of the CRD1 coding region. We also targeted the *tvb* start codon to achieve total disruption of *tvb* receptor protein production. We found that targeted loci were successfully modified to possess indel mutations, and most mutations occurred in regions neighboring protospacer-adjacent motif sequences, which is consistent with previous research (Figure 2C) [17].

Next, we cultured DF-1 clones harboring *tvb* mutations to obtain clones with homozygous genotypes (Additional file 1). To avoid misinterpretation due to mixed genotypes during the virus challenge experiment, we verified DF-1 genotypes by sequencing analysis of PCR products. In total, 21 single DF-1 clones from TVB#2-transfected DF-1 cells were established. Of these, 12 had indel mutations in *tvb*, of which 11 were deletions, and only 1 was an insertion (Table 2). As previous research has reported, our results showed that the deletions were mostly CRISPR/Cas9-mediated mutations [29]. Sequencing analysis showed that all DF-1 clones had bi-allelic mutations, which was also consistent with previous research (Additional files 2 and 3) [30, 31]. However, using TVB#1 we were able to obtain only DF-1 clones that had 1 bp insertions in the 5' region (see Additional file 2). The sequencing results for

TVA#1-transfected DF-1 cells suggested that more clones were required for analysis or that precise genome editing mediated by homologous recombination was required to obtain clones with mutations in ATG sequences.

To evaluate the viral susceptibility of established single DF-1 cells, the cells were infected with ALV subgroup B produced by replication-competent ALV long terminal repeat (LTR) using a splice acceptor (RCAS) vector. The RCAS vector used in the present study is replication-competent in avian cells, and the vector spreads rapidly and infects most cells in vitro within a short period of time [32]. Exploiting these characteristics, we successfully produced ALV subgroup B in DF-1 cells (Figure 1B). In the virus challenge experiments, single DF-1 clones with mutations (#2, #10, #13, #14, #17, #18, #19, #21, #22, #23, #25, #27 and #28) had significantly lower levels of GFP expression compared with WT DF-1 cells. This suggests that genetic modification of *tvb* affected ALV subgroup B susceptibility in DF-1 cells. However, in this paper, we could not get the absolute resistant against to ALV subgroup B. 5.9% (#10) was the least expression of GFP among the clones (Figure 3C). The results may come from different between genotype of chicken that has *tvb^r* and those of *tvb*-modified DF-1 clones. Analysis of deduced amino acid shows *tvb*-modified DF-1 clones have still 59th cysteine residue that is important in ALV subgroup B entry [7]. Precise modification of the DF-1 *tvb* gene to *tvb^r* genotypes may cause absolute resistant to the virus. Furthermore, the results can come from difference between in vivo and in vitro system. Previous report revealed that the chickens that have resistant to ALV subgroup A do not have any proliferation of sarcomas even after 42 dpi even 40% of their CEF express GFP at 7 dpi by ALV subgroup A infection [6]. The results suggest that there is difference between in vivo and in vitro validation. To identify resistance to ALV subgroup B, genome-edited chicken needs to be produced and validated comparing with the chickens that have *tvb^r* genotype.

Analysis of deduced amino acid sequences revealed that genetic modifications of *tvb* generated a premature stop codon in the CRD2 domain (Figure 4B). This suggested that the artificially generated stop codon plays a crucial role in ALV subgroup B entry into host cells, similar to virus-resistant WL CEFs [7]. Resistance to human immunodeficiency virus (HIV) infection is also associated with mutations in a host receptor, CCR5. Individuals who have a 32 bp deletion that creates a premature stop codon in the CCR5 receptor are resistant to HIV [33, 34]. Therefore, our results support the notion that amino acid substitutions, particularly those that generate premature stop codons in host receptors, can abolish the functions of these receptors in viral interactions.

Interestingly, DF-1 clone #16 contained 91.8% GFP-expressing cells, although *tvb* gene contained a 12 bp deletion. This suggests that the deletion of four amino acids from the 76th to 79th positions of the TVB receptor does not significantly alter viral susceptibility. Comparing this clone with clones #13 and #28, which possessed a 15 bp deletion, suggested that cysteine 80 and arginine 81 within the TVB receptor play an important role in ALV subgroup B entry into host cells. Indeed, cysteine residues in CRDs are crucial for viral entry in several organisms. For example, the attachment of herpes simplex virus (HSV), equine infectious anemia virus (EIAV), feline immunodeficiency virus (FIV) and rabies virus (RABV) to host cells is mediated by the CRDs of their specific TNF receptors (herpes virus entry mediator [TANFRSF14] for HSV and EIAV, Ox40 [CD134, TNFRSF4] for FIV and NTRp75 for RABV). Cysteine residues in these CRDs are highly conserved, and mutations in these residues cause conformational changes in the extracellular regions of the receptors, altering their affinity to ligands [35]. In avian species, a cysteine-to-tryptophan substitution in the low-density lipoprotein receptor-like region of TVA drastically reduces the binding affinity of ALV subgroup A; similarly, a cysteine-to-serine mutation at position 62 in the TVB$^{S3}$ receptor reduces susceptibility to ALV subgroup E [4, 36]. Collectively, the results of the present study and previous research suggest the importance of bisulfide bonds in CRDs mediated by cysteine residues. However, studies investigating the precise replacement of cysteine 80 by homologous recombination are required to provide further support for our hypothesis.

## Conclusion

In the present study, we demonstrated the feasibility of CRISPR/Cas9-mediated genome modification for engineering resistance to ALV subgroup B. We efficiently modified DF-1 chicken fibroblasts using the CRISPR/Cas9 system and confirmed that modified DF-1 cells acquired resistance to ALV subgroup B. These results indicate that generating premature stop codons in the CRDs of TVB receptors can alter viral susceptibility, and that cysteine residues forming bisulfide bonds in CRDs may play important roles in determining susceptibility to ALV subgroup B. Furthermore, our results show that the CRISPR/Cas9 system can be used to efficiently modify the avian genome and establish novel avian cell lines, including virus-resistant chicken cell lines, mediated by primordial germ cells with germline competency. Furthermore, we expect that this system will facilitate the study of virus-host interactions not only in avian species but also in humans, for example, HIV and its relationship with the human CCR5 co-receptor [33, 34].

## Additional files

**Additional file 1. Establishment of *tvb*-modified DF-1 clones.** (A) DF-1 cell morphology during *in vitro* culture. Scale bar = 50 μm. (B) Establishment of 21 individual DF-1 clones. Wild type (WT) DF-1 cells were used as the control. Scale bar = 200 μm.
**Additional file 2. Sequencing results of TVB#1-transfected DF-1 clones with chromatography.** Wild type (WT) DF-1 cells with *tvb*$^{s3}$ genotypes were used as the control. The red arrow indicates the guide RNA recognition site, and red rectangles indicate insertions in *tvb*.
**Additional file 3. Sequencing results of TVB#2-transfected DF-1 clones using chromatography.** Wild type (WT) DF-1 cells with *tvb*$^{s3}$ genotypes were used as the control. The red arrow indicates the guide RNA recognition site, and orange rectangles indicate specific single nucleotide polymorphisms in *tvb*.

## Abbreviations

CRDs: cysteine rich domains; ALV: avian leukosis virus; *tvb*: tumor virus locus B; *tva*: tumor virus locus A; *tvc*: tumor virus locus C; W38: tryptophan 38; CRISPR/Cas9: clustered regularly interspaced short palindromic repeats (CRISPR)/CRISPR-associated; DMEM: Dulbecco's minimum essential medium; FBS: fetal bovine serum; ABAM: antibiotic–antimycotic; WL: White Leghorn; CEF: chicken embryonic fibroblast; EDTA: ethylenediaminetetraacetic acid; dpi: days post-infection; SAS: the statistical analysis system; ANOVA: analysis of variance; WT: wild type; GFP: green fluorescent protein; TNFRSF10B: tumor necrosis factor receptor superfamily member 10B; DD: death domain; PAM: protospacer adjacent motif; LTR: long terminal repeat; RCAS: replication-competent ALV LTR with a splice acceptor; HIV: human immunodeficiency virus; EIAV: equine infectious anemia virus; FIV: feline immunodeficiency virus; RABS: rabies virus; HVEM: herpes virus entry mediator; LDLR: low-density lipoprotein receptor; PGC: primordial germ cell; gRNA: guide RNA.

## Competing interests

The authors declare that they have no competing interests.

## Authors' contributions

HJY participated in study design and coordination. LHJ participated in the design of the study, carried out the experiments, and wrote the first draft of the manuscript. LKY carried out the experiments. PYH and CHJ were involved in statistical analysis and data interpretation. YY and NV were involved in data interpretation and in writing the final versions of the manuscript. All authors read and approved the final manuscript.

## Acknowledgements

Not applicable.

## Author details

  Department of Agricultural Biotechnology, College of Agriculture and Life Sciences, and Research Institute of Agriculture and Life Sciences, Seoul National University, Seoul 08826, South Korea. 2 The Pirbright Institute, Woking, Pirbright, Surrey GU24 0NF, UK. 3 Institute for Biomedical Sciences, Shinshu University, Minamiminowa, Nagano 399-4598, Japan.

## Funding

This work was supported by a National Research Foundation of Korea (NRF) grant funded by the Korea government (MSIP) (No. 2015R1A3A2033826). Authors also acknowledge the funding support from the Royal Society International Professorships.

# References

1. Justice J 4th, Beemon KL (2013) Avian retroviral replication. Curr Opin Virol 3:664–669

2. Payne LN, Howes K, Gillespie AM, Smith LM (1992) Host range of *Rous sarcoma* virus pseudotype RSV(HPRS-103) in 12 avian species: support for a new avian retrovirus envelope subgroup, designated J. J General Virol 73:2995–2997

3. Payne LN, Nair V (2012) The long view: 40 years of avian leukosis research. Avian Pathol 41:11–19

4. Elleder D, Melder DC, Trejbalova K, Svoboda J, Federspiel MJ (2004) Two different molecular defects in the Tva receptor gene explain the resistance of two tvar lines of chickens to infection by subgroup A avian sarcoma and leukosis viruses. J Virol 78:13489–13500

5. Chen W, Liu Y, Li H, Chang S, Shu D, Zhang H, Chen F, Xie Q (2015) Intronic deletions of tva receptor gene decrease the susceptibility to infection by avian sarcoma and leukosis virus subgroup A. Sci Rep 5:9900

6. Reinišová M, Plachý J, Trejbalová K, Šenigl F, Kučerová D, Geryk J, Svoboda J, Hejnar J (2012) Intronic deletions that disrupt mRNA splicing of the tva receptor gene result in decreased susceptibility to infection by avian sarcoma and leukosis virus subgroup A. J Virol 86:2021–2030

7. Klucking S, Adkins HB, Young JA (2002) Resistance to infection by subgroups B, D, and E avian sarcoma and leukosis viruses is explained by a premature stop codon within a resistance allele of the tvb receptor gene. J Virol 76:7918–7921

8. Reinisová M, Senigl F, Yin X, Plachy J, Geryk J, Elleder D, Svoboda J, Federspiel MJ, Hejnar J (2008) A single-amino-acid substitution in the TvbS1 receptor results in decreased susceptibility to infection by avian sarcoma and leukosis virus subgroups B and D and resistance to infection by subgroup E in vitro and in vivo. J Virol 82:2097–2105

9. Elleder D, Stepanets V, Melder DC, Senigl F, Geryk J, Pajer P, Plachy J, Hejnar J, Svoboda J, Federspiel MJ (2005) The receptor for the subgroup C avian sarcoma and leukosis viruses, Tvc, is related to mammalian butyrophilins, members of the immunoglobulin superfamily. J Virol 79:10408–10419

10. Chai N, Bates P (2006) Na+/H+ exchanger type 1 is a receptor for pathogenic subgroup J avian leukosis virus. Proc Natl Acad Sci U S A 103:5531–5536

11. Kucerová D, Plachy J, Reinisová M, Senigl F, Trejbalová K, Geryk J, Hejnar J (2013) Nonconserved tryptophan 38 of the cell surface receptor for subgroup J avian leukosis virus discriminates sensitive from resistant avian species. J Virol 87:8399–8407

12. Jinek M, Chylinski K, Fonfara I, Hauer M, Doudna JA, Charpentier E (2012) A programmable dual-RNA—guided DNA endonuclease in adaptive bacterial immunity. Science 337:816–821

13. Hwang WY, Fu Y, Reyon D, Maeder ML, Tsai SQ, Sander JD, Peterson RT, Yeh JR, Joung JK (2013) Efficient genome editing in zebrafish using a CRISPR-Cas system. Nat Biotechnol 31:227–229

14. Tan W, Carlson DF, Lancto CA, Garbe JR, Webster DA, Hackett PB, Fahrenkrug SC (2013) Efficient nonmeiotic allele introgression in livestock using custom endonucleases. Proc Natl Acad Sci U S A 110:16526–16531

15. Wang H, Yang H, Shivalila CS, Dawlaty MM, Cheng AW, Zhang F, Jaenisch R (2013) One-step generation of mice carrying mutations in multiple genes by CRISPR/Cas-mediated genome engineering. Cell 153:910–918

16. Gao Y, Wu H, Wang Y, Liu X, Chen L, Li Q, Cui C, Liu X, Zhang J, Zhang Y (2017) Single Cas9 nickase induced generation of NRAMP1 knockin cattle with reduced off-target effects. Genome Biol 18:13

17. Oishi I, Yoshii K, Miyahara D, Kagami H, Tagami T (2016) Targeted mutagenesis in chicken using CRISPR/Cas9 system. Sci Rep 6:23980

18. Dimitrov L, Pedersen D, Ching KH, Yi H, Collarini EJ, Izquierdo S, van de Lavoir MC, Leighton PA (2016) Germline gene editing in chickens by efficient CRISPR-mediated homologous recombination in primordial germ cells. PLoS One 11:e0154303

19. Sakuma T, Nishikawa A, Kume S, Chayama K, Yamamoto T (2014) Multiplex genome engineering in human cells using all-in-one CRISPR/Cas9 vector system. Sci Rep 4:5400

20. Lee HJ, Lee HC, Kim YM, Hwang YS, Park YH, Park TS, Han JY (2016) Site-specific recombination in the chicken genome using Flipase recombinase–mediated cassette exchange. FASEB J 30:555–563

21. Park TS, Lee HJ, Kim KH, Kim JS, Han JY (2014) Targeted gene knockout in chickens mediated by TALENs. Proc Natl Acad Sci U S A 111:12716–12721

22. Ali Z, Abulfaraj A, Idris A, Ali S, Tashkandi M, Mahfouz MM (2015) CRISPR/Cas9-mediated viral interference in plants. Genome Biol 16:238

23. Hu W, Kaminski R, Yang F, Zhang Y, Cosentino L, Li F, Luo B, Alvarez-Carbonell D, Garcia-Mesa Y, Karn J, Mo X, Khalili K (2014) RNA-directed gene editing specifically eradicates latent and prevents new HIV-1 infection. Proc Natl Acad Sci U S A 111:11461–11466

24. Price AA, Sampson TR, Ratner HK, Grakoui A, Weiss DS (2015) Cas9-mediated targeting of viral RNA in eukaryotic cells. Proc Natl Acad Sci U S A 112:6164–6169

25. Suenaga T, Kohyama M, Hirayasu K, Arase H (2014) Engineering large viral DNA genomes using the CRISPR-Cas9 system. Microbiol Immunol 58:513–522

26. Zhen S, Hua L, Liu YH, Gao LC, Fu J, Wan DY, Dong LH, Song HF, Gao X (2015) Harnessing the clustered regularly interspaced short palindromic repeat (CRISPR)/CRISPR-associated Cas9 system to disrupt the hepatitis B virus. Gene Ther 22:404–412

27. Burkard C, Lillico SG, Reid E, Jackson B, Mileham AJ, Ait-Ali T, Whitelaw CB, Archibald AL (2017) Precision engineering for PRRSV resistance in pigs: macrophages from genome edited pigs lacking CD163 SRCR5 domain are fully resistant to both PRRSV genotypes while maintaining biological function. PLoS Pathog 13:e1006206

28. Khalili K, White MK, Jacobson JM (2017) Novel AIDS therapies based on gene editing. Cell Mol Life Sci 74:2439–2450

29. Varshney GK, Pei W, LaFave MC, Idol J, Xu L, Gallardo V, Carrington B, Bishop K, Jones M, Li M, Harper U, Huang SC, Prakash A, Chen W, Sood R, Ledin J, Burgess SM (2015) High-throughput gene targeting and phenotyping in zebrafish using CRISPR/Cas9. Genome Res 25:1030–1042

30. Jao LE, Wente SR, Chen W (2013) Efficient multiplex biallelic zebrafish genome editing using a CRISPR nuclease system. Proc Natl Acad Sci U S A 110:13904–13909

31. Wang X, Zhou J, Cao C, Huang J, Hai T, Wang Y, Zheng Q, Zhang H, Qin G, Miao X, Wang H, Cao S, Zhou Q, Zhao J (2015) Efficient CRISPR/Cas9-mediated biallelic gene disruption and site-specific knockin after rapid selection of highly active sgRNAs in pigs. Sci Rep 5:13348

32. Hughes SH (2004) The RCAS vector system. Folia Biol 50:107–119

33. Liu R, Paxton WA, Choe S, Ceradini D, Martin SR, Horuk R, MacDonald ME, Stuhlmann H, Koup RA, Landau NR (1996) Homozygous defect in HIV-1 coreceptor accounts for resistance of some multiply-exposed individuals to HIV-1 infection. Cell 86:367–377

34. Samson M, Libert F, Doranz BJ, Rucker J, Liesnard C, Farber CM, Saragosti S, Lapoumeroulie C, Cognaux J, Forceille C, Muyldermans G, Verhofstede C, Burtonboy G, Georges M, Imai T, Rana S, Yi Y, Smyth RJ, Collman RG, Doms RW, Vassart G, Parmentier M (1996) Resistance to HIV-1 infection in caucasian individuals bearing mutant alleles of the CCR-5 chemokine receptor gene. Nature 382:722–725

35. Kinkade A, Ware CF (2006) The DARC conspiracy—virus invasion tactics. Trends Immunol 27:362–367

36. Adkins HB, Blacklow SC, Young JA (2001) Two functionally distinct forms of a retroviral receptor explain the nonreciprocal receptor interference among subgroups B, D, and E avian leukosis viruses. J Virol 75:3520–3526

# 6

# Protecting effect of PrP codons M142 and K222 in goats orally challenged with bovine spongiform encephalopathy prions

C. Fast[1†], W. Goldmann[2†], P. Berthon[3†], K. Tauscher[1†], O. Andréoletti[4], I. Lantier[3], C. Rossignol[3], A. Bossers[5], J. G. Jacobs[5], N. Hunter[2], M. H. Groschup[1], F. Lantier[3] and J. P. M. Langeveld[5*]

## Abstract

Breeding towards genetic resistance to prion disease is effective in eliminating scrapie. In sheep, classical forms of scrapie have been eradicated almost completely in several countries by breeding programs using a prion protein (PrP) gene (*PRNP*) amino acid polymorphism. For goats, field and experimental studies have provided evidence for several amino acid polymorphisms that are associated with resistance to scrapie, but only limited data are available concerning the susceptibility of caprine *PRNP* genotypes to BSE. In this study, goat kids representing five *PRNP* genotypes based on three polymorphisms (M142, Q211 and K222 and the wild type I142, R211 and Q222) were orally challenged with bovine or goat BSE. Wild type goats were killed with clinical signs between 24–28 months post inoculation (mpi) to both challenges, and goats with genotype R/Q211 succumbed between 29–36 mpi. I/M142 goats developed clinical signs at 44–45 mpi and M/M142 goats remained healthy until euthanasia at 48 mpi. None of the Q/K222 goats showed definite clinical signs. Taken together the highest attack ratios were seen in wild type and R/Q211 goats, and the lowest in I/M142, M/M142 and Q/K222. In all genotype groups, one or more goats remained healthy within the incubation period in both challenges and without detectable PrP deposition in the tissues. Our data show that both the K222 and M142 polymorphisms lengthen the incubation period significantly compared to wild type animals, but only K222 was associated with a significant increase in resistance to BSE infection after oral exposure to both BSE sources.

## Introduction

Prion diseases or transmissible spongiform encephalopathies (TSEs) are caused by a unique infectious agent ("prion") characterised by an entirely proteinaceous nature with apparent absence of functional nucleic acids [1, 2]. Disease transmission is possible within and between mammalian host species. Pivotal for transmissibility is the host's prion protein (PrP) that in its normal state is a cell membrane protein (PrP$^C$) to which recently several potential functions have been ascribed either in receptor mediation or immunological quiescence [3, 4].

In prion diseases PrP$^C$ is converted into a stable "pathological" conformer (PrP$^{Sc}$), which is the diagnostic disease marker detectable in immunohistochemistry by its disease associated deposition patterns (PrP$^D$) and biochemically by its aggregation properties and protease resistance of its C-terminal core region (PrP$^{res}$) [5–7].

The emergence of bovine spongiform encephalopathy (BSE) in cattle and its subsequent transmission to humans as variant Creutzfeld–Jakob disease (vCJD) has proven that prion diseases represent a threat for man and other mammalian species [8, 9]. Goats represent the only other domestic ruminant species to be affected by BSE under field conditions [10–12]. Furthermore, goats are susceptible to classical scrapie although the disease occurs in Europe generally at 2–3 times lower prevalence than in sheep [13]. Susceptibility to TSE infection in sheep and goats has a strong genetic component that

*Correspondence: jan.langeveld@wur.nl
†C. Fast, W. Goldmann, P. Berthon and K. Tauscher contributed equally to the study
5 Wageningen BioVeterinary Research, Wageningen University & Research, Houtribweg 39, 8221RA Lelystad, The Netherlands
Full list of author information is available at the end of the article

potentially allows selection by breeding for resistance. The basis for this selection is the polymorphic character of the PrP amino acid sequence, because some of these PrP variants do not convert easily to PrP$^{Sc}$ [14]. Breeding towards resistance has been successfully accomplished for sheep in some EU countries using the Q171R amino acid polymorphism as selection target, helped by the fact that the R171 allele appears to be dominant with almost complete protection to natural scrapie in R/R171 homozygotes as well as in Q/R171 heterozygotes [13, 15, 16].

A review of genotype surveys conducted worldwide revealed that on average almost 40% of goat *PRNP* sequences showed some variation of the amino acid sequence compared to the wild type [17, 18]. Case control studies have narrowed the potential candidates for resistance-associated polymorphisms to six amino acid changes: M142, S146, D146, H154, Q211 and K222 (wild type I142, N146, R154, R211 and Q222) [19–25]. It should be noted that wild type and variant *PRNP* alleles vary in codon 240 either encoding S240 or P240. While the wild type allele appears to split on average equally between S240 and P240 sequences, some of the variant alleles have so far only been observed in one combination, for example K222-S240. Association of codon 240 with TSE resistance is most likely weak or absent [19–21, 26]. The occurrence and frequencies of these *PRNP* alleles are breed and region dependent [27–29]. The strong genetic resistance to classical scrapie conferred by the K222 allele was corroborated by studies in goats using intracerebral and oral scrapie challenges with isolates from Italy, the USA or France [30–32].

We have previously published an interim report on a study of an oral challenge in goats with caprine BSE [33]. Here we report the final and full results of this study in which caprine and bovine BSE isolates were inoculated orally into goats of five different genotypes which were homozygous wild type (wt/wt) and M/M142 or heterozygous I/M142, R/Q211 and Q/K222. The data provide convincing evidence that the K222 allele is the strongest protective factor in goats against BSE.

## Materials and methods

### Animals

Three different laboratories were involved in the challenges to exploit the available space: INRA Nouzilly, France (lab1), The Roslin Institute, UK (lab2) and FLI, Germany (lab3). Animal experimentation was performed according to European directive 2010/63/EU as well as in compliance with the respective national legislations in these countries (reference number for Germany LALLF

7221.3-2.5-001/05, Animal & Scientific Procedures Act 1986, UK). At INRA (France), all experiments were conducted in accordance with the guidelines of the European Council Directive (86/609) and approved by the local ethical committee; the animals were kept in Biosafety Level 3 confined housing (PFIE, UE-1277, INRA Centre Val de Loire, Nouzilly, France). Goat kids of different breeds were obtained after weaning from the following sources: for lab1 and lab3 through Francis Barillet (goat production at INRA Centre Val-de-Loire in Bourges Experimental Unit, INRA division of Animal Genetics) and for lab2 through acquisition from UK holdings and through artificial insemination of females from the Roslin Institute. The animals belonged to the following breeds: Alpine, Saanen, Boer, Toggenburg and their crosses. Animals had been bred and selected based on their *PRNP* genotype, they were either I/M142, M/M142, R/Q211, Q/K222 or homozygous wild type for any of these codons (wt/wt). In total 129 animals were used in this study (Table 1).

### Challenge and disease monitoring

Bovine and goat BSE brain materials were derived from clinically and PrP$^{Sc}$—positive confirmed cases. The cattle BSE homogenate for first passage was derived from a pool of two clinically affected UK BSE cases supplied by the VLA (now APHA, Weybridge, UK) (Table 1). The goat BSE homogenate for second passage was pooled brain material derived from three clinically and PrP$^{Sc}$ positive animals of wt/wt genotype following intracerebral challenge with cattle BSE [34]. Animals were orally challenged twice with 1 g of bovine BSE in 10 mL physiological saline solution with a 2 weeks interval (lab1, lab2) or only once with 1 g of goat BSE in 5 mL saline due to the lower amount of goat brain material available (lab2, lab3). During the incubation period, blood samples (lab1–3) as well as tonsil (lab1–3) and rectal (lab3) biopsies were taken on a regular scheme (Additional file 1). One to three animals per genotype were euthanized at first at pre-defined time points during the observation period. In addition goats were killed after showing consistently clinical signs typical for BSE (i.e. neurological disorders such as abnormalities in sensation and movement) or due to animal welfare reasons other than BSE. The last goats were killed due to animal welfare reasons other than BSE at 81 mpi. Seven unchallenged wt/wt goats (lab1 two, lab2 three, and lab3 two) and one unchallenged R/Q211 (lab3) shared the pens with challenged animals between 13 and 47 months of the inoculation period to control for horizontal transmission. At necropsy a wide range of tissue samples were harvested under TSE-sterile conditions.

**Table 1  Experimental setup in the different labs performing the goat oral challenge**

|  | lab1 | | lab2 | | lab3 |
|---|---|---|---|---|---|
| Experimental setup | 1st passage | | 2nd passage | | |
| Inoculum | Cattle BSE (UK) | | Goat BSE (gBSE-P12; wt/wt) | | |
| Inoculation | 2 × 1 g/goat, interval of 15 days | | 1 × 1 g/goat | | |
| Mode of inoculation | 10 mL/goat, (1:10 in glucose) | | | | 5 mL/goat, (1:5 in saline) |
| Age at inoculation | 3–4 months | 6–9 months | 6–9 months | | 6–7 months |
| Goat breed | Alpine, Saanen | Saanen, Boer, Toggenburg | | | Alpine–Saanen |
| Number of goats and genotype | | | | | |
| Total | 38 | 27 | 24 | | 40 |
| wt/wt | 12 | 12 | 11 | | 15 |
| I/M142 | | 10 | 11 | | |
| M/M142 | | 4 | | | |
| R/Q211 | 12 | | | | 11 |
| Q/K222 | 12 | | | | 11 |
| Controls | 2 (wt/wt) | 1 (wt/wt) | 2 (wt/wt) | | 3 (2 wt/wt, 1 R/Q211) |

BSE, bovine spongiform encephalopathy; UK, United Kingdom; gBSE-P12, identification number of goat brain pooled homogenate; wt/wt, homozygous wild type; I/M142, heterozygous isoleucine/methionine genotype at codon 142; M/M142, homozygous methionine genotype at codon 142; R/Q211, heterozygous arginine/glutamine genotype at codon 211; Q/K222, heterozygous glutamine/lysine genotype at codon 222.

## Antibody sources

PrP specific antibodies used and their sources were: Bar224, Sha31 and SAF84 [35], 6C2 and 12B2 [36, 37], R145 [38], F99/97.6.1 [39], P4 and L42 [40], and 6H4 [41]. R145 and F99/97.6.1 were epitope mapped by Pepscan analysis to the respective ovPrP sequences 223RESQ226 and 221YQRE224 following published methods [42].

## Histology and immunohistochemistry

The formalin fixed tissue samples were hematoxylin and eosin (H&E) stained and immunohistochemically (IHC) processed with well established procedures using PrP specific antibodies [38, 43, 44]. Methodological details are summarized in Additional file 1.

## Biochemical analysis for scrapie-BSE discrimination and in-depth TSE typing

Brain stem samples of all animals were further examined by Western blot for discrimination between classical scrapie and BSE (Additional file 1) as described

before [44–47]. Furthermore for in-depth TSE typing, triplex Western blot (triplex-WB) analyses were carried out as described before, using a mix of three antibodies, 12B2, Sha31 and either SAF84 or F99 after first immuno-complexing these respectively with Zenon labels Alexa 647, 555, and 488 [48]. These antibodies are markers: (1) for presence of the N-terminal epitope (12B2) typical for classical scrapie but absent in classical BSE, and CH1641 scrapie, (2) the core region of PrP$^{res}$ (Sha31), and (3) the presence of a second PrP$^{res}$ population covering the C-terminal PrP region between the Sha31 epitope (sequence 148YEDRYYRE155, ovine numbering) and the C-terminus of mature PrP which is only recognized by antibodies like SAF84 and F99 (respective epitope sequences 166YRPVDQY171 and 221YQRE224) and which fragment is characteristic for CH1641 scrapie and H-type BSE. For comparison, reference samples used were: C-type, H-type and L-type BSE from cattle, and small ruminant BSE, classical scrapie, and CH1641 scrapie (sheep and/or goat) were used as in previous publications [31, 49].

## Mouse bioassay

In lab1 and lab3 mouse bioassays were performed at 6 and 12 mpi with different tissues taken from respectively cattle BSE and goat BSE infected goats to test for the eventual presence of infectivity in the early stage of disease incubation. In doing so transgenic mice overexpressing ovine (in lab1 Tg338 and in lab3 TgshpIX) and bovine PrP (in lab 1 Tg110) were used. All mouse lines are known to be highly sensitive for the detection of prion infectivity of different origin including BSE (Tg110 in [33], the Tg338 and Tgshp IX in preparation by Nonno et al.). Additionally end-point titration experiments with a goat BSE isolate were done using Tg110 [33] and TgshpIX mice (lab 3, unpublished results), but data are not included here. The mice were intracerebrally inoculated (6–15 mice per sample, depending of the different lab schedules routinely done in France and Germany) with 20–30 µL of a 10% tissue homogenate diluted in physiological saline [45, 50, 51]. Subsequently all mice were clinically checked at least twice a week and either sacrificed due to animal welfare reasons or after 730 dpi at the latest. The mouse brains were subsequently tested for the presence of proteinase K resistant PrP$^{Sc}$ (PrP$^{res}$) by Western blot [44].

## Statistical analysis

Differences in incubation period lengths were analysed for statistical significance with Student's T test and significance for differences in distribution between healthy and disease animals by challenge and genotype groups were analysed with Fisher's Exact Test for a 2 × 2 Contingency Table with two-tailed probability (p).

## Results

Goat challenge results were classified in four health stage categories: (a) clinical—when consistent neurological signs pointing to a BSE infection were observed, (b) late preclinical—when no obvious clinical signs were observed but the animal appeared post mortem positive by IHC in the central nervous system (CNS), (c) early preclinical—when animals showed positivity by IHC in peripheral tissues but not yet in the CNS, and (d) healthy—without any of these markers. The occurrence of these categories in the time line after challenge of individual goats with their genotypes can be viewed in Additional file 2. Additionally, the time points mentioned below refer to the date of necropsy and subsequent prove of BSE infection by the detection of PrP$^D$ in the brain stem. However, it has to be born in mind that some of these goats displayed the first clinical signs up to 6–12 weeks before necropsy.

### Goat challenges: first passage (bovine BSE)

Sixty-two animals were challenged with bovine BSE in lab1 and lab2. The goats were in five *PRNP* genotype groups: wt/wt (n = 24), I/M142 (n = 10), M/M142 (n = 4), R/Q211 (n = 12) and Q/K222 (n = 12). Three unchallenged wild type animals were kept as contact controls (Table 1). In total 22 animals were affected by BSE, while 40 goats and the controls remained completely negative with observation periods up to 48 months post-inoculation (mpi) (Figure 1).

Clinical signs appeared in ten goats: five wt/wt goats at 25/26 mpi, three R/Q211 animals between 28–33 mpi

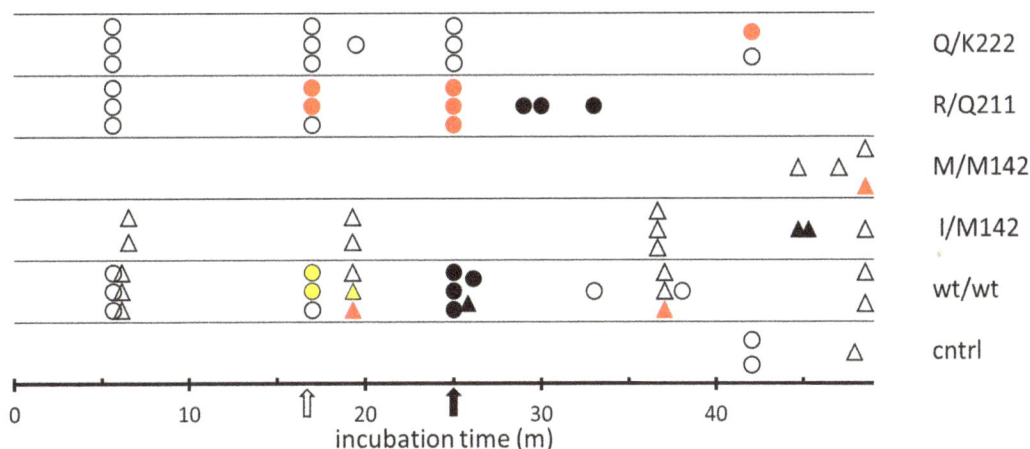

**Figure 1 Overview of the results of challenge with bovine BSE (1$^{st}$ passage) in goats with five different genotypes.** Each symbol represents an individual goat. Symbol colours: empty, yellow, red and black represents TSE negative, preclinical PrP$^D$ (positivity in peripheral sites), late preclinical (PrP$^D$ positivity in CNS, no clear clinical signs) and clinical cases (these are also PrP$^D$ positive in periphery and CNS). Symbol shapes represent location of experiment: circles, lab 1, triangles lab 2 (see also "Materials and methods" section). The two arrows under the X-axis: open and bold indicate respectively the month after inoculation at which respectively the first preclinical and clinical cases were observed.

and even later at 44/45 mpi in two I/M142 goats. All clinically affected animals were PrP$^D$ positive by immunohistochemistry (IHC) in the central nervous system (CNS) and peripheral tissues in various combinations (see below).

A further nine animals were in a late preclinical state at necropsy and revealed PrP$^D$ in brain stem as shown by IHC and/or biochemical analysis, but none of these goats showed clearly identifiable clinical signs typical for BSE. This group included two wt/wt goats sacrificed at 19 and 36 mpi, five R/Q211 goats sacrificed at 17 (n = 2) and 25 (n = 3) mpi, one Q/K222 goat killed at 43 mpi and one M/M142 goat killed at 48 mpi.

Another three wt/wt goats were in an early preclinical state at 17 (n = 2) and 19 (n = 1), revealing weak amounts of PrP$^D$ in different peripheral tissues only (see below). Samples from CNS and spleen from nine (3 wt/wt, 3 R/Q211, 3 Q/K222) healthy, BSE negative goats, which were culled at 6 mpi as part of the pathogenesis study, were examined by mouse bioassay using transgenic mouse lines Tg110 and Tg338. None of these mice showed clinical or pathological signs of a TSE infection.

The 40 non-affected animals were euthanized at various time points with the longest survival times in the different genotypes as follows: 48 mpi for 2 wt/wt, one I/M142 and one M/M142, and 43 mpi for one Q/K222 goat.

Because some animals were removed from the challenge groups at pre-defined post-inoculation times, attack ratios for preclinical, late preclinical and clinical animals 12 mpi and later were only considered for estimation. These ratios were not less than 56% in wt/wt, 25% in I/M142 goats, 25% in M/M142, 89% in R/Q211, and 11% in Q/K222 goats (Table 2). These values decreased for four genotypes when only clinical positive animals were included: 28% in wt/wt, 0% in M/M142, 33% in R/Q211 and 0% in Q/K222 goats.

**Table 2  Data concerning the effectiveness of the oral challenges in goats with bovine (1$^{st}$ passage) and caprine (2$^{nd}$ passage) BSE**

| Genotype | Numbers | | | Numbers from 12 mpi | | | | Inc. time clinical, mpi ±SD (n) |
|---|---|---|---|---|---|---|---|---|
| | Total | Before 12 mpi | After 12 mpi | Pre-clinical | Late preclinical | Clinical | Attack ratios affected/ total (%) + significance[a] | |
| bovBSE | | | | | | | | |
| wt | 24 | 6 | 18 | 3 | 2 | 5 | 10/18 (56%) | 25.2 ± 0.4 (5) |
| I/M142 | 10 | 2 | 8 | 0 | 0 | 2 | 2/8 (25%)** | 44.5 ± 0.7 (2) |
| M/M142 | 4 | 0 | 4 | 0 | 1 | 0 | 1/4 (25%) | NA |
| R/Q211 | 12 | 3 | 9 | 0 | 5 | 3 | 8/9 (89%) | 30.7 ± 2.1 (3) |
| Q/K222 | 12 | 3 | 9 | 0 | 1[b] | 0 | 1/9 (11%)** | NA |
| gtBSE | | | | | | | | |
| wt | 26 | 6 | 20 | 2 | 3 | 5 | 10/20 (50%) | 25.6 ± 1.5 (5) |
| I/M142 | 11 | 3 | 8 | 0 | 0 | 0 | 0/8 (0%)* | NA |
| R/Q211 | 11 | 4 | 7 | 1 | 0 | 3 | 4/7 (57%) | 34.3 ± 1.5 (3) |
| Q/K222 | 11 | 3 | 8 | 0 | 1[c] | 0 | 1/8 (13%)[c]* | NA |

| Genotype | Total | mpi | | Numbers from 12 mpi | | | | Inc. time clinical, mpi ±SD (n) |
|---|---|---|---|---|---|---|---|---|
| | | 1$^{st}$ clin case | Last clin case | Pre-clinical | Late preclinical | Clinical | Attack ratios affected/ total (%) + significance | |
| Combined challenges | | | | | | | | |
| wt | 50 | 24 | 28 | 5 | 5 | 10 | 20/38 (53%) | 25.4 ± 1.1 (10) |
| I/M142 | 21 | 44 | 45 | 0 | 0 | 2 | 2/16 (13%)** | 44.5 ± 0.7 (2) |
| M/M142 | 4 | NA | NA | NA | NA | NA | NA | NA |
| R/Q211 | 23 | 28 | 36 | 1 | 5 | 6 | 12/16 (75%) | 32.5 ± 2.6 (6) |
| Q/K222 | 23 | 43 | NA | 0 | 2 | 0 | 2/17 (12%)*** | NA |

NA, not applicable.

[a] Statistical data: compared to the wild type group. Fisher's exact test, *, **, and *** respectively $p < 0.05$, $p < 0.01$, $p < 0.001$.

[b] This Q/K222 goat was CNS- and muscle-positive.

[c] One Q/K222 case was CNS-positive, and psoas-muscle-positive but by mouse bioassay (Tg110) only [33]. If considered negative (by IHC) this group was statistically positive compared to the wild type group ($p < 0.05$).

## Goat challenges: second passage (goat BSE)

Fifty-nine goats were challenged with goat BSE in lab 2 and lab 3. They were in four *PRNP* genotype groups: wt/wt (n = 26), I/M142 (n = 11), R/Q211 (n = 11), and Q/K222 (n = 11) (Table 1). Four wildtype and one R/Q211 animals were kept as unchallenged contact controls. In total 15 animals were affected by a BSE infection, and 44 goats and the controls remained completely negative within the observation period up to 81 mpi (Figure 2).

Clinical signs appeared in eight goats: five wt/wt goats between 24 and 28 mpi, and three R/Q211 animals between 33–36 mpi. All clinically affected animals were PrP$^D$ positive by IHC in the CNS and in peripheral tissues in various combinations (for details see below).

Additional four animals were in a late preclinical state at necropsy revealing PrP$^D$ or infectivity in brain stem as shown by IHC. None of these goats showed clinical signs typical for BSE. This group included three wt/wt goats at 19, 24 and 36 mpi as well as one Q/K222 goat at 45 mpi (infectivity data from this goat are published in [33]).

Two wt/wt goats (12 and 25 mpi) and one R/Q211 goat (12 mpi) were in an early preclinical state, revealing weak amounts of PrP$^D$ in peripheral tissues only (for details see below). None of the I/M142 and Q/K222 goats showed clinical TSE signs.

Various samples from CNS (brain stem) and peripheral tissues (including samples from gut, lymphoreticular tissues as well as autonomous nervous system) from two healthy and BSE negative wt/wt goats, which were culled at 12 mpi as part of the pathogenesis study, were examined by mouse bioassay using transgenic mouse lines TgshpIX. None of these mice showed clinical or pathological signs of a TSE infection.

The 44 non-affected animals were euthanized at various time points with the longest survival times in the different genotypes as follows: 81 mpi for one wt/wt and one Q/K222 goat, 47 mpi for three I/M142 goats and 77 mpi for a R/Q211 goat.

Similar to the first passage BSE study, challenged animals 12 mpi and later were only considered for estimation of attack ratios. These attack ratios for preclinical, late preclinical and clinical animals together were not less than 50% in wt/wt, 0% in I/M142 goats, 57% in R/Q211, and 13% in Q/K222 goats (Table 2). Including only clinically positive animals reduced these values to 25% in wt/wt, 43% in R/Q211 and 0% in Q/K222 goats, while I/M142 goats remained unchanged.

## Statistical analysis

There was no statistically significant difference in the wild type challenge outcomes regarding the number of affected animals or the incubation period length of clinically affected goats between the two BSE isolates or between the three different laboratories. The small number of goats developing clinical disease made it difficult to analyse differences of incubation period length between genotypes.

Considering the period from 12 mpi, where the first preclinical signs appeared in the challenges (12mpi, in a wt and a R/Q211 goat), till the end of the experiments (see Figure 2) there were significant differences in attack ratios between wild type and QK222 groups in both challenges if only based on IHC observations (Table 2). The attack ratios values between wt and IM142 goats in goat BSE challenge were also statistically different (p < 0.05), but not after challenge with bovine BSE.

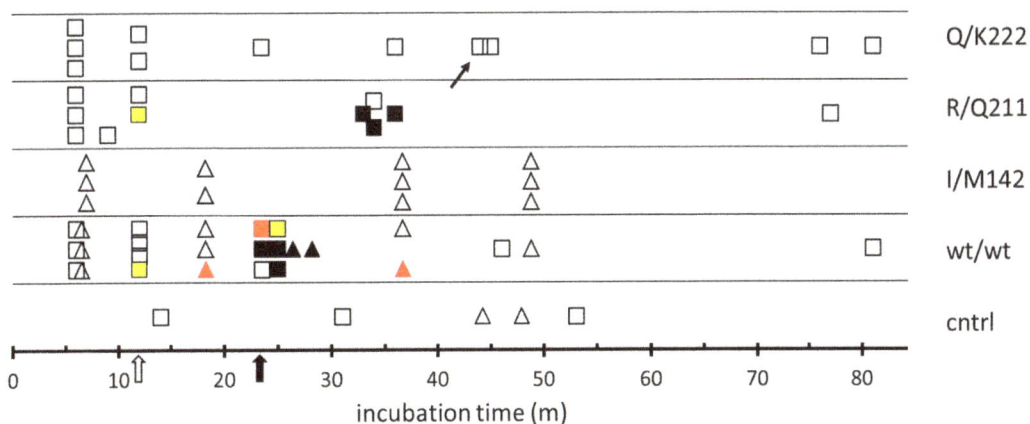

**Figure 2 Overview of the results of challenge with goat BSE (= 2$^{nd}$ passage) in goats with four different genotypes.** Each symbol represents an individual goat. Symbol colours and arrows are explained in Figure 1. Symbol shapes represent the laboratory of experiment: triangles lab 2, and squares lab 3. The two arrows under the X-axis: open and bold indicate respectively the month after inoculation at which respectively the first preclinical and clinical cases were observed. Small arrow near one Q/K222 symbol is reflecting the animal previously found weakly brain (only) positive in infectivity testing in Tg110 mice [33].

Furthermore, differences became also apparent when the observation period was divided into early (12–30 mpi) and late (> 30 mpi) phase and when both challenges were combined. In the early phase, infected animals were found only in wt/wt and R/Q211 goats at ratios of 18/25 (72%) and 7/11 (64%), respectively; no infected animals occurred in genotypes I/M142 (0/4) and Q/K222 (0/10). The difference between group I (wt/wt, R/Q211) and group II (I/M142, Q/K222) was highly significant ($p < 0.0001$).

The late phase showed no significant difference between group I and group II and all genotypes had infected animals. After 30 mpi, R/Q211 had a higher attack ratio of 5/7 (71%) than either wt/wt with 2/12 (17%) or I/M142 with 2/12 ($p = 0.03$), but the difference to Q/K222 (2/7) was not significant. While the minimal attack ratio for R/Q211 was unchanged between the two observation phases, wt/wt genotypes were significantly less likely to be infected ($p < 0.002$) once they had survived 30 mpi.

## Immunohistochemistry

There were no distinct differences between the animals from the first and the second passage, therefore the immunohistochemical results will be presented for all groups together (see Additional files 3 and 4 for further details in respectively first and second passage results).

In total 30 goats revealed a clear PrP$^D$ accumulation in the brain stem (CNS positive cases in Figure 3A). The degree of PrP$^D$ deposition was associated with the clinical state of the animal. Thus, goats being in a late preclinical state showed a weak (n = 1), mild (n = 5) and moderate (n = 4) PrP$^D$ accumulation; only one R/Q211 goat and one Q/K222 goat (Figure 3B) were severely affected. In contrast, animals with clear clinical signs mostly exhibited a severe PrP$^D$ deposition (n = 16) and more rarely a moderate accumulation (n = 2). In most cases PrP$^D$ accumulation was widespread and involved the whole brain stem, both grey and white matter. In animals with only mild PrP$^D$ accumulation, the most prominent depositions were seen in the dorsal motor nucleus of the vagus

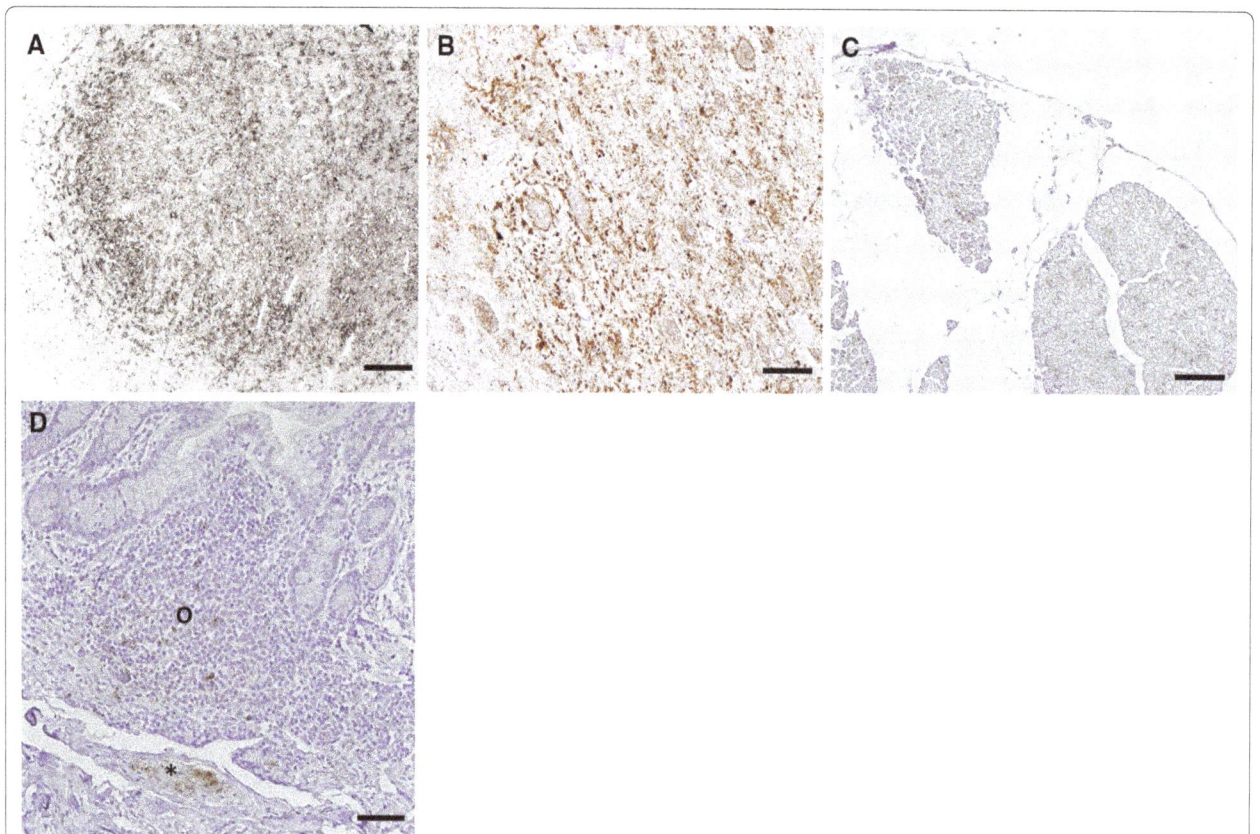

**Figure 3 PrP$^D$ accumulation in central and peripheral nervous tissues of BSE infected goats. A** Brain stem of a clinical goat BSE infected wt/wt goat, 24 mpi, showing a severe intra- and extracellular PrP$^D$ accumulation. Antibody 6C2, bar 50 μm. **B** Brain stem of the late preclinical cattle BSE infected Q/K222 goat, 43 mpi, showing a severe intra- and extracellular PrP$^D$ accumulation in the obex (DMNV). Antibody Bar224, bar 20 μm. **C** Spinal nerve of a clinical cattle BSE infected wt/wt goat, 25 mpi, showing moderate intra-axonal and intraglial PrP$^D$ accumulation. Antibody Bar224, bar 100 μm. **D** Ileum of a clinical cattle BSE infected wt/wt goat, 25 mpi, showing PrP$^D$ accumulation in neurons and glial cells of the enteric nervous system as well as intracellular in lymphoid cells of the ileal follicle. Antibody Bar224, bar 20 μm.

nerve (DMNV), the nucleus of the solitary tract, cuneate nucleus, hypoglossal nucleus, spinal tract nucleus and the olivary nuclei. Using antibodies specific for the PrP C-terminus which detect BSE associated $PrP^D$ very well [52], intraneuronal, intraglial and cell-membrane-associated/extracellular fine to coarse $PrP^D$ accumulations were seen in all brain areas examined.

Several peripheral lymphoreticular tissue samples were analysed for $PrP^D$ accumulation, amongst them were mesenterial lymph nodes (MesLn), tonsil, ileum including Peyer's patches (PP), rectal follicles (RAMALT), celiac and mesenteric ganglion complex (CMGC), ileal and rectal enteric nervous system (ENS), vagal nerve and brachial plexus, along with different skeletal muscles (Mm. oculomotorius, psoas major and semitendinosus) (Figure 4). The analysis of five wt/wt and one R/Q211 goat, which were negative in the brain

stem, revealed $PrP^D$ accumulations in the tonsil (n = 1), CMGC (n = 2) and ENS of the Ileum (n = 2) and in the ileal PP (n = 1).

The ileal ENS was the most frequently positive site (n = 8) in the twelve late preclinical goats, which had only mild to moderate amounts of $PrP^D$ in the brain stem. Only four animals showed a more widespread distribution of $PrP^D$ involving the rectal ENS (n = 1), MesLn (n = 2), ileal PP (n = 2) and tonsil (n = 2).

The positive Q/K222 goat (43 mpi) which was in a late preclinical state, showed a severe $PrP^D$ accumulation in the brain, but no involvement of the LRS (Figure 5). The only peripheral tissues slightly positive are rectal ENS and different muscles (M. oculomotorius, M. psoas major).

Clinically ill wt/wt and R/Q211 goats (n = 16) with moderate up to severe $PrP^D$ accumulation in the brain

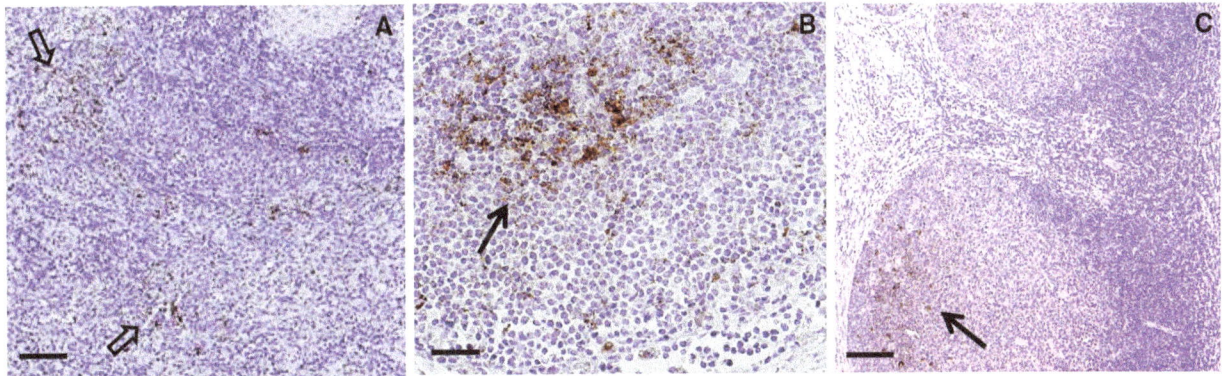

**Figure 4** **$PrP^D$ accumulation in lymphoreticular tissues of BSE infected goats. A** Spleen of a clinical cattle BSE infected wt/wt goat, 26 mpi. Antibody Bar224, bar 50 μm. **B** Mesenterial lymph node of a clinical cattle BSE infected R/Q211 goat, 30 mpi. Antibody bar 224, bar 20 μm. **C** Tonsil of a clinical cattle BSE infected I/M142 goat. Antibody R145, bar 50 μm. In all samples a mild to moderate $PrP^D$ accumulation in follicles and in the sinus of the spleen can be seen.

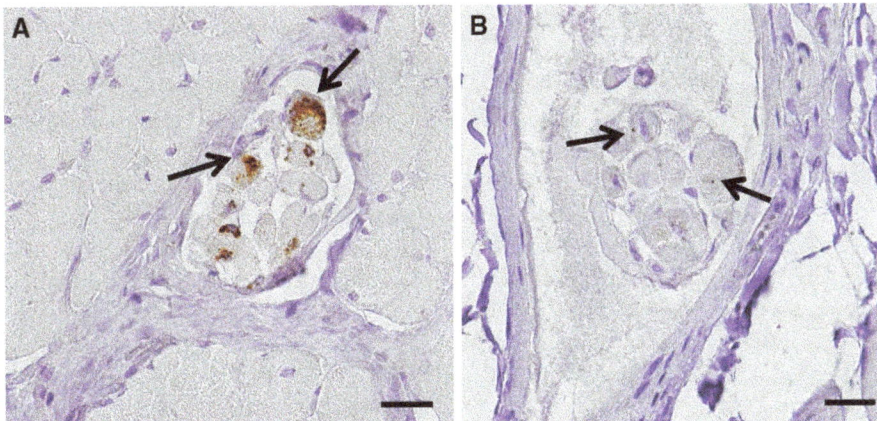

**Figure 5** **$PrP^D$ accumulation in different skeletal muscles. A** Ocular muscle of a Q/R211 goat infected with cattle BSE showing $PrP^D$ accumulation in muscle spindles, 28 mpi. Antibody Bar224, bar 20 μm. **B** Psoas muscle of a Q/K222 goat infected with cattle BSE showing weak $PrP^D$ accumulation in muscle spindles, 43 mpi. Antibody Bar224, bar 20 μm.

stem, revealed a more widespread distribution of $PrP^D$ in the LRS, ENS and different skeletal muscles with only five animals, in which $PrP^D$ accumulations were confined to the ENS and PP of the gut. Two animals even showed a positive reaction in peripheral nerves. More interestingly are the two I/M142 goats, both with severely affected brains. $PrP^D$ could be found in ileal ENS but not in the PP. Yet, one of these goats showed a mild $PrP^D$ deposition in tonsil follicles.

In tissues of the LRS the $PrP^D$ depositions were mostly confined to the follicles and rarely seen in the sinus. Reaction pattern seen is an intracellular fine to coarse granular staining in tingible body macrophages, follicular dendritic cells and few lymphocytes. Neuronal as well as glial cells were positive in the ENS (Figure 3), but in the CMGC only single neuronal cells showed a diffuse intracellular pattern. Single muscle spindles revealed a mild accumulation of $PrP^D$ (Figure 5).

### Discriminatory analysis and TSE typing

Positivity in brain stem of all goats was analysed in the three laboratories, each with their own methodology to discriminate C-type BSE from classical scrapie (data not shown). Furthermore, in samples from goats of all genotypes and both passage numbers the type of TSE was studied in more detail using as reference samples bovine C-type, H-type and L-type BSE, ovine and caprine BSE, classical scrapie, and CH1641 scrapie (Figure 6A). The low presence of 12B2 epitope (12B2/Sha31 signal ratio < 0.3), the glycoprofile expressed as the ratio between mono- and diglycosylated $PrP^{res}$ (< 0.4, using glycoform fractions of total $PrP^{res}$ in the Sha31 epitope detection) and the presence of only a single $PrP^{res}$ population pointed out that all positive samples did show the character of a C-type BSE infection (Figure 6B) [48, 49].

### Discussion

This oral challenge study in goats elucidates the significant protection conferred by the Q/K222 prion protein genotype against bovine and goat BSE infection administered through the oral route. There was no clear clinical case with this genotype in 17 challenged animals, although it has to be considered that both late-preclinical Q/K222 goat from the bovine and caprine BSE challenges might have developed clinical disease at some later stage. I/M142 heterozygous genotypes appeared to provide partial resistance, with two clinically positive cases. Including the M/M142 late-preclinical case, M142 is also clearly associated with lengthened incubation periods in BSE similar to scrapie challenges [31].

While the R/Q211 genotyped goats exhibited extended incubation periods of the clinical cases by about 5–9 months compared to the wild type goats in the two

BSE challenges, it appeared that there was also a difference in the susceptibility beyond 30 months post inoculation. In that late phase of the experiments, 2 out of 7 (29%) animals survived BSE challenge in the R/Q211 group only whereas in the wild type group 10 out of 12 (83%) animals showed no signs of BSE infection. Additional amino acid polymorphisms in *PRNP* can be excluded as reason for a survival difference between the two genotypes, therefore other genetic loci might be involved [53]. It is unlikely though to be solely due to breed or laboratory differences as discussed below.

This study has been conducted in three laboratories in parallel following similar protocols as much as possible, but with different breeds of different regional origins, and different age groups. Despite this set-up, which was logistically necessary to conduct a challenge study of 129 goat kids, significant differences were not observed between the laboratory groups as evidenced by a short mean incubation period and a narrow standard deviation ($25.4 \pm 1.1$, Table 2) for the ten clinical cases of the wild type groups. This finding is supported by the fact that the tissue distribution did not reveal any remarkable deviations between the different laboratories.

The goat kids used here were aged 3–9 months at challenge, depending on the lab involved. Previous findings in sheep and goats suggest that to achieve the highest attack rates in oral challenge, administration before weaning was important, possibly due to the developmental stage of the Peyer's patches in the intestine [34, 54–56]. Although the exact response to challenge for the early age range was not known for goat kids, challenge of the kids before weaning was planned but could not be implemented due to logistic problems in animal movements. Nevertheless, the mean attack rate of 53% for all wild type animals in this study was distinctly higher than the 21% reported before for BSE challenged lambs of the 3–6 month age range [54]. It might reflect a higher intrinsic susceptibility of goats for oral challenge than sheep, which may also explain that BSE has only been identified in this species in natural conditions [10–12]. Taken together the data do not imply large variation due to selection of various age groups and breeds, but we cannot completely rule out that the sensitivity in the challenges of the five genotypes was reduced through an age effect.

Considering the successful transmissions in the different genotypes, our data showed that clinical disease was appearing first in the wt/wt goats at 24–28 mpi with no differentiation between cattle BSE (first passage) and caprine BSE (second passage). This is rather surprising, as it has been shown previously that interspecies transmission of TSEs results in long incubation periods, which usually shorten on further passages [57]. In particular, this result seems to contradict previous observations

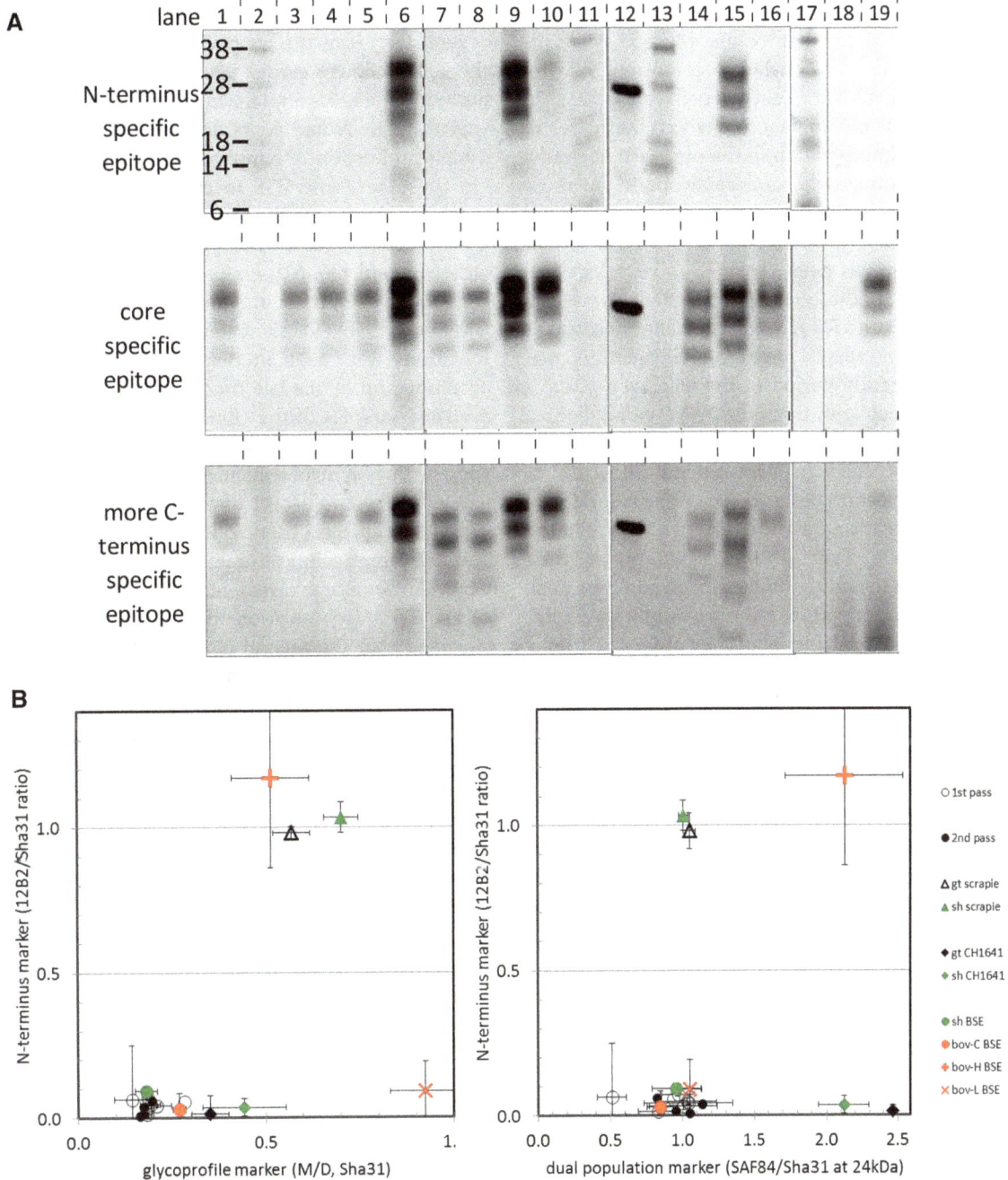

**Figure 6 Western blot: triplex Western blot analysis of goat BSE brain stem samples with three antibodies on one membrane.** Samples from orally challenged goats were analysed together with a set of different types of TSEs from goat, sheep and cattle to illustrate the classical BSE like character in the BSE-challenged goats. **A** Analysis with a mixture of three antibodies with different PrP specificities: N-terminus (12B2), core (Sha31) and C-terminus (SAF84, lanes 1–16; or F99, lanes 17–19). Lanes: 1, 3–5, 19 goat BSE material from respectively wt/wt 2nd pass, R/Q211 2nd pass, wt/wt 2nd pass, R/Q211 2nd pass, Q/K222 1st pass; lane 6, classical scrapie from i.c. challenged R/Q211 goat; lane 7, CH1641 scrapie from i.c. challenge in wt/wt sheep; lane 8 CH1641 scrapie from i.c. challenge in wt/wt goat; lane 9 natural scrapie from wt/wt sheep; lane 10 BSE from i.c. challenged wt sheep 1st pass; lanes 14–16 respectively bovine C-type BSE, H-type BSE and L type BSE; lane 18, non-challenged goat material. Applied tissue equivalents were 0.5 mg, or (in lanes 3, 4, 14–16 and 19) 1 mg. Lanes 2, 11, 13, and 17, mol mass markers are indicated with their kDa; in lane 12, 15 ng rec-ovine PrP (wt). For linear epitope specificities of the antibodies, see paragraph Biochemical analysis of the Methods section. **B** Dot plots showing the TSE-type markers of individual samples derived from the antibody signals of PrP$^{res}$ in triplex-WB. Each symbol represents the average signal ratio obtained from a triplicate analysis per individual sample (bars for the standard deviations). All orally challenged goats yield a typical C-BSE pattern for the markers N-terminus, glycoprofile and dual population independent of genotype and passage (1st or 2nd). The 12 analysed goat samples from the BSE challenges were: from 1st pass two wt/wt, two I/M142, three R/Q211, and one Q/K222 cases (open circles); from 2nd pass three wt/wt, and one R/Q211 cases (closed black circles).

in transgenic mice expressing bovine PrP (Tg110), in which sheep- or goat-passaged BSE would lead to shorter incubation times than bovine BSE [58, 59]. Differences between the two challenge conditions or titre of the challenge materials might have played a role. On the other hand, this phenomenon may well be the result of intracerebral administration in the mice, whereas BSE transmissibility through the oral route might be more dependent of host factors encountered in the LRS and ENS before entering the CNS [60]. However, a similar pattern of adaption has been observed in vitro by serial PMCA [60]. Overall, these results imply that passage of BSE through wt/wt and R/Q211 goats will not necessarily lead to a measurable adaptation of the BSE agent to goat. Overall, the incubation period of the wild type goats is very similar to sheep with the same *PRNP* genotype [54, 61–63].

The immunohistochemical data did not show differences between the genotypes or between the laboratories involved. More surprising are the results concerning the tissue distribution of PrP$^D$. This regards both the time course of the disease and the tissues involved. Even weak PrP$^D$ accumulations in peripheral tissue samples were not seen before 12 mpi and only in a single animal. Furthermore, late preclinical goats, which already have a mild to moderate accumulation of PrP$^D$ in the CNS, not only showed a minor involvement of peripheral tissue samples, but in most cases even a confinement of the PrP$^D$ accumulations to the Peyer's patches and enteric nervous system of the gut. Only a few animals revealed a mild PrP$^D$ positive staining reaction in other lymphoid tissues, i.e. tonsil and mesenteric lymph nodes. A more widespread distribution of PrP$^D$ in lymphoid tissues was only seen in a few clinical goats, late in the incubation period. This is in clear contrast to classical scrapie in sheep and goats as well as BSE in sheep [25, 44, 62, 64]. This unusual PrP$^D$ distribution pattern is reflected by examinations addressing the infectivity in peripheral tissue samples. As described by [33] and shown by results presented here none of the samples examined from goats early in the incubation period (6 and 12 mpi) revealed any signs of infectivity, neither in Tg110, Tg338 nor Tgshp IX. On the other hand similar to the results seen in immunohistochemistry a more widespread distribution of BSE infectivity was seen in different peripheral tissue samples of clinical goats among others the popliteal lymph node of goats with different genotype [33] and in the spleen of a wild type goat (lab 3, data not shown).

A French study showed that the time course of the scrapie pathogenesis is slightly prolonged in goats as compared to sheep [65]. However, the spread of the scrapie agent during the incubation time was quite similar [25, 44, 66]. This was also observed in BSE affected sheep

[61, 63]. PrP$^D$ accumulations are widespread with distinct PrP$^D$ depositions in follicles and neurons, involving several tissues of the lymphoreticular system as well as the autonomous nervous system early in the incubation period [25, 44, 61, 63, 66]. In other words TSE neuroinvasion in sheep and goats normally did not occur until a high proportion of lymphoid tissues was positive [66]. On the other hand BSE in cattle spreads almost solely along the autonomous nervous system, with Peyer's patches of the gut as the only lymphoid tissues regularly involved [36, 67]. Unfortunately, CMGC, as a representative sample for the autonomous nervous system, was not available for all goats. However, weak PrP$^D$ accumulations were seen in two preclinical goats, distinct accumulation in one late preclinical goat as well as in all available samples of the clinical goats (data not shown). Thus, the pathogenesis seen in our BSE infected goats, with no major involvement of the lymphoreticular system is more reminiscent of the disease in cattle. This is supported by the observation that one clinical I/M142 and two late preclinical (one Q/K222 and one M/M142) goats showed no involvement of the LRS at all, even with severe PrP$^D$ accumulation in the brain stem. It should be noted that the second clinical I/M142 goat revealed a slight staining reaction in rectal follicles and in tonsil. From this point, it remains a speculation what might be the reason behind this unusual distribution pattern in the LRS of BSE infections and, as described by others [66], some scrapie infected goats. There might be an inability of goat lymphoid tissues to accumulate certain PrP$^D$'s. On the other hand it is also conceivable that the low amounts of PrP$^D$ detectable in the LRS are due to better clearance abilities in those goats. The animal numbers here are too low to reach a conclusion on the extent to which this pattern is influenced by the genotype, but a similar pattern has been reported before [66].

The two I/M142 with clinical disease and the Q/K222 in the late preclinical state of infection showed incubation times at 44 mpi and 43 mpi, respectively. In the goat BSE challenges clinical signs were not recorded for any of the I/M142 and Q/K222 carriers, but a confirmation by IHC of PrP$^D$ in the CNS of an M/M142 goat at 48 mpi and by mouse bioassay of low level infectivity in the CNS of a Q/K222 goat at 45 mpi [33] (see arrow in Figure 2) was possible. Therefore, as shown previously for goat scrapie [24, 30, 31], not only the attack ratios but also the incubation periods of BSE in goats appeared influenced by these genotypes. Low attack rates leading to few infected animals and even fewer clinical cases with long incubation periods provides valuable data in support of a protective effect against BSE infection by the M142 and K222 variants. By necessity, our study was mostly conducted in heterozygous goats and both polymorphisms, M142 and

K222, showed a dominant phenotype as expected from goat scrapie studies and sheep TSE challenges [30, 31, 68]. Resistance to scrapie in the presence of either allele has been shown in many case–control studies and, due to the relative low genotype frequency of homozygotes, the association with resistance has been significant mostly for heterozygotes [15, 20, 32, 54]. The survival of the four M/M142 to 48 mpi without clinical disease suggests that homozygotes are at least as resistant to BSE as heterozygotes, which is also evident for scrapie [25]. Similar data for oral BSE exposure of K/K222 goats are still missing, but an attack ratio of 1/5 and an incubation period of 69 mpi for intracerebral inoculation with scrapie [31] combined with evidence that transgenic mice expressing only caprine K222 PrP were resistant to bovine BSE increases the likelihood that K/K222 goats will show significant resistance to BSE too [58]. Of course, this is crucial as breeding programs designed to increase the K222 allele frequency will inevitably lead to an increase in the number of homozygous K/K222 animals in goat populations. As a polymorphism that protects from scrapie and BSE, K222 is the strongest candidate for breeding programs for the eradication of TSEs from goats.

However, the K222 allele is not always available for TSE—resistance breeding, since it occurs in variable and often very low frequencies in the European goat population. It varies even within seemingly similar breeds depending on their geographical locations [17, 18, 27, 29]. Introduction of this variant into goat populations with an endemic scrapie problem may be worth considering. The use of alternative PrP polymorphisms associated with a protective effect at least for classical scrapie such as N146D and N146S may be possible for a restricted range of breeds [69, 70].

Our challenge data further strengthen the view that the caprine K222 allele is an attractive *PRNP* variant for TSE resistance breeding since it is not only strongly limiting the transmission of classical scrapie, but as is exemplified here it also has a protective effect against BSE infection.

## Additional files

Additional file 1. Summary of the immunohistochemical methods, bioassays and sampling applied in the different labs involved.

Additional file 2. Additional file tables A and B: overview of goats challenged with cattle BSE (first passage) and goatBSE (second passage).

Additional file 3. Summary of the immunohistochemical results obtained from the brain stem and different peripheral tissue samples from goats infected with Cattle BSE (first passage).

Additional file 4. Summary of the immunohistochemical results obtained from the brain stem and different peripheral tissue samples from goats infected with goat BSE (second passage).

**Competing interests**
The authors declare that they have no competing interests.

**Authors' contributions**
AB, OA and MHG oversaw the challenge experiments in the different laboratories; CF and KT performed the challenge experiments, tissue analyses and mouse bioassays at FLI; PB, IL, CR and FL performed the challenge experiments, tissue analyses and mouse bioassays at INRA-Nouzilly; WG and NH performed the challenge experiments and tissue analyses at Roslin; JGJ performed triplex-WB experiments. CF also collected all the data into a general data base. All authors were involved in the writing of the manuscript lead by JPML. All authors read and approved the final manuscript.

**Acknowledgements**
European project FOOD-CT-2006-36353 (GoatBSE), Dutch Ministry of Economic Affairs project WOT-01-002-001.01, the Biotechnology and Biological Sciences Research Council (strategic programme Grant BB/J004332/1 to The Roslin Institute) to WG and NH and Frederic Bouvier and his group from the INRA Experimental Unit of Bourges "La Sapinière" in France are thanked for the production and supply of experimental goats. We thank Dr. Francis Barillet (INRA, INRA, UR 631, Station d'amélioration géné tique des animaux, BP 52627, 31326 Castanet-Tolosan Cedex, France) for prodividing genotyped goats to CF and FL. We are grateful to the Experimental Infectiology Platform (PFIE, UE-1277, INRA Centre Val de Loire, Nouzilly, France) and the team working in the confinement unit. We are indebted to C. Rossignol and H. Le Roux for their excellent technical assistance in the management and treatment of samples. Dr. Lorenzo Gonzalez is recognized for his outstanding pathology work and comments to the manuscript. We are thankful to Dr. Susanne Niedermeyer for her excellent scientific and practical contribution in the animal experiments at FLI, Greifswald-Insel Riems, Germany. All animal keepers are acknowledged for the excellent care and handling of the experimental goats. Additionally Gesine Kreplin, James Foster, Paula Stewart, Kelly Ryan, and David Parnham are acknowledged for their outstanding technical assistance.

**Author details**
[1] Friedrich-Loeffler-Institut, Institute of Novel and Emerging Infectious Diseases, Greifswald-Insel Riems, Germany. [2] The Roslin Institute and Royal (Dick) School of Veterinary Studies, University of Edinburgh, Easter Bush, Midlothian, UK. [3] UMR 1282 ISP, Institut National de la Recherche Agronomique (INRA), University of Tours, 37380 Nouzilly, France. [4] INRA, UMR 1225, Interactions Hôtes Agents Pathogènes, Ecole Nationale Vétérinaire de Toulouse, Toulouse Cedex, France. [5] Wageningen BioVeterinary Research, Wageningen University & Research, Houtribweg 39, 8221RA Lelystad, The Netherlands.

**References**
1. Griffith JS (1967) Self-replication and scrapie. Nature 215:1043–1044
2. Prusiner SB (1982) Novel proteinaceous infectious particles cause scrapie. Science 216:136–144
3. Bakkebø MK, Mouillet-Richard S, Espenes A, Goldmann W, Tatzelt J, Tranulis MA (2015) The cellular prion protein: a player in immunological quiescence. Front Immunol 6:450
4. Küffer A, Lakkaraju AK, Mogha A, Petersen SC, Airich K, Doucerain C, Marpakwar R, Bakirci P, Senatore A, Monnard A, Schiavi C, Nuvolone M, Grosshans B, Hornemann S, Bassilana F, Monk KR, Aguzzi A (2016) The prion protein is an agonistic ligand of the G protein-coupled receptor Adgrg6. Nature 536:464–468
5. Schaller O, Fatzer R, Stack M, Clark J, Cooley W, Biffiger K, Egli S, Doherr M, Vandevelde M, Heim D, Oesch B, Moser M (1999) Validation of a western immunoblotting procedure for bovine PrP(Sc) detection and its use as a rapid surveillance method for the diagnosis of bovine spongiform encephalopathy (BSE). Acta Neuropathol 98:437–443

6.  Serban D, Taraboulos A, DeArmond SJ, Prusiner SB (1990) Rapid detection of Creutzfeldt–Jakob disease and scrapie prion proteins. Neurology 40:110–117

7.  van Keulen LJ, Schreuder BE, Meloen RH, Poelen-van den Berg M, Mooij-Harkes G, Vromans ME, Langeveld JP (1995) Immunohistochemical detection and localization of prion protein in brain tissue of sheep with natural scrapie. Vet Pathol 32:299–308

8.  Wells GA, Scott AC, Johnson CT, Gunning RF, Hancock RD, Jeffrey M, Dawson M, Bradley R (1987) A novel progressive spongiform encephalopathy in cattle. Vet Rec 121:419–420

9.  Will RG, Ironside JW, Zeidler M, Cousens SN, Estibeiro K, Alperovitch A, Poser S, Pocchiari M, Hofman A, Smith PG (1996) A new variant of Creutzfeldt–Jakob disease in the UK. Lancet 347:921–925

10. Eloit M, Adjou K, Coulpier M, Fontaine JJ, Hamel R, Lilin T, Messiaen S, Andreoletti O, Baron T, Bencsik A, Biacabe AG, Beringue V, Laude H, Le Dur A, Vilotte JL, Comoy E, Deslys JP, Grassi J, Simon S, Lantier F, Sarradin P (2005) BSE agent signatures in a goat. Vet Rec 156:523–524

11. Jeffrey M, Martin S, González L, Foster J, Langeveld JP, van Zijderveld FG, Grassi J, Hunter N (2006) Immunohistochemical features of PrP(d) accumulation in natural and experimental goat transmissible spongiform encephalopathies. J Comp Pathol 134:171–181

12. Spiropoulos J, Lockey R, Sallis RE, Terry LA, Thorne L, Holder TM, Beck KE, Simmons MM (2011) Isolation of prion with BSE properties from farmed goat. Emerg Infect Dis 17:2253–2261

13. EFSA (2014) Scientific Opinion on the scrapie situation in the EU after 10 years of monitoring and control in sheep and goats. EFSA J 12:3781

14. Bossers A, de Vries R, Smits MA (2000) Susceptibility of sheep for scrapie as assessed by in vitro conversion of nine naturally occurring variants of PrP. J Virol 74:1407–1414

15. Belt PB, Muileman IH, Schreuder BE, Bos-de Ruijter J, Gielkens AL, Smits MA (1995) Identification of five allelic variants of the sheep PrP gene and their association with natural scrapie. J Gen Virol 76:509–517

16. Hunter N, Bossers A (2006) The PrP genotype as a marker for scrapie susceptibility in sheep. In: Hörnlimann B, Riesner D, Kretzschmar H (eds) Prions in humans and animals. de Gruyter, Berlin, pp 640–647

17. EFSA (2017) Genetic resistance to transmissible spongiform encephalopathies (TSE) in goats. EFSA J 15(8):4962. doi:10.2903/j.efsa.2017.4962

18. Vaccari G, Panagiotidis CH, Acin C, Peletto S, Barillet F, Acutis P, Bossers A, Langeveld J, van Keulen L, Sklaviadis T, Badiola JJ, Andreoletti O, Groschup MH, Agrimi U, Foster J, Goldmann W (2009) State-of-the-art review of goat TSE in the European Union, with special emphasis on PRNP genetics and epidemiology. Vet Res 40:48

19. Acutis PL, Bossers A, Priem J, Riina MV, Peletto S, Mazza M, Casalone C, Forloni G, Ru G, Caramelli M (2006) Identification of prion protein gene polymorphisms in goats from Italian scrapie outbreaks. J Gen Virol 87:1029–1033

20. Barillet F, Mariat D, Amigues Y, Faugeras R, Caillat H, Moazami-Goudarzi K, Rupp R, Babilliot JM, Lacroux C, Lugan S, Schelcher F, Chartier C, Corbiere F, Andreoletti O, Perrin-Chauvineau C (2009) Identification of seven haplotypes of the caprine PrP gene at codons 127, 142, 154, 211, 222 and 240 in French Alpine and Saanen breeds and their association with classical scrapie. J Gen Virol 90:769–776

21. Billinis C, Panagiotidis CH, Psychas V, Argyroudis S, Nicolaou A, Leontides S, Papadopoulos O, Sklaviadis T (2002) Prion protein gene polymorphisms in natural goat scrapie. J Gen Virol 83:713–721

22. Bouzalas IG, Dovas CI, Banos G, Papanastasopoulou M, Kritas S, Oevermann A, Papakostaki D, Evangelia C, Papadopoulos O, Seuberlich T, Koptopoulos G (2010) Caprine PRNP polymorphisms at codons 171, 211, 222 and 240 in a Greek herd and their association with classical scrapie. J Gen Virol 91:1629–1634

23. Corbiere F, Perrin-Chauvineau C, Lacroux C, Costes P, Thomas M, Bremaud I, Martin S, Lugan S, Chartier C, Schelcher F, Barillet F, Andreoletti O (2013) PrP-associated resistance to scrapie in five highly infected goat herds. J Gen Virol 94:241–245

24. Goldmann W, Ryan K, Stewart P, Parnham D, Xicohtencatl R, Fernandez N, Saunders G, Windl O, González L, Bossers A, Foster J (2011) Caprine prion gene polymorphisms are associated with decreased incidence of classical scrapie in goat herds in the United Kingdom. Vet Res 42:110

25. González L, Martin S, Siso S, Konold T, Ortiz-Pelaez A, Phelan L, Goldmann W, Stewart P, Saunders G, Windl O, Jeffrey M, Hawkins SA, Dawson M, Hope J (2009) High prevalence of scrapie in a dairy goat herd: tissue distribution of disease-associated PrP and effect of PRNP genotype and age. Vet Res 40:65

26. Goldmann W, Martin T, Foster J, Hughes S, Smith G, Hughes K, Dawson M, Hunter N (1996) Novel polymorphisms in the caprine PrP gene: a codon 142 mutation associated with scrapie incubation period. J Gen Virol 77:2885–2891

27. Vitale M, Migliore S, La Giglia M, Alberti P, Presti VDML (2016) Scrapie incidence and PRNP polymorphisms: rare small ruminant breeds of Sicily with TSE protecting genetic reservoirs. BMC Vet Res 12:141

28. White S, Herrmann-Hoesing L, O'Rourke K, Waldron D, Rowe J, Alverson J (2008) Prion gene (PRNP) haplotype variation in United States goat breeds (Open Access publication). Gen Sel Evol 40:553–561

29. Windig JJ, Hoving RA, Priem J, Bossers A, van Keulen LJ, Langeveld JP (2016) Variation in the prion protein sequence in Dutch goat breeds. J Anim Breed Genet 133:366–374

30. Acutis PL, Martucci F, D'Angelo A, Peletto S, Colussi S, Maurella C, Porcario C, Iulini B, Mazza M, Dell'atti L, Zuccon F, Corona C, Martinelli N, Casalone C, Caramelli M, Lombardi G (2012) Resistance to classical scrapie in experimentally challenged goats carrying mutation K222 of the prion protein gene. Vet Res 43:8

31. Lacroux C, Perrin-Chauvineau C, Corbiere F, Aron N, Aguilar-Calvo P, Torres JM, Costes P, Bremaud I, Lugan S, Schelcher F, Barillet F, Andreoletti O (2014) Genetic resistance to scrapie infection in experimentally challenged goats. J Virol 88:2406–2413

32. White SN, Reynolds JO, Waldron DF, Schneider DA, O'Rourke KI (2012) Extended scrapie incubation time in goats singly heterozygous for PRNP S146 or K222. Gene 501:49–51

33. Aguilar-Calvo P, Fast C, Tauscher K, Espinosa JC, Groschup MH, Nadeem M, Goldmann W, Langeveld J, Bossers A, Andreoletti O, Torres JM (2015) Effect of Q211 and K222 PRNP polymorphic variants in the susceptibility of goats to oral infection with goat bovine spongiform encephalopathy. J Infect Dis 212:664–672

34. Foster JD, Hope J, Fraser H (1993) Transmission of bovine spongiform encephalopathy to sheep and goats. Vet Rec 133:339–341

35. Feraudet C, Morel N, Simon S, Volland H, Frobert Y, Creminon C, Vilette D, Lehmann S, Grassi J (2005) Screening of 145 anti-PrP monoclonal antibodies for their capacity to inhibit PrPSc replication in infected cells. J Biol Chem 280:11247–11258

36. Hoffmann C, Eiden M, Kaatz M, Keller M, Ziegler U, Rogers R, Hills B, Balkema-Buschmann A, van Keulen L, Jacobs JG, Groschup MH (2011) BSE infectivity in jejunum, ileum and ileocaecal junction of incubating cattle. Vet Res 42:21

37. Rigter A, Langeveld JP, Timmers-Parohi D, Jacobs JG, Moonen PL, Bossers A (2007) Mapping of possible prion protein self-interaction domains using peptide arrays. BMC Biochem 8:6

38. González L, Jeffrey M, Siso S, Martin S, Bellworthy SJ, Stack MJ, Chaplin MJ, Davis L, Dagleish MP, Reid HW (2005) Diagnosis of preclinical scrapie in samples of rectal mucosa. Vet Rec 156:846–847

39. Spraker TR, O'Rourke KI, Balachandran A, Zink RR, Cummings BA, Miller MW, Powers BE (2002) Validation of monoclonal antibody F99/97.6.1 for immunohistochemical staining of brain and tonsil in mule deer (Odocoileus hemionus) with chronic wasting disease. J Vet Diagn Investig 14:3–7

40. Harmeyer S, Pfaff E, Groschup MH (1998) Synthetic peptide vaccines yield monoclonal antibodies to cellular and pathological prion proteins of ruminants. J Gen Virol 79:937–945

41. Korth C, Stierli B, Streit P, Moser M, Schaller O, Fischer R, Schulz-Schaeffer W, Kretzschmar H, Raeber A, Braun U, Ehrensperger F, Hornemann S, Glockshuber R, Riek R, Billeter M, Wuthrich K, Oesch B (1997) Prion (PrPSc)-specific epitope defined by a monoclonal antibody. Nature 390:74–77

42. Slootstra JW, Puijk WC, Ligtvoet GJ, Langeveld JP, Meloen RH (1996) Structural aspects of antibody–antigen interaction revealed through small random peptide libraries. Mol Divers 1:87–96

43. Andreoletti O, Berthon P, Marc D, Sarradin P, Grosclaude J, van Keulen L, Schelcher F, Elsen JM, Lantier F (2000) Early accumulation of PrP(Sc) in gut-associated lymphoid and nervous tissues of susceptible sheep from a Romanov flock with natural scrapie. J Gen Virol 81:3115–3126

44. Niedermeyer S, Eiden M, Toumazos P, Papasavva-Stylianou P, Ioannou I, Sklaviadis T, Panagiotidis C, Langeveld JP, Bossers A, Kuczius T, Kaatz M, Groschup MH, Fast C (2016) Genetic, histochemical and biochemical studies on goat TSE cases from Cyprus. Vet Res 47:99

45. Le Dur A, Beringue V, Andreoletti O, Reine F, Lai TL, Baron T, Bratberg B, Vilotte JL, Sarradin P, Benestad SL, Laude H (2005) A newly identified type

of scrapie agent can naturally infect sheep with resistant PrP genotypes. Proc Natl Acad U S A 102:16031–16036

46. Martin S, González L, Chong A, Houston FE, Hunter N, Jeffrey M (2005) Immunohistochemical characteristics of disease-associated PrP are not altered by host genotype or route of inoculation following infection of sheep with bovine spongiform encephalopathy. J Gen Virol 86:839–848

47. Martin S, Jeffrey M, González L, Siso S, Reid HW, Steele P, Dagleish MP, Stack MJ, Chaplin MJ, Balachandran A (2009) Immunohistochemical and biochemical characteristics of BSE and CWD in experimentally infected European red deer (Cervus elaphus elaphus). BMC Vet Res 5:26

48. Jacobs JG, Sauer M, van Keulen LJ, Tang Y, Bossers A, Langeveld JP (2011) Differentiation of ruminant transmissible spongiform encephalopathy isolate types, including bovine spongiform encephalopathy and CH1641 scrapie. J Gen Virol 92:222–232

49. Langeveld JP, Jacobs JG, Erkens JH, Baron T, Andreoletti O, Yokoyama T, van Keulen LJ, van Zijderveld FG, Davidse A, Hope J, Tang Y, Bossers A (2014) Sheep prions with molecular properties intermediate between classical scrapie, BSE and CH1641-scrapie. Prion 8:296–305

50. Castilla J, Gutierrez Adan A, Brun A, Pintado B, Ramirez MA, Parra B, Doyle D, Rogers M, Salguero FJ, Sanchez C, Sanchez-Vizcaino JM, Torres JM (2003) Early detection of PrPres in BSE-infected bovine PrP transgenic mice. Arch Virol 148:677–691

51. Kupfer L, Eiden M, Buschmann A, Groschup MH (2007) Amino acid sequence and prion strain specific effects on the in vitro and in vivo convertibility of ovine/murine and bovine/murine prion protein chimeras. Biochim Biophys Acta 1772:704–713

52. Jeffrey M, Martin S, González L, Ryder SJ, Bellworthy SJ, Jackman R (2001) Differential diagnosis of infections with the bovine spongiform encephalopathy (BSE) and scrapie agents in sheep. J Comp Pathol 125:271–284

53. Lloyd S, Mead S, Collinge J (2011) Genetics of prion disease. Top Curr Chem 305:1–22

54. Hunter N, Houston F, Foster J, Goldmann W, Drummond D, Parnham D, Kennedy I, Green A, Stewart P, Chong A (2012) Susceptibility of young sheep to oral infection with bovine spongiform encephalopathy decreases significantly after weaning. J Virol 86:11856–11862

55. Ryder SJ, Dexter GE, Heasman L, Warner R, Moore SJ (2009) Accumulation and dissemination of prion protein in experimental sheep scrapie in the natural host. BMC Vet Res 5:9

56. St Rose SG, Hunter N, Matthews L, Foster JD, Chase-Topping ME, Kruuk LE, Shaw DJ, Rhind SM, Will RG, Woolhouse ME (2006) Comparative evidence for a link between Peyer's patch development and susceptibility to transmissible spongiform encephalopathies. BMC Infect Dis 6:5

57. Carp RI, Callahan SM (1991) Variation in the characteristics of 10 mouse-passaged scrapie lines derived from five scrapie-positive sheep. J Gen Virol 72:293–298

58. Aguilar-Calvo P, Espinosa JC, Pintado B, Gutierrez-Adan A, Alamillo E, Miranda A, Prieto I, Bossers A, Andreoletti O, Torres JM (2014) Role of the goat K222-PrP(C) polymorphic variant in prion infection resistance. J Virol 88:2670–2676

59. Espinosa JC, Andreoletti O, Castilla J, Herva ME, Morales M, Alamillo E, San-Segundo FD, Lacroux C, Lugan S, Salguero FJ, Langeveld J, Torres JM (2007) Sheep-passaged bovine spongiform encephalopathy agent exhibits altered pathobiological properties in bovine-PrP transgenic mice. J Virol 81:835–843

60. EFSA (2015) Scientific Opinion on a request for a review of a scientific publication concerning the zoonotic potential of ovine scrapie prions. EFSA J 13:4197

61. Bellworthy SJ, Dexter G, Stack M, Chaplin M, Hawkins SA, Simmons MM, Jeffrey M, Martin S, González L, Hill P (2005) Natural transmission of BSE between sheep within an experimental flock. Vet Rec 157:206

62. Saunders SE, Bartz JC, Bartelt-Hunt SL (2009) Prion protein adsorption to soil in a competitive matrix is slow and reduced. Environ Sci Technol 43:7728–7733

63. van Keulen LJ, Vromans ME, Dolstra CH, Bossers A, van Zijderveld FG (2008) Pathogenesis of bovine spongiform encephalopathy in sheep. Arch Virol 153:445–453

64. van Keulen LJ, Schreuder BE, Vromans MEW, Langeveld JP, Smits M (2000) Pathoegenesis of natural scrapie in sheep. Arch Virol 16:57–71

65. EFSA (2010) Scientific Opinion on BSE/TSE infectivity in small ruminant tissues. EFSA J 8:1875

66. González L, Martin S, Hawkins SA, Goldmann W, Jeffrey M, Siso S (2010) Pathogenesis of natural goat scrapie: modulation by host PRNP genotype and effect of co-existent conditions. Vet Res 41:48

67. Kaatz M, Fast C, Ziegler U, Balkema-Buschmann A, Hammerschmidt B, Keller M, Oelschlegel A, McIntyre L, Groschup MH (2012) Spread of classic BSE prions from the gut via the peripheral nervous system to the brain. Am J Pathol 181:515–524

68. Houston F, Goldmann W, Foster J, González L, Jeffrey M, Hunter N (2015) Comparative susceptibility of sheep of different origins, breeds and PRNP genotypes to challenge with bovine spongiform encephalopathy and scrapie. PLoS One 10:e0143251

69. Papasavva-Stylianou P, Kleanthous M, Toumazos P, Mavrikiou P, Loucaides P (2007) Novel polymorphisms at codons 146 and 151 in the prion protein gene of Cyprus goats, and their association with natural scrapie. Vet J 173:459–462

70. Papasavva-Stylianou P, Windl O, Saunders G, Mavrikiou P, Toumazos P, Kokoyiannis C (2011) PrP gene polymorphisms in Cyprus goats and their association with resistance or susceptibility to natural scrapie. Vet J 187:245–250

# 7

# RNA-seq comparative analysis of Peking ducks spleen gene expression 24 h post-infected with duck plague virulent or attenuated virus

Tian Liu[1,2], Anchun Cheng[1,2,3]*, Mingshu Wang[1,2,3]*, Renyong Jia[1,2,3], Qiao Yang[1,2,3], Ying Wu[1,2,3], Kunfeng Sun[1,2,3], Dekang Zhu[2,3], Shun Chen[1,2,3], Mafeng Liu[1,2,3], XinXin Zhao[1,2,3] and Xiaoyue Chen[2,3]

## Abstract

Duck plague virus (DPV), a member of alphaherpesvirus sub-family, can cause significant economic losses on duck farms in China. DPV Chinese virulent strain (CHv) is highly pathogenic and could induce massive ducks death. Attenuated DPV vaccines (CHa) have been put into service against duck plague with billions of doses in China each year. Researches on DPV have been development for many years, however, a comprehensive understanding of molecular mechanisms underlying pathogenicity of CHv strain and protection of CHa strain to ducks is still blank. In present study, we performed RNA-seq technology to analyze transcriptome profiling of duck spleens for the first time to identify differentially expressed genes (DEGs) associated with the infection of CHv and CHa at 24 h. Comparison of gene expression with mock ducks revealed 748 DEGs and 484 DEGs after CHv and CHa infection, respectively. Gene pathway analysis of DEGs highlighted valuable biological processes involved in host immune response, cell apoptosis and viral invasion. Genes expressed in those pathways were different in CHv infected duck spleens and CHa vaccinated duck spleens. The results may provide valuable information for us to explore the reasons of pathogenicity caused by CHv strain and protection activated by CHa strain.

## Introduction

After firstly reported in Netherlands at 1923, duck plague (DP) was rapidly spread around the world [1]. In China, the DP was not suspected until 1958 and the outbreak of DP results in a devastated hit to duck industries in China, one of the largest duck breeding countries in the world, due to DP's high mortality [2, 3]. The disease is caused by duck plague virus (DPV), a member of alphaherpesvirus subfamily, which is a double-stranded DNA virus composed with capsid, tegument and envelope [4]. DPV Chinese virulent strain (CHv), which was isolated from dead infected ducks in China, is highly pathogenic and could

induce massive petechial hemorrhages in parenchymal organ, lymphoid and digestive tract and causes massive ducks death [5–8]. To control this disease on duck farms, attenuated DPV vaccines, such as CHa, have been put into service against duck plague with billions of doses in China each year [9].

Compared to other Herpesviruses, the development of DPV researches, particularly in viral gene functions and virus-host interplay, undergoes a slow process. After the first reports of DPV highly virulent strain and attenuated strain genomes, the studies of gene structure and functions have been spring up. DPV highly virulent strain genes, such as capsid protein genes UL19, UL35 tegument protein genes UL16, UL51 and envelope glycoprotein genes like UL44, US7, US8 were well studied [10–16]. Furthermore, it has been reported that the five ORFs, including UL2, UL12, US10, UL47 and UL41, might represent DPV virulence factors [17]. However, although

*Correspondence: chenganchun@vip.163.com; mshwang@163.com
[1] Avian Disease Research Center, College of Veterinary Medicine, Sichuan Agricultural University, Wenjiang, Chengdu 611130, People's Republic of China
Full list of author information is available at the end of the article

exploring basic gene mechanisms of highly virulent DPV strains and attenuated DPV strains on genomic level is indeed helpful, it still lacks systemic and comprehensive studies on nature host duck biological processes when infect with DP virus. Performed works reported that DPV virulent strain conducted a latent infection following a primary infection in trigeminal ganglion and lymphoid tissues including PBL and spleen [18], whereas how the virus processes a latent infection and what the mechanisms of latency infection have not been clear. Meanwhile, although Yuan observed programmed cell death on lymphocytes after infection of highly virulent DPV strain, and the result indicated membrane proteins of DPV could alter characteristics of apoptotic cells in duck embryo fibroblast culture [19]. However, no further studies about DPV-induced apoptosis were observed. Moreover, as we all know, the processes for virus to entry into a cell is critical to initiate their whole life cycles, however, we have little information about DPV entry [20–22]. Although genes involved in other herpesvirus entry such as glycoprotein gB and gD were well studied, it is still a puzzle part that whether these genes are necessary in DPV entry or not [23, 24].

In this study, with the help of RNA-seq platform we explored a bioinformatics analysis on duck spleen gene expression for the first time after highly virulent DPV CHv strain and attenuated DPV CHa strain infection at post-infected 24 h. Previous study indicated that attenuated DPVs were rapid distribution and proliferation in duck's tissues 12 h post-inoculation, however, copies of attenuated DPV were dramatic decline in duck's tissues 24 h post-infection (hpi), which means that attenuated DPV could rapidly invoke host immune response and inhibit DPV proliferation in the early stage of inoculation [6]. Thus, 24 h was chosen as a samples collection time point to explore reasons of protection stimulated by attenuated DPV in short time after infection. In order to detect accurate biological differences from sequencing data, the setting of multiple biological replicates and the meticulous analysis of statistic were performed. Furthermore, high quality reads mapping was presented by using a paired-end mRNA sequencing approach. Eventually, 748 differentially expressed genes (DEGs) in CHv infected group and 484 DEGs in CHa vaccinated group were selected. Gene pathway analysis of DEGs highlighted several valuable biological processes involved in host immune response, cell apoptosis and viral invasion. Genes expressed in those pathways were different in CHv infected duck spleens and CHa vaccinated duck spleens. Overall, our findings generated in this work firstly provided a detailed view of global changes in duck spleen gene expression when infected with either highly virulent

DPV CHv strain or attenuated DPV CHa strain at 24 hpi and the results may provide valuable information for us to explore the reasons of pathogenicity caused by CHv strain and protection activated by CHa strain.

## Materials and methods
### Virus and experiment design
Highly virulence DPV CHv strain and attenuated modified vaccine DPV CHa strain used in this study were obtained from the Key Laboratory of Animal Disease and Human Health of Sichuan Province. Twenty-seven Peking ducklings were conducted from a DPV-free farm where vaccination against DPV was not implementation. Three experimental groups, including CHv infected group, CHa vaccinated group and normal saline intramuscular injected control group, were explored in this study. Each experimental group contained three biology repeats and each repeat included three ducks. CHv-infected and CHa-vaccinated groups were inoculated using intramuscular administration ($4.1 \times 10^8$ copies CHv and CHa, respectively). Ducks were euthanized to collect spleen samples at 24 hpi. The samples were rapidly kept in liquid nitrogen for further experiments.

### Library preparation for RNA-seq
Total RNA was isolated from spleen samples by TRIzol extraction (Invitrogen, CA, USA) following the manufacturer's instructions. RNA purity was checked by using the NanoPhotometer® spectrophotometer (IMPLEN, CA, USA) and its concentration was measured using Qubit® RNA Assay Kit in Qubit® 2.0 Flurometer (Life Technologies, CA, USA). RNA integrity was assessed using the RNA Nano 6000 Assay Kit of the Bioanalyzer 2100 system (Agilent Technologies, CA, USA). A total amount of 3 µg RNA per sample was used as input material for the RNA sample preparations. Sequencing libraries were generated using NEBNext® UltraTM RNA Library Prep Kit for Illumina® (NEB, USA) following manufacturer's recommendations and index codes were added to attribute sequences to each sample. Briefly, mRNA was purified from total RNA using poly-T oligo-attached magnetic beads. Fragmentation was carried out using divalent cations under elevated temperature in NEBNext First Strand Synthesis Reaction Buffer (5×). First strand cDNA was synthesized using random hexamer primer and M-MuLV Reverse Transcriptase (RNase H⁻). Second strand cDNA synthesis was subsequently performed using DNA Polymerase I and RNaseH were converted into blunt ends via exonuclease/polymerase activities. After adenylation of 3′ ends of DNA fragments, NEBNext Adaptors with hairpin loop structure were ligated to prepare for

hybridization. In order to select cDNA fragments of preferentially 150–200 bp in length, the library fragments were purified with AMPure XP system (Beckman Coulter, Beverly, USA). Then 3 μL USER Enzyme (NEB, USA) was used with size-selected, adaptor-ligated cDNA at 37 °C for 15 min followed by 5 min at 95 °C before PCR. Then PCR was performed with phusion high-fidelity DNA polymerase, universal PCR primers and index (X) primer. At last, PCR products were purified (AMPure XP system) and library quality was assessed on the Agilent Bioanalyzer 2100 system. The clustering of the index-coded samples was performed on a cBot Cluster Generation System using TruSeq PE Cluster Kit v3-cBot-HS (Illumia) according to the manufacturer's instructions. After cluster generation, the library preparations were sequenced on Hiseq-PE150 platform and 125 bp/150 bp paired-end reads were generated.

### Bioinformatics analysis of RNA-seq data

Clean reads were obtained to remove reads containing adapters, poly-N and low quality sequences in raw reads. Clean reads were calculated through Q20, Q30 and GC content to make sure data with high quality. All the downstream analyses were based on clean data with high quality. Paired-end clean reads were mapped to duck reference genome using TopHat v2.0.12. Reads numbers of each gene were counted through the HTSeq v0.6.1. In order to normalize the expression of each gene from different samples, FPKM (expected number of Fragments per kilobase of transcript sequence per Millions base pairs sequenced) was introduced. Genes with an expression level more than 1 FPKM were used for downstream analysis. To test the differential expression genes (DEGs) of two groups, CHv infected ducks and CHa vaccinated ducks (three biological replicates per group), the DESeq R package (1.18.0) was performed and genes with a $p$-value < 0.05 found by DESeq were assigned as differentially expressed.

### Gene ontology enrichment analysis

GOseq R package was used to perform gene ontology (GO) enrichment analysis of differential expression genes. GO terms with $p$-value < 0.05 were selected as significant enrichment.

### KEGG pathway analysis

KEGG is a database resource for understanding functions and utilities of the biological system, such as the cell, the organism and the ecosystem, from molecular-level information. We used KOBAS software to test the statistical enrichment of differential expression genes in KEGG pathways. KEGG pathways with $p$-value < 0.05 were selected as significant enrichment.

## Results

### Collection of duck spleen samples and construction of cDNA libraries after CHv and CHa infection

Transcriptome sequencing by RNA-seq was used to detect global changes of Peking duck spleen gene expression after CHv and CHa infection. Three experimental groups, including CHv infected group, CHa vaccinated group and normal saline intramuscular injected control group, were explored in this study. Each experimental group contained three biology repeats and each repeat included three ducks. Nine Peking duck spleen samples were collected and stored at liquid nitrogen until total RNA extraction and quality testing was done. Finally, nine cDNA libraries were performed.

### Differentially expressed genes after CHv and CHa infection

By using Hiseq-PE150 platform, a total of 571 million (571 134 310) raw data were produced across nine samples. To guarantee ideal results for following genomic mapping and differential gene change analysis, raw reads were filtered to remove low quality data with a total of 545 million (545 498 360) clean reads acquired, a mean of 61.23% of which mapped to duck reference genome (Table 1).

Heat map visually compares the whole level of different expression genes (DEGs) and classifies gene expression patterns in different treatment experimental groups under different experimental conditions. As showed in Figure 1A, notwithstanding genes harbored the same or similar expression pattern in CHv, CHa and control treatment groups, the regulation of gene expression was in an entirely different level. For exploring a global view on the change of duck gene expression between different experimental treatment groups, two paired comparisons (CHv vs control, CHa vs control) were performed. In all, RNA-seq analysis detected 748 and 484 genes, which were expressed at significantly different levels in CHv and CHa groups compared to control at a $p$ value < 0.05, respectively (Figure 1B). The purpose of this study is to explore differences of duck spleen gene expression at 24 h between high-virulence DPV CHv strain infected group and attenuated DPV CHa strain vaccinated group through high throughput RNA-seq analysis. In order to learn clearly and precisely about differentially expressed genes, venn analysis was utilized (Figure 1B) and there were three main parts of it. From the green part, there were 561 genes represented the numbers of genes only expressed in CHv infected ducks when compared to control and as for the red part, there were 297 DEGs that only expressed in CHa vaccinated ducks when compared to control. The intersection part with 187 DE genes were co-expressed genes in both CHv infected and CHa vaccinated groups when compared to control.

**Table 1  Number of reads of all bases detected using RNA-seq in DPV-infected and control ducks**

| Library | Number of raw reads | Number of clean reads | Number of uniquely mapped reads | Percentage of reads mapped (%) |
|---|---|---|---|---|
| CHv-1 | 61 196 398 | 58 437 658 | 35 429 191 | 60.63 |
| CHv-2 | 61 868 452 | 59 080 194 | 35 273 016 | 59.7 |
| CHv-3 | 69 529 094 | 66 485 428 | 40 823 382 | 61.4 |
| CHa-1 | 63 045 260 | 60 281 664 | 36 842 779 | 61.12 |
| CHa-2 | 61 100 482 | 58 372 142 | 36 312 302 | 62.21 |
| CHa-3 | 68 613 194 | 65 544 842 | 40 272 899 | 61.44 |
| Control-1 | 64 108 500 | 61 235 756 | 37 298 283 | 60.91 |
| Control-2 | 60 808 456 | 58 101 298 | 35 789 540 | 61.6 |
| Control-3 | 60 864 474 | 57 959 378 | 35 637 789 | 61.49 |
| Total | 571 134 310 | 545 498 360 | 333 679 181 | |

## Annotation of duck spleen DEGs based on GO analysis after CHv infection or CHa vaccination

To ensure differentially expressed genes function, gene ontology (GO) analysis was performed to categorize and annotate DEGs of all of three parts in Venn diagram into three groups including biological process (BP), cellular component (CC) and molecular function (MF), respectively. As shown in Table 2, a total of 2654 GO terms were assigned to DE genes only expressed in CHv infected group including 1806 BP terms, 511 MF terms and 341 CC terms. As for DE genes only expressed in CHa vaccinated group, a total of 1479 GO terms were annotated including 976 BP terms, 277 MF terms and 226 CC terms. Furthermore, DE genes expressed in both CHv infected group and CHa vaccinated group were categorized into GO terms with a total numbers of 1098 including 697 BP terms, 215 MF terms and 186 CC terms.

And then, in order to pick out the helpful and useful genes for further exploration, 30 significant GO terms were listed and each terms contained more than 2 genes (Figure 2). Top 30 GO terms were selected according $p$-value < 0.05. Top three significant GO terms of DEGs expressed in both CHv infected group and CHa vaccinated group were protein localization to centrosome (GO:0071539), smooth muscle contractile fiber (GO:0030485) and extracellular matrix structural constituent (GO:0005201). Top three significant GO terms of DEGs only expressed in CHv infected group were paraxial mesoderm formation (GO:0048341), MHC class I protein complex (GO:0042612) and transmembrane receptor protein tyrosine kinase adaptor activity (GO:0005068). Top three significant GO terms of DEGs expressed only in CHa vaccinated group were positive regulation of cellular extravasation (GO:0002693), clathrin coat of trans-Golgi network vesicle (GO:0030130) and dipeptidase activity (GO:0016805).

## Pathway analysis of DEGs based on KEGG after CHv and CHa infection

KEGG pathway analysis was used as a combination way to explore the function of DEGs. Top 20 enrichment KEGG pathways were listed in Figure 3 according to $p$ value < 0.05. Four functional categories were identified to potentially play important roles associated with CHv infection including phagosome, antigen processing and presentation, leukocyte transendothelial migration and Fc gamma R-mediated phagocytosis. Three functional categories were identified to potentially play important roles associated with CHa vaccination including cytokine–cytokine receptor interaction, antigen processing and presentation as well as phagosome. Three functional categories were identified to potentially play important roles associated with both CHv infection and CHa vaccination including ECM-receptor interaction, focal adhesion as well as protein digestion and absorption. Putative functional roles and interactions of these genes involved in mediating host response of ducks are discussed in detail.

## Discussion

Duck plague (DP) is a disease that has been reported to cause significant economic losses on duck farms per year in China [3]. Although attenuated vaccine inoculation is an effective way for preventing this disease on duck industries, the potential risk of live attenuated vaccines of virulence return has raised more and more concern. Furthermore, the lack of effective therapeutic tools is another worry to control this disease spreading, indicating that it is urgent to not only give a deeply insight into pathogenesis mechanism of DPV highly pathogenic strain, but also give a profound understanding of protective mechanism of DPV attenuated vaccine strain. From our results, we performed RNA-seq technology for the

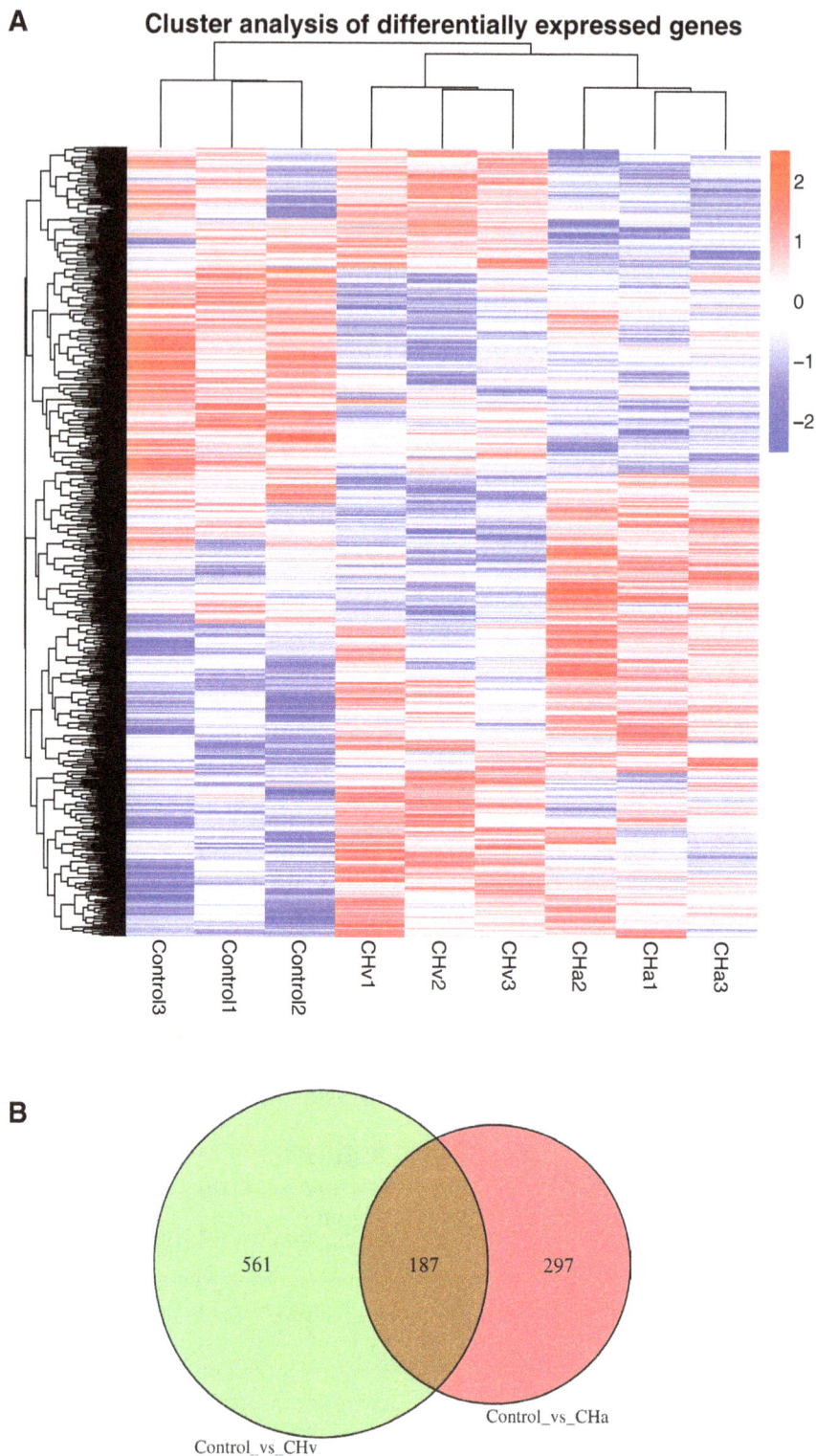

**Figure 1 Differentially expressed genes in different experimental conditions.** Heatmap is used to classify gene expression patterns under different experimental conditions and Venn diagram displays a global view on the numbers of differentially expressed genes. **A** Genes with similar expressed patterns were clustered and showed above in the heatmap. Intensity of color indicates gene expression levels that were normalized according to $\log_{10}$ (FPKM + 1) values. Red color represent high expression level genes and blue color represent low expression level genes. The three major clusters represent CHv infected duck group, CHa vaccinated ducks group and control group. **B** The overlap of differentially expressed genes of CHv vs Control and CHa vs Control. The number in the diagram indicated gene number refers to each comparison.

**Table 2  A summary of GO term numbers after CHv and CHa infection**

|  | GO terms-BP | GO terms-MF | GO terms-CC | Total terms |
|---|---|---|---|---|
| DEGs only express in CHv | 1806 | 511 | 341 | 2658 |
| DEGs only express in CHa | 976 | 277 | 226 | 1479 |
| DEGs expressed in CHv and CHa | 697 | 215 | 186 | 1098 |

first time and explored important information about host-viral interaction at post 24 h infection in which the ducks were infected by DPV highly pathogenic strain CHv and DPV attenuated vaccine strain CHa.

### Antigen processing and presentation

Cytotoxic T lymphocytes (CTLs) recognized virus-derived peptides presenting by MHC class I and MHC class II at cell surface is a critical immune monitor system and this high sensitive antigen processing and presentation system also becomes a prime target to escape host immune surveillance deployed by many viruses, particularly large DNA virus like herpesvirus [25]. Thus, antigen processing and presentation pathway annotated by KEGG analysis evoked our strong interests.

From results, we got differentially expressed genes related to antigen processing and presentation in KEGG pathway (Table 3). It was no surprise that at 24 hpi, duck spleen genes expression related to antigen processing and presentation had been changed when ducks infected no matter by CHv strain or by CHa strain. However, the results showed that there was huge diversity on the types of differentially expressed genes. CHv infection resulted in genes differential expression located to both MHC class I and MHC class II pathway, however, as for CHa infection, specific gene expression only changed in MHC class II pathway. Furthermore, from the results we could find that the MHC class II genes expressed were up-regulated in CHv infection group whereas down-regulated in CHa vaccinated group. It means that under the experiment condition in this study, the antigen processing and presentation process presented by highly virulence DPV strain CHv and attenuated DPV strain CHa is totally different in vivo.

Virus antigens are degraded by proteasome in cytosolic origin in MHC class I presentation pathway and then are translocated into the endoplasmic reticulum (ER) by Transporter associated with Antigen Processing (TAP) to load onto newly synthesis MHC class I molecules [26]. In the ER, the MHC class I molecule is assembled from a heavy chain and a light chain called $\beta_2$-microglobulin ($\beta_2$m) [27]. The peptide inserts itself deep into the MHC class I peptide-binding groove and then ensure the stability of the complex [27]. The fully assembled molecule loaded with virus protein segments then release from

the ER and travels via the Golgi apparatus to the plasma membrane for antigen processing and preparation to CD8$^+$ T cells [28]. From our results, in CHv infected group, genes correlated to MHC class I molecule composition, such as MHC1 and $\beta_2$m, and antigen processing transporters, such as TAP1 and TAP2, are up-regulated (Table 3). However, in CHa vaccinated group, only the expression of $\beta_2$m gene was changed. Previous studies reported that herpesviruses could target each steps of MHC class I antigen presenting pathway to evade host immune response. A large number of proteins are encoded by herpesviruses to disturb MHC I antigen presentation and then prevent elimination of the target cell by CTLs. The mRNA of MHC class I high chain is degraded by host shut-off protein of herpes simplex virus (HSV) and bovine herpes virus (BHV-1) [29, 30]. Furthermore, immature MHC class I molecules are directed into cytosol from ER with the use of US10 protein of human cytomegalovirus (HCMV) and finally degraded by proteinase [31]. Moreover, with the help of ICP47, HSV could inhibit the transport of peptides through TAP [32]. Thus, we conclude that there may be some critical mechanisms used by DPV CHa strain to evade MHC class I molecules identify and presentation and then finally evade immune response.

Although MHC class I and MHC class II are similar in presenting virus antigen peptides to CD8$^+$ and CD4$^+$, the basic antigen presentation pathways of them are extremely diverse [28]. Firstly, these molecules have different cell distributions. MHC class I molecules are expressed at kinds of nucleated cells, however, MHC class II molecules are specifically found at antigen presenting cells (APCs), such as dendritic cells macrophages and B cells [33]. Unlike the source of viruses degraded in MHC class I molecules presentation pathway, virus protein presented in MHC II pathway is degraded in endosome. As for MHC class II molecules, after assembling with the transmembrane chains and the invariant chain (Ii, also named CD74) in the ER, MHC class II is transported to the MHC class II compartment (MIIC). In this part, Ii is digested by endosomal proteases such as asparaginyl endopeptidase (APE) and then leave a residual class II-associated Ii peptide (CLIP) occupying the peptide-binding groove of the MHC class II molecules [34]. In the MIIC, the CLIP fragment is displaced by viral

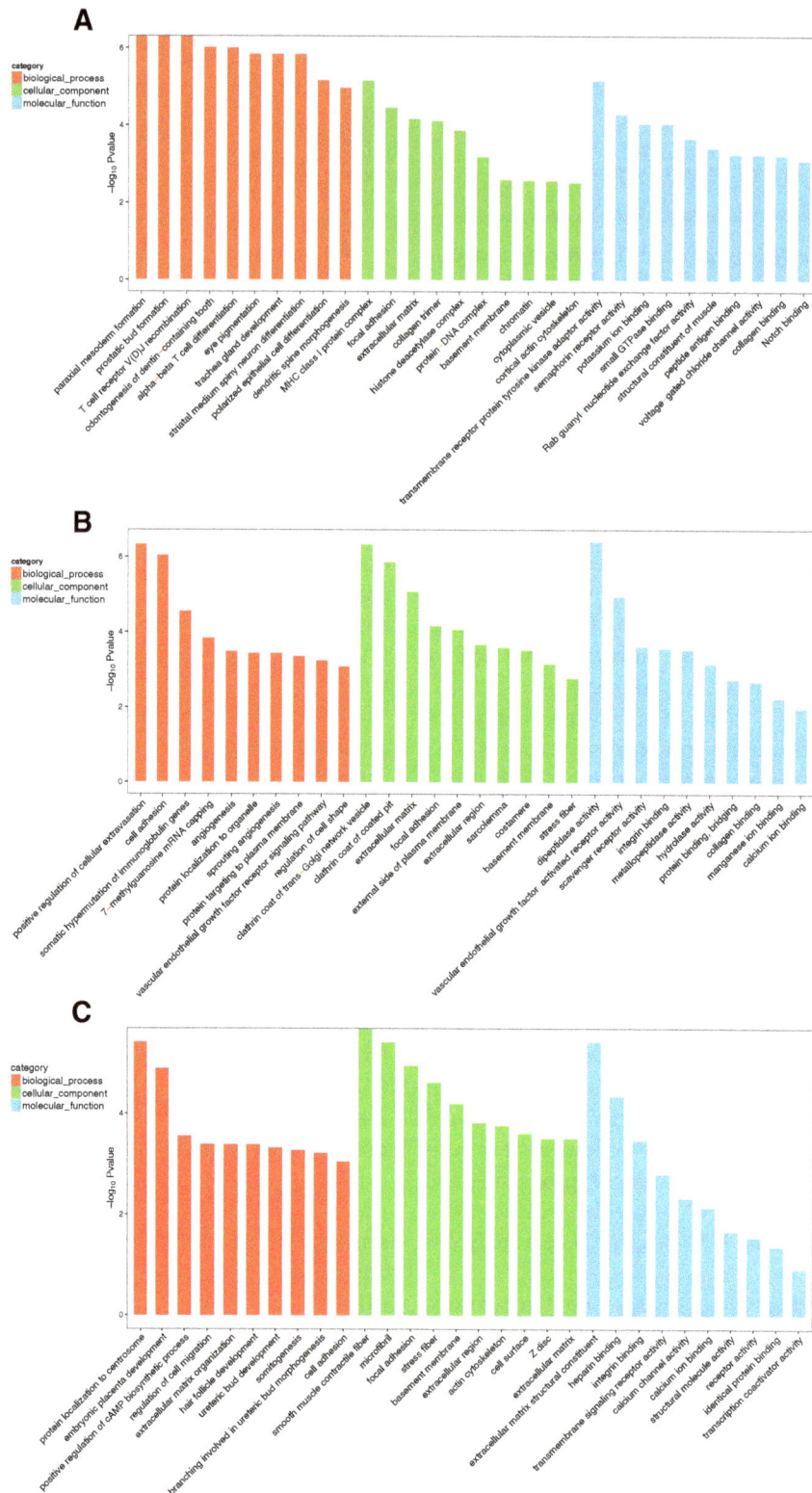

**Figure 2 Top 30 Gene ontology (GO) terms of DEGs expressed in CHv infected or CHa vaccinated group.** GO-terms were processed under three categories including cellular component (CC), molecular function (MF) and biological process (BP). Top 30 GO terms were selected according p-value < 0.05 **A** GO annotation of DEGs expressed only in CHv infected group **B** GO annotation of DEGs expressed only in CHa vaccinated group **C** GO annotation of DEGs expressed in both CHv infected group and CHa vaccinated group.

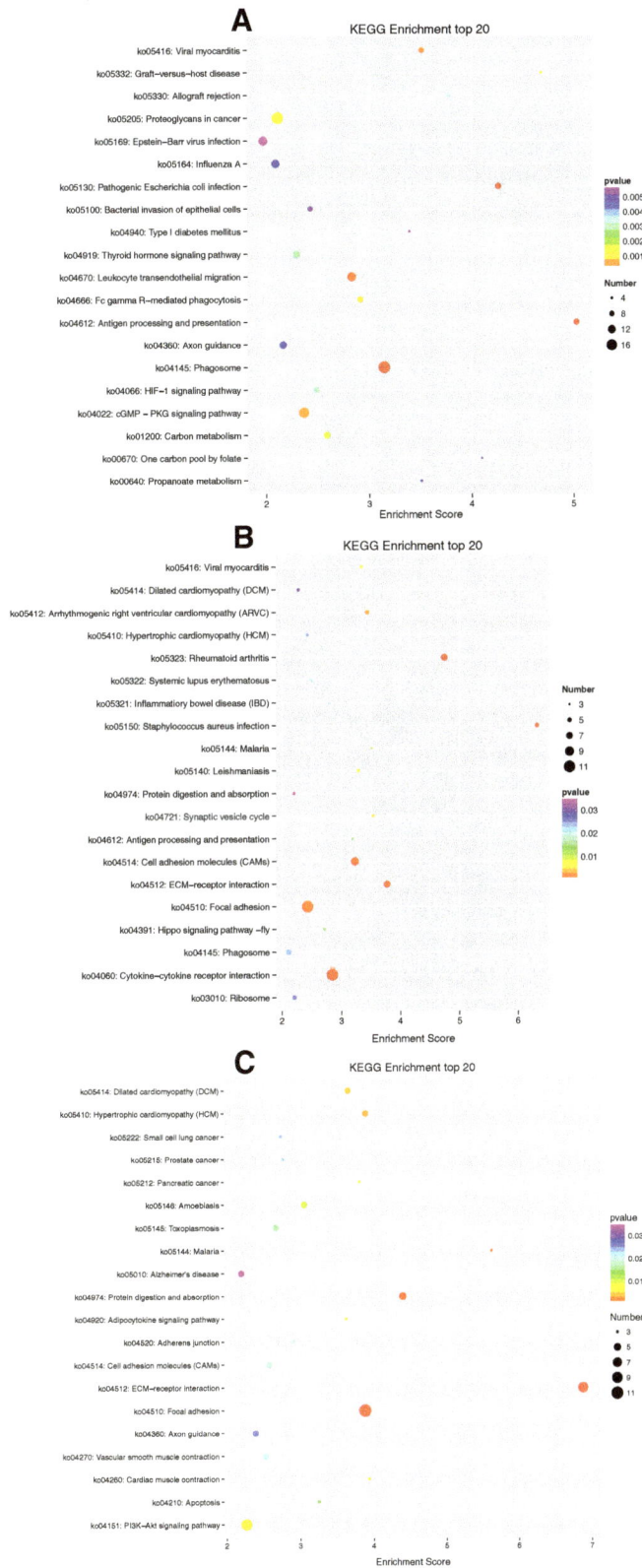

**Figure 3  Top 20 KEGG pathways in CHv infected or CHa vaccinated group. A** KEGG pathways of DEGs expressed in CHv infected group. **B** KEGG pathways of DEGs expressed in CHa vaccinated group. **C** KEGG pathways of DEGs expressed after CHv and CHa infection.

**Table 3　Genes listed involved in multiple cell biological processes after CHv and CHa infection**

| Gene ID | Gene name | Gene description | Source of DEGs |
|---|---|---|---|
| Antigen processing and presentation | | | |
| MHC-1 pathway | | | |
| 101797502 | MHC1 | Major histocompatibility complex, class I | CHv vs control |
| 101797680 | TAP1 | ATP-binding cassette, subfamily B (MDR/TAP), member 2 | CHv vs control |
| 101797091 | TAP2 | ATP-binding cassette, subfamily B (MDR/TAP), member 3 | CHv vs control |
| 101799108 | β2m | Beta-2-microglobulin | CHv vs control and CHa vs control |
| MHC-II pathway | | | |
| 101801019 | LGMN | Legumain | CHv vs control |
| 101803352 | CD74 | CD74 antigen | |
| 101804125 | MHC2 | Major histocompatibility complex, class II | CHv vs control and CHa vs control |
| 101803864 | GILT | Gamma-inducible protein 30 | |
| Cytokine-cytokine receptor interaction | | | |
| 101799854 | IFNGR1 | Interferon gamma receptor 1 | CHv vs control |
| 101794299 | CSF2RB | Cytokine receptor common subunit beta | CHv vs control |
| 101791761 | SF18 | Tumor necrosis factor receptor superfamily member 18 | CHv vs control |
| 101799587 | PDGFRB | Platelet-derived growth factor receptor beta | CHv vs control |
| 101801232 | SF21 | Tumor necrosis factor receptor superfamily member 21 | CHv vs control |
| 101795038 | CX3CL1 | C-X3-C motif chemokine 1 | CHa vs control |
| 101790039 | CCL19 | C–C motif chemokine 19 | CHa vs control |
| 101802287 | TGFB3 | Transforming growth factor beta-3 | CHa vs control |
| 101793182 | CNTFR | Granulocyte–macrophage colony-stimulating factor receptor alpha | CHa vs control |
| 101797327 | FLT1 | FMS-like tyrosine kinase 1 | CHa vs control |
| 101792543 | FLT4 | FMS-like tyrosine kinase 4 | CHa vs control |
| 101795963 | IL22RA2 | Interleukin 22 receptor alpha 2 | CHa vs control |
| 101802521 | IL15 | Interleukin 15 | CHv vs control and CHa vs control |
| 101803777 | TNFSF13B | Tumor necrosis factor ligand superfamily member 13B | CHv vs control and CHa vs control |
| 101797830 | EGFR | Epidermal growth factor receptor | CHv vs control and CHa vs control |
| Apoptosis | | | |
| 101803461 | PIK3CB | Phosphatidylinositol-4,5-bisphosphate 3-kinase catalytic subunit alpha/beta/delta | CHv vs control |
| 101793887 | IL3RB | Cytokine receptor common subunit beta | CHv vs control |
| 101801064 | IKKA | Inhibitor of nuclear factor kappa-B kinase subunit alpha | CHv vs control and CHa vs control |
| 101794069 | CASP6 | Caspase 6 | CHv vs control and CHa vs control |
| Viral invasion | | | |
| Cell surface-related receptor | | | |
| 101796910 | HSPG2 | Heparan sulfate proteoglycan 2 | CHv vs control |
| 101791819 | HS3ST5 | Heparan sulfate glucosamine 3-O-sulfotransferase 5 | CHv vs control |
| Cell cytoskeletal-related protein | | | |
| 101805015 | TUBA1C | Tubulin alpha-1C chain | CHv vs control |
| 101805212 | TUBA1B | Tubulin alpha-1B chain | CHv vs control |
| 101801170 | KIF14 | Kinesin protein KIF14 | CHa vs control |
| 101793497 | ACTA2 | Actin, aortic smooth muscle | CHv vs control |
| 101792376 | ACTG2 | Actin, gamma-enteric smooth muscle | CHv vs control and CHa vs control |
| 101790019 | AFAP1L2 | Actin filament-associated protein 1-like 2 | CHv vs control and CHa vs control |
| 101799368 | MYL9 | Myosin light chain 9 | CHv vs control and CHa vs control |
| 101803563 | MYH11 | Myosin heavy chain 11 | CHa vs control |
| Inner nuclear membrane-related protein | | | |
| 101797969 | LMNA | Lamin A/C | CHv vs control and CHa vs control |

protein segment through participation of the H2-DM chaperone [35]. The MHC II molecules then traffic to the plasma membrane and present virus peptides to CD4$^+$ cells [35]. From our results, extreme diversity of different genes expression of MHC-II pathway has been present in CHv infection group and CHa vaccinated group (Table 3). The expression of genes related to basic composition of MHC-II like CD74 was up-regulated in CHv infected group which means the infection of CHv strain processes the potential to be presented to CD4$^+$ cells and then evoke duck adaptive immune response in 24 hpi. Yet, genes like MHC2 and GILT related to CHa vaccinated group were down-regulated. GILT, a gamma-interferon inducible lysosomal thiol reductase, could catalyze antigenic disulfide bond reduction in endocytosis pathway and this function is essential in MHC-II antigen processing [36]. From our results, we conclude that in order to evade immune response, CHa depressed the expression of GILT and escape the degradation of disulfide bond. It may be an effective way for CHa to avoid identification by CD4$^+$ cells. Meanwhile, we also found that, no matter in CHv infected group or CHa vaccinated group, the expression of Class II Transcriptional Activator (CIITA) gene was down-regulated. Previous works reported that, CIITA is a co-activator and tightly controls expression of all components of MHC-II at the transcriptional level, such as MHC-II and Ii [37]. It means that CIITA plays an important role in MHC-II antigen processing in both CHv and CHa infection.

From this part, we conclude that CHv could be present by MHC-I and MHC-I as well as identified by both CD8$^+$ T cells and CD4$^+$ T cells, and as for CHa, there may be some critical ways to escape the immunosurveillance at 24 h post DPV infection.

## Cytokine–cytokine receptor interaction

Cytokines are soluble extracellular proteins or glycoproteins including chemokines, interferons (IFN), interleukins (IL), lymphokines, and tumor necrosis factors (TNF) [38]. Cytokines play crucial roles in many cell biological processes. They are engaged in humoral and cell-based immune responses, cell growth, differentiation, maturation, death, angiogenesis and homeostasis [38]. Through binding through corresponding cytokines receptors, cytokines transmit signals from outside into inside of cells. In cells, through phosphorylation and dephosphorylation events, signal transduction pathways are activated [38]. In our results, from cytokine–cytokine receptor KEGG pathway, we found that the expression of many important cytokines and cytokine receptors genes were changed in CHv infected or CHa vaccinated group. For example, the expression of IFN-γ receptor IFNGR1, the common receptor CSF2RB of IL3,

IL5 as well as tumor necrosis factors receptor SF18 were depressed after CHv infection. The expression of PDG-FRB genes involved in tyrosine kinase receptors and SF21 related to TNF receptors were increased in CHv infected group. Meanwhile, CX3CL1 and CCL19 chemotactic factor as well as transforming growth factor TGFB3 were up-regulated in CHa vaccinated group. Cytokines receptors including IL-6 receptor CNTFR as well as tyrosine kinase receptors FLT1 and FLT4 were also increased after CHa vaccination. Yet, the expression of IL22 receptor, IL22RA2 was down regulation in CHa vaccination. Furthermore, the expression of IL15 and TNFSF13B were down regulation and epidermal growth factor (EGF) receptor EGFR was up regulation in both CHv and CHa infected group. Some significant genes related to viral immune evasion were picked out and performed detailed illustrations.

Viral invasion of a host cell triggers immune responses and the major protection against viral infection implemented by host is activation of the interferon (IFN)-mediated antiviral pathway. IFNs, one of a family of cytokines, contain two subtypes including type I IFNs (IFN-α and IFN-β) and type II IFN (IFN-γ). IFN-α/β is responsible for the recognition and clearance of virus as the first innate immune defense. IFN-γ is produced by activate T cells and nature kill (NK) cells. It is involved in many biological processes including immunosurveillance and cell-mediated immune response [39]. From our results, we found that the expression of IFN-γ receptor IFNGR1 was down-regulated after CHv infection. It has been reported that Kaposi's sarcoma-associated herpesvirus (KSHV) has been shown to inhibit the function of IFN-γ through depressing the expression of IFNGR1 with the help of K3 and K5 protein [40]. Similarly, another herpesvirus, Epstein–Barr virus (EBV), also block the process of IFN response through down regulation of the IFN-γ receptor gene expression by BZLF1 [41]. It means that just like another herpesvirus, highly virulence DPV CHv strain suppress both cytokines-induced and cell-mediated immunity response through depressing the expression of IFN-γ receptor. It may be an efficient way for CHv to avoid host immune control.

Chemokines are pivotal regulatory factors on the aspects of the accumulation, activation and movement of leukocytes into inflamed cells [38]. CX3CL1 is a cell surface-expressed chemokine and plays a distinct role in several aspects of leukocyte activation and motion during inflammation and viral infection [42]. KSHV encodes CX3CL1 receptor homologs protein US28 to prevent the function of CX3CL1 and then serve the immune evasion purpose [42]. In CHa vaccinated group, CX3CL1 gene was increased in expression. We conclude that CXC3L1 may perform an important role no matter in host immune defense or in viral immune evasion during CHa infection. Further studies need to be done to uncover the exact functions of CXC3L1 in CHa infection.

Nature killing (NK) cells are Innate Lymphoid Cells (ILC) and are capable of killing virus-infected cells in the early stage of infections. IL15, type I cytokines, possesses a pivotal biological activity in stimulating NK cells and controlling various aspects of NK cell immunologic surveillance process [43]. For instance, previous studied reported that IL15 stimulated NK cells cytotoxicity and then severely depress human herpesvirus-6 (HHV-6) expression [44]. This study showed that IL-5 gene expression was reduced after CHv and CHa infection. It means that depression of the expression of IL15 may be an effective way for DPV to evade NK cell immunologic monitor at 24 hpi.

## Apoptosis
Cells infected with viruses would occur apoptosis to protect other cells from infection and reduce production of new virus from these infected cells [45]. Therefore, in order to survive long enough in cells, viruses have evolved apoptotic inhibitory mechanisms. Successful inhibitory mechanisms alter host cell signaling pathways to govern cell survival and the viral life cycle.

Viruses selectively inhibit apoptotic pathways through blocking the synthetic processes such as depressing the synthesis of pro-apoptotic protein like caspases and p53 or the expression of anti-apoptotic protein like Bcl-2 [46, 47]. Furthermore, PI3K-Akt, an important anti-apoptosis signaling pathway, is commonly exploited by viruses to regulate cell survival [48]. Our results showed that the genes expression in PI3K-Akt signaling pathway was changed in CHv infected group (Table 3). It means that PI3K-Akt signaling pathway may be a key mechanism for highly virulence DPV CHv strain to regulate anti-apoptosis.

Phosphatidylinositol 3-kinase (PI3K) phosphorylates the lipid substrate $PtdIns(4,5)P_2$ to $PtdIns(3,4,5)P_3$ on the plasma membrane [49]. The phosphorylated lipid acts as a second messenger to activate Akt protein on plasma membrane. Activated Akt phosphorylates a number of target proteins, including transcription factor like NF-κB and pro-apoptotic protein caspase-9 and then lead to suppression of apoptosis [50]. Previous studied reported that PIK3/Akt pathway is also utilized by herpesvirus to maintain cellular survival and viral replication. For example, herpes simplex virus I (HSV-1) induced the phosphorylation of Akt and glycogen synthase kinase 3 (GSK-3) to regulate apoptosis and viral gene expression [48]. From our results, the PIK3CB gene expression was down-regulated after the infection of CHv. PIK3CB, one of the four catalytic subunits of PI3K, plays an important role in cell

growth [51]. It means that regulating the expression of PIK3CB may be useful for CHv to anti-apoptosis. Furthermore, some other genes were also found related to apoptosis. IKKA, one of subunits of IkB kinase complex (IKK), from our results, was down regulated in both CHv infected group and CHa vaccinated group. The IKKA is necessary for IkB phosphorylation and NF-kB activation [52]. Moreover, the expression of CASP6, apoptosis-related cysteine protease, was also depressed in CHv infected group and CHa vaccinated group [53]. It means that IKKA and CASP6 genes play a critical role in modulating cell apoptosis in highly virulence CHv infected group and attenuated CHa vaccinated group.

## Viral invasion
With no autonomous metabolic and motile capacity, viruses must rely on host cells to achieve genome replication, protein synthesis and structural assembling [54]. In order to finish above processes, viruses must suffer from four steps of cell entry processes that is adsorption to the cell surface, penetration, intracellular transport and egress from nucleus [55].

Adsorption to the cell surface is regarded as a prelude to viral infection and cell surface specific structures serve as viral binding locus. Heparan sulfate proteoglycans (HSPGs) are glycoproteins and participate many biological systems, and one of the important roles for HSPGs is adsorption receptors and facilitates viruses concentrated on the cell surface. HSPGs are the first receptor for many herpes viruses entry process, such as HSV, varicella zoster virus (VZV) and pseudorabies virus (PRV), to attach around host cell surface through their envelope glycoproteins like gB and/or gC [56, 57]. However, the types of adsorption receptors of DPV on duck cells surface and the specific interactive envelope proteins of DPV have not been reported in recent years. In our results, the different gene expression of HSPG2 gene was detected in CHv infected ducks indicating that HSPG perhaps plays an important role in the cell surface adsorption process of DPV (Table 3). Interestingly, although Yong reported that DPV glycoproteins gC played an important role in the initial adsorption on chicken embryo fibroblasts (CEF) cell surface, however, they detected that HSPGs was not interactive sites to DPV gC [58]. Therefore, it is necessary to perform further experiments to explore the functions of HSPGs on the process of DPV entry and the types of DPV glycoprotein interacted with HSPGs.

The next necessary step for enveloped viral entry is penetration reaction and this membrane fusion process is promoted by cues of specific envelope-membrane receptor bindings [54]. Specific cellular receptors participated in penetration process of herpes virus, such as HSV, fall into three classes, and one of important receptors are specific sites in heparan sulphate catalyzed by certain heparan sulfate glucosamine 3-O-sulfotransferase (HS3ST) [59]. Nevertheless, so far there are still no relevant reports paid attention on the types of envelope-membrane binding receptors when ducks infected by DPV. In our study, we detected that the expression of HS3ST genes HS3ST5 was changed in CHv infected ducks (Table 3). It suggests that for highly virulence strain of DPV, HS3ST protein may exercise as the same functions as other herpes virus.

In order to finish viral replication, assembly and maturation, intracellular complexes of virus utilize host intracellular cytoskeletal components and move from cell periphery to synthesis sites [54]. After assembly and maturation in cell, viral particles move from cell center to the cell membrane [54, 60]. Microtubules and actins, two important parts of cell cytoskeleton, play significant roles in herpesvirus transport within cells [61]. For example, microtubules provide long-distance transport for HSV with the assistance of their motor protein, kinesin. Our results showed that the expression of two types of alpha-tubulin (TUBA1C and TUBA1B) gene, whose products are basic components of microtubules, was changed in CHv infected ducks. Notably, the expression of kinesin-related genes were also found changed in CHa vaccinated ducks. N-type kinesin, one of a microtubules-binding plus-end-directed motors, could transport viral particles from their replication and transcription sites to cell membrane [62]. KIF1A, one of a member of N-types of kinesins, plays a key role in HSV transport, and its co-localization with herpes simplex virus II (HSV-2) UL56 protein were also reported [61]. In our study, a N-types kinesin gene KIF14 was detected different expression in CHa infected ducks (Table 3). It suggests that CHa strain could rely on important motors of microtubules to finish its cellular long-distance movement just like other herpes virus. In addition to microtubules, another medium, actin filament, is essential for herpesvirus to finish short-range transport [61]. It also contains fast-growing plus-ends and slow-growing minus-ends to link cell center and cell surface [61]. Myosin is a crucial motor to mediate the movement of HSV along actin filaments [61]. Our results also found the expression of some actin-related genes and myosin-related genes to give expression changes in both CHv and CHa infected duck (Table 3), indicating that short-distance transport is an important way to complete intercellular movement process of DPV and some relevant proteins are also used to finish this process.

Although the mechanisms by which DPV interacts with cell surface receptor to achieve viral adsorption, membrane fusion and motors have not been clearly studied, several significant genes related to DPV invasion were detected in this results and it may provide an initial view and supply a foundational data support for future experimental researches in DPV invasion aspect.

## Abbreviations

DPV: duck plague virus; CHv: DPV Chinese virulent strain; CHa: attenuated DPV vaccines; HSV: herpes simplex virus; BHV-1: bovine herpes virus; HCMV: human cytomegalovirus; KSHV: Kaposi's sarcoma-associated herpesvirus; EBV: Epstein–Barr virus; HHV-6: human herpesvirus-6; VZV: varicella zoster virus; PRV: pseudorabies virus; DEGs: differentially expressed genes; GO: gene ontology; BP: biological proces; CC: cellular component; MF: molecular function; CTLs: cytotoxic T lymphocytes; ER: endoplasmic reticulum; $\beta_2m$: $\beta_2$-microglobulin; TAP: transporter associated with Antigen Processing; APCs: antigen presenting cells; MIIC: MHC class II compartment; APE: asparaginyl endopeptidase; CLIP: class II-associated Ii peptide; CIITA: class II transcriptional activator; IFN: interferon; IL: interleukin; TNF: tumor necrosis factors; EGF: epidermal growth factor; ILC: innate lymphoid cell; PI3K: phosphatidylinositol 3-kinase; GSK-3: glycogen synthase kinase 3; HS3ST: heparan sulfate glucosamine 3-O-sulfotransferase.

## Competing interests

The authors declare that they have no competing interests.

## Authors' contributions

AC and MW conceived and designed the experiments; TL performed the experiments; TL, RJ, QY, YW, KS, DZ, SC, ML, XZ and XC analyzed the data and contributed analysis tools; TL wrote the paper. All authors read and approved the final manuscript.

## Acknowledgements

This research was supported by the National Key Research and Development Program of China (2016YFD0500800), China Agricultural Research System (CARS-42-17) and Special Fund for Key Laboratory of Animal Disease and Human Health of Sichuan Province (2016JPT0004).

## Animal ethics

The animal studies were approved by Institutional Animal Care and Use Committee of Sichuan Agricultural University, Sichuan, China and followed the National Institutes of Health guidelines for the performance of animal experiments.

## Author details

[1] Avian Disease Research Center, College of Veterinary Medicine, Sichuan Agricultural University, Wenjiang, Chengdu 611130, People's Republic of China. [2] Institute of Preventive Veterinary Medicine, Sichuan Agricultural University, Wenjiang, Chengdu 611130, People's Republic of China. [3] Key Laboratory of Animal Disease and Human Health of Sichuan Province, Wenjiang, Chengdu 611130, People's Republic of China.

## References

1. Converse KA, Kidd GA (2001) Duck plague epizootics in the United States, 1967-1995. J Wildl Dis 37:347–357
2. Hansen WR (2008) Duck virus enteritis. In: Gough RE (ed) Duck plague, vol 4. Blackwell Publishing Professional, Hoboken

3.  Wang G, Qu Y, Wang F, Hu D, Liu L, Li N, Yue R, Li C, Liu S (2013) The comprehensive diagnosis and prevention of duck plague in northwest Shandong province of China. Poult Sci 92:2892–2898

4.  Roizmann B, Desrosiers R, Fleckenstein B, Lopez C, Minson A, Studdert M (1992) The family Herpesviridae: an update. Arch Virol 123:425–449

5.  Dhama K, Kumar N, Saminathan M, Tiwari R, Karthik K, Kumar MA, Palanivelu M, Shabbir MZ, Malik YS, Singh RK (2017) Duck virus enteritis (duck plague)—a comprehensive update. Vet Q 37:57–80

6.  Qi X, Yang X, Cheng A, Wang M, Guo Y, Jia R (2009) Replication kinetics of duck virus enteritis vaccine virus in ducklings immunized by the mucosal or systemic route using real-time quantitative PCR. Res Vet Sci 86:63–67

7.  Qi X, Yang X, Cheng A, Wang M, Zhu D, Jia R, Luo Q, Chen X (2009) Intestinal mucosal immune response against virulent duck enteritis virus infection in ducklings. Res Vet Sci 87:218–225

8.  Guo Y, Shen C, Cheng A, Wang M, Zhang N, Chen S, Zhou Y (2009) Anatid herpesvirus 1 CH virulent strain induces syncytium and apoptosis in duck embryo fibroblast cultures. Vet Microbiol 138:258

9.  Yang X, Qi X, Cheng A, Wang M, Zhu D, Jia R, Chen X (2010) Intestinal mucosal immune response in ducklings following oral immunisation with an attenuated duck enteritis virus vaccine. Vet J 185:199–203

10. Cai MS, Cheng AC, Wang MS, Chen WP, Zhang X, Zheng SX, Pu Y, Lou KP, Zhang Y, Sun L et al (2010) Characterization of the duck plague virus UL35 gene. Intervirology 53:408–416

11. Chang H, Cheng A, Wang M, Zhu D, Jia R, Liu F, Chen Z, Luo Q, Chen X, Zhou Y (2010) Cloning, expression and characterization of gE protein of duck plague virus. Virol J 7:120

12. Li L, Cheng A, Wang M, Xiang J, Yang X, Zhang S, Zhu D, Jia R, Luo Q, Zhou Y (2011) Expression and characterization of duck enteritis virus gI gene. Virol J 8:1–9

13. Lian B, Xu C, Cheng A, Wang M, Zhu D, Luo Q, Jia R, Bi F, Chen Z, Zhou Y, Yang Z, Chen X (2010) Identification and characterization of duck plague virus glycoprotein C gene and gene product. Virol J 7:1–11

14. Dai B, Cheng A, Wang M (2012) Bioinformatics Analysis and characteristics of UL19 protein of duck plague virus. Appl Mech Mater 236–237:55–60

15. He Q, Yang Q, Cheng A, Wang M, Xiang J, Zhu D, Jia R, Luo Q, Chen Z, Zhou Y, Chen X (2011) Expression and characterization of UL16 gene from duck enteritis virus. Virol J 8:413

16. Shen CJ, Cheng AC, Wang MS, Guo YF, Zhao LC, Wen M, Xie W, Xin HY, Zhu DK (2009) Identification and characterization of the duck enteritis virus UL51 gene. Arch Virol 154:1061–1069

17. Wu Y, Cheng A, Wang M, Yang Q, Zhu D, Jia R, Chen S, Zhou Y, Wang X, Chen X (2012) Complete genomic sequence of Chinese virulent duck enteritis virus. J Virol 86:5965

18. Shawky S, Schat KA (2002) Latency sites and reactivation of duck enteritis virus. Avian Dis 46:308–313

19. Guiping Y, Anchun C, Mingshu W, Xiaoying H, Yi Z, Fei L (2007) Preliminary study on duck enteritis virus-induced lymphocyte apoptosis in vivo. Avian Dis 51:546–549

20. Tawar RG, Schuster C, Baumert TF (2016) HCV receptors and virus entry. In: Miyamura T, Lemon S, Walker C, Wakita T (eds) Hepatitis C virus, I. Springer, Tokyo, pp 81–103

21. Jardetzky TS, Lamb RA (2014) Activation of paramyxovirus membrane fusion and virus entry. Curr Opin Virol 5:24–33

22. Vanderlinden E, Naesens L (2013) Emerging antiviral strategies to interfere with influenza virus entry. Med Res Rev 34:301–339

23. Perelygina L, Patrusheva I, Vasireddi M, Brock N, Hilliard J (2015) B virus (Macacine herpesvirus 1) glycoprotein D is functional but dispensable for virus entry into macaque and Human skin cells. J Virol 89:5515–5524

24. Chesnokova LS, Ahuja MK, Hutt-Fletcher LM (2014) Epstein–Barr virus glycoprotein gB and gH/gL can mediate fusion and entry in trans, and heat can act as a partial surrogate for gH/gL and trigger a conformational change in gB. J Virol 88:12193–12201

25. Horst D, Verweij MC, Davison AJ, Ressing ME, Wiertz EJ (2011) Viral evasion of T cell immunity: ancient mechanisms offering new applications. Curr Opin Immunol 23:96–103

26. Reits E, Griekspoor A, Neijssen J, Groothuis T, Jalink K, Veelen PV, Janssen H, Calafat J, Drijfhout JW, Neefjes J (2003) Peptide diffusion, protection, and degradation in nuclear and cytoplasmic compartments before antigen presentation by MHC Class I. Immunity 18:97–108

27. Ardeniz Ö, Unger S, Onay H, Ammann S, Keck C, Cianga C, Gerçeker B, Martin B, Fuchs I, Salzer U et al (2015) β2-Microglobulin deficiency causes a complex immunodeficiency of the innate and adaptive immune system. J Allergy Clin Immunol 136:392–401

28. Neefjes J, Jongsma ML, Paul P, Bakke O (2011) Towards a systems understanding of MHC class I and MHC class II antigen presentation. Nat Rev Immunol 11:823–836

29. Powers CJ, Früh K (2008) Signal peptide-dependent inhibition of MHC class I heavy chain translation by rhesus cytomegalovirus. PLoS Pathog 4:e1000150

30. Koppers-Lalic D, Rijsewijk FA, Verschuren SB, van Gaans-Van den Brink JA, Neisig A, Ressing ME, Neefjes J, Wiertz EJ (2001) The UL41-encoded virion host shutoff (vhs) protein and vhs-independent mechanisms are responsible for down-regulation of MHC class I molecules by bovine herpesvirus 1. J Gen Virol 82:2071–2081

31. Park B, Spooner E, Houser BL, Strominger JL, Ploegh HL (2010) The HCMV membrane glycoprotein US10 selectively targets HLA-G for degradation. J Exp Med 207:2033–2041

32. Cresswell P, Ackerman AL, Giodini A, Peaper DR, Wearsch PA (2005) Mechanisms of MHC class I-restricted antigen processing and cross-presentation. Immunol Rev 207:145–157

33. Paul P, van den Hoorn T, Jongsma ML, Bakker MJ, Hengeveld R, Janssen L, Cresswell P, Egan DA, van Ham M, Ten Brinke A, Ovaa H, Beijersbergen RL, Kuijl C, Neefjes J (2011) A genome-wide multidimensional RNAi screen reveals pathways controlling MHC class II antigen presentation. Cell 145:268–283

34. Cresswell P, Roche PA (2014) Invariant chain-MHC class II complexes: always odd and never invariant. Immunol Cell Biol 92:471–472

35. Kenneth M, Casey W (2017) Janeway's immunobiology. Garland Science. http://www.garlandscience.com/product/isbn/9780815344452 ?fromSearchResults=fromSearchResults, https://scholar.google.com/ scholar?hl=zh-CN&q=Janeway%27s+Immunobiology+&btnG=&lr=. Accessed 28 Mar 2017

36. Huang WS, Duan LP, Huang B, Zhou LH, Liang Y, Tu CL, Zhang FF, Nie P, Wang T (2015) Identification of three IFN-γ inducible lysosomal thiol reductase (GILT)-like genes in mud crab Scylla paramamosain with distinct gene organizations and patterns of expression. Gene 570:78–88

37. Reith W, Leibundgutlandmann S, Waldburger JM (2005) Regulation of MHC class II gene expression by the class II transactivator. Nat Rev Immunol 5:793–806

38. Turner MD, Nedjai B, Hurst T, Pennington DJ (2014) Cytokines and chemokines: at the crossroads of cell signalling and inflammatory disease. Biochim Biophys Acta 1843:2563–2582

39. Pestka S, Krause CD, Walter MR (2004) Interferons, interferon-like cytokines, and their receptors. Immunol Rev 202:8–32

40. Li Q, Means R, Lang S, Jung JU (2007) Downregulation of gamma interferon receptor 1 by Kaposi's sarcoma-associated herpesvirus K3 and K5. J Virol 81:2117–2127

41. Morrison TE, Mauser A, Wong A, Ting JP, Kenney SC (2001) Inhibition of IFN-gamma signaling by an Epstein–Barr virus immediate-early protein. Immunity 15:787–799

42. Mclean KA, Holst PJ, Martini L, Schwartz TW, Rosenkilde MM (2004) Similar activation of signal transduction pathways by the herpesvirus-encoded chemokine receptors US28 and ORF74. Virology 325:241–251

43. Marçais A, Cherfils-Vicini J, Viant C, Degouve S, Viel S, Fenis A, Rabilloud J, Mayol K, Tavares A, Bienvenu J, Gangloff YG, Gilson E, Vivier E, Walzer T (2014) The metabolic checkpoint kinase mTOR is essential for IL-15 signaling during the development and activation of NK cells. Nat Immunol 15:749–757

44. Arena A, Merendino RA, Bonina L, Iannello D, Stassi G, Mastroeni P (2004) Role of IL-15 on monocytic resistance to human herpesvirus 6 infection. New Microbiol 23:105–112

45. Goodkin ML, Morton ER, Blaho JA (2015) Herpes simplex virus infection and apoptosis. Int Rev Immunol 23:141–172

46. Maruzuru Y, Koyanagi N, Takemura N, Uematsu S, Matsubara D, Suzuki Y, Arii J, Kato A, Kawaguchi Y (2016) p53 is a host cell regulator during herpes simplex encephalitis. J Virol 90:6738–6745

47. Kvansakul M, Hinds MG (2015) The Bcl-2 family: structures, interactions and targets for drug discovery. Apoptosis 20:136–150

48. Hsu MJ, Wu CY, Chiang HH, Lai YL, Hung SL (2010) PI3K/Akt signaling mediated apoptosis blockage and viral gene expression in oral epithelial cells during herpes simplex virus infection. Virus Res 153:36–43

49. Eramo MJ, Mitchell CA (2016) Regulation of PtdIns(3,4,5)P3/Akt signalling by inositol polyphosphate 5-phosphatases. Biochem Soc Trans 44:240–252

50. Cooray S (2004) The pivotal role of phosphatidylinositol 3-kinase-Akt signal transduction in virus survival. J Gen Virol 85:1065–1076

51. Lin Z, Zhou P, von Gise A, Gu F, Ma Q, Chen J, Guo H, van Gorp PR, Wang DZ, Pu WT (2014) Pi3kcb links Hippo-YAP and PI3K-AKT signaling pathways to promote cardiomyocyte proliferation and survival. Circ Res 116:35–45

52. Hinz M, Scheidereit C (2014) The IκB kinase complex in NF-κB regulation and beyond. EMBO Rep 15:46–61

53. Wu H, Che X, Zheng Q, Wu A, Pan K, Shao A, Wu Q, Zhang J, Hong Y (2014) Caspases: a molecular switch node in the crosstalk between autophagy and apoptosis. Int J Biol Sci 10:1072–1083

54. Marsh M, Helenius A (2006) Virus entry: open sesame. Cell 124:729–740

55. Greber UF, Way M (2006) A superhighway to virus infection. Cell 124:741–754

56. Sarrazin S, Lamanna WC, Esko JD (2011) Heparan sulfate proteoglycans. Cold Spring Harb Perspect Biol 3:pii:a004952

57. Rue CA, Ryan P (2002) Characterization of pseudorabies virus glycoprotein C attachment to heparan sulfate proteoglycans. J Gen Virol 83:301–309

58. Hu Y, Liu X, Zou Z, Jin M (2013) Glycoprotein C plays a role in the adsorption of duck enteritis virus to chicken embryo fibroblasts cells and in infectivity. Virus Res 174:1–7

59. Spear PG (2004) Herpes simplex virus: receptors and ligands for cell entry. Cell Microbiol 6:401–410

60. Taylor MP, Koyuncu OO, Enquist LW (2011) Subversion of the actin cytoskeleton during viral infection. Nat Rev Microbiol 9:427–439

61. Lyman MG, Enquist LW (2009) Herpesvirus interactions with the host cytoskeleton. J Virol 83:2058–2066

62. Dodding MP, Way M (2011) Coupling viruses to dynein and kinesin-1. EMBO J 30:3527–3539

# 8

# Neutralizing immune responses induced by oligomeric H5N1-hemagglutinins from plants

Hoang Trong Phan[1,2], Thuong Thi Ho[1,2], Ha Hoang Chu[2], Trang Huyen Vu[2], Ulrike Gresch[1] and Udo Conrad[1*]

## Abstract

Plant-based transient expression is an alternative platform to produce hemagglutinin-based subunit vaccines. This production system provides not only fast and effective response in the context of a pandemic but also enables the supply of big volume vaccines at low cost. Crude plant extracts containing influenza hemagglutinin are considered to use as vaccine sources because of avoidance of related purification steps resulting in low cost production allowing veterinary applications. Highly immunogenic influenza hemagglutinins are urgently required to meet these pre-conditions. Here, we present a new and innovative way to generate functional H5 oligomers from avian flu hemagglutinin in planta by the specific interaction of S·Tag and S·Protein. A S·Tag was fused to H5 trimers and this construct was transiently co-expressed in planta with S·Protein-TPs which was multimerized by disulfide bonds via cysteine residues in tailpiece sequences (TP) of IgM antibody. Multimerized S·Protein-TPs serve as bridges/molecular docks to combine S·Tag-fused hemagglutinin trimers to form very large hemagglutinin H5 oligomers. H5 oligomers in the plant crude extract were highly active in hemagglutination resulting in high titers. Immunization of mice with two doses of plant crude extracts containing H5 oligomers after storage for 1 week at 4 °C caused strong immune responses and induced neutralizing specific humoral immune responses in mice. These results allow for the development of cheap influenza vaccines for veterinary application in future.

## Introduction

Influenza A viruses, negative-stranded enveloped orthomyxoviruses, are among the most serious respiratory pathogens. They cause severe and potentially fatal illnesses [1]. Highly pathogenic avian flu influenza viruses are expected to cause the next global pandemic threat due to their relative easy spread by avian hosts and their ability to directly infect humans [2]. During several H5N1 outbreaks, very large direct and indirect impacts on poultry and tourist industries in South-East Asia were observed [3]. Recently, highly pathogenic avian influenza viruses (HPAI) A (H5N8) caused outbreaks in South Korea, China and Japan and were actually reported in many European countries as well as in the US and Canada (for an review, see [4]). Therefore, the development of an effective and cheap vaccination strategy to protect poultry is necessary. This should include high efficacy of the vaccine, easy and sure production strategies and an efficient way to handle distribution and application. Here, subunit vaccines from plants, which have the general advantages of low production cost, ease of scale up, low infrastructure cost, high stability and long shelf life are in the focus [5]. Transient expression in tobacco plants has been developed as a very fast and efficient method to produce therapeutic proteins in plants (for a review, see [6]). A recently developed strategy is the production of virus-like particle (VLP)-based vaccines in the tobacco species *N. benthamiana*, by transient expression and downstream processing steps that include several filtrations, diafiltrations, continuous flow centrifugations and tangential flow filtration, or, alternatively, chromatographic methods [7, 8]. The production of VLP's is accompanied by several constraints such as high down-stream cost and/or low expression levels. We produced trimeric H5

*Correspondence: conradu@ipk-gatersleben.de
[1] Leibniz Institute of Plant Genetics and Crop Plant Research (IPK), Gatersleben, Germany
Full list of author information is available at the end of the article

hemagglutinins in the endoplasmic reticulum of plant leaf cells. An artificially designed trimerization domain (GCN4-pII, [9]) was used to achieve stable trimers of H5 hemagglutinins from plants [10]. The purified trimers were shown to be active in a hemagglutination assay and also induced neutralizing humoral immune responses as shown by mouse immunization and hemagglutination inhibition assays. We also developed a suitable cheap and efficient purification system from plant extracts by using ELPylation [11].

In the current article we wanted to check, if a further increase of the size of H5 multimers could improve the induction of immune responses. Because hemagglutinin forms trimers in its' native structure on the surface of viruses we planned to keep the trimers as a basic structure of the oligomers. Further oligomerization should be caused by S·Tag–S·Protein interaction. Bovine pancreatic ribonuclease A, 124 amino acids in length, is cleaved by the protease subtilisin. The cleavage product consists of two tightly associated fragments: S-peptide (residues 1–20) and S·Protein (residues 21–124). Only residues 1–15 of S-peptide were found to be necessary to complex specifically with S·Protein. This shorter fragment is named as "S15" or the "S·Tag" sequence [12]. High-affinity interaction between S·Protein and S·Tag of bovine pancreatic ribonuclease A was recently developed as target for protein purification [12] or for drug delivery [13]. We applied this technology to generate H5 oligomers. To achieve this goal, a S·Tag was fused to H5 trimers and this construct was transiently co-expressed with different multimeric variants of S·Protein in planta.

These variants are based on different structures that support the multimerization of S·Protein, as GCN4 (dimerization), GCN4-pII (trimerization) [9] and tailpiece (TP) from IgM [14] (dimerization, Figure 1). Multimerized S·Proteins serve now as bridges/molecular docks to combine S·Tag-fused hemagglutinin trimers to form hemagglutinin oligomers (Figure 1). Furthermore, we wanted to proof, if neutralizing immune responses could also be achieved by immunization with plant crude extracts, thus minimizing the down-stream cost. Enlargement of immunogenic trimers to oligomers was successfully proven to enhance immunogenicity by inducing neutralizing antibodies. Here we showed that crude plant extracts containing H5 oligomers could induce specific and strong immune responses against H5 hemagglutinin in mice.

## Materials and methods
### Construction of plant expression vectors

The DNA sequences corresponding to aa 2–564 of the hemagglutinin of A/duck/Viet Nam/TG24-01/2005 (H5N1) strain and aa 21–124 of S·Protein (UniProtKB

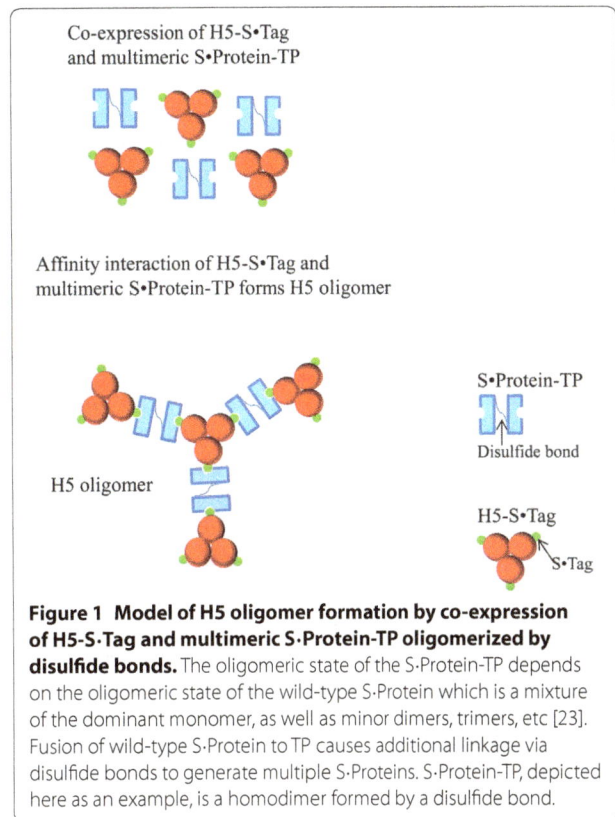

Figure 1 **Model of H5 oligomer formation by co-expression of H5-S·Tag and multimeric S·Protein-TP oligomerized by disulfide bonds.** The oligomeric state of the S·Protein-TP depends on the oligomeric state of the wild-type S·Protein which is a mixture of the dominant monomer, as well as minor dimers, trimers, etc [23]. Fusion of wild-type S·Protein to TP causes additional linkage via disulfide bonds to generate multiple S·Proteins. S·Protein-TP, depicted here as an example, is a homodimer formed by a disulfide bond.

Accession Numbers: Q14RX0 and P61823, respectively) were synthesized commercially (GENECUST EUROPE, Luxembourg) and provided in pUC57 vectors designated pUC57-H5TG and pUC57-S·Protein. To express the wild-type S·Protein, the DNA sequence coding for S·Protein was cloned into pRTRA-35S-H5pII [10] at the BamHI and NotI sites to form a recombinant vector designated pRTRA-S·Protein. To multimerize S·Protein, DNA sequences coding for S·Protein were introduced into pRTRA vectors, which contain trimerization (GCN4-pII) or dimerization (GCN4 wild-type) domains [9], or a tail piece of mouse IgM antibody that forms disulfide bonds via its cysteine residues; the resulting vectors were pRTRA-His-S·Protein-GCN4pII, pRTRA-His-S·Protein-GCN4wt, and pRTRA-S·Protein-TP, which were used for expression of S·Protein-pII, S·Protein-GCN4, S·Protein-TP, respectively (Figure 2). An S·Tag sequence was inserted into pRTRA-H5TG-GCNpII to produce the pRTRA-H5TG-GCNpII-S·Tag vector, which was used for expression of trimeric H5-S·Tag. Five expression cassettes constructed in pRTRA vectors (pRTRA-S·Protein, pRTRA-His-S·Protein-GCN4wt, pRTRA-His-S·Protein-GCN4pII, pRTRA-S·Protein-TP, pRTRA-H5TG-GCNpII-S·Tag) (Figure 2) were cloned into the pCB301 shuttle vector [15] at HindIII restriction sites. The pCB301 shuttle vectors were introduced into the *Agrobacterium* pGV2260 strain.

### *Agrobacterium* infiltration

Agrobacterium infiltration for expression of recombinant proteins was described in detail by Phan and Conrad, 2016 [16], and is briefly described here. *Agrobacteria* harboring the shuttle vectors for the expression of recombinant proteins (Figure 2) and the plant vector for expression of HcPro, which is a suppressor of gene silencing that has been found to enhance the expression levels of recombinant proteins in plant cells [17, 18] were precultivated separately in LB medium with 50 µg/mL kanamycin, 50 µg/mL carbenicillin and 50 µg/mL rifampicin overnight at 28 °C and 140 rpm. The precultures were added to a new LB culture containing the appropriate antibiotics. After 24 h of cultivation, bacteria were harvested by centrifugation (4000*g*, 30 min, 4 °C) and resuspended in infiltration buffer (10 mM 2-(N-morpholino) ethanesulfonic acid (MES), 10 mM MgSO4, pH 5.6). *Agrobacteria* harboring the shuttle vector for the expression of recombinant protein and the plant vector for the expression of HcPro were combined and diluted in infiltration buffer to a final OD600 of 1.0. *N. benthamiana*

plants (6–8 weeks old) were infiltrated by completely submerging each plant in an *Agrobacterium*-containing cup standing inside a desiccator. Vacuum was applied for 2 min and then quickly released. The plants were then placed in the greenhouse at 21 °C, 16 h light per day. Five days after infiltration, leaf samples were harvested and stored at −80 °C. Two agrobacterial strains were mixed and combined with HcPro strain to co-express H5-S·Tag and S·Protein variants. *Agrobacteria* were then diluted in the infiltration buffer, and were used for vacuum infiltration described above.

### Total soluble protein extraction

Five days after vacuum infiltration of *Agrobacterium*, 20 g of leaf samples were harvested, ground in liquid nitrogen and homogenized in 60 mL of PBS buffer (pH 7.4) using a commercial blender. The extracts were clarified by centrifugation (16 200 *g*, 30 min, 4 °C). Total soluble protein contents of clear plant extracts were determined by Bradford assay [19].

Protein concentrations of all plant extracts were diluted to 3 µg/µL. A H5-S·Tag plant extract was then combined with a single S·Protein variant plant extract in equal volume. The mixtures were rotated at 4 °C for 1 h and used

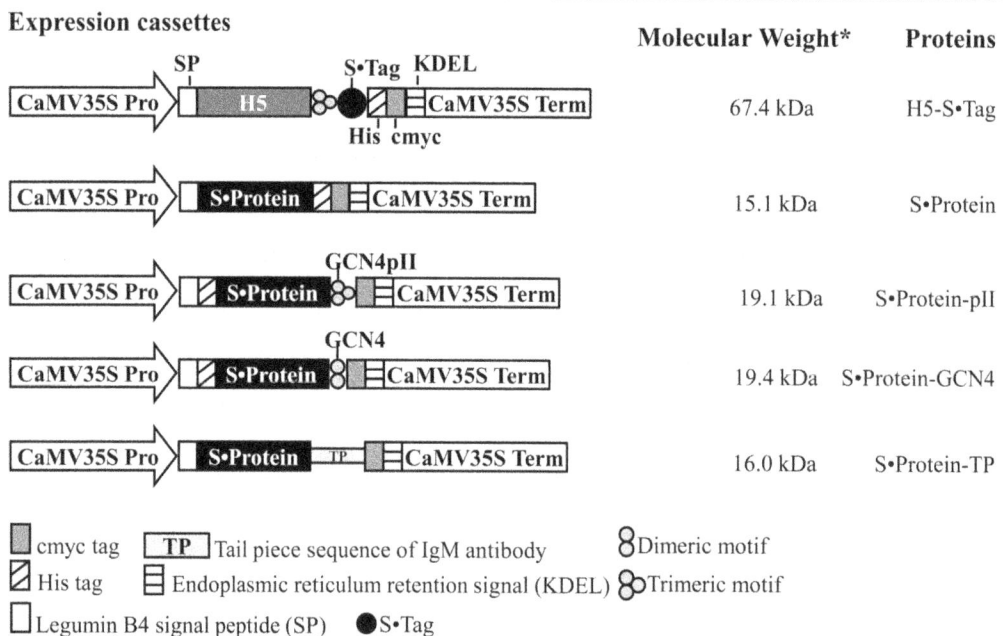

**Figure 2 Expression cassettes for the in planta production of H5-S·Tag and S·Protein fusion proteins.** The ectodomain of hemagglutinin (H5) was trimerized by c-terminal fusion of trimeric motif (GCN4pII) [10]. While wild-type S·Protein was either expressed alone or multimerized by fusion with different oligomeric motifs, such as trimerization (GCN4-pII, S·Protein-pII) and dimerization (GCN4 wild-type, S·Protein-GCN4) domains [9], and a mouse tailpiece (TP) element of mouse IgM (S·Protein-TP). Each of recombinant proteins was fused to a c-myc tag to allow for downstream detection by Western blot, a His tag (except for S·Protein-TP) to facilitate their purification by IMAC. The legumine B4 signal peptide and the KDEL motif were used to promote transgene products retention in the endoplasmic reticulum. CaMV35S Pro: cauliflower mosaic virus 35S ubiquitous promoter; CaMV 35S Term: cauliflower mosaic virus 35S terminator; Asterisk: the molecular weight of proteins was calculated for unglycosylated monomers.

for hemagglutination assay. H5 oligomer or H5-S·Tag in crude plant extracts was semi-quantified by Western blotting. A series of known concentrations of the anti TNFα-nanobody-ELP standard protein [20] was used to construct blot signal intensities. Hemagglutinin contents in the plant crude extracts were determined by comparing their blot signal intensities and blot signal intensities of the standard protein.

### SDS-PAGE and Western blotting

Extracted plant proteins, purified proteins, or an anti TNFα-nanobody-ELP standard protein [20] were separated by reducing SDS-PAGE (10% polyacrylamide) and then electrotransferred to nitrocellulose membranes. The Western blotting procedure was carried out using monoclonal anti-c-myc antibodies following the protocol described by Gahrtz and Conrad [21]. Sheep anti-mouse IgG, horseradish peroxidase-linked whole antibody was used as the secondary antibody (secondary antibodies, GE Healthcare UK limited, Little Chalfont Buckinghamshire, UK) followed by enhanced chemiluminescence-based detection (ECL). A total of 10 ng of the IMAC and SEC purified hemagglutinin was separated by reducing SDS-PAGE (10% polyacrylamide) and electrotransferred to nitrocellulose membranes. To detect H5-specific mouse antibodies, ten mouse sera from each group were mixed, and the membranes were incubated with the respective mixtures (200 times dilution). Specific signals were detected as described above.

### Protein purification by IMAC

Five days after vacuum infiltration of *Agrobacterium*, leaf samples were harvested, frozen in liquid nitrogen and homogenized using a commercial blender. Total proteins were extracted in 50 mM Tris buffer (pH 8.0). The extracts were clarified by centrifugation (75 600 $g$, 30 min, 4 °C) and then filtrated through paper filters. The clarified extracts were mixed with Ni–NTA agarose resin that had been washed twice with water beforehand. After mixing for 30 min at 4 °C, the mixture was added to a chromatography column. Thereafter, the column was extensively washed (50 mM $NaH_2PO_4$, 300 mM NaCl, 30 mM imidazole, pH 8.0). Recombinant proteins were then eluted from the column with elution buffer (50 mM $NaH_2PO_4$, 300 mM NaCl, 125 mM Imidazole, pH 8.0), put into dialysis bags, concentrated in PEG 6000 and dialyzed against PBS.

### Purification of H5 oligomer using *Galanthus nivalis* (GLN)-linked agarose

Frozen leaf samples (40 g) were homogenized in liquid nitrogen. Total soluble proteins were extracted in PBS (137 mM NaCl, 2.7 mM KCl, 10 mM $Na_2HPO_4$, 1.8 mM $KH_2PO_4$, pH 7.5). The extract was centrifuged twice

(75 600 $g$, 30 min, 4 °C) and mixed with 10 mL of GLN resin that had been washed twice with water and once with PBS. After mixing at 4 °C for 30 min, the mixture was applied to a chromatography column. Thereafter, the column was washed two times with 30 mL PBS. The recombinant protein was then eluted from the column with 10 mL elution buffer (137 mM NaCl, 2.7 mM KCl, 10 mM $Na_2HPO_4$, 1.8 mM $KH_2PO_4$, 200 mM α-methyl mannoside, pH 7.4). The protein solution was dialyzed against PBS at 4 °C overnight and concentrated using PEG 6000. The protein products were loaded on Superose™ 6 increase 10/300GL.

### Size exclusion chromatography

A total of 34 μg protein/0.5 mL of purified H5 oligomers and H5-S·Tag, respectively, were loaded onto a Superose™ 6 increase 10/300GL column (GE Healthcare). The high molecular weight kit contains standard proteins with molecular weights in the range of 44–2000 kDa, which were loaded onto the column to estimate the molecular weight of the proteins of interest. Five hundred microliters per fraction were collected for hemagglutination test and Western blot analysis.

For ELISA, affinity-purified trimeric hemagglutinin was used as an antigen for the plate coating and was further purified via the Superose™ 6 increase 10/300GL column with starting concentrations of 1.25 mg in 0.5 mL.

### Mouse immunization

The hemagglutinin contents (H5 oligomer and H5-S·Tag) in plant extracts were semi-quantified by Western blotting. Plant extracts containing 100 ng of either H5 oligomers or H5-S·Tag were selected for mouse immunization. In the control groups, a plant extract containing S·Protein-TP and a non-transformed plant extract that had the same amount of total soluble protein as plant extracts containing H5 oligomers and H5-S·Tag were used. All plant extracts were formulated with the Emulsigen®-D adjuvant (MVP Technologies, 4805 G Street, Omaha, NE 68117, USA) at 20% final concentration. Seven–nine-week-old male C57/Bl6/J mice (Charles River Laboratories, Research Models and Services, Germany GmbH; twelve per group) were subcutaneously immunized with Emulsigen®-D adjuvant-formulated plant extracts at days 0, 14 and 28. One week after the 2nd and 3rd immunizations, mice were bled via the retro-orbital sinus. Mouse sera were collected individually for hemagglutination inhibition and ELISA tests.

### Hemagglutination test and hemagglutination inhibition assay

The hemagglutination test was based on a standard protocol [22]. The dilution that induced complete hemagglutination was defined as one hemagglutination unit (HAU). The HI assay was performed similarly based on a standard procedure [22]. Because of unavailability of the A/duck/Viet Nam/TG24-01/2005 (H5N1) virus in an inactivated form, the heterologous inactivated virus strain rg A/swan/Germany/R65/2006(H5N1) was used for HI assay. The deduced hemagglutinin amino acid sequence similarity of both strains is 96%. A 25 µL aliquot of serum from a single mouse was placed in the first well of a microtiter plate containing 25 µL PBS, and two-fold serial dilutions were made across the row of 8 wells. A 25 µL volume containing 4 HAU of the inactivated rg A/swan/Germany/R65/2006(H5N1) virus was added to the reaction and incubated at 25 °C for 30 min. Then, 25 µL of 1% chicken red blood cells was added, and the plates were incubated at 25 °C for 30 min. The HI titer is presented as the reciprocal of the highest dilution of serum that could completely inhibit hemagglutination.

## Indirect ELISA

Microtiter plates (ImmunoPlateMaxisorp, Nalgen Nunc International, Roskilde, Denmark) were coated with 100 µL of 0.5 µg/mL of IMAC- and SEC-purified hemagglutinin trimers in phage PBS (100 mM NaCl, 32 mM $Na_2HPO_4$, 17 mM $Na_2HPO_4$, pH 7.2) and incubated overnight at room temperature. After blocking with 3% (w/v) bovine serum albumin (BSA), 0.05% (v/v) Tween20 in PBS (PBST) for 2 h, 100 µL of the specific dilution ($6 \times 10^{-4}$) was applied and incubated at 25 °C for 1 h. Plates were washed 5 times with PBST, incubated with alkaline phosphatase-conjugated rabbit anti-mouse IgG diluted (2000 times) in 1% (w/v) BSA and washed again. The enzymatic substrate, p-nitrophenyl phosphate (pNPP) in 0.1 M diethanolamine-HCl (pH 9.8) was added, and the absorbance signal was measured at 405 nm after a 1 h incubation at 37 °C.

## Statistical analysis

Statistical analyses of HI data and ELISA results were performed using Mann–Whitney Rank-Sum test and T test (ELISA) in Sigma Plot software. p-values < 0.05 were defined as significant.

## Results

### Recombinant hemagglutinin-S·Tag fusion proteins and S·Protein variants are produced in planta

Trimeric hemagglutinin containing S·Tag and S·Protein variants were designed and expressed in planta, to generate influenza hemagglutinin oligomers based on the specific interaction of bovine S·Protein and the S·Tag (Figure 1). We fused the S·Tag (15 amino acid in length) c-terminally to the artificial trimerization domain (GCN4-pII) of the H5 hemagglutinin. This trimerization domain was proven to stabilize influenza hemagglutinin as trimers in planta [10]. An ubiquitous plant promoter (CaMV35S), a signal peptide and an endoplasmic reticulum (ER) retention signal (KDEL) allow for the production and accumulation of trimers in the ER of leaf cells after transient expression (Figure 2). The accumulation of such trimers has been analyzed by Western blot via the c-myc tag after separation of plant crude extracts at denaturing conditions in a SDS gel.

A band corresponding to H5-S·Tag could be identified (Figure 3B, H5-S·Tag, lane 6).

We constructed an expression vector, that allows for the production of potentially multimeric wild-type S·Protein [23] in the plant ER (Figure 2) and performed transient expression experiments in N. benthamiana leaves. The analysis of crude extracts of these leaves by Western blot after separation at denaturing conditions revealed a major band that corresponds to a S·Protein monomer (Figure 3B, S·Protein, lane 7).

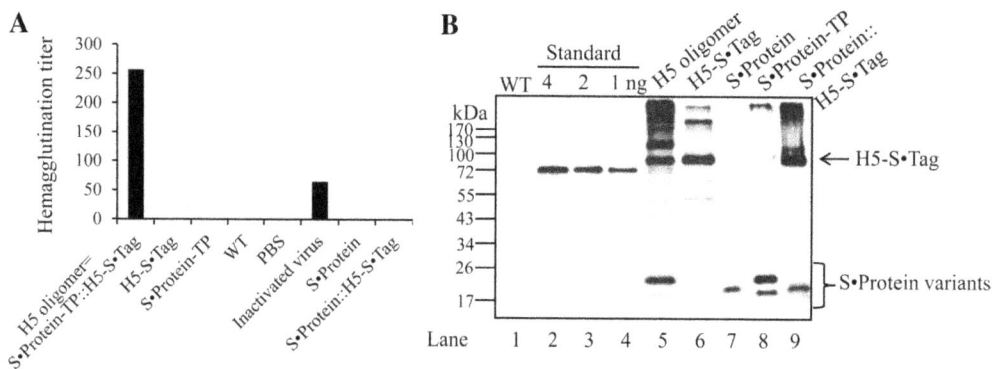

**Figure 3 Hemagglutinin oligomers from plants. A** Hemagglutination titers of plant extracts and inactivated virus rg A/swan/Germany/R65/2006(H5N1). WT wild-type N. benthamiana; PBS phosphate-buffered saline. **B** Hemagglutinin derivatives and S·Protein derivatives (30 µg total soluble protein/land) in plant extracts analyzed by anti-c-myc tag Western blot. Standard: anti-TNFalpha-nanobody-ELP [34]; S·Protein::H5-S·Tag: co-expression; H5 oligomer: S·Protein-TP::H5-S·Tag: co-expression.

H5-S·Tag and S·Protein constructs were co-expressed in the ER of leaf cells. After co-infiltration of *N. benthamiana* with the appropriate *Agrobacterium* strains, leaf crude extracts were analyzed by Western blot after separation at denaturing conditions. Two major bands, reflecting H5-S·Tag and S·Protein, each corresponding in size to the molecular weights of the single expressed proteins were detected (Figure 3B, S·Protein::S·Tag, lane 9).

To multimerize the wild-type S·Protein, trimerization (GCN4-pII), dimerization (GCN4 wild-type) domains [9], or a tail piece of mouse IgM antibody that forms disulfide bonds via its cysteine residues were fused to the wild-type S·Protein C-terminally (Figure 2). Resulting recombinant proteins were S·Protein-pII, S·Protein-GCN4, and S·Protein-TP, respectively (Figure 2). Expression of these single recombinant S·Protein variants and co-expression with trimeric H5-S·Tag was always confirmed by Western blot analyses presented partially in Figure 3B and in Additional file 1 and summarized in Tables 1 and 2. Notably, hemagglutinin, S·Protein and the TP element contain five [24], one [25], and one [14] N-glycosylation sites, respectively. This influences the mobility in SDS gels and therefore, higher molecular weights in appearance will be detected (Figure 3B, Additional file 1). In general, all recombinant proteins were expressed in plants.

## Screening for an optimal hemagglutinin oligomerization tool

The hemagglutination assay is based on the ability of influenza hemagglutinin to bind sialic acid receptors presented on the surface of chicken red blood cells. Cross-linkages between influenza hemagglutinin and red blood cell cause the formation of a lattice called hemagglutination. In the hemagglutinin oligomers (Figure 1), cross-linkages between hemagglutinin trimers were already built via S·Protein and S·Tag interaction, while influenza trimers lack these linkages. Therefore, when hemagglutinin oligomers were mixed with given amount of red blood cells, high hemagglutination titers will be expected compared with those of trimeric hemagglutinin. This assay was used to screen for formation of hemagglutinin oligomers in plant crude extracts. The hemagglutination titers caused by the plant crude extracts containing single H5-S·Tag or S·Protein, as well as co-expressed proteins (H5-S·Tag and S·Protein) were all very low (Figure 3A; Table 2). We hypothesized that the wild-type S·Protein was not being sufficiently multimerized. Therefore, we fused different oligomerization motifs, such as the trimerization motif GCN4-pII, the dimerization motif GCN4 wild-type [9] and a tailpiece (TP) element of mouse IgM to the c-terminal end of the S·Protein sequence to multimerize the S·Protein. TP elements are responsible for the interchain connections between constant parts of single

**Table 1  Expression and functionality profiles of recombinant influenza hemagglutinin and S·Protein variants**

| Proteins | Protein expression confirmed by Western blot | Hemagglutination unit (HAU) | |
|---|---|---|---|
| | | Plant extracts containing each single recombinant protein | Combination with H5-S·Tag in vitro |
| H5-S·Tag | (+) | 0 | |
| S·Protein | (+) | 0 | 0 |
| S·Protein-pII | (+) | 0 | 0 |
| S·Protein-GCN4 | (+) | 0 | 0 |
| S·Protein-TP | (+) | 0 | 0 |

Each single protein was transiently expressed in plants. The expression of proteins was confirmed by Western blot. Plant extracts containing S·Protein variants were combined with the H5-S·Tag containing plant extract in vitro. Mixtures were rotated at 4 °C for 1 h. The oligomer formation of all variants was investigated by hemagglutination assay. (+): expression of a single protein confirmed by Western blot.

**Table 2  Expression and functionality profiles of recombinant influenza hemagglutinin and S·Protein variants**

| Proteins | Protein expression confirmed by Western blot | Hemagglutination unit (HAU) |
|---|---|---|
| | | Co-expression with H5-S·Tag in plants in vivo |
| S·Protein | (++) | 4 |
| S·Protein-pII | (++) | 0 |
| S·Protein-GCN4 | (++) | 2 |
| S·Protein-TP | (++) | 256 |

Two proteins (one of the S·Protein variants and H5-S·Tag) were co-expressed transiently in plants. The expression of both proteins (++) was confirmed by Western blot. The oligomer formation of all variants was investigated by hemagglutination assay.

IgM chains to penta- or hexamers via disulfide bridges [14] (Figures 1 and 2). The principal plant expression constructs coding for S·Protein-pII, S·Protein-GCN4 and S·Protein-TP are shown in Figure 2. The plant expression has been tested by a transient assay in *N. benthamiana*. Each single crude extract was analyzed by a hemagglutination assay but no hemagglutination activity could be measured (Table 1). These S·Protein variants (S·Protein-pII, S·Protein-GCN4, and S·Protein-TP, respectively), were co-expressed with H5-S·Tag. In parallel, extracts containing the single S·Protein variants, were each mixed in vitro with extracts containing H5-S·Tag. These extracts respectively mixtures were tested in hemagglutination assays. Only the variant co-expression of S·Protein-TP with H5-S·Tag (named as H5 oligomers) was found to cause a very high hemagglutination titer of 256 (Figure 3A; Table 2). All other variants, including the S·Protein-TP with H5-S·Tag mixtures conducted in vitro, did not cause increased hemagglutination titers (Tables 1 and 2). The analysis of H5 oligomer extracts, H5-S·Tag extracts and S·Protein-TP extracts by Western blot revealed major bands of expected sizes (Figure 3B, lanes 5, 6 and 8). Notably, the co-expression of H5-S·Tag and S·Protein-TP had no significant effect on the accumulation of hemagglutinin (Figure 3B). Hemagglutinin was accumulated in plants with around 0.2% of total soluble proteins estimated by Western blot (data not shown).

### Formation of H5 oligomers in planta but not in vitro

The H5-S·Tag protein contains a His tag, whereas S·Protein-TP does not contain this tag. Both proteins contain the c-myc tag (Figure 2). Therefore, we could analyze by co-purification if the H5-S·Tag protein interacts with S·Protein-TP. For this purpose H5 oligomers were purified by immobilized metal affinity chromatography (IMAC). The purified products were then analyzed by Western blot. Both H5-S·Tag and S·Protein-TP (without 6 × His) were detected (Figure 4). The co-purification of the S·Protein-TP indicated specific interaction of this protein with the H5-S·Tag. The further characterization of the potential oligomers was done at native conditions, thus keeping the oligomeric structure intact. Purified H5 oligomers and purified H5-S·Tag were separated by size exclusion chromatography (SEC) and the hemagglutination titer of every fraction was estimated. High hemagglutination titers were observed in fractions A3 to A8 of H5 oligomers. The highest molecular weight (fraction A3, 2000 kDa) corresponds to the highest hemagglutination titer (Figure 5A). The analysis of H5-S·Tag by SEC did not show high molecular weights or high hemagglutination titers (Figure 5A). The fractions of H5 oligomers were separated by SDS-PAGE and analyzed in parallel with fractions of H5-S·Tag (without S·Protein-TP) by Western

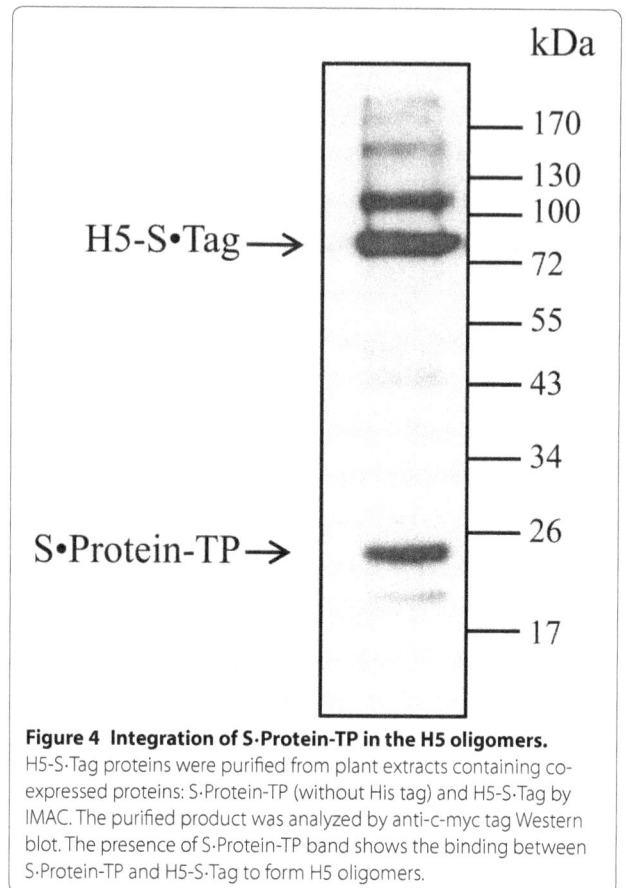

**Figure 4 Integration of S·Protein-TP in the H5 oligomers.**
H5-S·Tag proteins were purified from plant extracts containing co-expressed proteins: S·Protein-TP (without His tag) and H5-S·Tag by IMAC. The purified product was analyzed by anti-c-myc tag Western blot. The presence of S·Protein-TP band shows the binding between S·Protein-TP and H5-S·Tag to form H5 oligomers.

blot. This analysis showed that very high molecular weight hemagglutinins (> 700–2000 kDa, fractions A7–A3) were exclusively achieved in H5 oligomer extracts after co-expression of H5-S·Tag and S·Protein-TP, but not after expression of a single component (Figures 5A and B). This result indicated that the H5 oligomers were a mixture of oligomers which are made from different numbers of H5-S·Tag and S·Protein-TP incorporated into the complexes (Figure 1). Based on calculated size of trimeric H5-S·Tag (200 kDa), and the size of H5 oligomer determined by SEC, the number of trimeric H5-S·Tag integrated in H5 oligomers ranged from 1 to 8.

The protein expression of each S-tagged H5 trimers and S·Protein-TP in different plants and the in vitro combination of the extracts caused hemagglutination titers of 0 (Table 1), although production of the different components at the expected molecular weights was shown by Western blot (Figure 5B, summarized in Tables 1 and 2). The low hemagglutination titers reflect that hemagglutinin oligomers were not formed in vitro. As shown in previous studies, functionally active S·Protein was only yielded in the presence of the S·Tag. Obviously, the S·Tag serves as a template for proper folding of S·Protein [12,

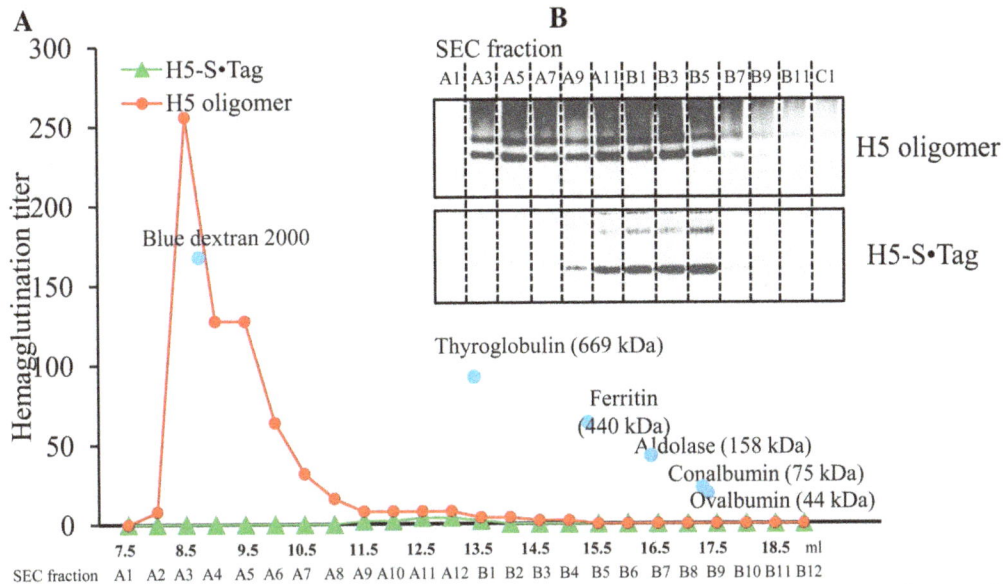

**Figure 5 Oligomeric H5 formation, as demonstrated by size exclusion chromatography, hemagglutination and Western blot analyses.** IMAC-purified H5 oligomers or H5-S·Tag (each 34 µg in 0.5 mL) were separated on Superose™ 6 increase 10/300 GL, and the fractions were analyzed by hemagglutination assay (**A**) and Western blot (**B**).

13, 26]. We suppose, that S·Protein-TP is expressed in an inactive form in the absence of H5-S·Tag and therefore it does not interact with H5-S·Tag in vitro. Exclusively, the co-expression of H5-S·Tag and S·Protein-TP caused high hemagglutination titers as well as very high molecular weights by production in planta in the ER, thus allowing folding and oligomerization by closure of disulfide bridges. This variant presents a new and innovative way to generate functional H5 oligomers in planta.

### H5 oligomers are highly immunogenic

The immunogenicity of the H5 oligomers was tested in comparison to the immunogenicity of the components H5-S·Tag and S·Protein-TP by immunization of mice. Each 12 C57Bl6/J mice were immunized with either wild-type plant crude extracts or crude extracts

containing H5 oligomers, H5·S·Tag trimers or S·Protein-TP, respectively (Figure 6). Crude extracts were chosen, because animal vaccine development should fit into the economical demands of mass immunizations in chicken, especially in terms of minimized down-stream processing. The resulting antibody-dependent humoral immune responses were firstly tested against purified hemagglutinin H5 in Western blot (Figure 7). Specific antibodies against purified hemagglutinin H5 have been detected after 2 and 3 immunizations by plant extracts containing H5 oligomers and, to a lower extend, after immunizations by H5-S·Tag. After 3 immunizations, much stronger bands were visible. The immune responses in the sera of each 12 mice per group have been measured against purified hemagglutinin H5 by an indirect ELISA. Whereas no immune response against hemagglutinin

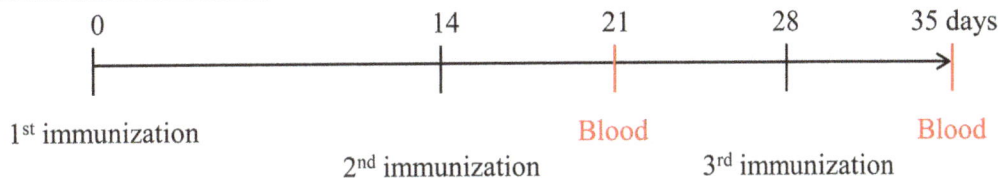

**Figure 6 Mouse immunization and bleeding schedule.** Each mouse was immunized either with crude extracts containing 0.1 µg (H5 oligomer or H5-S·Tag) formulated with the Emulsigen®-D adjuvant at 20% final concentration (two experimental groups) or with *N. benthamiana* wild type leaf extracts or S·Protein-TP leaf extracts formulated with the Emulsigen®-D adjuvant at 20% final concentration (negative control groups). Comparable leaf protein amounts were in applied to each mouse. Twelve mice per group were vaccinated with the formulated vaccines at days 0, 14 and 28. One week after the 2nd and 3rd immunizations, mice were bled via the retro-orbital sinus.

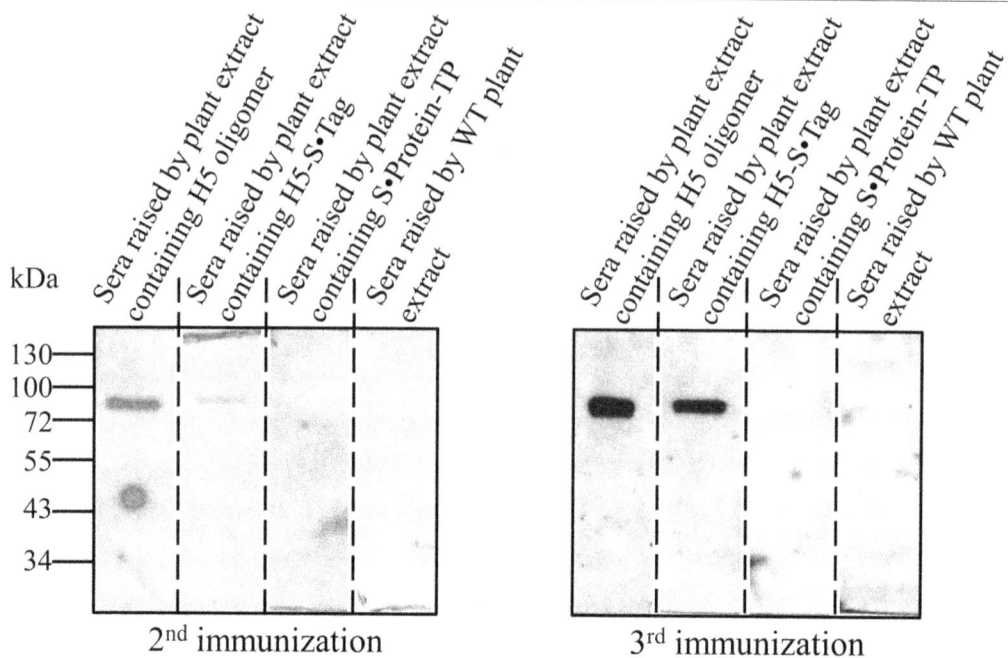

**Figure 7  Strong and specific immune responses induced by H5 oligomers compared to trimers in mice analyzed by Western blot.**
H5 specific binding of antibodies from mixtures of 10 sera raised against corresponding plant extracts as demonstrated by Western blot. Identical serum dilutions (200 times dilution) of each group were used to recognize 10 ng of the H5 hemagglutinin.

H5 was, as expected, detected after immunization with crude extracts containing S·Protein-TP or wild-type crude extracts, specific binding to purified hemagglutinin H5 was measured after immunization with H5 oligomer and H5-S·Tag crude extracts (Figures 8A and C). The immunogenicity of H5 oligomers was significantly higher, especially after three immunizations with a $p$ value of 0.008 (Figure 8C). Hemagglutination inhibition (HI) assays were performed to measure, if neutralizing antibodies could be induced. Because the A/duck/Viet Nam/TG24-01/2005 (H5N1) virus was unavailable in an inactivated form, the heterologous inactivated virus strain rg A/swan/Germany/R65/2006(H5N1) was used instead for the HI assay. The deduced hemagglutinin amino acid sequence similarity of both strains is 96%. HI assays showed that neutralizing antibodies inhibiting hemagglutination were produced in mice by immunization with H5 oligomer crude extracts and with H5-S·Tag crude extracts (vaccine groups) after 2nd immunization, and their HI geometric mean titres (HI GMTs) were 13.5 and 5.3, respectively (Figure 8B). The neutralizing antibody response was significantly better after immunization two times with H5 oligomer extracts compared to the sera of mice immunized two times with H5-S·Tag trimer extracts ($p < 0.001$, Figure 8B). This comparison shows the neutralization enhancing effect of oligomerization. In mice vaccinated two times with wild-type plant

crude extracts and S·Protein-TP crude extracts (negative control groups), most of the mouse sera caused low HI titres. The HI GMTs of these groups were 1.8 and 1.5, respectively. These HI GMTs were much lower than those of sera from mice vaccinated with H5 oligomer and H5-S·tag (trimer) crude extracts. A fourfold increase in HI GMTs was observed in sera from mice vaccinated with H5 oligomer crude extracts compared to sera from mice immunized with S·Protein-TP crude extracts and wildtype crude extracts. A fourfold increase in HI titres is associated with two-fold decrease in the risk of infection [27] and defined as seroconversion [28]. Following the third immunization, the HI GMTs of vaccine groups were higher than after the second immunization, especially in the sera derived from mice vaccinated with H5 oligomer crude extracts (Figures 8B–D). The HI GMTs of these mice were 53.8 and 10.7, while the negative control sera HI titres were as low as 1.3 and 1.7. Again, neutralizing antibody titres induced by the H5 oligomer crude extracts were significantly higher than those induced by H5-S·Tag crude extracts (Figure 8D). A fourfold increase in HI titres was now observed in the both vaccine groups compared to sera from mice immunized with S·Protein-TP crude extracts and wild-type crude extracts.

We conclude that plant crude extracts containing H5 oligomers are more immunogenic than the trimeric H5-S·Tag containing extracts as measured by an

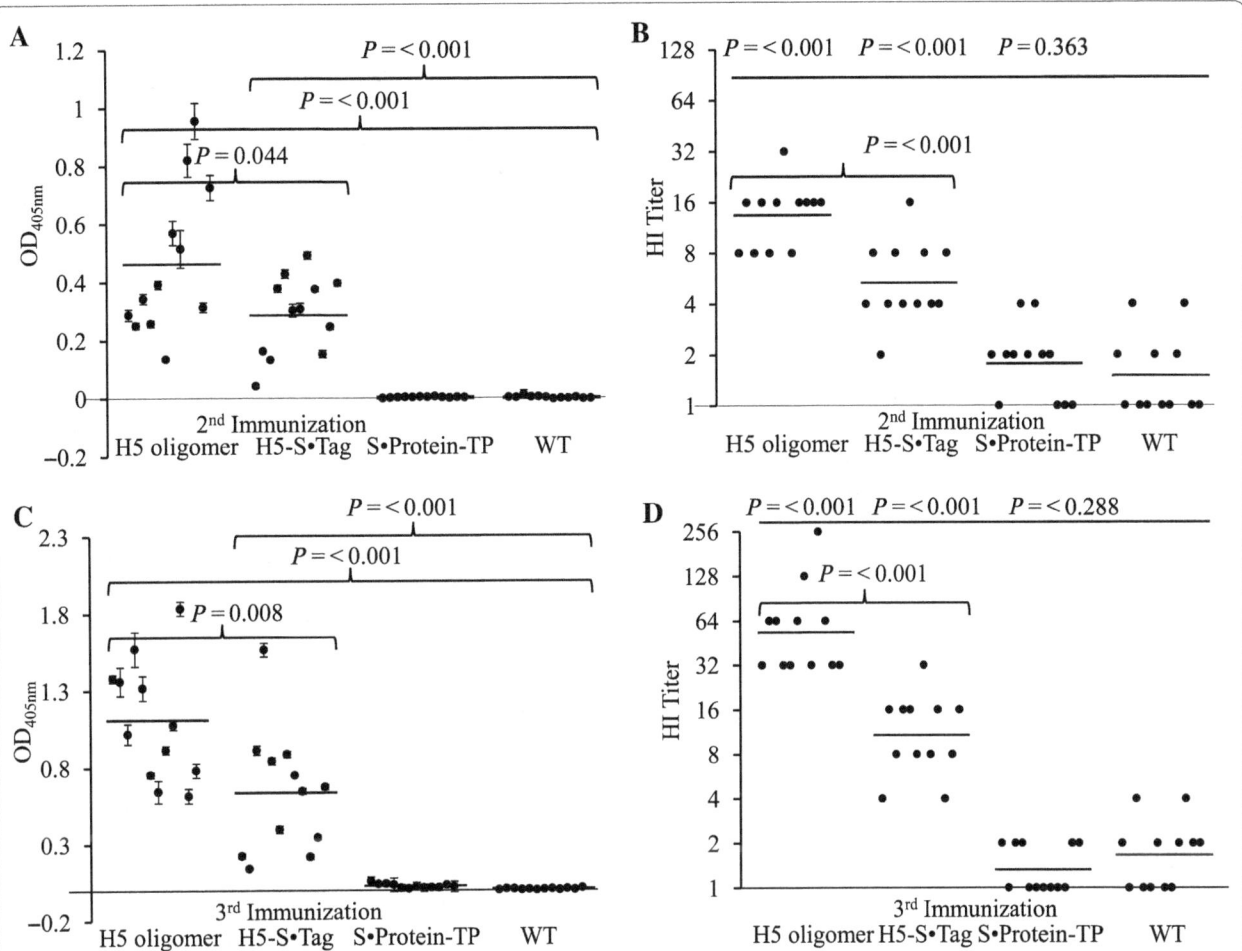

**Figure 8 Immunological characterization of H5 oligomer, H5-S·Tag and S·Protein-TP extracts compared to wild-type extracts. A, B** Antibody responses after the 2nd immunization. Measurement of antibody responses raised by injection of different extracts into mice after two immunizations by indirect ELISA (**A**) and hemagglutination inhibition assay (**B**). **C, D** Antibody responses after the 3rd immunization. Measurement of antibody responses raised by injection of different extracts into mice after three immunizations by indirect ELISA (**C**) and hemagglutination inhibition assay (**D**). *P*-value. A single dot represents the ELISA result from a single serum sample measured in five parallels. Standard deviations are given. Bars are the mean of each test group. Measurement of hemagglutination inhibition titers of sera raised against the extracts mentioned above. A single dot represents the hemagglutinin titer of the single serum sample, and bars are the geometric mean titre of each test group.

indirect ELISA. H5 oligomers induce neutralizing antibodies to a significantly higher extend compared to trimeric H5-S·Tag vaccines. The stability of H5 derivatives in crude extracts is important for the feasibility of the concept. The immunogenic extracts were stored at 4 °C for 1 week without loss of antigen content, as revealed by Western blot and hemagglutination titer (see Additional file 2).

## Discussion

The transient expression system has emerged as an alternative platform to produce influenza subunit vaccine candidates because of its capacity to be easily scaled up and because of the rapid production process [7, 29]. The

method of infiltration of plant leaves with *Agrobacteria* harboring the transgene is a robust and technologically simple method [30]. Two major approaches have been developed to efficiently express influenza vaccine candidates: expression of hemagglutinin ectodomains from swine flu H1N1 strains [31] or from avian flu H5N1 strains [10] and production of enveloped hemagglutinins as VLPs [7, 8, 29]. All plant-made hemagglutinin ectodomains tested to date were expressed as soluble monomeric [10, 32] as well as trimeric proteins stabilized by trimeric motifs [10, 31]. Artificially trimerized hemagglutinin ectodomains without S·Tag fusion, mimicking hemagglutinin homotrimers on the viral surface, enhanced immunogenicity, induced neutralizing antibodies [10] and reduced the necessary vaccine doses [31]. In the actual study, trimeric hemagglutinin fused with S·Tag (H5-S·Tag) in crude extracts was confirmed again to induce neutralizing antibodies (Figures 8B and D). Here, we present a strategy to produce hemagglutinin trimer-based antigen oligomers. This concept is based on the specific interaction of bovine S·Protein and the S·Tag, both of them are cleavage products of ribonuclease A by the proteinase subtilisin [12]. The trimerization by a specific domain (GCN4-pII motif [9, 10]) served as a founding structure of putative oligomers to design basic structures resembling native hemagglutinin homotrimers (see above). These hemagglutinin trimers should be further multimerized by interaction of an S·Tag fused to hemagglutinin with S·Proteins via co-expression of both proteins in the ER of plant cells. S·Proteins themselves are expected to consist of a mixture of monomeric, dimeric, trimeric and tetrameric proteins (or even more), as could be concluded from a previous study using ribonuclease A [33] (reviewed by [23]). Obviously, this was not sufficient to produce oligomeric H5 in the ER of plant cells (Tables 1 and 2). The fusion of dimerization and trimerization domains to the C-terminus of the S·Proteins and the subsequent co-expression in the plant cell ER (Figures 3A and B) also did not induce oligomers in high concentrations as could be concluded from low hemagglutination titers (Figure 3A; Tables 1 and 2). However, the plant extracts achieved after co-expression of H5-S·Tag and S·Protein-TP (containing the TP sequence at the c terminus) showed significantly increased hemagglutination titers compared to hemaglutination titers induced by H5-S·Tag or S·Protein-TP, respectively (Figures 3A and B; Table 2). This could be explained by the different structures of dimerization or, trimerization motives and disulfide bonds. The dimerization and trimerization domains are parallel, coiled coil structures [9] which can force their fusion partners to dimerize or trimerize in their fixed angles. However, the disulfide bonds formed by cysteine residues in the TP elements are flexible joins allowing S·Protein-TPs to fold correctly into an active form and allowing S·Protein-TPs to bend, twist, and flex into an optimal position to bind H5-S·Tag to finally form oligomers.

We conclude, that large oligomers were built. When a tail piece sequence was fused to wild-type S·Protein, monomeric, dimeric, trimeric or tetrameric S·Protein-TP joined with themselves or with others to generate multimerized S·Protein-TP via disulfide bonds. The plant ER, containing protein disulphide isomerases, is the perfect compartment for these processes. The resulting multimeric S·Protein-TPs have multiple valences to bind trimeric H5-S·Tag proteins to form H5 oligomers. This process is partially presented in Figure 1. In fact, H5 oligomers are a mixture of different numbers of H5-S·Tag and S·Protein-TP incorporated into the complexes (Figures 1, 4 and 5). Larger complexes cause higher hemagglutination titers (Figure 5). These large complexes cause improved neutralizing immune responses as shown by higher hemagglutination inhibition titers (Figure 8B and D). The low $p$ values ($p \leq 0.001$) comparing the HI titers after immunizations with either H5 oligomer or H5-S·Tag after 2 and 3 immunizations document the significance of these differences. Other crucial prerequisites for the successful development of a veterinary vaccine against avian flu are speed and practicability. *Agrobacterium* infiltration systems allow for the production of large amounts of proteins only a few days after finishing the cloning procedure, and thus, this concept generally shares speed and convenience [34]. The lack of down-stream processing effort also fits into the general timeline demands for flu vaccines [19]. Down-stream cost for recombinant expression systems can represent up to 80% of the overall processing cost [35]. These high downstream costs are a major bottleneck limiting the commercial production of plant-based pharmaceuticals [36]. Thus, the successful use of crude extracts for immunization as performed in the actual study can significantly lower down-stream cost. This is essentially important for veterinary vaccines, where cost have to be low to fit into economical parameters of animal-based production [37]. The principles shown and discussed here will generally allow for the development of low cost vaccines with unlimited scalability as precautions for veterinary immunotherapies [5]. In the actual paper, we use a synthetic biology approach to combine different principles of protein–protein interaction from different organisms to design an innovative vaccine concept in plants [38].

## Additional files

**Additional file 1. Expression of recombinant proteins in plants.**
**Hemagglutinin derivatives and S·Protein derivatives (30 μg total soluble protein/lane) in plant extracts analyzed by anti-c-myc tag Western blot.** S·Protein-pII::H5-S·Tag: co-expression; S·Protein-GCN4::H5-S·Tag: co-expression; S·Protein-pII, S·Protein-GCN4, and H5-S·Tag: single expression; WT: wild-type *N. benthamiana*.

**Additional file 2. Stability of H5 oligomers in plant crude extracts.**
(A) Western blot analysis of each 20 μL of H5 oligomers stored as crude extracts on ice. (B) H5 oligomer stability after storage of crude extracts on ice measured by hemagglutination in comparison to inactivated virus and negative control (PBS).

**Competing interests**
The authors declare that they have no competing interests.

**Authors' contributions**
HTP, HHC, THV and UC conceived the study and designed the experiments. TTH, UG and HTP performed experiments. UC, HTP and TTH wrote the manuscript with the input of all other authors. All authors read and approved the final manuscript.

## Acknowledgements

We thank J. Veits from FLI Riems for providing inactivated influenza viruses and U. Apel and H. Ziebell, JKI Quedlinburg for help with the animal experiments. The help of E. Stöger, BOKU Vienna and E. Sorge, IPK, in critical reading the manuscript is also gratefully acknowledged. This work was supported by the Federal Ministry of Education and Research-BMBF, Germany, 031A283 and by the Ministry of Science and Technology-MOST, Vietnam, NĐT.07.GER.15.

## Author details

[1] Leibniz Institute of Plant Genetics and Crop Plant Research (IPK), Gatersleben, Germany. [2] Institute of Biotechnology, Hanoi, Vietnam.

## References

1. Cox RJ, Brokstad KA, Ogra P (2004) Influenza virus: immunity and vaccination strategies. comparison of the immune response to inactivated and live, attenuated influenza vaccines. Scand J Immunol 59:1–15

2. Yen HL, Webster RG (2009) Pandemic influenza as a current threat vaccines for pandemic influenza. In: Compans RW, Orenstein WA (eds) vaccines for pandemic influenza. Springer, Berlin Heidelberg, pp 3–24

3. Food and Agriculture Organization of the united nations (2005) A global strategy for the progressive control of highly pathogenic avian influenza. http://www.fao.org/avianflu/documents/hpaiglobalstrategy31oct05.pdf

4. European Centre for Disease Prevention and Control (2016) Outbreak of highly pathogenic avian influenza A(H5N8) in Europe. https://ecdc.europa.eu/en/publications-data/rapid-risk-assessment-outbreaks-highly-pathogenic-avian-influenza-ah5n8-europe-18

5. Topp E, Irwin R, McAllister T, Lessard M, Joensuu JJ, Kolotilin I, Conrad U, Stöger E, Mor T, Warzecha H, Hall JC, McLean MD, Cox E, Devriendt B, Potter A, Depicker A, Virdi V, Holbrook L, Doshi K, Dussault M, Friendship R, Yarosh O, Yoo HS, MacDonald J, Menassa R (2016) The case for plant-made veterinary immunotherapeutics. Biotechnol Adv 34:597–604

6. Chen Q, Lai H, Hurtado J, Stahnke J, Leuzinger K, Dent M (2013) Agroinfiltration as an effective and scalable strategy of gene delivery for production of pharmaceutical proteins. Adv Tech Biol Med 1:103

7. D'Aoust MA, Lavoie PO, Couture MMJ, Trépanier S, Guay JM, Dargis M, Mongrand S, Landry N, Ward BJ, Vézina LP (2008) Influenza virus-like particles produced by transient expression in *Nicotiana benthamiana* induce a protective immune response against a lethal viral challenge in mice. Plant Biotechnol J 6:930–940

8. Landry N, Ward BJ, Trépanier S, Montomoli E, Dargis M, Lapini G, Vézina LP (2010) Preclinical and clinical development of plant-made virus-like particle vaccine against avian H5N1 influenza. PLoS One 5:e15559

9. Harbury P, Zhang T, Kim P, Alber T (1993) A switch between two-, three-, and four-stranded coiled coils in GCN4 leucine zipper mutants. Science 262:1401–1407

10. Phan HT, Pohl J, Floss DM, Rabenstein F, Veits J, Le BT, Chu HH, Hause G, Mettenleiter T, Conrad U (2013) ELPylated haemagglutinins produced in tobacco plants induce potentially neutralizing antibodies against H5N1 viruses in mice. Plant Biotechnol J 11:582–593

11. Phan HT, Conrad U (2011) Membrane-based inverse transition cycling: an improved means for purifying plant-derived recombinant protein-elastin-like polypeptide fusions. Int J Mol Sci 12:2808

12. Raines RT, McCormick M, Van Oosbree TR, Mierendorf RC (2000) The S-tag fusion system for protein purification. In: Thorner J, Emr SD, Abelson JN (eds) Methods in enzymology, Academic Press, pp.362–376

13. Backer MV, Gaynutdinov TI, Aloise R, Przekop K, Backer JM (2002) Engineering S-protein fragments of bovine ribonuclease A for targeted drug delivery. Protein Expr Purif 26:455–461

14. Müller R, Gräwert MA, Kern T, Madl T, Peschek J, Sattler M, Groll M, Buchner J (2013) High-resolution structures of the IgM Fc domains

reveal principles of its hexamer formation. Proc Natl Acad Sci U S A 110:10183–10188

15. Xiang C, Han P, Lutziger I, Wang K, Oliver DJ (1999) A mini binary vector series for plant transformation. Plant Mol Biol 40:711–717

16. Phan HT, Conrad U (2016) Plant-based vaccine antigen production. In: Brun A (ed) Vaccine technologies for veterinary viral diseases: methods and protocols. Springer New York, New York, pp 35–47

17. Sudarshana MR, Plesha MA, Uratsu SL, Falk BW, Dandekar AM, Huang TK, McDonald KA (2006) A chemically inducible cucumber mosaic virus amplicon system for expression of heterologous proteins in plant tissues. Plant Biotechnol J 4:551–559

18. Conley AJ, Joensuu JJ, Jevnikar AM, Menassa R, Brandle JE (2009) Optimization of elastin-like polypeptide fusions for expression and purification of recombinant proteins in plants. Biotechnol Bioeng 103:562–573

19. Bradford MM (1976) A rapid and sensitive method for the quantitation of microgram quantities of protein utilizing the principle of protein-dye binding. Anal Biochem 72:248–254

20. Conrad U, Plagmann I, Malchow S, Sack M, Floss DM, Kruglov AA, Nedospasov SA, Rose-John S, Scheller J (2011) ELPylated anti-human TNF therapeutic single-domain antibodies for prevention of lethal septic shock. Plant Biotechnol J 9:22–31

21. Gahrtz M, Conrad U (2009) Immunomodulation of plant function by in vitro selected single-chain Fv intrabodies. Methods Mol Biol 483:289–312

22. World Organization for Animal Health (2004) Highly pathogenic avian influenza, in manual of diagnostic tests and vaccines for terrestrial animals (mammals, birds, and bees). Paris: World Organization for Animal Health (OIE), pp. 259–269. http://www.oie.int/en/international-standard-setting/terrestrial-manual/access-online/

23. Libonati M, Gotte G (2004) Oligomerization of bovine ribonuclease A: structural and functional features of its multimers. Biochem J 380:311–327

24. Zhang S, Sherwood RW, Yang Y, Fish T, Chen W, McCardle JA, Jones RM, Yusibov V, May ER, Rose JK, Thannhauser TW (2012) Comparative characterization of the glycosylation profiles of an influenza hemagglutinin produced in plant and insect hosts. Proteomics 12:1269–1288

25. Reid GE, Stephenson JL, McLuckey SA (2002) Tandem mass spectrometry of ribonuclease A and B: N-linked glycosylation site analysis of whole protein ions. Anal Chem 74:577–583

26. Kato I, Anfinsen CB (1969) On the stabilization of ribonuclease S-protein by ribonuclease S-peptide. J Biol Chem 244:1004–1007

27. Benoit A, Beran J, Devaster JM, Esen M, Launay O, Leroux-Roels G, McElhaney JE, Oostvogels L, van Essen GA, Gaglani M, Jackson LA, Vesikari I, Legrand C, Tibaldi F, Innis BL, Dewé W (2015) Hemagglutination inhibition antibody titers as a correlate of protection against seasonal A/H3N2 Influenza Disease. Open Forum Infect Dis 2:ofv067–ofv067

28. Hsu JP, Zhao X, Chen MIC, Cook AR, Lee V, Lim WY, Tan L, Barr IG, Jiang L, Tan CL, Phoon MC, Cui L, Lin R, Leo YS, Chow VT (2014) Rate of decline of antibody titers to pandemic influenza A (H1N1-2009) by hemagglutination inhibition and virus microneutralization assays in a cohort of seroconverting adults in Singapore. BMC Infect Dis 14:414

29. D'Aoust MA, Couture MMJ, Charland N, Trépanier S, Landry N, Ors F, Vézina LP (2010) The production of hemagglutinin-based virus-like particles in plants: a rapid, efficient and safe response to pandemic influenza. Plant Biotechnol J 8:607–619

30. Komarova TV, Baschieri S, Donini M, Marusic C, Benvenuto E, Dorokhov YL (2010) Transient expression systems for plant-derived biopharmaceuticals. Expert Rev Vaccines 9:859–876

31. Shoji Y, Jones RM, Mett V, Chichester JA, Musiychuk K, Sun X, Tumpey TM, Green BJ, Shamloul M, Norikane J, Bi H, Hartman CE, Bottone C, Stewart M, Streatfield SJ, Yusibov V (2013) A plant-produced H1N1 trimeric hemagglutinin protects mice from a lethal influenza virus challenge. Hum Vaccin Immunother 9:553–560

32. Shoji Y, Farrance CE, Bi H, Shamloul M, Green B, Manceva S, Rhee A, Ugulava N, Roy G, Musiychuk K (2009) Immunogenicity of hemagglutinin from A/Bar-headed Goose/Qinghai/1A/05 and A/Anhui/1/05 strains of H5N1 influenza viruses produced in *Nicotiana benthamiana* plants. Vaccine 27:3467–3470

33. Gotte G, Vottariello F, Libonati M (2003) Thermal aggregation of ribonuclease A: a contribution to the understanding of the role of 3D domain swapping in protein aggregation. J Biol Chem 278:10763–10769

34. Rybicki EP (2010) Plant-made vaccines for humans and animals. Plant Biotechnol J 8:620–637

35. Hassan S, Van Dolleweerd CJ, Ioakeimidis F, Keshavarz-Moore E, Ma JKC (2008) Considerations for extraction of monoclonal antibodies targeted to different subcellular compartments in transgenic tobacco plants. Plant Biotechnol J 6:733–748

36. Hussack G, Grohs BM, Almquist KC, McLean MD, Ghosh R, Hall JC (2010) Purification of plant-derived antibodies through direct immobilization of affinity ligands on cellulose. J Agric Food Chem 58:3451–3459

37. Floss DM, Conrad U (2013) Plant molecular pharming, veterinary applications plant molecular pharming veterinary applications. In: Christou P (ed) Sustainable food production. Springer New York, New York, pp 1358–1365

38. Patron NJ, Orzaez D, Marillonnet S, Warzecha H, Matthewman C, Youles M, Raitskin O, Leveau A, Farré G, Rogers C, Smith A, Hibberd J, Webb AAR, Locke J, Schornack S, Ajioka J, Baulcombe DC, Zipfel C, Kamoun S, Jones JDG, Kuhn H, Robatzek S, Van Esse HP, Sanders D, Oldroyd G, Martin C, Field R, O'Connor S, Fox S, Wulff B, Miller B, Breakspear A, Radhakrishnan G, Delaux PM, Loqué D, Granell A, Tissier A, Shih P, Brutnell TP, Quick WP, Rischer H, Fraser PD, Aharoni A, Raines C, South PF, Ané JM, Hamberger BR, Langdale J, Stougaard J, Bouwmeester H, Udvardi M, Murray JAH, Ntoukakis V, Schäfer P, Denby K, Edwards KJ, Osbourn A, Haseloff J (2015) Standards for plant synthetic biology: a common syntax for exchange of DNA parts. New Phytol 208:13–19

# 9

# Global proteomic profiling of *Yersinia ruckeri* strains

Gokhlesh Kumar[1]*[ID], Karin Hummel[2], Timothy J. Welch[3], Ebrahim Razzazi-Fazeli[2] and Mansour El-Matbouli[1]

## Abstract

*Yersinia ruckeri* is the causative agent of enteric redmouth disease (ERM) of salmonids. There is little information regarding the proteomics of *Y. ruckeri*. Herein, we perform whole protein identification and quantification of biotype 1 and biotype 2 strains of *Y. ruckeri* grown under standard culture conditions using a shotgun proteomic approach. Proteins were extracted, digested and peptides were separated by a nano liquid chromatography system and analyzed with a high-resolution hybrid triple quadrupole time of flight mass spectrometer coupled via a nano ESI interface. SWATH-MS technology and sophisticated statistical analyses were used to identify proteome differences among virulent and avirulent strains. GO annotation, subcellular localization, virulence proteins and antibiotic resistance ontology were predicted using bioinformatic tools. A total of 1395 proteins were identified in the whole cell of *Y. ruckeri*. These included proteases, chaperones, cell division proteins, outer membrane proteins, lipoproteins, receptors, ion binding proteins, transporters and catalytic proteins. In virulent strains, a total of 16 proteins were upregulated including anti-sigma regulatory factor, arginine deiminase, phosphate-binding protein PstS and superoxide dismutase Cu–Zu. Additionally, several virulence proteins were predicted such as Clp and Lon pro-teases, TolB, PPIases, PstS, PhoP and LuxR family transcriptional regulators. These putative virulence proteins might be used for development of novel targets for treatment of ERM in fish. Our study represents one of the first global proteomic reference profiles of *Y. ruckeri* and this data can be accessed via ProteomeXchange with identifier PXD005439. These proteomic profiles elucidate proteomic mechanisms, pathogenicity, host-interactions, antibiotic resistance ontology and localization of *Y. ruckeri* proteins.

## Introduction

Enteric redmouth disease (ERM) is one of the most important bacterial diseases of salmonids and causes significant economic losses in the aquaculture industry worldwide. ERM can affect fish from all age classes and appears as a more chronic condition in older and larger fish. The disease is caused by *Yersinia ruckeri*, a Gram-negative rod-shaped enterobacterium [1, 2]. *Y. ruckeri* enters the fish via the secondary gill lamellae and from there spreads to the blood and internal organs [3]. Clinical signs of the disease include exophthalmia, darkening of the skin in addition to subcutaneous hemorrhages in and around the mouth and throat. The spleen is often enlarged and can be almost black in color and the lower intestine can become reddened and filled with an opaque,

yellowish fluid [1, 2]. Focal areas of necrosis can be present in the organs (spleen, kidney and liver). Degenerated renal tubules, glomerular nephritis and a marked increase in melano-macrophages may be observed in the kidney of infected fish [1, 2, 4]. Several virulence factors of *Y. ruckeri* have been identified such as extra-cellular products and Yrp1. Extra-cellular products have been shown to reproduce the clinical signs of the disease [5]. The 47 kDa metalloprotease Yrp1 is necessary for virulence and degrades fibronectin, actin and myosin of the fish [6].

Strains of *Y. ruckeri* have been categorized into two biotypes: biotype 1 strains are motile and lipase positive, while biotype 2 strains are negative for these phenotypes [2, 7]. Previously, the majority of epizootic outbreaks in salmonids were caused by biotype 1 strains which could be easily controlled by vaccination with a bacterin vaccine [5]. Nevertheless, biotype 2 strains have recently emerged and have been responsible for outbreaks in

*Correspondence: Gokhlesh.Kumar@vetmeduni.ac.at
[1] Clinical Division of Fish Medicine, University of Veterinary Medicine, Veterinärplatz 1, 1210 Vienna, Austria
Full list of author information is available at the end of the article

both naive and vaccinated fish, thereby suggesting that biotype 2 strains may be less sensitive to the traditional ERM vaccine which is made from a biotype 1 strain [8, 9]. This relationship between vaccine failure and emergence of biotype 2 has led to the hypothesis that the loss of the flagellum is essential for resistance to immersion vaccination [9, 10]. However, bivalent or biotype 2 vaccines provide good protection against the biotype 2 strains [2, 11].

Whole genome sequences of *Y. ruckeri* strains have been annotated and can now be used for comparative genomic analysis of strains and other research purposes [12]. Global proteomic identification and comparative analysis of *Y. ruckeri* strains are required to create a proteomic map, understanding proteomic biology, proteomic changes and proteomic differences between strains. Little is known about the proteomics of *Y. ruckeri*. Outer membrane protein and whole cell protein patterns of *Y. ruckeri* isolates were described using SDS-PAGE and 2D-PAGE [11, 13, 14]. Reference proteome maps of many bacteria including *Y. pestis* have been created, and this work is leading to an understanding of the virulence mechanisms and the regulatory networks used by pathogenic bacteria [15]. However, for fish pathogens, in-depth proteomic analysis is not yet well established.

In our previous study, we compared two culture conditions of *Y. ruckeri* strains and focused only on proteins expressed in response to iron-limited culture conditions [16]. In this study, we identified, quantified and analyzed the global proteomic profiles of *Y. ruckeri* strains grown under standard culture conditions using a shotgun proteomic approach. Furthermore, we predicted virulence proteins and antibiotic resistance ontology in the proteome of *Y. ruckeri*.

## Materials and methods
### Bacterial strains
Two biotype 1 (SP-05 and CSF007-82) and two biotype 2 (7959-11 and YRNC-10) *Y. ruckeri* strains were used in the present study. These four strains were isolated from rainbow trout (*Oncorhynchus mykiss*) and all are serotype 01. Strains SP-05 and 7959-11 originated from Austria and the other two strains, CSF007-82 and YRNC-10, originated from the USA. Virulence for rainbow trout was determined previously using an experimental challenge model. Strains CSF007-82, 7959-11 and YRNC-10 were virulent [17, 18] and strain SP-05 was not virulent (Authors unpublished data). The antimicrobial susceptibility of strains was tested using routine clinical laboratory susceptibility methods employing antimicrobial discs [(enrofloxacin (5 μg), florfenicol (30 μg), tetracycline (30 μg), amoxicillin (10 μg), oxolinic acid (2 μg), trimethoprim–sulfamethoxazole (25 μg), flumequine (30 μg) and doxycycline (30 μg)].

## Culture conditions
The culture conditions and growth yield of *Y. ruckeri* strains have been previously described [16]. Briefly, a single colony of each strain was used to inoculate duplicate 5 mL tryptic soy broth cultures. Duplicate starter cultures of each strain ($OD_{600}$ 0.10) were then used to inoculate 25 mL tryptic soy broth cultures and grown overnight at 22 °C until the late log phase. The yield of CSF007-82, 7959-11 and YRNC-10 strains ($OD_{600}$ 1.62) were similar to each other but the yield of SP-05 strain was slightly lower ($OD_{600}$ 1.32) compared to the other three strains [16]. Cells were harvested and washed three times with sterile phosphate buffered saline containing bacterial protease inhibitor cocktail.

## Protein extraction and digestion
The protein extraction procedures used have been previously described [16]. Briefly, bacterial cells were resuspended in denaturing lysis buffer (7 M urea, 2 M thiourea, 4% 3-[(3-cholamidopropyl)dimethyl-ammonio]-1-propane sulfonate and 1% dithiothreitol) containing bacterial protease inhibitor cocktail. Cells were then sonicated on ice and cellular debris removed by centrifugation. Protein digestion was performed using the standard two-step in-solution digestion protocol for Trypsin/LysC mix according to the user manual (Promega) and digested samples were acidified.

## Nano LC–MS/MS analysis
Tryptic peptides were separated by a nano liquid chromatography system (Dionex Ultimate 3000 RSLC) and analyzed with a high-resolution hybrid triple quadrupole time of flight mass spectrometer (TripleTOF 5600+, Sciex) coupled via a nano-ESI interface. Preconcentration and desalting of samples were accomplished with a 5 mm Acclaim PepMap μ-Precolumn (Dionex). Details of the LC–MS/MS procedure were described previously [16]. Briefly, 370 ng of digested protein were used per injection and peptide separation was performed on a 25 cm Acclaim PepMap C18 column with a flow rate of 300 nL/min. The gradient started with 4% mobile phase B (80% acetonitrile with 0.1% formic acid) and increased to 35% B over 120 min. MS1 survey scans were collected in the range of 400–1500 mass-to-charge ratio (m/z). The 25 most intense precursors with charge state 2–4, which exceeded 100 counts per second, were selected for fragmentation for 250 ms. MS2 product ion scans were collected in the range of 100–1800 m/z for 110 ms. Precursor ions were dynamically excluded from reselection for 12 s.

For quantitative measurements, data independent sequential window acquisition of all theoretical spectra (SWATH) technology based on MS2 quantification was used [19, 20]. Peptides from biological and technical replicates were fragmented in 35 fixed fragmentation windows of 20 Dalton (Da) in the range of 400–1100 Da with an accumulation time of 50 ms in TOF MS mode and 80 ms in product ion mode. The nano-HPLC system was operated by Chromeleon 6.8 (Dionex) and the MS by Analyst Software 1.6 (Sciex).

## Data analysis

Database searches of raw files of data dependent acquisition were carried out with Protein Pilot Software version 5.0 (Sciex). UniProt database (Released 10_2016) was restricted to *Y. ruckeri*. Mass tolerance in MS mode was set with 0.05 and 0.1 Da in MS/MS mode for the rapid recalibration search as well as 0.0011 Da in MS and 0.01 Da in MS/MS mode for the final search. The following sample parameters were applied: trypsin digestion, cysteine alkylation set to iodoacetamide and the search effort set was to rapid identification. False discovery rate analysis was performed using the integrated tools in ProteinPilot. The global false discovery rate (FDR) was set to < 1% on the protein level, peptide level as well as spectra level. Information dependent data acquisition identification results were used to create the SWATH ion library with the MS/MS (ALL) with SWATH Acquisition Micro-App 2.0 in PeakView 2.2 (both Sciex). Peptides were chosen based on a FDR rate < 1%, excluding shared and modified peptides. Up to six peptides per protein and up to 6 transitions per peptide were used. MarkerView 1.2.1 (Sciex) was used for calculation of peak areas of SWATH samples after retention time alignment and normalization using total area sums. The resulting protein lists were then used for visualization of data after principal component analysis (PCA) in form of loading plots and score plots to get a first impression of the overall data structure and to assess variability between technical and biological replicates.

Differentially expressed proteins were determined by statistical analysis in R programming language [21]. Raw peak areas after normalization to total area sums were $\log_2$-transformed to approach a normal distribution. On a logarithmic scale, technical replicates were aggregated by arithmetic mean before application of statistical tests. This procedure is equivalent to the application of a hierarchical model in the subsequent ANOVA, as the same number of technical replicates was measured per biological replicate. Differential expression of proteins in each strain was assessed using one-way ANOVA for each protein. To adjust for multiple testing, the method of Benjamini and Hochberg [22] was used to control the FDR. Differences were considered significant if adjusted $p$-values were smaller than the significance level of $\alpha = 0.001$. For those proteins, Tukey's honest significant difference

method was applied as post hoc test to assess the significance of the pairwise comparisons. Protein expression was considered differential if the adjusted $p$-value was below $\alpha$ and the absolute fold change was at least three (fold change $< -3$ or $> +3$).

## GO annotation and prediction of virulent proteins

Venn diagrams were used to show the differences between protein lists originating from different strains [23]. Gene ontology annotation of all identified proteins was classified using the software tool for researching annotations of proteins [24]. Subcellular localization of proteins was predicted by PSORTb version 3.0 [25]. Virulence proteins were predicted by a method based on bi-layer cascade Support Vector Machine using Virulent-Pred [26].

## Antibiotic resistance ontology and their validation

Antibiotic resistance ontology was identified using a comprehensive antibiotic resistance database [27]. The antibiotic resistance phenotypes predicted by in silico analysis were validated using the disc diffusion technique and minimal inhibitory concentration (MIC) determination [28, 29]. The antimicrobial commercial Oxoid discs (µg disc/mL, Thermo Scientific): gentamicin (10 µg), polymyxin B (300 UI), erythromycin (15 µg), rifampin (5 µg), novobiocin (5 µg) and mupirocin (5 µg) were applied to inoculated Mueller–Hinton agar (Thermo Scientific) in triplicate. In parallel, MIC ranges for the same antibiotics were determined using microtiter plates and solutions of antibiotics prepared from powders of known potencies (Sigma-Aldrich). All plates were incubated for 48 h at 22 °C. The diameter of the inhibition halo of antimicrobial discs and lowest concentration of antibiotic that inhibited visible growth of bacteria were defined and categorized as susceptible or resistant (Additional file 1) as previously using standard methods [28, 29].

## Results
### Protein identification

A total of 1395 proteins in the whole cell of *Y. ruckeri* were identified (Additional file 2). The number of proteins identified in each strain was 1193 for SP-05, 1263 for CSF007-82, 1244 for 7959-11 and 1208 for YRNC-10. The list of identified proteins in each strain is given in Additional file 3. Forty-six proteins in SP-05, 43 proteins in CSF007-82, 31 proteins in 7959-11 and 13 proteins in YRNC-10 were uniquely identified (Figure 1). PCA score plots of all strains suggested that strain SP-05 differs from the other three strains (CSF007-82, 7959-11 and YRNC-10) but the latter three strains showed minor proteomic differences (Additional file 4). The list of uniquely identified proteins in each strain is given in Additional file 5.

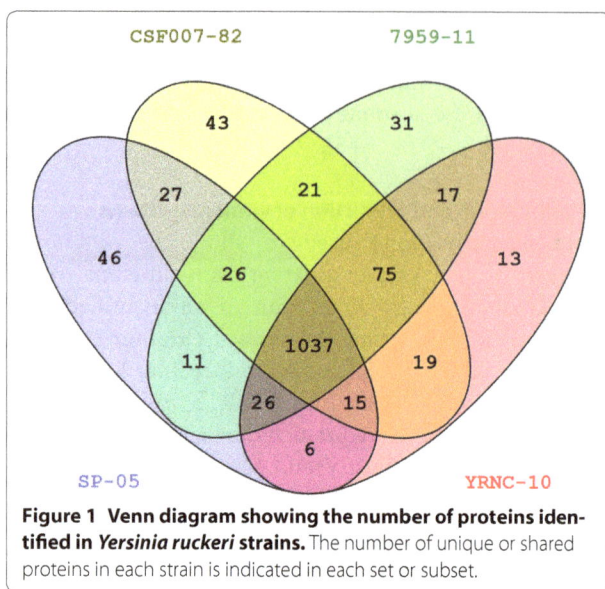

**Figure 1 Venn diagram showing the number of proteins identified in *Yersinia ruckeri* strains.** The number of unique or shared proteins in each strain is indicated in each set or subset.

## Protein quantification

Sophisticated statistical evaluation revealed a total number of 36 differentially expressed proteins within the four analyzed *Y. ruckeri* strains. Of these, 16 were upregulated (SP-05 strain versus the other strains) (Table 1) and 20 were downregulated (Additional file 6). As can be seen in Table 1, upregulated proteins were related to iron ion homeostasis, regulation of transcription, transporter activity and metabolic processes. Similarly, downregulated proteins were related to flagellar motility, phosphotransferase system, glycolysis and metabolic processes. We observed upregulation of two proteins: phosphoenolpyruvate (> 25.1-fold) and asparagines synthase (4.3-fold) in biotype 2 strains [biotype 1 strain (CSF007-82) versus biotype 2 strains (7959-11 and YRNC-10)] but saw no significant expression differences between biotype 2 strains (7959-11 versus YRNC-10).

## GO annotation and subcellular localization of proteins

The identified proteins were associated with cellular process, metabolic process, regulation, localization and response to stimulus (Figure 2A). Proteins were localized in the cytoplasm, plasma membrane, ribosome, macromolecular complex, nucleus, chromosome and others (Figure 2B). Proteins involved in catalytic activity and binding were the most abundant among those identified proteins, 51 and 39%, respectively (Figure 2C). The identified proteins were predicted in the cytoplasmic space (67%), unknown (16%), cytoplasmic membrane (8%), periplasmic space (6%), outer membrane (2%) and extracellular space (1%) (Figure 3). The unknown group included proteins with multiple subcellular and unknown localizations.

## Virulence proteins and antibiotic resistance ontology

Several predicted virulence proteins were identified: HtrA protease, protein TolB, peptidyl-prolyl cis–trans isomerase, UvrY response regulator, chaperone protein fimC, lipoprotein NlpD, putative exported protein, MltA-interacting protein, superoxide dismutase Cu–Zn, PhoP, LuxR and AsnC family transcriptional regulators (Table 2 and Additional file 7).

We also predicted antibiotic resistance ontology in 12 antibiotic classes (Table 3) in the proteome of *Y. ruckeri*, which contains 14 proteins such as bacterial regulatory protein (cyclic AMP receptor protein), membrane fusion protein of the resistance-nodulation-division (RND) family multidrug efflux pump, bifunctional polymyxin resistance protein ArnA and RND efflux system inner membrane transporter CmeB.

## Antimicrobial susceptibility test

Strains of *Y. ruckeri* were susceptible to enrofloxacin, florfenicol, tetracycline, amoxicillin, oxolinic acid, trimethoprim–sulfamethoxazole, flumequine and doxycycline (data not shown). Additional file 1 shows the diameter of the inhibition zone and MIC of antimicrobial agents used for validation of antibiotic resistance ontology. Novobiocin and mupirocin discs displayed no inhibition zone against *Y. ruckeri* strains, while strains showed intermediate susceptibility to gentamicin and polymyxin B. *Y. ruckeri* strains were resistant to erythromycin (MIC = 1024 µg/mL), rifampin (MIC = 32 µg/mL), novobiocin (MIC = 16–32 µg/mL) and mupirocin (MIC = 32–64 µg/mL). Three antibiotic resistance ontologies: novobiocin, mupirocin and erythromycin were fully consistent with the proteomic data such as cys regulon transcriptional activator CysB, alanine tRNA ligase and isoleucine-tRNA ligase.

## Discussion

Here we identify global proteomic reference profiles of *Y. ruckeri* strains (PXD005439) grown under standard culture conditions. These global proteomic profiles help us to understand the physiology, protein biology, virulence factors, host-interactions, localization and antibiotic resistance of *Y. ruckeri*. The total number of proteins identified was 1395 in *Y. ruckeri* (Additional file 2). These included proteases, chaperones, cell division proteins, outer membrane proteins, chromosome partitioning proteins and transporters. Proteins have been classified into different functional categories such as biological process and molecular function (Figure 2) and this information will be useful for further studies in the direction of extracellular (flagellin and flagellar hook-associated protein), interaction with cells (invasin and manganese ABC transporter, periplasmic-binding protein SitA), antioxidant

**Table 1 Fold changes of differentially expressed proteins of *Yersinia ruckeri* strains compared to each other**

| UniProt accession number | Protein | Function | SP-05 vs CSF007-82 | SP-05 vs 7959-11 | SP-05 vs YRNC-10 | CSF007-82 vs 7959-11 | CSF007-82 vs YRNC-10 | 7959-11 vs YRNC-10 |
|---|---|---|---|---|---|---|---|---|
| A0A085U6V7_YERRU | Bacterioferritin | Ferric iron binding | 6.8* | 5.7* | 6.5* | −1.2 | −1.0 | 1.1 |
| A0A085U4B6_YERRU | DNA protection during starvation protein | Iron ion homeostasis | 3.2* | 3.8* | 1.9 | 1.2 | −1.7 | −2.1 |
| A0A085U5L5_YERRU | Anti-sigma factor antagonist | Regulation of transcription | 3.6* | 3.7* | 3.8* | 1.0 | 1.1 | 1.0 |
| A0A085U5L7_YERRU | Anti-sigma regulatory factor | Serine/threonine kinase activity | 3.9* | 3.9* | 4.3* | −1.0 | 1.1 | 1.1 |
| A0A085UBQ1_YERRU | Arginine deiminase | Arginine catabolic process | 5.7* | 5.2* | 5.8* | −1.1 | 1.0 | 1.1 |
| A0A085U6O5_YERRU | Amino acid transporter | Transporter activity | 4.3* | 4.2* | 4.0* | −1.0 | −1.1 | −1.0 |
| A0A085U8U0_YERRU | Phosphate-binding protein PstS | Phosphate ion transmembrane transport | 3.0 | 3.1* | 3.4* | 1.0 | 1.1 | 1.1 |
| A0A0A5FQB4_YERRU | Superoxide dismutase Cu–Zn | Superoxide dismutase activity | 2.8 | 3.2* | 3.4* | 1.2 | 1.2 | 1.1 |
| A0A0A5FMC5_YERRU | Arginine decarboxylase, catabolic | Amino acid metabolic process | 7.9* | 6.5* | 6.2* | −1.2 | −1.3 | −1.0 |
| A0A085UBP8_YERRU | Glutamate decarboxylase | Glutamate metabolic process | 10.4* | 8.5* | 6.8* | −1.2 | −1.5 | −1.3 |
| A0A0A8VE52_YERRU | Glutaminase | Glutamine metabolic process | 6.7* | 6.5* | 8.2* | −1.0 | 1.2 | 1.3 |
| A0A085U745_YERRU | Glucose-1-phosphate adenylyltransferase | Glycogen biosynthetic process | 5.3* | 5.0* | 3.8* | −1.1 | −1.4 | −1.3 |
| A0A085UBM7_YERRU | 3-Oxoacyl-ACP reductase | Oxidoreductase | 6.2* | 6.1* | 6.8* | −1.0 | 1.1 | 1.1 |
| A0A085U7G0_YERRU | Uncharacterized protein | Unknown | 9.1* | 7.9* | 9.5* | −1.2 | 1.0 | 1.2 |
| A0A085UBQ0_YERRU | Uncharacterized protein | Unknown | 5.0* | 4.9* | 4.3* | −1.0 | −1.2 | −1.2 |
| A0A085U732_YERRU | Putative exported protein | Unknown | 2.9 | 2.9 | 3.4* | 1.0 | 1.2 | 1.2 |

ANOVA was performed for UniProt database searches.

* Denotes statistically significant difference according to Tukey's honest significant difference post hoc test with FDR-adjusted $p < 0.001$ and fold change < −3 or > +3.

(thioredoxin reductase and glutathione amide-dependent peroxidase) and molecular transducer (methyl-accepting chemotaxis protein) activity. The identification of predicted virulence proteins (Table 2; Additional file 7) and antibiotic resistance ontology (Table 3) contributes to our understanding of this pathogen and will aid in the rational design of novel treatment strategies for ERM disease.

Biotype 2 strains showed minor proteomic differences among each other (Additional file 4). However, the Austrian biotype 1 strain (SP-05) showed major proteomic differences when compared to the USA biotype 1 strain (CSF007-82) and biotype 2 strains (7959-11 and YRNC-10). These major differences may be due to the slightly lower yield and growth rate of SP-05 strain compared to the other three strains (CSF007-82, 7959-11 and YRNC-10) or its avirulent nature toward the fish.

Sixteen upregulated proteins were identified in virulent *Y. ruckeri* strains using a sophisticated statistical analysis (avirulent SP-05 strain versus virulent strains). We found strong upregulation of bacterioferritin (5.7- to 6.8-fold) and DNA protection during starvation protein (3.2- to 3.8-fold) in *Y. ruckeri* strains. However, iron dependent proteins (bacterioferritin and iron-sulfur cluster assembly scaffold protein IscU) were downregulated (−3-fold) in *Y. ruckeri* strains in response to iron-limited culture conditions [16]. The phosphate-binding protein PstS is a high affinity phosphate binding protein of the Pst transport system and has been shown to be involved in pathogenesis, invasion and biofilm formation of many bacteria [30]. Superoxide dismutase Cu–Zn is an important for oxidative stress and has been shown to contribute to the pathogenicity of many bacteria [31]. Arginine

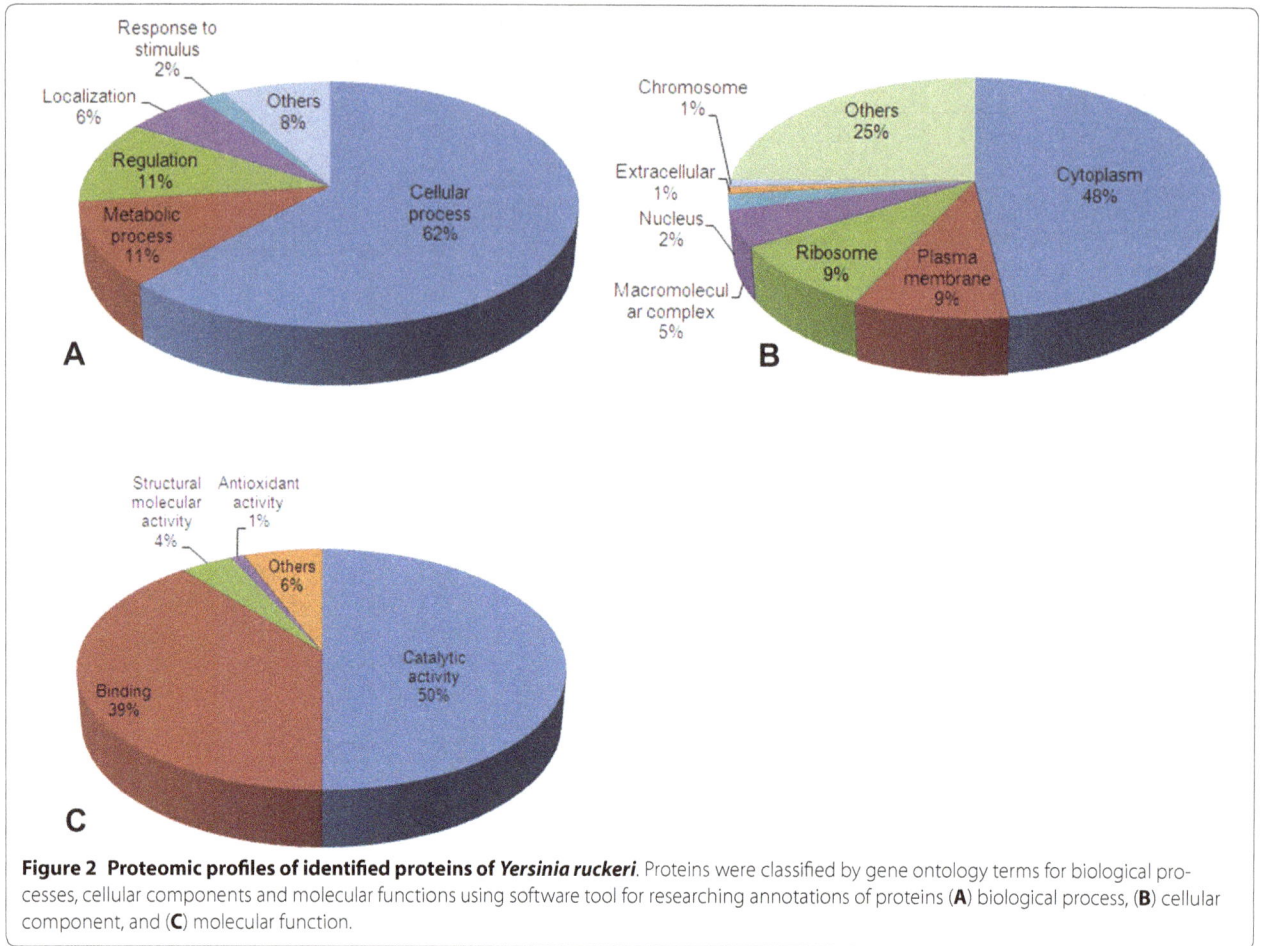

**Figure 2 Proteomic profiles of identified proteins of *Yersinia ruckeri*.** Proteins were classified by gene ontology terms for biological processes, cellular components and molecular functions using software tool for researching annotations of proteins (**A**) biological process, (**B**) cellular component, and (**C**) molecular function.

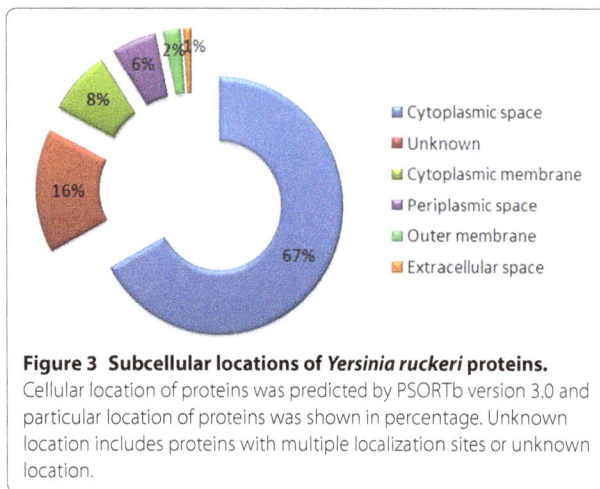

**Figure 3 Subcellular locations of *Yersinia ruckeri* proteins.** Cellular location of proteins was predicted by PSORTb version 3.0 and particular location of proteins was shown in percentage. Unknown location includes proteins with multiple localization sites or unknown location.

deiminase protects bacterial cells against the damaging effects of acidic environments and enhances the ability of cells to survive in acidic extracellular conditions [32]. We observed strong upregulation of phosphate-binding protein PstS (> 3-fold), superoxide dismutase Cu–Zn (3.3- to 3.4-fold) and arginine deiminase (5.2- to 5.8-fold) in *Y. ruckeri* strains. Based on the results of the present study, it appears that upregulated proteins (avirulent strain versus virulent strains) such as PstS, SOD-Cu–Zn and arginine deiminase may be involved in the establishment of disease inside the host and the survival of *Y. ruckeri* during the infection process.

Several proteases such as HtrA, Lon, carboxy-terminal, signal peptidase I, La Type II, HslUV, pyrrolidone–carboxylate, FtsH, protease III, Clp, protease 4, putative protease, peptidase B, T and M37 were identified. These proteases were serine, threonine, cysteine, metalloproteinase and ATP-dependent type proteases, and belonged to the C15, M16, M17, M20B, M23, S16, S26, S41A, S49, U32, AAA ATPase and Clp families including PDZ domains. Proteases play critical roles in the invasion of host tissues, contribute to virulence and damage host tissue during infection [33]. The Yrp1 protease of *Y. ruckeri* has been implicated in the hydrolysis of different matrix and muscle proteins of fish and vaccination with Yrp1 elicits a strong protection against the development of

**Table 2  Lists of important virulence proteins of *Yersinia ruckeri***

| Protein | Function | Cascade of SVMs and PSI-BLAST, score |
| --- | --- | --- |
| Gene expression modulator/haemolysin expression modulating protein | Haemolysin expression | 1.0520 |
| HtrA protease | Serine-type endopeptidase activity | 0.5097 |
| Outer membrane stress sensor protease DegQ serine protease | Serine-type endopeptidase activity | 1.0012 |
| Anti-sigma regulatory factor | Protein serine/threonine kinase activity | 0.9363 |
| Beta-barrel assembly-enhancing protease | Chaperone and a metalloprotease | 1.0339 |
| BarA-associated response regulator UvrY | Regulation of transcription | 0.9837 |
| Peptidyl-prolyl cis–trans isomerase | Protein folding | 0.9128 |
| PhoP family transcriptional regulator | Regulation of transcription | 1.0898 |
| LuxR family transcriptional regulator | Regulation of transcription | 1.0031 |
| AsnC family transcriptional regulator | Regulation of transcription | 0.7053 |
| RNA-binding protein Hfq | Regulation of transcription | 1.0260 |
| Anti-sigma factor antagonist | Regulation of transcription | 0.9804 |
| Attachment invasion locus protein | Invasion | 1.0123 |
| Invasin | Cell adhesion | 1.0130 |
| Superoxide dismutase Cu–Zn | Superoxide dismutase activity | 1.0003 |
| Molybdenum ABC transporter periplasmic molybdenum-binding protein ModA | Transporter activity | 0.8399 |
| DcrB protein | Required for phage C1 adsorption | 1.0009 |
| Methyl-accepting chemotaxis protein I | Chemotaxis | 0.9279 |
| Methyl-accepting chemotaxis protein III | Chemotaxis | 0.9922 |

Proteins were predicted by a method based on bi-layer cascade support vector machine using VirulentPred.

**Table 3  Details of antibiotic resistance ontology of *Yersinia ruckeri***

| Protein | Antibiotic resistance ontology | Bit score |
| --- | --- | --- |
| Bacterial regulatory, crp family protein (cyclic AMP receptor protein) | Fluoroquinolone (enrofloxacin), beta-lactam (amoxicillin), Macrolide (erythromycin) | 431.409 |
| Cys regulon transcriptional activator CysB | Aminocoumarin (novobiocin) | 620.928 |
| Copper-sensing two-component system response regulator CpxR | Aminoglycoside (gentamicin), aminocoumarin (novobiocin) | 389.808 |
| Alanine tRNA ligase | Aminocoumarin | 1487.63 |
| Transcription repair-coupling factor | Fluoroquinolone | 1938.7 |
| Dihydropteroate synthase | Sulfonamide | 440.654 |
| Membrane fusion protein of RND family multidrug efflux pump | Fluoroquinolone, beta-lactam, Macrolide, Rifampin, Chloramphenicol, Tetracycline, Aminocoumarin | 548.125 |
| Beta-lactamase | beta-lactam (amoxicillin) | 608.601 |
| Outer membrane channel protein | Fluoroquinolone, beta-lactam, Macrolide, Rifampin, Chloramphenicol, Tetracycline, Aminocoumarin | 689.878 |
| Elongation factor Tu | Elfamycin | 583.178 |
| Bifunctional polymyxin resistance protein ArnA | Polymyxin B | 951.814 |
| DNA gyrase subunit A | Fluoroquinolone | 751.895 |
| RND efflux system inner membrane transporter CmeB | Fluoroquinolone, tetracycline | 751.125 |
| Isoleucine-tRNA ligase | Mupirocin | 219.55 |

Antibiotic resistance ontology was predicted in the proteome of *Y. ruckeri* using a comprehensive antibiotic resistance database.

enteric redmouth disease [6]. Additionally, the Clp and Lon pro-teases have been shown to have a role in the regulation of the type III secretion systems (T3SS) in various bacterial pathogens. The T3SS forms a needle-like structure in several Gram negative bacteria that allows direct transfer of bacterial virulence factors into the cytoplasm of host cells. The T3SS has been linked to flagellum biosynthesis [34]. We also identified flagellar biosynthesis proteins (FliC, FliG, FliH and FliN), flagellar hook proteins (FlgD, FlgE and FlgK), flagellar brake protein

YcgR, flagellar motor protein MotB and pilus assembly protein PilW in *Y. ruckeri*. FliC and FliH flagellar proteins have been linked with pathogenesis in the fish pathogen, *Edwardsiella tarda* [35]. Additionally, the *Y. ruckeri* flagellin protein has been shown to elicit a robust innate immune response and protect fish against biotype 1 and biotype 2 *Y. ruckeri* strains [36]. More research on the role of proteases and T3SS in *Y. ruckeri* virulence is needed to more fully understand the pathogenicity of *Y. ruckeri*.

We also identified other important virulence proteins such as the UvrY response regulator, peptidyl-prolyl cis–trans isomerase (PPIases), TolB, PhoP and LuxR family transcriptional regulators. UvrY is a response regulator of the BarA-UvrY two-component system and has been shown to be involved in the pathogenesis of *Y. ruckeri*, probably through its regulation of both the invasion of epithelial cells and protection against oxidative stress induced by immune cells [37]. PPIases are FKBP domain-containing ubiquitous folding proteins and have been reported as virulence factors in several bacterial pathogens [38]. Upregulation of FKBP-type peptidyl-prolyl cis–trans isomerases has been observed in iron-starved biotype 2 *Y. ruckeri* strains [16], which may be involved in virulence of *Y. ruckeri*. PhoP is part of a two component system and is important for bacterial survival and replication in macrophages [39]. TolB is the periplasmic component of the Tol–Pal system and is important for antibiotic resistance and pathogenicity in Gram negative pathogens and has been suggested as a suitable candidate for the development of novel drugs against *Pseudomonas aeruginosa* [40]. The LuxR transcriptional regulator is a key player in quorum sensing and affects survival, virulence, antibiotic biosynthesis and biofilm formation of bacteria [41].

A number of chaperone proteins (CbpA, ClpB, DnaK, DnaJ, fimC, HscA, HscB, HtpG, skp, SurA, ProQ), an acid stress chaperone HdeB, universal stress protein E, cold shock (CspC and CspE) and a phage shock protein were identified in *Y. ruckeri*. Bacterial pathogens produce a number of chaperone proteins for survival during changing environments and stress conditions [42]. Some chaperone proteins have also been implicated in bacterial virulence [43]. DnaK chaperone protein plays a role in protein folding and interacts with ClpB in reactivating proteins which have become aggregated after heat shock [44]. The DnaK/DnaJ chaperone machinery and ClpB have been shown to be involved in the invasion of epithelial cells and survival within macrophages of the host, leading to systemic infection of *Salmonella enterica* and *Francisella tularensis* in mice [43, 45]. Upregulation of ClpB, HtpG and universal stress protein A have been observed in *Flavobacterium psychrophilum*

during in vivo growth in fish and were suggested to play an important role in the pathogenesis of *F. psychrophilum* [46]. Based on these data, we suggest that some chaperone proteins may be important for in vivo survival and pathogenesis of *Y. ruckeri*.

A number of cell division proteins (BolA, DedD, DamX, FtsA, FtsE, FtsH, FtsP, FtsZ, ZapA, ZapB and ZapD), chromosome partitioning proteins (ParA, ParB, MukB and MukE) and biosynthesis proteins (iscR, MraZ, basR/pmrA, IF-1, IF-3, S2-S21, L1-L6, RsmA-RsmC and RsmG-RsmI) were identified. The FtsZ and ParA proteins have been identified as potential drug targets against clinically important bacterial pathogens [47]. Protein synthesis (transcriptional and translational) proteins have been targeted for inhibition of bacterial pathogens [48]. However, cell division and chromosome partitioning proteins may act as new drug targets for *Y. ruckeri*. Additionally, we predicted 12 antibiotic resistance classes (Table 3) in the *Y. ruckeri* proteome, particularly for cys regulon transcriptional activator CysB, bifunctional polymyxin resistance protein ArnA, copper-sensing two-component system response regulator CpxR and isoleucine-tRNA ligase. We observed intermediate susceptibility of aminoglycoside (gentamicin, MIC = 4–8 μg/mL) and polymyxin B (MIC = 4 μg/mL) antibiotics against *Y. ruckeri* strains. Similar results were previously reported in French *Y. ruckeri* isolates with aminoglycoside (gentamicin) [49] and greatest variation (MIC = 2–512 μg/mL) in antibiotic sensitivity of polymyxin B was reported among *Y. ruckeri* strains [50]. These higher MIC values suggest that *Y. ruckeri* strains may harbor acquired or intrinsic resistance mechanisms to aminoglycosides and polymyxin B. Additionally, our *Y. ruckeri* strains were highly resistant to erythromycin (MIC = 1024 μg/mL) and rifampin (MIC = 32 μg/mL), consistent with observations by Calvez et al. [49] and Stock et al. [51], who found *Y. ruckeri* strains to be resistant to erythromycin (MIC = 32–64 μg/mL) and rifampin (MIC = 8–16 μg/mL). Erythromycin and novobiocin discs did not show inhibition zone against the Chinese *Y. ruckeri* strain H01 [52]. Similarly, we did not observe any inhibition zone of novobiocin and mupirocin discs against the *Y. ruckeri* strains examined. Inherent resistance to erythromycin and rifampin has been described for the other *Yersinia* species (*Y. enterocolitica*, *Y. mollaretii* and *Y. aldovae*) [51]. Our results support these findings and suggest that *Y. ruckeri* strains might also be resistant to novobiocin and mupirocin. Moreover, two efflux pumps of the RND family were identified. This family is widespread among Gram negative bacteria and, in Enterobacteriaceae such as *E. coli*, contributes to the intrinsic resistance against several antibiotics, including macrolide and novobiocin [53]. This is consistent with our present results that found

*Y. ruckeri* to be resistant to both antibiotics. Finally, it is important to note that the antimicrobial agents used to validate the results of our antibiotic resistance ontology are generally not approved for use in aquaculture. *Y. ruckeri* strains are susceptible to commonly applied antimicrobial agents such as florfenicol and oxytetracycline to treat fish diseases [49].

The outer membrane proteins (OmpA, OmpC, OmpF and OmpW), outer membrane assembly factors (BamA, BamB, BamC, BamD and BamE), outer membrane lipoproteins (Blc, pcp, RcsF, LolB, LolD, Omp16, RcsF and YfeY), lipoproteins (NlpD, NlpE and NlpI) and lipopolysaccharide biosynthesis proteins (LptA, LptD and LptE) were identified. These proteins play an important role in pathogen-host interactions and pathogenicity [54]. Additionally, OMPs help in resisting host defense mechanisms and have been shown to confer protection in fish [54, 55]. The outer membrane assembly factor YeaT and OmpC have been shown to induce a strong immune response and protect *Labeo rohita* and *Japanese flounder* against *Edwardsiella tarda* infection [56, 57].

In conclusion, our study provides the first global proteomic profiles of *Y. ruckeri* and this work will provide a better understanding of the physiology, proteomic biology, proteomic changes, virulence mechanisms and localization of *Y. ruckeri* proteins. The most commonly expressed proteins such as SOD-Cu–Zn and PstS might be useful to develop a single vaccination protocol or single drug therapy for both biotype 1 and biotype 2 strains. Additionally, proteins associated with virulence and antigenicity such as Clp and Lon pro-teases, TolB, PPIases, PhoP and LuxR family transcriptional regulators may be used for the construction of novel vaccines for yersiniosis in fish. The comprehensive data set generated in this study will serve as a reference proteome for future studies such as protein–protein interaction and network analysis.

## Data deposition

Shotgun proteomics data have been deposited in the ProteomeXchange Consortium (http://proteomecentral.proteomexchange.org) via the PRIDE partner repository [58] with the dataset identifier PXD005439.

## Additional files

**Additional file 1. Antimicrobial susceptibility of *Yersinia ruckeri* strains.** Antibiotic susceptibility was determined using the disc diffusion technique on Mueller–Hinton agar and minimal inhibitory concentration was determined with the same antibiotics using micro dilution on microtiter plates. The diameter of the inhibition halo and lowest concentration of antibiotic that inhibited visible growth of bacteria was defined after incubation 48 h at 22 °C. Novobiocin and mupirocin discs displaced no inhibition zone against *Y. ruckeri* strains. Note: I = intermediate and R = resistant.

**Additional file 2. Details of total identified proteins of *Yersinia ruckeri*.** Number of proteins was identified at false discovery rate 1% with more than one peptide.

**Additional file 3. Details of identified proteins of *Yersinia ruckeri* strains.** Number of proteins was identified at false discovery rate 1% with more than one peptide.

**Additional file 4. Principal component analysis of *Yersinia ruckeri* strains.** The score plots show that strain SP-05 differs from the three strains (CSF007-82, 7959-11 and YRNC-10) but the latter three strains showed minor proteomic differences.

**Additional file 5. Lists of uniquely identified proteins in each strain of *Yersinia ruckeri*.** Forty-six proteins in SP-05, 43 proteins in CSF007-82, 31 proteins in 7959-11 and 13 proteins in YRNC-10 were uniquely identified.

**Additional file 6. Fold changes of differentially down regulated proteins of *Yersinia ruckeri* strains compared to each other.** ANOVA was performed for UniProt database searches. * Denotes statistically significant difference according to Tukey's honest significant difference post hoc test with false discovery rate-adjusted $p$-value < 0.001 and fold change < −3 or > +3.

**Additional file 7. Lists of virulence proteins of *Yersinia ruckeri*.** Proteins were predicted by a method based on bi-layer cascade support vector machine using VirulentPred.

## Abbreviations

ERM: enteric redmouth disease; LC–MS: liquid chromatography–mass spectrometry; TOF: triple quadrupole time of flight; FDR: false discovery rate; SWATH: sequential window acquisition of all theoretical spectra; IDA: information dependent data acquisition; PCA: principal component analysis.

## Competing interests

The authors declare that they have no competing interests.

## Authors' contributions

GK and MEM conceived and designed the experiment. GK performed the experiment. KH, GK and ERF performed the LC–MS/MS. GK analyzed the data and drafted the manuscript. TJW, ERF and MEM revised the manuscript. All authors read and approved the final manuscript.

## Acknowledgements

This study was funded by the Austrian Science Fund (FWF) Project No. P 27489-B22 to Gokhlesh Kumar. We are thankful to Mag. Katharina Nöbauer and Dipl.-Biol. Sarah Schlosser for their technical assistance.

## Author details

[1] Clinical Division of Fish Medicine, University of Veterinary Medicine, Veterinärplatz 1, 1210 Vienna, Austria. [2] VetCore Facility for Research/Proteomics Unit, University of Veterinary Medicine, Vienna, Austria. [3] National Center for Cool and Cold Water Aquaculture, Kearneysville, USA.

## References

1. Horne MT, Barnes AC (1999) Enteric redmouth disease (*Yersinia ruckeri*). In: Woo PTK, Bruno DW (eds) Fish diseases and disorders. Viral, bacterial and fungal infections. CABI Publishing, Wallingford, pp 445–477
2. Kumar G, Menanteau-Ledouble S, Saleh M, El-Matbouli M (2015) *Yersinia ruckeri*, the causative agent of enteric redmouth disease in fish. Vet Res 46:103

3.  Ohtani M, Villumsen KR, Strøm H, Raida MK (2014) 3D Visualization of the initial *Yersinia ruckeri* infection route in rainbow trout (*Oncorhynchus mykiss*) by optical projection tomography. PLoS One 9:e89672

4.  Tobback E, Decostere A, Hermans K, Ryckaert J, Duchateau L, Haesebrouck F, Chiers K (2009) Route of entry and tissue distribution of *Yersinia ruckeri* in experimentally infected rainbow trout *Oncorhynchus mykiss*. Dis Aquat Org 84:219–228

5.  Romalde JL, Toranzo AE (1993) Pathological activities of *Yersinia ruckeri*, the enteric redmouth (ERM) bacterium. FEMS Microbiol Lett 112:291–300

6.  Fernández L, Lopez JR, Secades P, Menendez A, Marquez I, Guijarro JA (2003) In vitro and in vivo studies of the Yrp1 protease from *Yersinia ruckeri* and its role in protective immunity against enteric red mouth disease of salmonids. Appl Environ Microbiol 69:7328–7335

7.  Davies RL (1991) Outer membrane protein profiles of *Yersinia ruckeri*. Vet Microbiol 26:125–140

8.  Austin DA, Robertson PAW, Austin B (2003) Recovery of a new biogroup of *Yersinia ruckeri* from diseased rainbow trout (*Oncorhynchus mykiss*, Walbaum). Syst Appl Microbiol 26:127–131

9.  Welch TJ, Verner-Jeffreys DW, Dalsgaard I, Wiklund T, Evenhuis JP, Cabrera JA, Hinshaw JM, Drennan JD, LaPatra SE (2011) Independent emergence of *Yersinia ruckeri* biotype 2 in the United States and Europe. Appl Environ Microbiol 77:3493–3499

10. Fouz B, Zarza C, Amaro C (2006) First description of non-motile *Yersinia ruckeri* serovar I strains causing disease in rainbow trout, *Oncorhynchus mykiss* (Walbaum), cultured in Spain. J Fish Dis 29:339–346

11. Tinsley JW, Lyndon AR, Austin B (2011) Antigenic and cross-protection studies of biotype 1 and biotype 2 isolates of *Yersinia ruckeri* in rainbow trout, *Oncorhynchus mykiss* (Walbaum). J Appl Microbiol 111:8–16

12. Nelson MC, LaPatra SE, Welch TJ, Graf J (2015) Complete genome sequence of *Yersinia ruckeri* strain CSF007-82, etiologic agent of red mouth disease in salmonid fish. Genome Announc 3:e01491–e01494

13. Coquet L, Cosette P, Dé E, Galas L, Vaudry H, Rihouey C, Lerouge P, Junter GA, Jouenne T (2005) Immobilization induces alterations in the outer membrane protein pattern of *Yersinia ruckeri*. J Proteome Res 4:1988–1998

14. Bystritskaya E, Stenkova A, Chistuylin D, Chernysheva N, Khomenko V, Anastyuk S et al (2016) Adaptive responses of outer membrane porin balance of *Yersinia ruckeri* under different incubation temperature, osmolarity, and oxygen availability. Microbiologyopen 5:597–603

15. Zhou L, Ying W, Han Y, Chen M, Yan Y, Li L, Zhu Z, Zheng Z, Jia W, Yang R, Qian X (2012) A proteome reference map and virulence factors analysis of *Yersinia pestis* 91001. J Proteom 75:894–907

16. Kumar G, Hummel K, Ahrens M, Menanteau-Ledouble S, Welch TJ, Eisenacher M, Razzazi-Fazeli E, El-Matbouli M (2016) Shotgun proteomic analysis of *Yersinia ruckeri* strains under normal and iron-limited conditions. Vet Res 47:100

17. Evenhuis JP, Lapatra SE, Verner-Jeffreys DW, Dalsgaard I, Welch TJ (2009) Identification of flagellar motility genes in *Yersinia ruckeri* by transposon mutagenesis. Appl Environ Microbiol 75:6630–6633

18. Welch TJ, Wiens GD (2005) Construction of a virulent, green fluorescent protein-tagged *Yersinia ruckeri* and detection in trout tissues after intraperitoneal and immersion challenge. Dis Aquat Organ 67:267–272

19. Domon B, Aebersold R (2006) Mass spectrometry and protein analysis. Science 312:212–217

20. McQueen P, Spicer V, Schellenberg J, Krokhin O, Sparling R, Levin D, Wilkins JA (2015) Whole cell, label free protein quantitation with data independent acquisition: quantitation at the MS2 level. Proteomics 15:16–24

21. R Core Team (2015) R: a language and environment for statistical computing. R foundation for statistical computing, Vienna. R version 3.2.2. https://www.R-project.org/. Accessed 8 Mar 2016

22. Benjamini Y, Hochberg Y (1995) Controlling the false discovery rate: a practical and powerful approach to multiple testing. J R Stat Soc B 57:289–300

23. Oliveros JC (2007) VENNY. An interactive tool for comparing lists with Venn Diagrams. http://bioinfogp.cnb.csic.es/tools/venny/index.html. Accessed 28 Nov 2016

24. Bhatia VN, Perlman DH, Costello CE, McComb ME (2009) Software tool for researching annotations of proteins: open-source protein annotation software with data visualization. Anal Chem 81:9819–9823

25. Yu NY, Wagner JR, Laird MR, Melli G, Rey S, Lo R, Dao P, Sahinalp SC, Ester M, Foster LJ, Brinkman FS (2010) PSORTb 3.0: improved protein subcellular localization prediction with refined localization subcategories and predictive capabilities for all prokaryotes. Bioinformatics 26:1608–1615

26. Garg A, Gupta D (2008) VirulentPred: a SVM based prediction method for virulent proteins in bacterial pathogens. BMC Bioinform 9:62

27. McArthur AG, Waglechner N, Nizam F, Yan A, Azad MA, Baylay AJ et al (2013) The comprehensive antibiotic resistance database. Antimicrob Agents Chemother 57:3348–3357

28. CLSI (2006) Methods for antimicrobial disk susceptibility testing of bacteria isolated from aquatic animals; approved guideline. CLSI document VET03-A. Clinical and Laboratory Standards Institute, Wayne, PA, USA. https://clsi.org/standards/products/packages/vet03pk/. Accessed 23 Mar 2017

29. CLSI (2006) Methods for broth dilution susceptibility testing of bacteria isolated from aquatic animals; approved guideline. CLSI document VET04-A. Clinical and Laboratory Standards Institute, Wayne, PA, USA. https://clsi.org/standards/products/veterinary-medicine/documents/vet04/. Accessed 23 Mar 2017

30. Jacobsen SM, Lane MC, Harro JM, Shirtliff M, Mobley HL (2008) The high-affinity phosphate transporter Pst is a virulence factor for *Proteus mirabilis* during complicated urinary tract infection. FEMS Immunol Med Microbiol 52:180–193

31. Fang FC, DeGroote MA, Foster JW, Bäumler AJ, Ochsner U, Testerman T, Bearson S, Giárd JC, Xu Y, Campbell G, Laessig T (1999) Virulent *Salmonella typhimurium* has two periplasmic Cu, Zn-superoxide dismutases. Proc Natl Acad Sci U S A 96:7502–7507

32. Xu B, Yang X, Zhang P, Ma Z, Lin H, Fan H (2016) The arginine deiminase system facilitates environmental adaptability of *Streptococcus equi* ssp. zooepidemicus through pH adjustment. Res Microbiol 167:403–412

33. Frees D, Brøndsted L, Ingmer H (2013) Bacterial proteases and virulence. Subcell Biochem 66:161–192

34. Fernández L, Prieto M, Guijarro JA (2007) The iron- and temperature-regulated haemolysin YhlA is a virulence factor of *Yersinia ruckeri*. Microbiology 153:483–489

35. Zhou D, Galán J (2001) *Salmonella* entry into host cells: the work in concert of type III secreted effector proteins. Microbes Infect 3:1293–1298

36. He Y, Xu T, Fossheim LE, Zhang XH (2012) FliC, a flagellin protein, is essential for the growth and virulence of fish pathogen *Edwardsiella tarda*. PLoS One 7:e45070

37. Dahiya I, Stevenson RMW (2010) The UvrY response regulator of the BarA-UvrY two-component system contributes to *Yersinia ruckeri* infection of rainbow trout (*Oncorhynchus mykiss*). Arch Microbiol 192:541–547

38. Ünal CM, Steinert M (2014) Microbial Peptidyl-Prolyl *cis/trans* Isomerases (PPIases): virulence factors and potential alternative drug targets. Microbiol Mol Biol Rev 78:544–571

39. Groisman EA, Chiao E, Lipps CJ, Heffron F (1989) *Salmonella typhimurium* phoP virulence gene is a transcriptional regulator. Proc Natl Acad Sci U S A 86:7077–7081

40. Lo Sciuto A, Fernández-Piñar R, Bertuccini L, Iosi F, Superti F, Imperi F (2014) The periplasmic protein TolB as a potential drug target in *Pseudomonas aeruginosa*. PLoS One 9:e103784

41. Alonso-Hearn M, Eckstein TM, Sommer S, Bermudez LE (2010) A *Mycobacterium avium* subsp. paratuberculosis LuxR regulates cell envelope and virulence. Innate Immun 16:235–247

42. Neckers L, Tatu U (2008) Molecular chaperones in pathogen virulence: emerging new targets for therapy. Cell Host Microbe 4:519–527

43. Takaya A, Tomoyasu T, Matsui H, Yamamoto T (2004) The Dnak/Dnaj chaperone machinery of *Salmonella enterica* serovar typhimurium is essential for invasion of epithelial cells and survival within macrophages, leading to systemic infection. Infect Immun 72:1364–1373

44. Lund PA (2001) Microbial molecular chaperones. Adv Microb Physiol 44:93–140

45. Meibom KL, Dubail I, Dupuis M, Barel M, Lenco J, Stulik J, Golovliov I, Sjöstedt A, Charbit A (2008) The heat-shock protein ClpB of *Francisella tularensis* is involved in stress tolerance and is required for multiplication in target organs of infected mice. Mol Microbiol 67:1384–1401

46. LaFrentz BR, LaPatra SE, Call DR, Wiens GD, Cain KD (2009) Proteomic analysis of *Flavobacterium psychrophilum* cultured in vivo and in iron-limited media. Dis Aquat Organ 87:171–182

47. Nisa S, Blokpoel MC, Robertson BD, Tyndall JD, Lun S, Bishai WR, O'Toole R (2010) Targeting the chromosome partitioning protein ParA in tuberculosis drug discovery. J Antimicrob Chemother 65:2347–2358

48. Hong W, Zeng J, Xie J (2014) Antibiotic drugs targeting bacterial RNAs. Acta Pharm Sin B 4:258–265

49. Calvez S, Gantelet H, Blanc G, Douet DG, Daniel P (2014) *Yersinia ruckeri* biotypes 1 and 2 in France: presence and antibiotic susceptibility. Dis Aquat Organ 109:117–126

50. De Grandis SA, Stevenson RM (1985) Antimicrobial susceptibility patterns and R plasmid-mediated resistance of the fish pathogen *Yersinia ruckeri*. Antimicrob Agents Chemother 27:938–942

51. Stock I, Henrichfreise B, Wiedemann B (2002) Natural antibiotic susceptibility and biochemical profiles of *Yersinia enterocolitica*-like strains: *Y. bercovieri*, *Y. mollaretii*, *Y. aldovae* and "*Y. ruckeri*". J Med Microbiol 51:56–69

52. Shaowu L, Di W, Hongbai L, Tongyan L (2013) Isolation of *Yersinia ruckeri* strain H01 from farm-raised amur sturgeon *Acipenser schrencki* in China. J Aquat Anim Health 25:9–14

53. Nikaido H, Takatsuka Y (2009) Mechanisms of RND multidrug efflux pumps. Biochim Biophys Acta 1794:769–781

54. Seltman G, Holst O (2002) The bacterial cell wall. Springer, Berlin, pp 9–40

55. Kumar G, Rathore G, Sengupta U, Singh V, Kapoor D, Lakra WS (2007) Isolation and characterization of outer membrane proteins of *Edwardsiella tarda* and its application in immunoassays. Aquaculture 272:98–104

56. Kumar G, Rathore G, El-Matbouli M (2014) Outer membrane protein assembly factor YaeT (omp85) and GroEL proteins of *Edwardsiella tarda* are immunogenic antigens for *Labeo rohita* (Hamilton). J Fish Dis 37:1055–1059

57. Fuguo L, Xiaoqian T, Xiuzhen S, Jing X, Wenbin Z (2016) *Edwardsiella tarda* outer membrane protein C: an immunogenic protein induces highly protective effects in Flounder (*Paralichthys olivaceus*) against Edwardsiellosis. Int J Mol Sci 17:1117

58. Vizcaíno JA, Csordas A, del-Toro N, Dianes JA, Griss J, Lavidas I, Mayer G, Perez-Riverol Y, Reisinger F, Ternent T, Xu QW, Wang R, Hermjakob H (2016) 2016 update of the PRIDE database and related tools. Nucleic Acids Res 44:D447–D456

# 10

# Molecular and virulence characterization of highly prevalent *Streptococcus agalactiae* circulated in bovine dairy herds

Maoda Pang[1], Lichang Sun[1], Tao He[1], Hongdu Bao[1], Lili Zhang[1], Yan Zhou[1], Hui Zhang[1], Ruicheng Wei[1], Yongjie Liu[2] and Ran Wang[1*]

## Abstract

Bovine mastitis caused by *Streptococcus agalactiae* continues to be one of the major veterinary and economic issues in certain areas of the world. The more prevalent *S. agalactiae* strains that cause bovine mastitis in China dairy farms belong to a number of bovine-adapted sequence types (STs) ST67, ST103 and ST568. However, it is unknown why these STs can emerge as highly prevalent clones in bovine dairy farms. Here, to determine if a variety of virulence characteristics were associated with these highly prevalent STs, the molecular and virulence characterization of 116 strains isolated from bovine, human, fish and environment were analyzed. Our data showed that all bovine-adapted strains could be assigned to capsular genotype Ia or II, and carried pilus island 2b, and lactose operon. Importantly, we demonstrated that the growth ability in milk, biofilm formation ability and adhesion ability to bovine mammary epithelial cells (BMECs) were significantly higher for all bovine-adapted strains compared to strains from other origins. Additionally, ST103 and ST568 strains exhibited significantly higher hemolytic activity and cytotoxicity than ST67 strains. In conclusion, our study provides substantial evidence for the hypothesis that the virulence characteristics including efficient growth in milk, elevated biofilm formation ability, together with strong adhesion ability might have favored the high prevalence of the STs in the bovine environment, whereas the hemolytic activity and cytotoxicity were not the crucial characteristics.

## Introduction

*Streptococcus agalactiae* is a gram-positive bacterium that has been considered as an important pathogen frequently associated with mastitis in bovine [1], neonatal meningitis in human [2] and meningoencephalitis in fish [3]. In large animals, bovine mastitis is the dominant health disorder leading to severe milk loss, and is responsible for significant financial losses in the dairy industry [4, 5]. An eradication has been implemented since 1960s to reduce the incidence of *S. agalactiae* mastitis in several European countries [6, 7]. However, in last several years,

*S. agalactiae* mastitis reemerged and the occurrence frequency has increased again in Denmark, Norway and other Scandinavian countries [6, 7]. In other countries, especially in China, *S. agalactiae* has become one of the most frequently detected pathogens in cows diagnosed with subclinical mastitis [8]. Globally, bovine mastitis infected by *S. agalactiae* is still prevalent in many dairy farms worldwide [6].

Over the last decades, numerous studies have been conducted to investigate the molecular epidemiology [8–11] and genomic diversity of *S. agalactiae* [6, 12–14]. Studies using multilocus sequence typing (MLST) have shown that *S. agalactiae* belongs to corresponding sequence types (STs) with different host specificities [11, 15]. It has been reported that the prevalent strains circulated in China dairy farms are predominantly assigned to the bovine-adapted STs ST67, ST103 and ST568 [8]. ST67 belonging to clonal complex (CC) 67 has previously

*Correspondence: ranwang@jaas.ac.cn
[1] Key Laboratory of Control Technology and Standard for Agro-product Safety and Quality, Key Lab of Food Quality and Safety of Jiangsu Province-State Key Laboratory Breeding Base, Institute of Food Safety and Nutrition, Jiangsu Academy of Agricultural Sciences, No. 50 Zhongling Street, Nanjing 210014, China
Full list of author information is available at the end of the article

been considered to be the common ST among bovine isolates [16], and have been found in many countries including Brazil [17], France, the UK [18] and the USA [19]. ST103 was occasionally isolated from dairy cows in Brazil according to previous studies [17, 20], however, ST103 has emerged as a highly prevalent ST in bovine herds in Norway [7] and Denmark [11]. Both ST103 and ST568 belong to CC103, since ST568 is a single-locus variant (SLV, in which one allele differs from the ST) of ST103. To date, although ST568 was only detected in China, it was observed in high frequencies [8]. For human, isolates cluster five major CCs CC1, CC10, CC17, CC19 and CC23, which are separately from bovine isolates [12]. In fish farms, ST7 strains are found to be the major cause of streptococcosis outbreaks [13]. *S. agalactiae* was also observed in pond water [21], sediment [21] and feeding equipment [7], but no CCs were reported to be prevalent in specific environmental samples. Except for MLST analysis, comparative genomics has provided a comprehensive understanding of the distinct dynamic among *S. agalactiae* strains isolated from bovine, human and fish [6, 12–14]. The key role that horizontal gene transfer plays in the evolution of the bovine *S. agalactiae* strains has been highlighted [6, 12, 14]. It has been reported that human isolates are dominated to be few tetracycline resistant clones, and the acquisition of integrative and conjugative elements harbouring *tet*(M) may lead to the expansion of CC17 clones that then contributes to the increase of neonatal infections [12]. However, it is unknown why or how the bovine-adapted strains emerged as highly prevalent clones in dairy farms, and the mechanism of pathogenesis of these strains still remain limited.

Previous studies have shown that specific STs or strains often associate with the virulence characteristics which can contribute to their infection in host organisms [22–24]. Since the bovine-adapted STs (ST67, ST103 and ST568) are specifically responsible for the majority of *S. agalactiae* mastitis, it indicates that they may harbor some specific virulence characteristics which permit them to cause bovine mastitis and be prevalent within the bovine environment. Therefore, in this study, we sought to identify the virulence characteristics required for *S. agalactiae* infection in bovine mastitis, with the ultimate goal of elucidating the mechanisms underlying pathogenesis.

## Materials and methods
### Isolates collection and identification
A total of 116 *S. agalactiae* strains including 84 bovine strains and 32 reference strains isolated from human, fish and environment (soil, pond water and pond sediment) were collected in this study. The information (accession NO. in GenBank, biological resource, geographic resource and date of isolation) about the 116 strains is provided in Additional file 1. All bovine strains were recovered from milk samples taken from cows presenting clinical or subclinical mastitis between March 2011 and June 2016 from 14 bovine dairy farms in China. The 14 bovine dairy farms were located in eight cities, and were not epidemiologically related. Six bovine isolates belonging to the same STs were randomly taken from each dairy farms.

For isolation of bovine *S. agalactiae*, we diagnosed the bovine mastitis firstly. The clinical mastitis was determined through visual investigation by herd veterinarians, while the subclinical mastitis was evaluated using milk somatic cell counts (SCC) calculated by Fossomatic 5000TM automatic equipment (Foss Electric). Subclinical mastitis was suspected when SCC were greater than 1 000 000 cells/mL, but with no inflammation of the udder. Before the collection of milk samples, each teat was disinfected with swabs soaked in 70% ethyl alcohol, and the foremilk was discarded. Then, 20 mL milk from quarters with clinical or subclinical mastitis were collected, and 1 mL of milk sample was inoculated into 5 mL Todd-Hewitt broth (THB, BD Difco) and incubated at 37 °C for 6 h. After enrichment, the samples were streaked on Todd-Hewitt agar (THA, BD Difco) and incubated at 37 °C for 18 h. Subsequently, single colonies suspected to be *S. agalactiae* were isolated and the bacterial DNA was extracted using Bacterial DNA Kit (Omega). *S. agalactiae* were further identified by PCR amplification of 16S ribosomal DNA (rDNA) with universal primers 27F/1492R [25], and the sequence of 16S rDNA were deposited in GenBank (https://www.ncbi.nlm.nih.gov/genbank/).

### Genotypic characterization and phylogenetic analysis
Multilocus sequence typing was performed as previously described [26]. Briefly, seven housekeeping genes *adhP*, *pheS*, *atr*, *glnA*, *sdhA*, *glcK* and *tkt* from each strain were submitted to the *S. agalactiae* MLST database (http://pubmlst.org/sagalactiae/) to determine their identity against existing alleles. Each gene fragment was translated into a distinct allele, and each strain was classified into its ST by the combination of the alleles of the seven housekeeping genes. New STs that differed from the pre-existing STs were assigned new numbers and the data were deposited in the MLST database. The eBURST V3 program (http://eburst.mlst.net) was then used to identify the eBURST groups of 1148 STs deposited in *S. agalactiae* MLST database based on sharing of 6 out of 7 alleles using standard eBURST methodology [27]. The capsular genotypes Ia to IX of *S. agalactiae* were identified by a multiplex PCR assay developed by the previous study [28]. For phylogenetic analysis, the seven

housekeeping genes previously sequenced were aligned and concatenated using MEGA7 (http://www.megasoftware.net/). Then, the phylogenetic tree was constructed using the neighbor-joining method on a set of 1000 bootstrap replicates [29].

## Distribution of virulence factors in *S. agalactiae*

A total of ten virulence genes *scpB*, *lmb*, *cylE*, *hylB*, *gapC*, *cspA*, *dltA*, *fbsA*, *fbsB* and *bibA*, and three pili genes designated as pilus island 1 (PI-1), PI-2a and PI-2b were detected according to previous study [21]. The examined virulence genes could be classified as being associated with bacterial adhesion and colonization (PI-1, PI-2a, PI-2b, *dltA*, *fbsA*, *fbsB*, *bibA* and *lmb*), bacterial invasion (*cspA*, *gapC* and *hylB*), immune evasion (*scpB*), toxin production (*cylE*), and metabolic adaptation (lactose operon) [5, 21]. The primers used to detect the lactose operon which referred to *lacABCDFEGX* [30] were newly designed in this study from conserved regions of *S. agalactiae* ATCC13813 and NEM316 using primer premier 6.24 (http://www.premierbiosoft.com/). All primers used in this study are listed in Additional file 2.

## Measurement of growth ability

The growth ability of each strain in milk was determined using the drop plate method [31]. In brief, cultures of each strain grown in THB for 6 h were adjusted to an optical density (OD) of 0.5 at 600 nm and then diluted 1:100 in 2 mL of sterile milk. The sterile milk inoculated with phosphate-buffered saline (PBS) was used as the negative control. Then, the inoculated milk was grown on a shaking incubator (80 rpm) at 37 °C for 12 h. For each time point, serial dilutions of milk were made in PBS and plated (100 µL in duplicate for each of the dilutions) on THA. After incubation for 24 h, colonies on THA were counted and the bacterial concentration was calculated. Experiments were carried out in triplicate and each independent experiment consisted of three technical replicates.

The growth ability of each strain in THB was determined as previously described [32] with some modifications. Briefly, cultures of strains grown in THB for 6 h were adjusted to an OD of 0.5 at 600 nm and then diluted 1:100 in 1 mL of THB. Every 200 µL of the inoculated cultures and blanks containing THB alone were injected into 96-well plates (Corning). Each growth condition was replicated in four wells and cultured at 37 °C. The growth of each strain was examined by measuring the absorbance of the cultures at 600 nm using a microplate reader (infinite M200 PRO, Tecan). The results are shown as the $OD_{600}$ obtained at each time point, normalized against the background OD of THB alone. Each independent experiment was repeated in triplicate.

## Measurement of biofilm formation ability

The biofilm formation ability of *S. agalactiae* strains were evaluated by crystal violet staining using 96-well plates as described previously [33], with some modifications. Bacteria grown in THB for 6 h were normalized to an $OD_{600}$ of 0.5 and then diluted 1:1000 in THB. The THB alone was used as the negative control. Two hundred microliters of inoculated THB was added to each well of 96-well plate and the plates were incubated statically at 37 °C. After incubated for 24 h, suspensions were discarded and the plates were washed with PBS thrice to remove planktonic cells. Subsequently, the surface-combined biofilms were fixed with methanol for 20 min. After discarding the methanol and drying at 37 °C, each well was stained with 200 µL of 1% (wt/vol) crystal violet solution for 15 min. Then, the plates were washed with PBS thrice to remove unbound dye. To quantify the biofilm biomass, the bound dye was redissolved in 200 µL of ethyl alcohol and a microplate reader was taken for each sample at $OD_{595}$. Each strain was repeated in eight wells, and the assay was repeated in four independent occasions. The mature biofilm formed by *S. agalactiae* strains were also observed as described previously [34]. Briefly, 2 mL of the prepared 1:1000 dilution was added to each well of a 6-well plate (Corning) that contained a pre-sterilized microscopic glass slide as the substratum for biofilm growth. After incubation at 37 °C for 24 h for biofilm development, the planktonic bacterial cells on the glass slides were removed by washed using PBS. Then, 10 µL of Alexa Fluor 488 (Invitrogen) was added to each glass slide with a final concentration of 10 µg/mL and incubated in dark for 20 min. After washing triplicate using PBS, the biofilm formed on the slide was observed by Ultra View VOX (PerkinElmer).

## Measurement of hemolytic activity

The *S. agalactiae* strains were cultured on commercial Columbia blood agar plates (KeMaJia) for 24 h to determine their hemolytic phenotype firstly. Then, the hemolytic activity of all strains were measured using culture filtrates of bacteria cultured for 18 h as described previously [35]. In brief, every 200 µL of culture filtrates, which were adjusted to per mL of cell filtrate per $1 \times 10^9$ CFU, were added to the well of a 96-well plate. Subsequentially, additions of 100 µL 2% sheep red blood cells (SRBCs) were added to the 96-well plate. The plate was incubated statically at 37 °C for 1 h, and then placed in 4 °C refrigerator for 12 h. Aliquots (100 µL) of normal saline and 1% (vol/vol) Triton-X 100 were added to an equal volume of 2% SRBCs as negative and positive controls, respectively. At the end of incubation at 4 °C, every 100 µL aliquot of supernatant was taken from each well to a new 96-well plate after centrifuged at 800 *g* for 10 min, and the OD of supernatant was measured at 540 nm. Hemolytic activity of each strain was reported as $(A - A_0/A_{max} - A_0) \times 100$, whereas $A_0$ is the absorbance caused by the background hemolysis occurring during incubation with normal saline, and $A_{max}$ is the absorbance at 100% hemolysis after incubation with 1% Triton X-100 [36].

### Measurement of cytotoxicity

The release of lactate dehydrogenase (LDH) was used to determine the cytotoxic effect of *S. agalactiae* strains against bovine mammary epithelial cells (BMECs) using the CytoTox 96 Non-Radioactive Cytotoxicity Assay (Promega). In brief, BMECs cultured in 96-well plates were infected with 100 μL aliquots of bacterial suspensions at multiplicity of infection (MOI) of 1, 10 and 100 separately. BMECs lysed with the lysis solution were used as the positive control (100% cytotoxicity), whereas non-infected BMECs and bacteria alone were used as negative controls. The 96-well plates were centrifuged at 800 *g* for 10 min to move the bacteria to the surface of each monolayer before incubated for 3 h at 37 °C in 5% $CO_2$. The plates were centrifuged again at 800 *g* for 10 min after incubation and 50 μL supernatant of each well was removed to new plates to determine the release of LDH by measuring $OD_{490}$. Ultimately, percent cytotoxicity of each strain was calculated through the formula provided by the manufacturer's instructions.

### Adhesion assay

Adhesion assay was performed according to the method described previously [37] with the following modifications. Cultures of each strain grown in THB for 6 h were harvested, washed twice with sterile PBS, and then resuspended in minimum essential medium (MEM, Yocon). BMECs cultured in 24-well plates (Corning) were infected with 500 μL aliquots of bacterial suspensions at an MOI of 100. The 24-well plates were centrifuged at 800 *g* for 10 min to move the bacteria to the surface of each monolayer before incubated for 2 h at 37 °C in 5% $CO_2$. After incubation, the supernatants from each well were recovered and BMEC monolayers were washed thrice with PBS to obtain non-adherent bacterial suspensions. Subsequently, BMEC monolayers were trypsinized using 0.25% Trypsin–EDTA and further lysed with Triton X-100 at a final concentration of 0.1% (vol/vol) to obtain the adherent bacterial cells. The number of adherent bacterial cells and non-adherent bacterial cells from the supernatants were determined by plating serial dilutions on THA and counting the colonies after incubation for 24 h. The adhesion ability of *S. agalactiae* strains were expressed as percentage of adherent bacterial cells relative to the total number of adherent and non-adherent

bacterial cells. Independent experiments were performed in triplicate.

### Statistical analysis

Continuous variables of virulence characteristics among different groups or subgroups were analyzed by analysis of variance (ANOVA), followed by Turkey's and Dunnett's T3 multiple comparison tests with $P < 0.05$ considered to be statistically significant, while $P < 0.01$ was considered to be an extremely significant difference. Error bars presented in the figures represent standard deviations of multiple replicate experiments. Data were collected and analyzed using Microsoft Excel (version 2010, Microsoft Corp.), GraphPad Prism (version 6.0, GraphPad Software Inc.) and SPSS Statics (version 22.0, SPSS Inc.).

### Results

#### Genotypic characterization and phylogenetic analysis

The genotypic characteristics of the 116 *S. agalactiae* strains were analyzed using MLST and molecular capsular type (MCT). A total of 15 STs were identified, and the 84 bovine isolates were assigned to three STs, which were ST67 (n = 30), ST103 (n = 30) and ST568 (n = 24), respectively. The human isolates belonged to ST17, ST19, ST23, ST110 and ST337, while the fish isolates used in this study all belonged to ST7. Each of the environmental isolates was classified into a separate ST and three new STs (ST1090, ST1091 and ST1092) were identified based on new combinations of allele profiles. To illustrate the relationship between the 15 STs obtained from this study and the existing STs in *S. agalactiae* MLST database, an eBURST population snapshot was generated (Figure 1A, Additional file 3). The eBURST analysis showed these STs could be grouped as 10 groups and 57 singletons, and the large groups included a number of major subgroups that used to separate CCs. The bovine isolates were grouped in CC67 and CC103 (ST103 and its SLV ST568), and human isolates were grouped in CC17, CC19 (ST19 and its SLV ST110), CC23 and CC337. However, CC23 formed a distinct group, which was not related to CC17, CC19 or CC337. The fish isolates were grouped in CC7 (ST7). For environmental isolates, ST1090, ST1091 and ST1092 were identified as three singletons, while ST58, ST226 and ST592 were grouped in CC103, CC314 and CC22, respectively.

To further investigate the phylogenetic relationship of the 116 *S. agalactiae* strains, a phylogenetic tree based on the seven housekeeping genes was constructed. As shown in Figure 1B, the phylogenetic tree could be classified into three clades. Clade I was the largest cluster which including ST58, ST103 and ST568. Clade II was consisted of

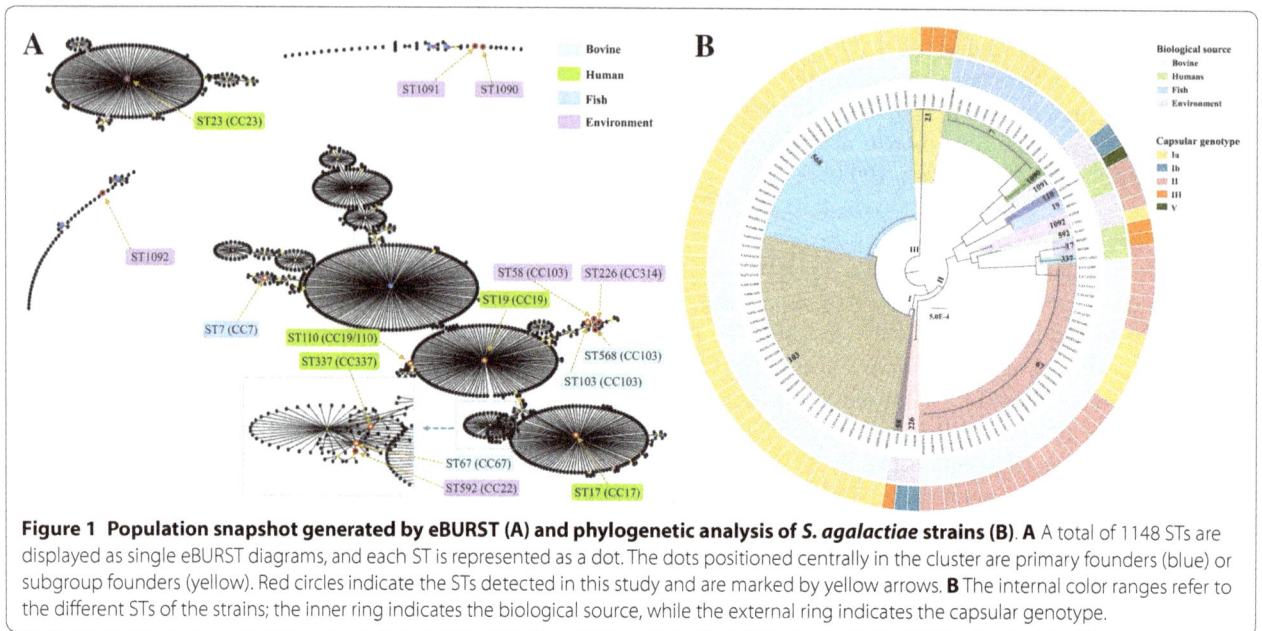

**Figure 1 Population snapshot generated by eBURST (A) and phylogenetic analysis of *S. agalactiae* strains (B).** **A** A total of 1148 STs are displayed as single eBURST diagrams, and each ST is represented as a dot. The dots positioned centrally in the cluster are primary founders (blue) or subgroup founders (yellow). Red circles indicate the STs detected in this study and are marked by yellow arrows. **B** The internal color ranges refer to the different STs of the strains; the inner ring indicates the biological source, while the external ring indicates the capsular genotype.

strains isolated from different origins, while Clade III was only consisted of four human isolates (ST23). To obtain further information on the genotypic heterogeneity of the individual STs, the capsular genotype was also analyzed. All strains belonging to ST7, ST103 and ST568 were assigned to capsular genotype Ia, whereas the ST67 strains were assigned to capsular genotype Ia or II. The capsular genotypes of human and environmental isolates were more diverse, which were consisted of Ia, Ib, II, III and V.

### Distribution of virulence factors in *S. agalactiae*

To determine whether *S. agalactiae* differed in virulence characteristics, an array of virulence genes were examined among the 116 strains. As shown in Figure 2, the examined virulence genes *hylB*, *gapC*, *cspA*, *dltA*, *fbsA*, *fbsB* and *bibA* were observed in all analyzed strains, while lactose operon (Lac), PI-1, PI-2a, PI-2b, *scpB*, *lmb* and *cylE* were responsible for the variety of virulence gene profiles. All the 84 bovine isolates belonged to virulence genotype Lac$^+$PI-1$^-$PI-2a$^-$PI-2b$^+$scpB$^-$lmb$^-$cylE$^+$, and all fish isolates belonged to virulence genotype Lac$^-$PI-1$^-$PI-2a$^-$PI-2b$^+$scpB$^+$lmb$^-$cylE$^+$. PI-2b was present in 100% of the bovine and fish isolates, whereas PI-1 and PI-2a were completely missing from those isolates. By contrast, PI-1 and PI-2a could be detected in human and environmental isolates. However, the virulence factors *scpB*, *lmb* and lactose operon distributed diversely in human and environmental strains. Most of the human isolates carried *scpB* and *lmb* genes, whereas only one isolate, ATCC13813, carried the lactose operon.

In addition, *cylE* was found in all examined strains except for human isolate ATCC13813.

### Growth ability

According to the origins, the 116 *S. agalactiae* strains were classified into four groups which were bovine, human, fish and environment, respectively. To determine whether there were significant differences among the bovine isolates belonging to different STs, they were further classified into three subgroups ST67, ST103 and ST568. The growth ability of all strains in milk were determined and being compared among different groups or subgroups. As depicted in Figure 3A, after cultured for 6 h, the bacterial concentration of bovine group was significantly higher than that of human, fish and environmental groups ($P < 0.01$). The concentration of each bovine subgroups cultured in milk was higher than $3.1 \times 10^8$ CFU/mL, whereas none of the other groups was higher than $9.3 \times 10^6$ CFU/mL. After cultured for 12 h, the bovine group increased further and showed an average bacterial concentration as high as $5.5 \times 10^9$ CFU/mL. Similarly, bacterial concentrations of human, fish and environmental groups also increased, however, their concentrations were still significantly lower than that of bovine group ($P < 0.01$). Additionally, it was observed the bacterial concentration of subgroup ST67 was lower than subgroups ST103 and ST568, but without significant difference ($P > 0.05$). Unlike in milk, less variations were observed when *S. agalactiae* were cultured in THB. There was no significant difference in bacterial growth between bovine and environmental groups, when they

Molecular and virulence characterization of highly prevalent Streptococcus agalactiae circulated...

113

| Origin | [a]Number | ST | [b]Cps | [c]Lac | Virulence gene | | | | | | | | | | | | |
|---|---|---|---|---|---|---|---|---|---|---|---|---|---|---|---|---|---|
| | | | | | PI-1 | PI-2a | PI-2b | *scpB* | *lmb* | *cylE* | *hylB* | *gapC* | *cspA* | *dltA* | *fbsA* | *fbsB* | *bibA* |
| Bovine | 6 | 67 | Ia | + | − | − | + | − | − | + | + | + | + | + | + | + | + |
| Bovine | 24 | 67 | II | + | − | − | + | − | − | + | + | + | + | + | + | + | + |
| Bovine | 30 | 103 | Ia | + | − | − | + | − | − | + | + | + | + | + | + | + | + |
| Bovine | 24 | 568 | Ia | + | − | − | + | − | − | + | + | + | + | + | + | + | + |
| Human | 2 | 17 | III | − | + | − | + | + | + | + | + | + | + | + | + | + | + |
| Human | 2 | 19 | II | − | + | − | − | + | + | + | + | + | + | + | + | + | + |
| Human | 1 | 23 | Ia | − | − | + | − | + | + | + | + | + | + | + | + | + | + |
| Human | 3 | 23 | III | − | + | + | − | + | + | + | + | + | + | + | + | + | + |
| Human | 1 | 110 | V | − | + | − | − | + | + | + | + | + | + | + | + | + | + |
| Human | 1 | 337 | II | + | − | − | + | − | − | + | + | + | + | + | + | + | + |
| Fish | 13 | 7 | Ia | − | − | − | + | − | − | + | + | + | + | + | + | + | + |
| Environment | 1 | 58 | III | + | + | + | − | + | − | + | + | + | + | + | + | + | + |
| Environment | 2 | 226 | Ib | − | + | − | − | + | − | + | + | + | + | + | + | + | + |
| Environment | 1 | 592 | Ia | − | + | + | − | − | + | + | + | + | + | + | + | + | + |
| Environment | 1 | 1090 | Ia | − | − | − | + | − | − | + | + | + | + | + | + | + | + |
| Environment | 2 | 1091 | Ib | + | + | + | − | + | + | + | + | + | + | + | + | + | + |
| Environment | 2 | 1092 | II | − | − | − | + | − | + | + | + | + | + | + | + | + | + |

**Figure 2 Distribution of virulence factors in *S. agalactiae*.** Only the representative genotypes were shown in the figure. [a]Number represents the number of strains belonging to the same genotype; [b]Cps and [c]Lac represent the capsular genotype and lactose operon, respectively; The symbols "+" and "−" represent the presence or absence of virulence factors, respectively.

were cultured in THB (Figure 3B). Moreover, the average bacterial growth of human and fish groups were even higher than that of bovine group after cultured for 12 h.

### Biofilm formation ability

The ability of each strain to form a biofilm was evaluated using crystal violet staining. As shown in Figure 4A, there were significant differences between bovine group and other three groups ($P < 0.01$). The subgroup ST103 formed the strongest biofilm, whereas fish group formed weakest biofilm. Furthermore, it was observed that although subgroup ST67 formed weaker biofilms compared to subgroups ST103 and ST568 ($P < 0.01$), subgroup ST67 could form much stronger biofilms than human, fish and environment groups ($P < 0.01$). However, it is noticeable that some human isolates, such as strains NZY014 and NYD001 belonging to ST23 could form a strong biofilm. The matured biofilms of representative strains NJPK1406 and GD201008-001, which belonged to ST103 and ST7 respectively, were observed using CLSM. As shown in Figure 4, the bovine isolate NJPK1406 formed structured multilayered aggregates of surface-adherent bacteria resembling a strong mature biofilm (Figure 4B), whereas the fish isolate GD201008-001 did not (Figure 4C).

### Hemolytic activity

As shown in Figure 5A, different hemolytic phenotypes of *S. agalactiae* were observed after cultured on Columbia blood agar plates. Most of the strains belonging to subgroups ST103 and ST568 showed the complete hemolytic rings (Figure 5A), whereas ST67 strains predominantly showed weak hemolytic rings (Figure 5B). However, fish group and some strains of human and environmental groups showed incomplete hemolytic rings (Figure 5C). To further compare the hemolytic activity among different groups, the hemolytic activity was evaluated using a SRBCs lysis assay. Our result showed the hemolytic activity of each strain measured using culture filtrates was relatively low. As shown in Figure 5D, the hemoglobin released from SRBCs by most of the *S. agalactiae* strains were not greater than 50% of the value of the positive control. The subgroups ST103 and ST568 showed similar hemolytic activity with the hemolysis around 48.3%, whereas subgroup ST67 showed an average of 18.3% hemolysis. The fish group exhibited significantly lower hemolysis than bovine group ($P < 0.01$). Unlikely, no significant differences were found when human and environmental groups were compared to bovine group. In particular, the hemolytic activity of human strains were diverse with the lysis rate ranging from 2 to 68%.

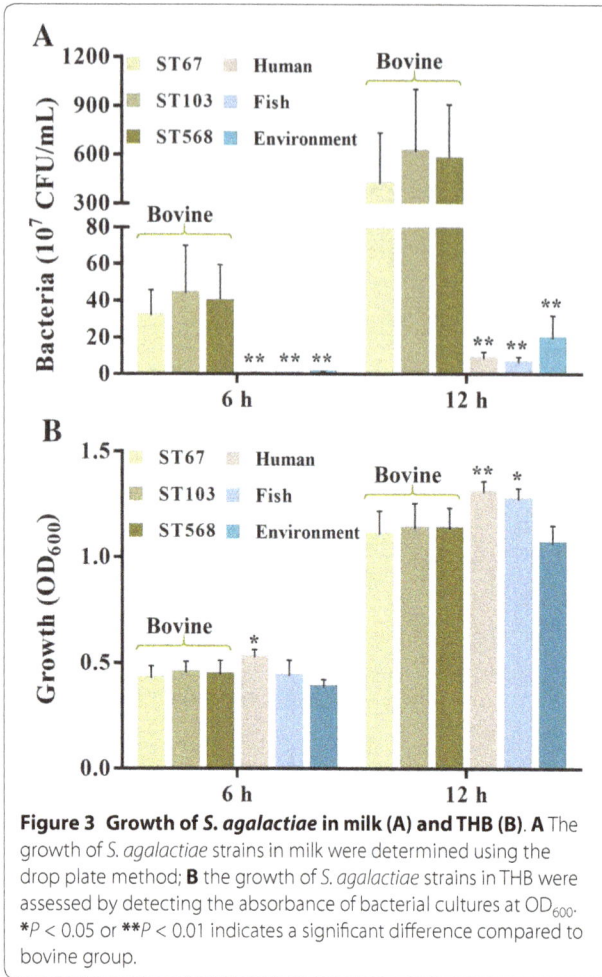

**Figure 3  Growth of *S. agalactiae* in milk (A) and THB (B). A** The growth of *S. agalactiae* strains in milk were determined using the drop plate method; **B** the growth of *S. agalactiae* strains in THB were assessed by detecting the absorbance of bacterial cultures at $OD_{600}$. **\***$P < 0.05$ or **\*\***$P < 0.01$ indicates a significant difference compared to bovine group.

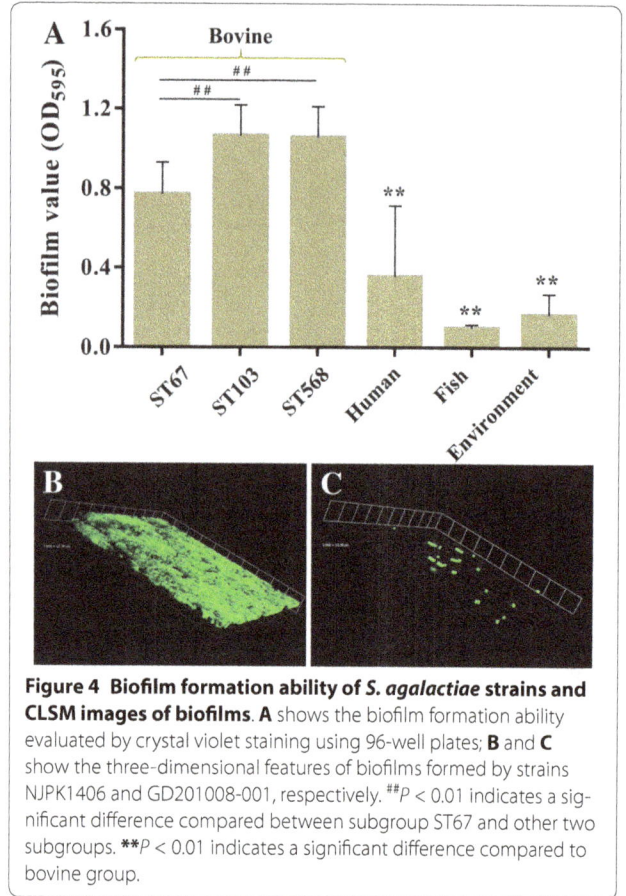

**Figure 4  Biofilm formation ability of *S. agalactiae* strains and CLSM images of biofilms. A** shows the biofilm formation ability evaluated by crystal violet staining using 96-well plates; **B** and **C** show the three-dimensional features of biofilms formed by strains NJPK1406 and GD201008-001, respectively. **##**$P < 0.01$ indicates a significant difference compared between subgroup ST67 and other two subgroups. **\*\***$P < 0.01$ indicates a significant difference compared to bovine group.

## Cytotoxicity to BMECs

To determine the cytotoxic effect of each *S. agalactiae* strain against BMECs, LDH release was examined, and the percent cytotoxicity was calculated. As depicted in Figure 6A, all groups were found to be cytotoxic to BMECs in a concentration-dependent manner, the cytotoxic effect become stronger along with the increase of MOI. No obvious cytotoxic effect of any group was found when MOI was 1. When at an MOI of 10, the percent cytotoxicity of fish group was significantly higher than bovine group ($P < 0.01$), whereas the percent cytotoxicity of environmental group was significantly lower than bovine group ($P < 0.01$). Significant differences were also found when subgroup ST67 was compared to subgroup ST103 or ST568 ($P < 0.05$), however, there was no significant difference between bovine and human groups on the cytotoxic effect. Furthermore, a similar result was also found when at an MOI of 100.

## Adhesion ability to BMECs

The adhesion ability of *S. agalactiae* strains to BMECs were evaluated. As shown in Figure 6B, all examined strains were able to adhere to BMECs after co-cultured for 2 h. However, there were significant differences between bovine group and other three groups. It showed that three bovine subgroups exhibited the strongest adhesion ability with the percent of adherent bacterial cells varying from 10.6 to 12.7%, whereas fish group showed the weakest adhesion ability. All of the bovine subgroups showed 100-fold higher levels of adherence than fish group ($P < 0.01$). Similarly, the adhesion ability of bovine group was also significantly higher than environmental group ($P < 0.01$). However, the adhesion ability of human strains were not uniformity, some strains such as NZY014 and NYD001 exhibited an adherence rate up to 12.1%, whereas adherence rates of other strains were lower than 3.2%.

## Discussion

Bovine mastitis caused by *S. agalactiae* continues to be one of the major veterinary and economic issues worldwide [6], representing a particularly prevalent problem

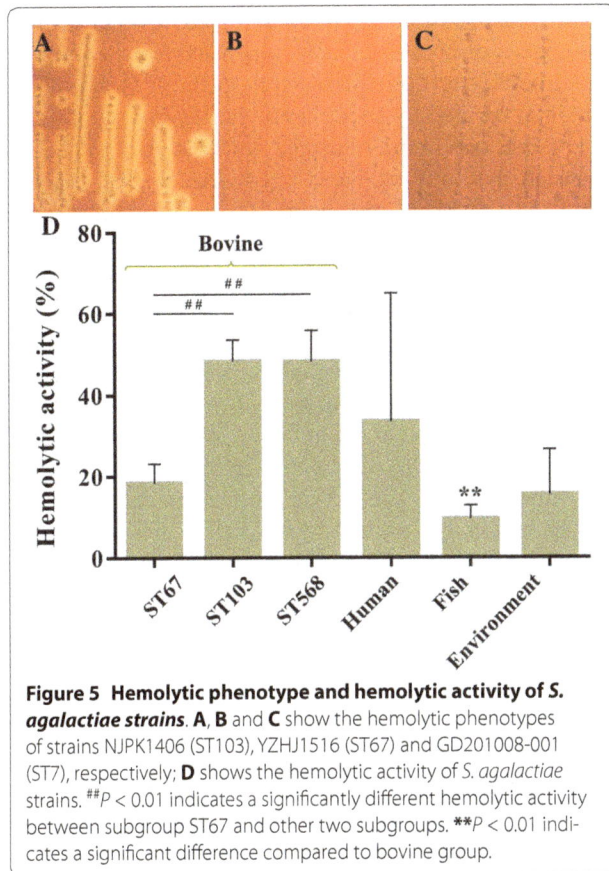

**Figure 5 Hemolytic phenotype and hemolytic activity of *S. agalactiae* strains. A, B** and **C** show the hemolytic phenotypes of strains NJPK1406 (ST103), YZHJ1516 (ST67) and GD201008-001 (ST7), respectively; **D** shows the hemolytic activity of *S. agalactiae* strains. $^{\#\#}P < 0.01$ indicates a significantly different hemolytic activity between subgroup ST67 and other two subgroups. $^{**}P < 0.01$ indicates a significant difference compared to bovine group.

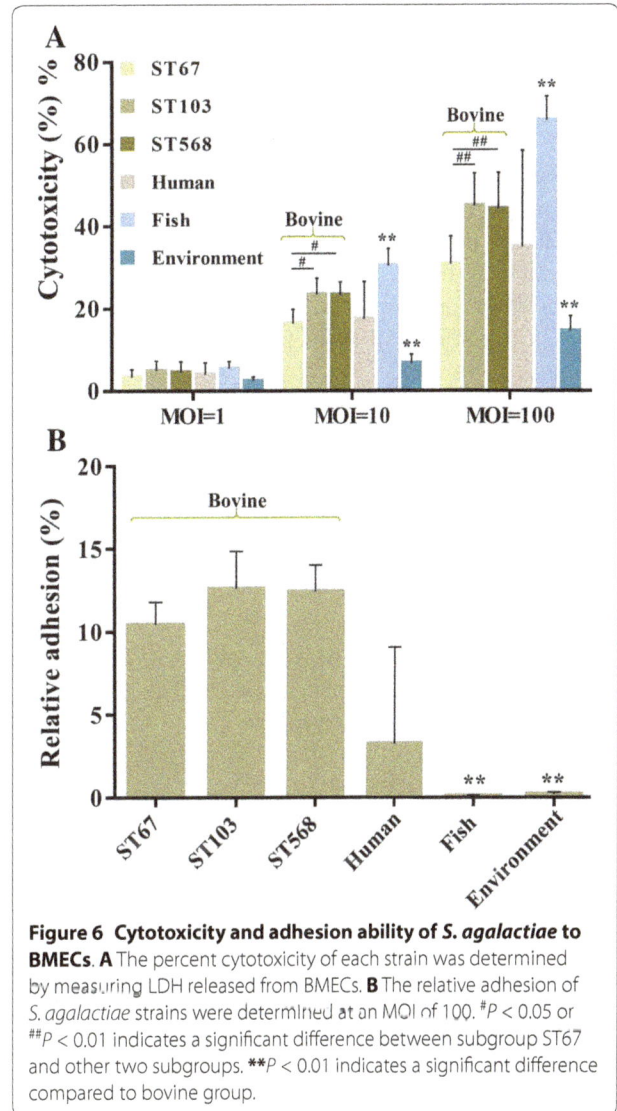

**Figure 6 Cytotoxicity and adhesion ability of *S. agalactiae* to BMECs. A** The percent cytotoxicity of each strain was determined by measuring LDH released from BMECs. **B** The relative adhesion of *S. agalactiae* strains were determined at an MOI of 100. $^{\#}P < 0.05$ or $^{\#\#}P < 0.01$ indicates a significant difference between subgroup ST67 and other two subgroups. $^{**}P < 0.01$ indicates a significant difference compared to bovine group.

in China [8]. In this study, we investigated the molecular characterization of 116 *S. agalactiae* strains isolated from bovine, human, fish and environment. Moreover, to identify the virulence characteristics of bovine-adapted strains which may confer them with ability to colonize and cause bovine mastitis, the virulence characteristics including growth ability in milk, biofilm formation ability, hemolytic activity, cytotoxic and adhesion to BMECs were analyzed.

To analyze the genotypic characteristics of the 116 strains, MLST, eBURST and phylogenetic analysis were used in this study. The results obtained from eBURST and phylogenetic analysis were similar. In general, the more alleles were identical, the STs would be more closer in the phylogenetic tree. The phylogenetic analysis showed bovine ST103 and ST568 formed a subclade, while bovine ST67 formed a subclade with human ST17 and ST337. It was also noted that human ST23 formed a clade which was clearly distinct to human ST17 and ST19. These results indicated that the STs which prevalent in specific animals may be genetically diverse. Notably, ST67 was the triple locus variants of ST17 and it has been proposed that ST17 and ST67 emerged from a common bovine ancestor [18]. However, our results showed

bovine ST67 and human ST17 differed in the presence of lactose operon, PI-1, PI-2a, PI-2b, *scpB* and *lmb*. Thus, in agreement with Sorensen's opinion [16], our data also suggested that human ST17 and bovine ST67 were distantly related. Since ST67, ST103 and ST568 were highly prevalent in bovine herds, it is intriguing to know which ST is more possible to cause clinical mastitis. However, since only few of the bovine strains were isolated from clinical cases (Additional file 1), the frequency analysis of STs linked with clinical or subclinical cases could not provide substantial data to determine which ST could cause a more severe infection, and this will be further investigated in our future work. Moreover, our results showed that MLST-based grouping did not correspond to grouping of strains based on MCT. The identical ST may be assigned to different capsular genotype, whereas the identical capsular genotype, such as genotype Ia, could be shared by various STs. This may be attributed to the lack of correlation between the two grouping methods since MLST is based on highly conserved housekeeping genes, whereas MCT is based on the horizontal transfer of capsular genes, which is likely to be supported by the acquired fitness or driven by the host immune response [9, 37].

To obtain more insight about the virulence factors of *S. agalactiae* strains, an array of virulence genes were screened (Figure 2). The result that *dltA*, *fbsA*, *fbsB*, *bibA*, *cspA*, *gapC* and *hylB* were found in all strains, suggesting they were conserved in *S. agalactiae* strains. The remaining seven virulence factors *lmb*, *scpB*, *cylE*, PI-1, PI-2a, PI-2b and lactose operon were responsible for the variety of virulence gene profiles among the examined strains. The absence of *lmb* and *scpB* in bovine and fish isolates suggests the activities of laminin-binding proteins and C5a peptidase may not be linked with their pathogenicity in bovine and fish. Similar to the findings of previous studies [8, 19], our data also showed that all bovine strains only carried PI-2b. Since previous works have reported that pilus-based vaccines can be used to prevent infections caused by *S. agalactiae* [38], the conserved PI-2b might be considered as a potential vaccine candidate for the development of subunit vaccines against bovine mastitis.

Successful survival and growth are requirements for bacteria to colonize the epithelial barrier, to produce virulence factors, and finally to transmit themselves to other hosts or the environment [39, 40]. To survive and colonize in the bovine mammary gland, it is of great importance for *S. agalactiae* to proliferate efficiently in milk. Importantly, we observed that all bovine isolates grew much faster than strains isolated from human, fish and environment (Figure 3A). After cultured for 6 h, the bacterial concentration of bovine group was higher than 100-folder compared to that of human and fish groups. However, the strains isolated from different origins showed less variation in THB (Figure 3B). After cultured for 12 h, the bacterial growth of human and fish groups were even higher than that of bovine group. These data suggest that growth ability in milk might contribute to the better adaptation for bovine isolates to the bovine herds. It has been reported that lactose operon can facilitate the metabolism of lactose [5], and the concentration of lactose contained in bovine milk can up to 5% [41]. Additionally, it was found that lactose operon was conserved in all bovine isolates. These data suggest that the ability of bovine isolates to grow rapidly in milk may attribute to the presence of lactose operon in bovine isolates. However, it should be noted that even some human and environmental isolates also carried lactose operon, they still grew much slower than bovine isolates in milk.

These results indicate there might be some other genetic differences in bovine isolates except for lactose operon, which could contribute to the growth ability in milk.

Biofilm formed by bacteria are usually described as "a structured community formed by bacteria themselves enclosed in a self-produced polymeric matrix" [42]. In the mammary gland, the biofilm-like communities could facilitate microbial survival by enhancing resistance to antibiotics and clearance by host defense mechanisms [43, 44]. Our study showed the biofilm formation ability of bovine group was significantly stronger than that of other groups ($P < 0.01$). In addition, a positive correlation was found between biofilm formation and adherence to BMECs. The adhesion ability of bovine group to BMECs was also significantly stronger than other groups except for human group. For *Streptococcus* spp., the adhesion ability of bacterial cells to BMECs are important for the bacteria to colonize the lactating mammary gland despite the flow of milk, which results in excretion of planktonic bacterial cells [45]. Therefore, it is reasonable to speculate that the strong biofilm formation and adhesion abilities allow bovine-adapted isolates to colonize and persist in bovine mammary gland, where it is able to survive for long periods leading to chronic and subclinical mastitis. Previous studies have demonstrated that pili play important roles in biofilm formation and adhesion to epithelial cells [46–48], and the adherence could be inhibited by PI-2b protein-specific antiserum significantly [49]. Interestingly, our study shows that all bovine isolates carrying PI-2b alone exhibited strong biofilm formation and adhesion abilities, however, all fish isolates which also only carried PI-2b did not form intact biofilms and could hardly adhere to BMECs. This finding raises the question of whether PI-2b plays any role in the infection of fish *S. agalactiae*, which needs to further study.

The hemolytic activity and cytotoxicity of *S. agalactiae* strains were also examined in the present study. It was demonstrated that bovine group exhibited higher hemolytic activity than fish and environmental groups. However, there were striking differences between subgroup ST67 and subgroups ST103 and ST568 ($P < 0.01$), whereas there were no significant differences when subgroup ST67 was compared to other groups. Similar to hemolytic activity, subgroup ST67 also showed significantly lower cytotoxicity towards BMECs compared to both subgroups ST103 and ST568. These data suggest the hemolytic activity and cytotoxicity might not be the essential abilities for the infection of bovine-adapted *S. agalactiae*. However, the fish group exhibited significantly higher cytotoxicity than other groups, even though fish isolates showed the lowest hemolytic activity. These findings raised the intriguing question of the fish isolates could be highly cytotoxic to BMECs, but with extremely

Molecular and virulence characterization of highly prevalent Streptococcus agalactiae circulated...

117

lower hemolytic activity. Conversely, it was reported that *S. agalactiae* strains with high hemolytic activity, were not cytotoxic to host cells [50]. Therefore, it is likely that differences underlying host–pathogen interaction at the cell–cell interface or unique virulence factors expressed in bacterial cells, may contribute to the cytotoxicity of fish isolates towards host cells.

Taken together, our study demonstrated that bovine isolates differed in the expression of some virulence-associated phenotypes compared to other isolates. In particular, bovine isolates all carried PI-2b and lactose operon, showed efficiently growth in milk, elevated biofilm formation ability and adhesion ability. Recently, studies have proposed that the evolutionary drove for bacteria to develop pathogenic characteristics was to access the nutrient resources that animals provided [39, 51]. For *S. agalactiae*, lethal outbreaks of ST7 strains have occurred in the fish farms in Asia, including China, Thailand and Kuwait [13], while ST17 strains has been well known as a hypervirulent clone occurred in pregnant women and newborns [52]. However, the bovine mastitis caused by *S. agalactiae* is usually chronic and subclinical, with intermittent episodes of clinical mastitis [53], and no available data in literature reported bovine isolates could be lethal for bovine. Generally, *S. agalactiae* is considered as a contagious pathogen which can readily be spread from the infected quarters to other quarters of the same cow, or from cow to cow [54]. Once the *S. agalactiae* strains could colonize and survive in bovine mammary gland, they could obtain nutrient-rich sources from milk to proliferate, and the harmful effect to bovine were long-term cumulative and might not be crucial. Therefore, we speculate that efficient growth in milk, elevated biofilm formation ability, together with strong adhesion ability might play key roles in the colonization and persistence in bovine mammary gland, whereas the hemolytic activity and cytotoxicity were not essential for the infection.

In conclusion, this study is a first step towards the elucidation of virulence strategies specific to the prevalent *S. agalactiae* STs. Although bovine ST67 were genetically diverse compared to ST103 and ST568, they harbored the similar virulence characteristics including growth ability in milk, biofilm formation ability and adhesion ability. The improved knowledge of the phenotypic characteristics of the prevalent strains is of crucial importance in the study of mastitis pathogenesis and would be valuable for the development of *S. agalactiae* control and treatment strategies. The ST-specific virulence characteristics permitting rapid colonization and persistence might explain why these STs could cause bovine mastitis and become prevalent within the bovine environment. However, the roles of these virulence characteristics in vivo and the host immune response merit further study.

## Abbreviations
*S. agalactiae*: *Streptococcus agalactiae*; ST: sequence type; BMECs: bovine mammary epithelial cells; MLST: multilocus sequence typing; CC: clonal complex; SLV: single-locus variant; SCC: somatic cell counts; rDNA: ribosomal DNA; THB: Todd-Hewitt broth; THA: Todd-Hewitt agar; PI: pilus island; Lac: lactose operon; OD: optical density; PBS: phosphate-buffered saline; SRBCs: sheep red blood cells; LDH: lactate dehydrogenase; MOI: multiplicity of infection; MEM: minimum essential medium; ANOVA: analysis of variance; MCT: molecular capsular type.

## Competing interests
The authors declare that they have no competing interests.

## Authors' contributions
Designed the experiment: MP and RW. Performed the experiment: MP, LS, TH, HB, LZ, YZ, HZ and RW. Analysis of data: MP, LS and TH. Drafted the manuscript: MP, RW and YL. Coordination of research: HZ and RW. All authors read and approved the final manuscript.

## Acknowledgements
This work was supported by Foundation of Jiangsu Academy of Agricultural Sciences (028046111673), Natural Science Foundation of Jiangsu Province (BK20170600, BK20160585 and BK20160577), Jiangsu Agricultural Science and Technology Foundation (CX(16)1060) and National agricultural product quality and safety risk assessment (GJGP201701203 and GJGP201700704). The authors thank Prof. Hongjie Fan, Nanjing Agricultural University, for providing a number of *S. agalactiae* strains. This work was also supported by Jiangsu Collaborative Innovation Center of Meat Production and Processing, Quality and Safety Control, Nanjing, China.

## Author details
[1] Key Laboratory of Control Technology and Standard for Agro-product Safety and Quality, Key Lab of Food Quality and Safety of Jiangsu Province-State Key Laboratory Breeding Base, Institute of Food Safety and Nutrition, Jiangsu Academy of Agricultural Sciences, No. 50 Zhongling Street, Nanjing 210014, China. [2] College of Veterinary Medicine, Nanjing Agricultural University, No. 1 Weigang, Nanjing 210095, China.

## References
1. Agger JF, Priou C, Huda A, Aagaard K (1994) Risk factors for transmission of *Streptococcus agalactiae* infection between Danish dairy herds: a case control study. Vet Res 25:227–234
2. Lyhs U, Kulkas L, Katholm J, Waller KP, Saha K, Tomusk RJ, Zadoks RN (2016) *Streptococcus agalactiae* serotype IV in humans and cattle, Northern Europe1. Emerg Infect Dis 22:2097–2103
3. Pereira UP, Mian GF, Oliveira IC, Benchetrit LC, Costa GM, Figueiredo HC (2010) Genotyping of *Streptococcus agalactiae* strains isolated from fish, human and cattle and their virulence potential in Nile tilapia. Vet Microbiol 140:186–192
4. Gonen E, Nedvetzki S, Naor D, Shpigel NY (2008) CD44 is highly expressed on milk neutrophils in bovine mastitis and plays a role in their adhesion to matrix and mammary epithelium. Vet Res 39:29
5. Richards VP, Choi SC, Pavinski Bitar PD, Gurjar AA, Stanhope MJ (2013) Transcriptomic and genomic evidence for *Streptococcus agalactiae* adaptation to the bovine environment. BMC Genomics 14:920
6. Almeida A, Alves-Barroco C, Sauvage E, Bexiga R, Albuquerque P, Tavares

F, Santos-Sanches I, Glaser P (2016) Persistence of a dominant bovine lineage of group B *Streptococcus* reveals genomic signatures of host adaptation. Environ Microbiol 18:4216–4229

7. Jørgensen HJ, Nordstoga AB, Sviland S, Zadoks RN, Sølverød L, Kvitle B, Mørk T (2016) *Streptococcus agalactiae* in the environment of bovine dairy herds–rewriting the textbooks? Vet Microbiol 184:64–72

8. Yang Y, Liu Y, Ding Y, Yi L, Ma Z, Fan H, Lu C (2013) Molecular characterization of *Streptococcus agalactiae* isolated from bovine mastitis in Eastern China. PLoS One 8:e67755

9. Gherardi G, Imperi M, Baldassarri L, Pataracchia M, Alfarone G, Recchia S, Orefici G, Dicuonzo G, Creti R (2007) Molecular epidemiology and distribution of serotypes, surface proteins, and antibiotic resistance among group B streptococci in Italy. J Clin Microbiol 45:2909–2916

10. Shome BR, Bhuvana M, Mitra SD, Krithiga N, Shome R, Velu D, Banerjee A, Barbuddhe SB, Prabhudas K, Rahman H (2012) Molecular characterization of *Streptococcus agalactiae* and *Streptococcus uberis* isolates from bovine milk. Trop Anim Health Prod 44:1981–1992

11. Zadoks RN, Middleton JR, McDougall S, Katholm J, Schukken YH (2011) Molecular epidemiology of mastitis pathogens of dairy cattle and comparative relevance to humans. J Mammary Gland Biol Neoplasia 16:357–372

12. Da Cunha V, Davies MR, Douarre PE, Rosinski-Chupin I, Margarit I, Spinali S, Perkins T, Lechat P, Dmytruk N, Sauvage E, Ma L, Romi B, Tichit M, Lopez-Sanchez MJ, Descorps-Declere S, Souche E, Buchrieser C, Trieu-Cuot P, Moszer I, Clermont D, Maione D, Bouchier C, McMillan DJ, Parkhill J, Telford JL, Dougan G, Walker MJ, DEVANI Consortium, Holden MTG, Poyart C, Glaser P (2014) *Streptococcus agalactiae* clones infecting humans were selected and fixed through the extensive use of tetracycline. Nat Commun 5:4544

13. Kayansamruaj P, Pirarat N, Kondo H, Hirono I, Rodkhum C (2015) Genomic comparison between pathogenic *Streptococcus agalactiae* isolated from Nile tilapia in Thailand and fish-derived ST7 strains. Infect Genet Evol 36:307–314

14. Richards VP, Lang P, Bitar PD, Lefébure T, Schukken YH, Zadoks RN, Stanhope MJ (2011) Comparative genomics and the role of lateral gene transfer in the evolution of bovine adapted *Streptococcus agalactiae*. Infect Genet Evol 11:1263–1275

15. Fischer A, Liljander A, Kaspar H, Muriuki C, Fuxelius HH, Bongcam-Rudloff E, de Villiers EP, Huber CA, Frey J, Daubenberger C, Bishop R, Younan M, Jores J (2013) Camel *Streptococcus agalactiae* populations are associated with specific disease complexes and acquired the tetracycline resistance gene *tetM* via a Tn916-like element. Vet Res 44:86

16. Sørensen UB, Poulsen K, Ghezzo C, Margarit I, Kilian M (2010) Emergence and global dissemination of host-specific *Streptococcus agalactiae* clones. MBio 1:e00178–10

17. Carvalho-Castro GA, Silva JR, Paiva LV, Custodio DAC, Moreira RO, Mian GF, Prado IA, Chalfun-Junior A, Costa GM (2017) Molecular epidemiology of *Streptococcus agalactiae* isolated from mastitis in Brazilian dairy herds. Braz J Microbiol 48:551–559

18. Bisharat N, Crook DW, Leigh J, Harding RM, Ward PN, Coffey TJ, Maiden MC, Peto T, Jones N (2004) Hyperinvasive neonatal group B *streptococcus* has arisen from a bovine ancestor. J Clin Microbiol 42:2161–2167

19. Springman AC, Lacher DW, Waymire EA, Wengert SL, Singh P, Zadoks RN, Davies HD, Manning SD (2014) Pilus distribution among lineages of group B *streptococcus*: an evolutionary and clinical perspective. BMC Microbiol 14:159

20. Oliveira IC, de Mattos MC, Pinto TA, Ferreira-Carvalho BT, Benchetrit LC, Whiting AA, Bohnsack JF, Figueiredo AM (2006) Genetic relatedness between group B *streptococci* originating from bovine mastitis and a human group B *Streptococcus* type V cluster displaying an identical pulsed-field gel electrophoresis pattern. Clin Microbiol Infect 12:887–893

21. Kayansamruaj P, Pirarat N, Katagiri T, Hirono I, Rodkhum C (2014) Molecular characterization and virulence gene profiling of pathogenic *Streptococcus agalactiae* populations from tilapia (*Oreochromis* sp.) farms in Thailand. J Vet Diagn Invest 26:488–495

22. Budd KE, Mitchell J, Keane OM (2016) Lineage associated expression of virulence traits in bovine-adapted *Staphylococcus aureus*. Vet Microbiol 189:24–31

23. Giannouli M, Antunes LC, Marchetti V, Triassi M, Visca P, Zarrilli R (2013) Virulence-related traits of epidemic *Acinetobacter baumannii* strains belonging to the international clonal lineages I-III and to the emerging genotypes ST25 and ST78. BMC Infect Dis 13:282

24. Tassi R, McNeilly TN, Sipka A, Zadoks RN (2015) Correlation of hypothetical virulence traits of two *Streptococcus uberis* strains with the clinical manifestation of bovine mastitis. Vet Res 46:123

25. Weisburg WG, Barns SM, Pelletier DA, Lane DJ (1991) 16S ribosomal DNA amplification for phylogenetic study. J Bacteriol 173:697–703

26. Jones N, Bohnsack JF, Takahashi S, Oliver KA, Chan MS, Kunst F, Glaser P, Rusniok C, Crook DW, Harding RM, Bisharat N, Spratt BG (2003) Multilocus sequence typing system for group B *streptococcus*. J Clin Microbiol 41:2530–2536

27. Feil EJ, Li BC, Aanensen DM, Hanage WP, Spratt BG (2004) eBURST: inferring patterns of evolutionary descent among clusters of related bacterial genotypes from multilocus sequence typing data. J Bacteriol 186:1518–1530

28. Imperi M, Pataracchia M, Alfarone G, Baldassarri L, Orefici G, Creti R (2010) A multiplex PCR assay for the direct identification of the capsular type (Ia to IX) of *Streptococcus agalactiae*. J Microbiol Methods 80:212–214

29. Kumar S, Stecher G, Tamura K (2016) MEGA7: molecular evolutionary genetics analysis version 7.0 for bigger datasets. Mol Biol Evol 33:1870–1874

30. Ferretti JJ, McShan WM, Ajdic D, Savic DJ, Savic G, Lyon K, Primeaux C, Sezate S, Suvorov AN, Kenton S, Lai HS, Lin SP, Qian Y, Jia HG, Najar FZ, Ren Q, Zhu H, Song L, White J, Yuan X, Clifton SW, Roe BA, McLaughlin R (2001) Complete genome sequence of an M1 strain of *Streptococcus pyogenes*. Proc Natl Acad Sci USA 98:4658–4663

31. Herigstad B, Hamilton M, Heersink J (2001) How to optimize the drop plate method for enumerating bacteria. J Microbiol Methods 44:121–129

32. Pang M, Jiang J, Xie X, Wu Y, Dong Y, Kwok AH, Zhang W, Yao H, Lu C, Leung FC, Liu Y (2015) Novel insights into the pathogenicity of epidemic *Aeromonas hydrophila* ST251 clones from comparative genomics. Sci Rep 5:9833

33. Stepanovic S, Vukovic D, Dakic I, Savic B, Svabic-Vlahovic M (2000) A modified microtiter-plate test for quantification of staphylococcal biofilm formation. J Microbiol Methods 40:175–179

34. Du H, Pang M, Dong Y, Wu Y, Wang N, Liu J, Awan F, Lu C, Liu Y (2016) Identification and characterization of an *Aeromonas hydrophila* oligopeptidase gene *pepF* negatively related to biofilm formation. Front Microbiol 7:1497

35. Pang M, Xie X, Dong Y, Du H, Wang N, Lu C, Liu Y (2017) Identification of novel virulence-related genes in *Aeromonas hydrophila* by screening transposon mutants in a *Tetrahymena* infection model. Vet Microbiol 199:36–46

36. Papazafiri P, Avlonitis N, Angelou P, Calogeropoulou T, Koufaki M, Scoulica E, Fragiadaki I (2005) Structure-activity relationships of antineoplastic ring-substituted ether phospholipid derivatives. Cancer Chemother Pharmacol 56:261–270

37. Cieslewicz MJ, Chaffin D, Glusman G, Kasper D, Madan A, Rodrigues S, Fahey J, Wessels MR, Rubens CE (2005) Structural and genetic diversity of group B *streptococcus* capsular polysaccharides. Infect Immun 73:3096–3103

38. Margarit I, Rinaudo CD, Galeotti CL, Maione D, Ghezzo C, Buttazzoni E, Rosini R, Runci Y, Mora M, Buccato S, Pagani M, Tresoldi E, Berardi A, Creti R, Baker CJ, Telford JL, Grandi G (2009) Preventing bacterial infections with pilus-based vaccines: the group B *streptococcus* paradigm. J Infect Dis 199:108–115

39. Rohmer L, Hocquet D, Miller SI (2011) Are pathogenic bacteria just looking for food? Metabolism and microbial pathogenesis. Trends Microbiol 19:341–348

40. Staib L, Fuchs TM (2014) From food to cell: nutrient exploitation strategies of enteropathogens. Microbiology 160:1020–1039

41. Silanikove N, Leitner G, Merin U (2015) The interrelationships between lactose intolerance and the modern dairy industry: global perspectives in evolutional and historical backgrounds. Nutrients 7:7312–7331

42. Costerton JW, Stewart PS, Greenberg EP (1999) Bacterial biofilms: a common cause of persistent infections. Science 284:1318–1322

43. Melchior MB, Fink-Gremmels J, Gaastra W (2006) Comparative assessment of the antimicrobial susceptibility of *Staphylococcus aureus* isolates from bovine mastitis in biofilm versus planktonic culture. J Vet Med B Infect Dis Vet Public Health 53:326–332

44. Rosini R, Margarit I (2015) Biofilm formation by *Streptococcus agalactiae*: influence of environmental conditions and implicated virulence factors. Front Cell Infect Microbiol 5:6

45. Leigh JA (1999) *Streptococcus uberis*: a permanent barrier to the control of bovine mastitis? Vet J 157:225–238

46. Konto-Ghiorghi Y, Mairey E, Mallet A, Duménil G, Caliot E, Trieu-Cuot P, Dramsi S (2009) Dual role for pilus in adherence to epithelial cells and biofilm formation in *Streptococcus agalactiae*. PLoS Pathog 5:e1000422

47. Lauer P, Rinaudo CD, Soriani M, Margarit I, Maione D, Rosini R, Taddei AR, Mora M, Rappuoli R, Grandi G, Telford JL (2005) Genome analysis reveals pili in Group B *Streptococcus*. Science 309:105

48. Papasergi S, Brega S, Mistou MY, Firon A, Oxaran V, Dover R, Teti G, Shai Y, Trieu-Cuot P, Dramsi S (2011) The GBS PI-2a pilus is required for virulence in mice neonates. PLoS One 6:e18747

49. Sharma P, Lata H, Arya DK, Kashyap AK, Kumar H, Dua M, Ali A, Johri AK (2013) Role of pilus proteins in adherence and invasion of *Streptococ-cus agalactiae* to the lung and cervical epithelial cells. J Biol Chem 288:4023–4034

50. Leclercq SY, Sullivan MJ, Ipe DS, Smith JP, Cripps AW, Ulett GC (2016) Pathogenesis of *Streptococcus* urinary tract infection depends on bacterial strain and beta-hemolysin/cytolysin that mediates cytotoxicity, cytokine synthesis, inflammation and virulence. Sci Rep 6:29000

51. de Lorenzo V (2015) *Pseudomonas aeruginosa*: the making of a pathogen. Environ Microbiol 17:1–3

52. Brzychczy-Wloch M, Gosiewski T, Pawlik D, Szumala-Kakol A, Samead A, Heczko PB (2012) Occurrence of the hypervirulent ST-17 clone of *Streptococcus agalactiae* in pregnant women and newborns. Przegl Epidemiol 66:395–401 (in Polish)

53. Keefe GP (1997) *Streptococcus agalactiae* mastitis: a review. Can Vet J 38:429–437

54. Thompson-Crispi K, Atalla H, Miglior F, Mallard BA (2014) Bovine mastitis: frontiers in immunogenetics. Front Immunol 5:493

# 11

# Control of endemic swine flu persistence in farrow-to-finish pig farms: a stochastic metapopulation modeling assessment

Charlie Cador[1,3]* ⓘ, Mathieu Andraud[1,3], Lander Willem[2] and Nicolas Rose[1,3]

## Abstract

Swine influenza viruses (swIAVs) are known to persist endemically in farrow-to-finish pig farms, leading to repeated swine flu outbreaks in successive batches of pigs at a similar age (mostly around 8 weeks of age). This persistence in European swine herds involves swIAVs from European lineages including $H1_{av}N1$, $H1_{hu}N2$, H3N2, the 2009 H1N1 pandemic virus and their reassortants. The specific population dynamics of farrow-to-finish pig farms, the immune status of the animals at infection-time, the co-circulation of distinct subtypes leading to consecutive or concomitant infections have been evidenced as factors favouring swIAV persistence within herds. We developed a stochastic meta-population model representing the co-circulation of two distinct swIAVs within a typical farrow-to-finish pig herd to evaluate the risk of reassortant viruses generation due to co-infection events. Control strategies related to herd management and/or vaccination schemes (batch-to-batch or mass vaccination of the sow herd and vaccination of growing pigs) were implemented to assess their relative efficacy regarding viral persistence. The overall probability of a co-infection event for France, possibly leading to reassortment, was evaluated to 16.8%. The export of consecutive piglets batches was identified as the most efficient measure facilitating swIAV infection fade-out. Although some vaccination schemes (batch-to-batch vaccination) had a beneficial effect in breeding sows by reducing the persistence of swIAVs within this subpopulation, none of vaccination strategies achieved swIAVs fade-out within the entire farrow-to-finish pig herd.

## Introduction

Swine influenza A viruses (swIAVs) are polymorphic enveloped single-stranded RNA viruses from the *Orthomyxoviridae* family widespread in pig-production units throughout the world [1]. These viruses are of great economic importance for the swine industry because of their involvement as a major co-factor of porcine respiratory disease complex [2, 3] and being also responsible in some cases for severe pulmonary distress leading to growth retardations. In the past, mainly sporadic outbreaks, affecting a large part of the herd population in a relatively short time-interval but with short-term consequences at the herd scale, were reported. However, in recent years endemic forms of influenza infections have been increasingly documented with a global persistence of swIAV viruses at the herd scale, systematically affecting successive batches of growing pigs [4, 5]. As such, the burden of respiratory diseases in growing pigs due to bacterial co-infections is increasing and causes alarming use of antibiotics.

Three main subtypes have been circulating in swine populations worldwide: H1N1, H1N2 and H3N2 [6–8]. Those subtypes permanently evolve, ending in different lineages containing genetic components derived from both avian and human influenza A strains. To date, endemic swIAVs persistence in European swine herds includes $H1_{av}N1$, $H1_{hu}N2$, H3N2, the 2009 H1N1 pandemic virus and their reassortants. Weak cross-immunity between subtypes and the rapid spread of swIAVs within herds might cause multiple, and possibly concomitant, infections in one animal [4, 8, 9]. Co-infection events

*Correspondence: charlie.cador@farmapro.fr
[1] Swine Epidemiology and Welfare Research Unit, French Agency for Food, Environmental and Occupational Health & Safety (ANSES), BP 53, 22440 Ploufragan, France
Full list of author information is available at the end of the article

can lead to the emergence of reassortant viruses, potentially more pathogenic for animals and/or transmissible to humans, and are therefore recognized as a main threat for veterinary and public health [10–15].

Although the understanding of swIAVs transmission in pig populations is clearly pivotal to manage the risk of spillover to humans, Dorjee and collaborators highlighted the gap of knowledge on influenza dynamics at the pig farm-level [16]. Combining epidemiological, viral and immunological characteristics of swIAVs, mathematical models are comprehensive tools to analyze how the population dynamics and immunity influence the dynamics of influenza A virus infections [17–20]. To date, four modeling studies focusing on swIAV dynamics in swine production units have been published. Reynolds et al. [19] developed a deterministic model to assess the impact of vaccination strategies (e.g. mass and pre-farrowing vaccination) on the spread of influenza A infection in breeding and finishing herds based on parameter estimations from experimental conditions. Unless the vaccine and spreading strains were fully homologous, no vaccination strategy was able to eradicate the virus. This result is consistent with field observations where vaccination has only limited effect on the infection dynamics at the herd scale. Vaccination is commonly performed in breeding animals with two main objectives: the reduction of clinical expression in gestating sows and further delivery of maternally-derived antibodies (MDAs) for clinical protection of the offspring. Although the first objective is globally achieved, a recent study by Cador et al. [17] highlighted an ambiguous role of MDAs on the transmission dynamics. The presence of maternal immunity in young piglets was evidenced to extend the duration of the epidemics within batches, which in turn favored the transmission of the infection from batch to batch increasing therefore the persistence of swIAV at the population level. Pitzer et al. [18] used a stochastic model to analyze critical herd sizes for swIAV persistence according to herd type and management practices (variation of the between-birth interval and between two introductions of finishers) and showed that the swIAV was able to persist in relatively small populations. White et al. [20] recently proposed a stochastic model representing the infection dynamics of swIAV in a typical US farrow-to-wean production unit. The authors evaluated intervention strategies based on different vaccination schemes, biosecurity measures and management options and confirmed the role of piglets in swIAV persistence in breeding herds. These four modeling studies highlight the complex relationship between population dynamics, immunity and transmission dynamics of swIAV among a pig population, considering only one subtype.

Co-circulation of different swIAV subtypes within one swine herd is regularly observed in field conditions [4, 5] but has not yet been covered in modeling studies to date. Such phenomenon could increase the likelihood of virus persistence at the herd level triggering the risk of co-infection, possibly leading to reassortant viruses. In the present study we extended the stochastic event-based metapopulation model from Cador et al. [17] to represent co-circulation of two swIAVs in different farrow-to-finish pig farm settings in order to identify drivers responsible for viruses persistence at the herd level. The model was also used to assess the risk of co-infection events and to evaluate the impact of control strategies on the transmission dynamics and persistence of swIAVs at the herd scale based on (1) the implementation of different vaccination schemes and (2) the concurrent export of weaning piglet batches.

## Materials and methods
### Model structure
#### Population dynamics
Two subpopulations—breeding sows and growing pigs—are considered. Animals are subdivided into batches according to their physiological state (breeding sows) or age (growing pigs). The breeding sows iterate through three physiological states (service [32 days], gestation [82 days], lactation [26 days]), while growing pigs pass through three stages (lactation [21 days], nursery [51 days] and fattening [105 days]). Batches of animals are managed independently and housed in facilities according to their physiological or growing stage. Breeding sows' facilities are divided in rooms containing batches having the same physiological stage. Growing pigs' facilities are divided in rooms containing one single batch of animals with movements occurring at fixed times according to all-in-all-out management policy at the room level. Direct physical contacts between batches of sows and growing pigs only occur in the farrowing room, during the lactating stage. More information and a flow diagram of the farrow-to-finish pig farm can be found in Cador et al. [17]. The model was implemented in Matlab (MATLAB 2012b, TheMathWorks, Inc., Natick, Massachusetts, United States).

The original model considered one batch-rearing (denominated BR thereafter) management with seven batches (7-BR system) and was extended to account for several BR systems commonly used in the field [21]. Each BR system leads to specific population dynamics and herd structure with different numbers of batches and corresponding rooms in the different facilities of the herd (Table 1). Thus, in the BR systems with short between-batch intervals (10- and 20-BR systems; 2 or

**Table 1 Modifications of the herd structure according to the BR (batch-rearing) systems (from: Agriculture chamber of Brittany Region, 2017 [21])**

| | Values | | | | |
|---|---|---|---|---|---|
| BR systems (number of batches) | 4 | 5 | 7 | 10 | 20 |
| Total number of productive sows | 192 | 245 | 203 | 430 | 620 |
| Proportion of herds according to the BR system | 0.12 | 0.21 | 0.48 | 0.10 | 0.09 |
| Duration of a sow reproductive cycle (days) | 140 | 140 | 147[a] | 140 | 140 |
| Number of sows per batch | 48 | 49 | 29 | 43 | 31 |
| Number of piglets per batch | 576 | 588 | 348 | 516 | 372 |
| Interval between two successive batches of sows and pigs (days) | 35 | 28 | 21 | 14 | 7 |
| Number of batches in service room | 1 | 2 | 2 | 3 | 5 |
| Number of batches in gestating room | 3 | 3 | 4 | 6 | 12 |
| Number of farrowing rooms | 1 | 1 | 2 | 2 | 4 |
| Number of nursery rooms | 2 | 2 | 2 | 4 | 7 |
| Number of finishing rooms | 3 | 4 | 6 | 9 | 18 |

[a] In the 7-BR system, weaning occurs at 28 days of age (21 days in the other BR systems). Then, the duration of a sow reproductive cycle is 7-day longer.

1 week-interval, respectively), a high number of batches are housed in the same facility at the same time.

*Epidemiological model*

Starting from a susceptible-infected-recovered-susceptible (SIRS) model, the epidemiological model in this study also accounts for specific features such as maternally-derived antibodies (MDAs) in neonates (lower susceptibility to infection) and sequential or concurrent infections with two different subtypes. The infectious process is ruled by the Gillespie's direct algorithm [22], where each random event corresponds to a health transition of a single animal. Due to the fast-acting transmission between individuals, the batch was selected as epidemiological unit. No efficient cross-protection after sequential infections by two different subtypes has been evidenced neither in field nor experimental conditions [4, 8]. Therefore, no cross-protection has been implemented in the model allowing the animals to be co-infected by the two viral subtypes simultaneously or consecutively. swIAV infection states and health transitions are presented in Figure 1, denoting the swIAV subtypes by subscripts 1 and 2. Subsequent infections are explicitly included in the model to represent realistic durations of shedding periods and the development of strain-specific immunity. Animals can be infected by the second subtype while still shedding the first subtype ($I_{1-2}$ or $I_{2-1}$ classes) or after recovery from the first subtype given the absence of cross-immunity ($Y_2$ or $Y_1$ classes). Strain-specific immunity durations were assumed gamma-distributed with a mean duration of 180 days [17]. Sows infected by a second subtype ($Y_2$ or $Y_1$ classes) and recovered from the first one ($R_1$ or $R_2$ classes) are assumed to develop an immune response regarding the second strain ($R_{1-2}$ or

$R_{2-1}$). The duration of dual immunity was restricted to 90 days after which immunity to the first subtype waned while specific immunity to the second strain persisted for 90 days (total immunity duration of 180 days). In consequence, breeding animals can be reinfected by the same subtype after waning immunity (Figure 1). Given the short lifespan of growing pigs (180 days), the loss of immunity towards a specific subtype with a subsequent re-infection by the same virus was deemed extremely unlikely. Hence, growing pigs were assumed to experiment only one infection for each subtype and develop specific immunity lasting for their economic lifespan. Waning of active and maternal immunity is represented by the stage approach [23–25]. The piglets' immune status after colostrum intake is determined by the health states of the farrowing sows (denoted with superscript $i$). Recovered sows ($R_1^i$, $R_2^i$, $R_{1-2}^i$, $R_{2-1}^i$ and $R^i$) give birth to $M^i$ piglets; $Y_1$ and $Y_2$ sows to $M^{i=1}$ piglets and $S$, $I_1$, $I_2$, $I_{1-2}$ and $I_{2-1}$ sows to fully susceptible piglets $S$. Piglets with MDAs ($M^i$ classes) were assumed to be partially protected against infection through a reduced susceptibility [26]. This protective factor was considered strain-specific based on the proportion of farrowing sows immune to each subtype.

Merging this epidemiological model with the population dynamics resulted in an event-driven epidemiological stochastic model embedded in specific population dynamics.

**Implementation of vaccination in the swIAV infectious model**

The trivalent vaccine used in European countries covers the majority of the circulating strains in Europe [27]. In our model, vaccination provides partial protection

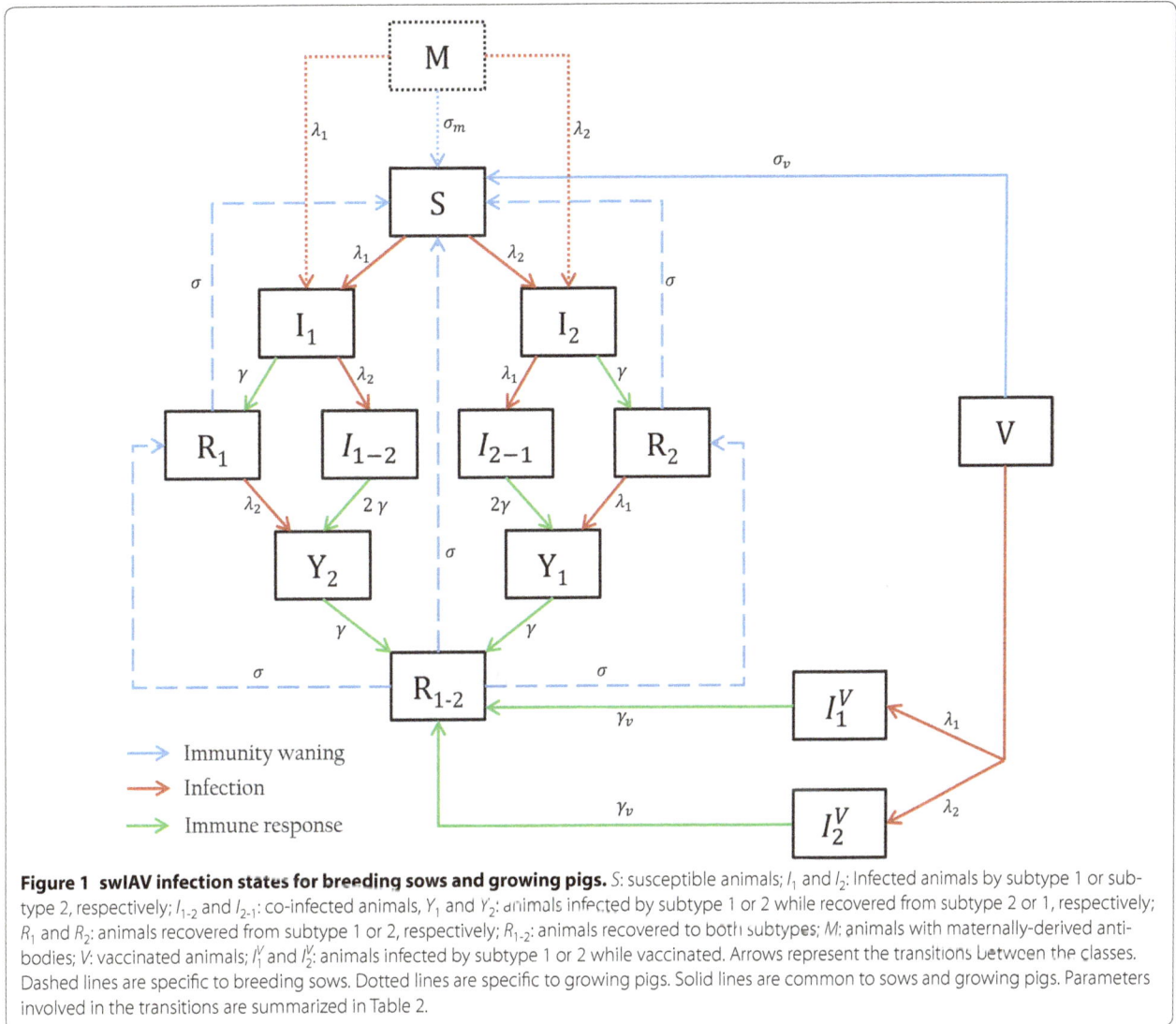

**Figure 1 swIAV infection states for breeding sows and growing pigs.** $S$: susceptible animals; $I_1$ and $I_2$: Infected animals by subtype 1 or subtype 2, respectively; $I_{1-2}$ and $I_{2-1}$: co-infected animals, $Y_1$ and $Y_2$: animals infected by subtype 1 or 2 while recovered from subtype 2 or 1, respectively; $R_1$ and $R_2$: animals recovered from subtype 1 or 2, respectively; $R_{1-2}$: animals recovered to both subtypes; $M$: animals with maternally-derived antibodies; $V$: vaccinated animals; $I_1^V$ and $I_2^V$: animals infected by subtype 1 or 2 while vaccinated. Arrows represent the transitions between the classes. Dashed lines are specific to breeding sows. Dotted lines are specific to growing pigs. Solid lines are common to sows and growing pigs. Parameters involved in the transitions are summarized in Table 2.

against the two circulating subtypes and is ineffective when applied to actively shedding animals ($I$ and $Y$ classes) because the immunity onset is established after 7 days at least after primary vaccination (RESPIPORC FLU3, summary of product characteristics, [28]). Vaccinated susceptible and immune animals ($S$ and $R$ classes, respectively) develop vaccine-induced immunity against both viral subtypes and are represented by $V$ classes. Waning of vaccine-induced immunity was assumed gamma-distributed and modeled using 7-exponential classes (stage approach). Vaccinated pigs have a reduced swIAV transmission probability and a lower shedding period [29]. In addition, piglets with high antibody levels ($M^{i=1}$ to $M^{i=3}$ stages) were assumed not to react to vaccination due to interference between passive- and vaccine-induced immunity in young piglets [30]. Conversely, the

vaccination of piglets with lower antibody levels ($M^{i=4}$ to $M^{i=7}$ stages) induced an increased duration of the vaccine-induced immunity according to the antibody decay of the piglets. Vaccinated animals are assumed to experience at most one infection by either subtype after which a long-lasting immunity to both subtypes is established until slaughter age [31].

### Force of infections
As swIAV transmission occurs mainly through pig-to-pig contact and the exposure to contaminated aerosols, the force of infection applied to each animal includes (1) the direct transmission from infected animals within the room and (2) the indirect transmission through airborne route from infected animals within the entire facility. Subtype-specific forces of infection are calculated

combining direct and indirect transmission routes. Parameter definitions and values are provided in Table 2.

The within-room direct transmission force of infection $\lambda_i^{direct}(t, r)$ for subtype $i$, at time $t$ in room $r$ is defined as:

$$\lambda_i^{direct}(t,r) = \frac{\beta(I_i(t,r) + I_{ji}(t,r) + I_{ij}(t,r) + Y_i(t,r)) + \beta_v I_i^v(t,r)}{N_r}, \quad j \neq i.$$

$I_i$ represents the number of animals infected by subtype $i$ only, $I_{ij}$ and $I_{ji}$ the number of animals infected by both subtypes simultaneously (accounting for the sequence of infections) and $Y_i$ the number of animals infected by subtype $i$ while immune against $j$. $I_i^v$ corresponds to the number of animals infected by subtype $i$ while vaccinated. $\beta$ and $\beta_v$ denote the related transmission rates per day for non-vaccinated and vaccinated pigs, respectively. Transmission rates for both subtypes are assumed to be the same.

The between-room airborne force of infection $\lambda_i^{indirect}(t, r)$ for subtype $i$, at time $t$ in room $r$ is expressed from the total prevalence of infected animals by subtype $i$ at time $t$ in neighbouring rooms $r'$:

$$\lambda_i^{indirect}(t,r) = \beta_{air} \frac{\sum_{r' \neq r} \left(I_i(t,r') + I_{ji}(t,r') + I_{ij}(t,r') + Y_i(t,r') + I_i^v(t,r')\right)}{\sum_{r' \neq r} N_{r'}}.$$

Here, $\beta_{air}$ denotes the transmission rate by airborne route and $N_{r'}$ the total number of pigs in the other rooms $r'$ of the same facility. This airborne force of infection is also applied to susceptible animals during transfer from one facility to another [17].

Therefore, the global force of infection $\lambda(t, r)$ for a given subtype $i$ at time $t$ in room $r$ is:

$$\lambda_i(t,r) = \lambda_i^{direct}(t,r) + \lambda_i^{indirect}(t,r).$$

The force of infection for animals with MDAs is assumed to be $\varepsilon * \lambda_i(t, r)$ using a reduced susceptibility factor $\varepsilon$ [26].

### Initialisation and study design

Subtypes were introduced separately with a lag-time of 20 weeks. The first subtype was introduced in a fully susceptible and demographically stable herd by the importation of a shedding gilt during the replacement process in the first batch between the farrowing and service room. Assuming no cross-immunity between the two subtypes, the population remained fully susceptible to the second subtype. Introduction of the second subtype was performed as described for the first subtype. Simulations were run for 5 years after the second virus introduction. For each scenario, 200 simulations are performed to capture the variability induced by stochastic processes while keeping a reasonable simulation time.

### Impact of the BR system on swIAV persistence

The impact of the different BR systems has been evaluated regarding the time to swIAVs fade-out and the probability of co-infection events. The latter risk was approximated as the proportion of days with co-infections on the total number of days with infected animals for each BR system (daily probability of co-infection). Finally, the global probability of co-infection events was assessed by combining the proportion of simulations with co-infections with the daily probability of co-infection

### Table 2  Parameters used in the swIAV infection dynamics model (Figure 1)

| Rate | Event | Sources | Value |
|------|-------|---------|-------|
| $\beta$ | Direct transmission rate | Cador et al. [26] | 2.43 |
| $\gamma$ | Recovery rate for infected animals (days$^{-1}$) | Rose et al. [4] | 1/8.5 |
| $\beta_{air}$ | Between-batch transmission rate | Cador et al. [17] | 0.1 |
| $\varepsilon$ | Susceptibility to infection for piglets having MDAs | Cador et al. [26] | 0.39 |
| $\sigma$ | Immunity waning (days$^{-1}$) | Cador et al. [17] | 1/180 |
| $\sigma_m$ | Loss of maternal immunity (days$^{-1}$) | Cador et al. [26] | 1/70 |
| $\beta_v$ | Transmission rate due to vaccine-immune infected animals | Romagosa et al. [29] | 0.28 |
| $\gamma_v$ | Recovery rate for infected-vaccinated animals (days$^{-1}$) | Romagosa et al. [29] | 1/4.0 |
| $\sigma_v$ | Vaccine immunity waning (days$^{-1}$) | Projected from Cador et al. [26] | 1/105 |

occurrence, weighted by the relative proportion of each BR system in the population in France [21].

## Implementation of control strategies

We tested 13 different combinations of vaccination schemes and piglet batch export. Each scenario has been simulated for two extreme BR systems in terms of batch population-size and time interval between batches (5- and 20-BR).

### Vaccination

Vaccination is implemented 3 months after the introduction of the second subtype.

In the present study, three vaccination schemes were considered:

- *Batch-to-batch vaccination of the breeding sows.* Vaccination is implemented in the gestating room 15 days before farrowing on all animals from the batch expecting to farrow. Hence vaccination time is ruled by the physiological status of the sows and the different batches are desynchronized in terms of boost vaccine immunity. This vaccine strategy aims at inducing a high antibody level in colostrum (pre-farrowing vaccination) and further transfer to piglets.
- *Mass vaccination of the breeding sows.* Vaccination is implemented every 3 or 4 months for all breeding sows present in service, gestating and farrowing rooms at the same time, in order to reduce infection pressure in breeding sow facilities.
- *Batch-to-batch vaccination of the breeding sows and growing pigs.* In addition to batch-to batch vaccination of the sows, growing pig vaccination is implemented in the five first batches entering the nursery from the beginning of the vaccination program to reduce the infection pressure in growing pig facilities. The same scenario was also tested on the five first batches entering the finishing rooms.

### Export of batches of weaned piglets

Batch export is implemented 3 months after the introduction of the second subtype. We tested the export of one batch of weaned piglets at a regular interval (every 24 weeks). The time interval between 2 exports was chosen to represent the export of a whole batch of weaned piglets to an external wean-to-finish site reared on an all-in all-out principle. The export of consecutive batches (2 or 4 batches according to the BR system) has also been tested.

### Statistical analysis of scenarios outputs

The efficiency of the different control strategies was evaluated as regards the probability of swIAVs fade-out within the herd. Time to swIAVs fade-out was studied using survival analysis comparing survival curves corresponding to different strategies using log-rank test. When conditions of proportional hazards assumption were met, a Cox-proportional hazard model was used to estimate Hazard ratios (HR) and compare control scenarios to the baseline (no measure implemented).

## Results

### Description of simulations after introduction of the two subtypes

Virus introduction via an infectious gilt (on D0 and D140) caused an initial peak in the number of infected sows due to the fully susceptible population (Figure 2). Transmission events to growing pigs occurred in the farrowing site, triggering the virus spread into the nursery and the finishing facilities. After an initial large outbreak in growing pigs and breeding animals, virus persistence was observed at the herd level due to the constant introduction of susceptible animals and immunity decay. However, sporadic fade-out periods were alternatively observed in growing pig and breeding sow subpopulations. These periods remained of relatively short durations due to virus transfer from one subpopulation to the other during between-facility movements (example at D780 in Figure 2).

In growing pigs and at the batch level, swIAVs infections of piglets occurred on successive batches at a similar age (i.e. around weaning). Consecutive batches showed similar outbreaks (Figure 3, three consecutive batches reared in a 10-BR system) however different patterns could be observed regarding the co-circulation of subtypes: (a) the infection by the subtype *i* closely followed by the infection by subtype *j* (or vice versa), allowing co-infections of the piglets during a short overlapping time-interval (Figure 3A); (b) the strict concomitant infections by the subtypes *i* and *j*, inducing a moderate number of infections by each subtype separately but a great number of co-infected piglets (Figure 3B); (c) the infection by the subtype *i* in young piglets followed by the infection of subtype *j* a few months later in finishing rooms, inducing two distinct outbreaks (Figure 3C). In each scenario, between 60 and 75% of the piglets were infected at the epidemic peak.

### Impact of the BR system on swIAVs dynamics
#### Impact of the BR system on the global within-herd persistence

Survival analysis of swIAV persistence at the herd level showed a low probability of infection fade-out up to 5 years after introduction (Figure 4). In the absence of external reintroduction and for all BR systems, at least one swIAV subtype was found to persist for more than

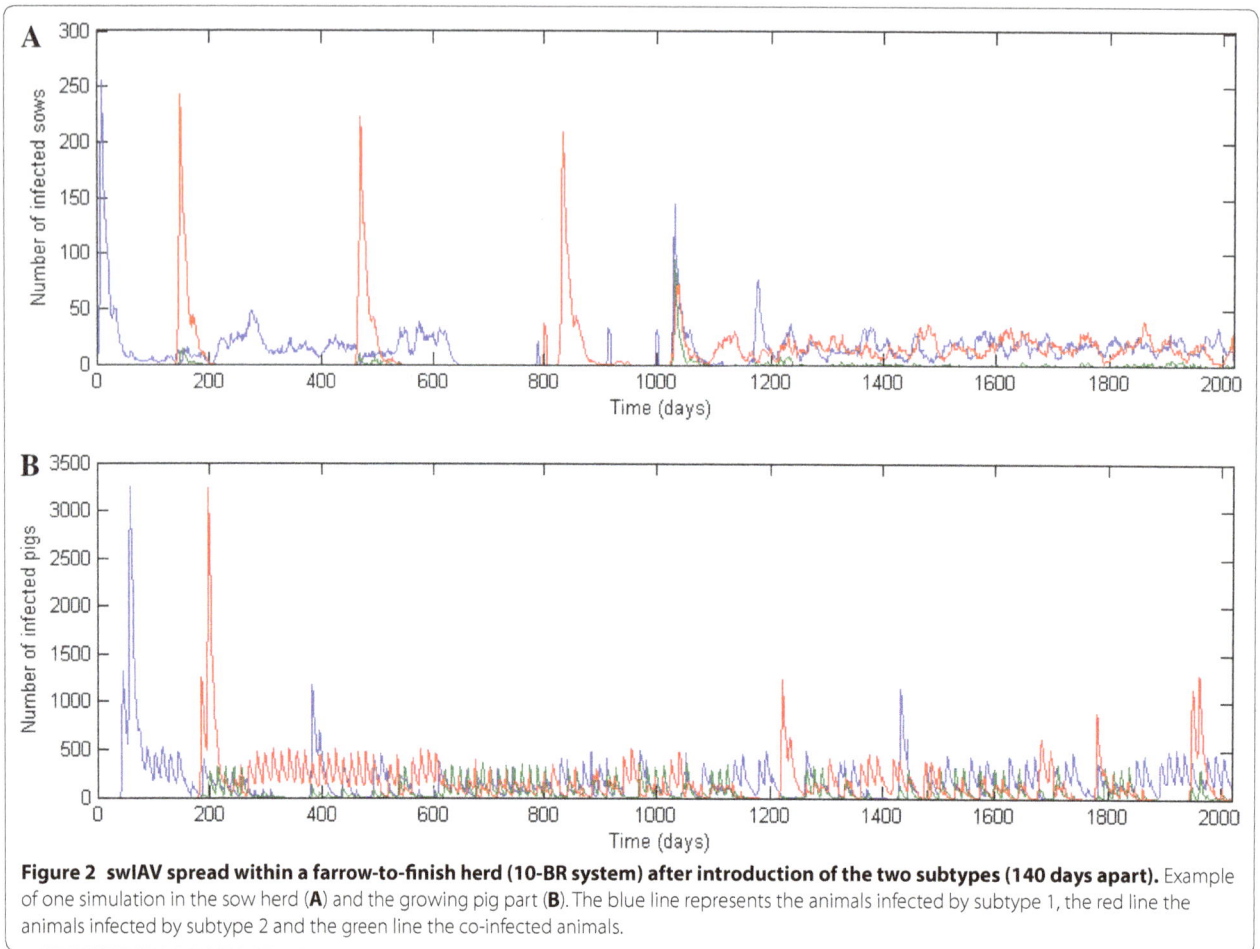

**Figure 2 swIAV spread within a farrow-to-finish herd (10-BR system) after introduction of the two subtypes (140 days apart).** Example of one simulation in the sow herd (**A**) and the growing pig part (**B**). The blue line represents the animals infected by subtype 1, the red line the animals infected by subtype 2 and the green line the co-infected animals.

3 years with a probability of 60% whatever the BR system. Differences between BR systems were however significant ($p < 0.001$, log-rank test). For BR systems with short intervals between batches (10 and 20 batches with a 14- and 7-days interval respectively), we observed a systematic endemic persistence. For these BR systems, only 8 out of 400 simulations showed stochastic fade-out before virus transmission while the infectious process lasted up to 5 years (simulation time) in all the other simulations (Table 3). Coinfections in growing pigs occurred in 84% of the 200 simulations in herds managed according to 10 and 20 batch-rearing systems.

The two BR systems with the largest between-batch intervals (4- and 5-BR with a 35- and 28-days interval respectively) showed similar behavior with a 10% fade-out probability in the first months after introduction followed by a slow decay of persistence probability throughout the simulation-time. While displaying a higher fade-out probability than the other BR systems in the two first months after introduction due to the longest in-between batches intervals, the average probability

of persistence after 5 years was evaluated to 61 and 86% for herd managed according to 4- and 5-BR systems, respectively. Forty-five to 46% of simulations resulted in coinfection events in growing pigs, reducing the probability of coinfection by 1.8 when compared to intensive batch-rearing systems (10-BR and 20-BR). The co-circulation of both subtypes was nevertheless still more frequent than the circulation of a unique subtype in these BR systems. The 7-BR system (21-day interval) showed an intermediate behavior regarding the coinfections events at the herd level, occurring in 49% of simulations (Table 3). Although swIAVs were more likely to persist during the first year after introduction compared to the 4- and 5-BR systems, the 7-BR system showed a continuous decay over time reaching the lowest probability of swIAV persistence after 5 years post-introduction (35% on average; data not shown). The order of subtype introduction did not have any effect with similar proportions of the simulations showing the circulation of only the first or the second subtype, irrespectively of the BR system (Table 3).

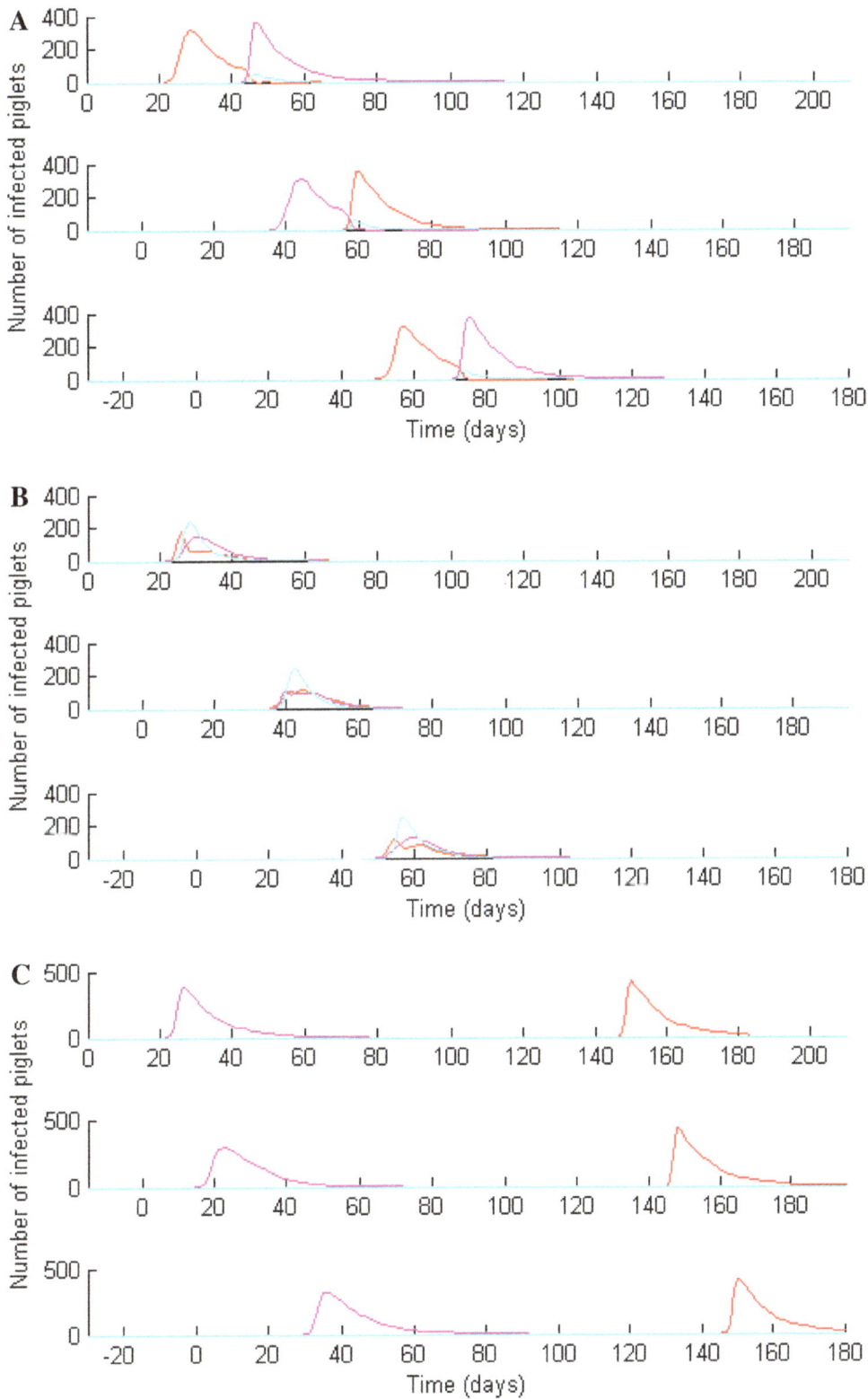

**Figure 3  Evidence of different patterns of swIAV co-circulation within growing pigs leading to partial and total concomitant infections (A, B), or consecutive infections (C).** Example of simulations carried out in the 10-BR system.

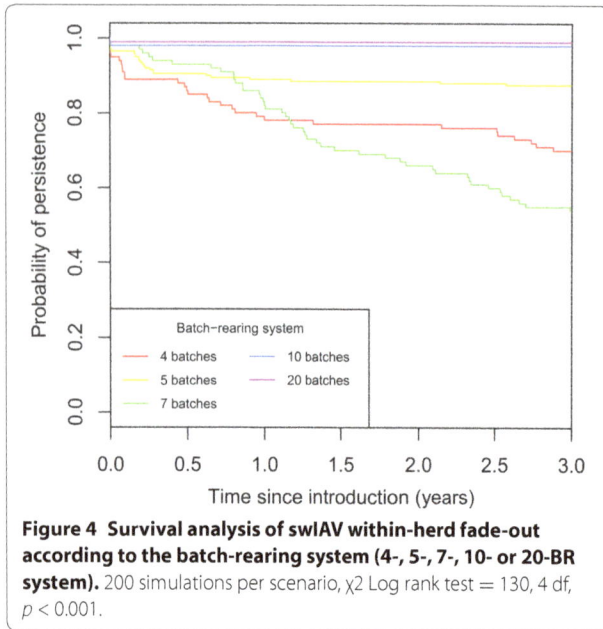

**Figure 4  Survival analysis of swIAV within-herd fade-out according to the batch-rearing system (4-, 5-, 7-, 10- or 20-BR system).** 200 simulations per scenario, χ2 Log rank test = 130, 4 df, p < 0.001.

### Assessment of the frequency of co-infection events according to the BR system

Co-circulation of both subtypes can lead to co-infections (green lines, Figure 2). The BR system had a significant impact on the presence of co-circulations at the herd level and co-infection at the individual level (Table 3). Likewise, the probability of co-infection events was significantly different between the BR systems (Kruskal–Wallis test, p < 0.001) (Figure 5). As such, the median occurrence of co-infections was 5.4, 8.1 and 16.4% for the 4-, 5- and 7-BR systems, respectively, compared to 58.8 and 91.9% in the 10- and 20-BR systems. The 10-BR system presented the highest dispersion in the occurrence of co-infections. When accounting for the relative proportion of each BR system in the French pig herd populations, the overall probability of a co-infection event possibly leading to reassortment was 16.8%.

### Evaluation of control measures

*Impact of vaccination on swIAVs persistence in breeding sows*

The implementation of vaccination 3 months after the introduction of the second subtype induced a significant rise of fade-out probability in breeding sows in the 5-BR system while having no impact on the persistence in breeding sows reared in 20-BR systems (see Additional file 1).

In the 5-BR system, all vaccination schemes significantly increased swIAV fade-out probability (HR = 4.3 [3.1–5.9] for batch-to-batch vaccination, HR = 1.6 [1.2–2.1] for mass vaccination, Cox proportional hazard model, p values < 0.05). No significant difference was observed in regards with mass vaccination schedule (3 or 4 month-interval) and outputs from these two vaccination schemes have been merged for further analyses. Batch-to-batch vaccination led to a rapid decrease of swIAV persistence probability a few months after implementation while the mass vaccination had a limited impact at that time. Mass vaccination reduced swIAV persistence probability at regular intervals but was still less efficient in sows 4 years after introduction compared to the batch-to-batch vaccination.

*Impact of vaccination on swIAV persistence at the herd level*

Although vaccination increased swIAV fade-out probability in breeding sows, the effect on the global persistence of swine flu was not reflected at the herd level. In the 5-BR system, although a global difference was found between the tested scenarios (Figure 6), when each vaccination strategies was compared to the reference 'No control measures', no significant differences were found (Cox proportional hazard model, p > 0.05). Vaccination strategies had no impact on global swIAV persistence in the 20-BR system (data not shown).

*Impact of the association of vaccination and batch export on swIAV persistence at the herd level*

In the 5-BR system, the export of piglet batches in vaccinated herds increased the probability of swIAV

**Table 3  Summary statistics (percentage of simulations) of the circulation pattern in growing pigs (no virus spread after introduction, spread of each subtype alone, spread of both subtypes with co-infection events, 5 batch-rearing (BR) systems, 200 simulations per BR system)**

|  | No virus spread | First subtype only (%) | Second subtype only (%) | Both subtypes (with co-infection events) (%) |
|---|---|---|---|---|
| 4-BR system | 11 | 23 | 19 | 47 (45) |
| 5-BR system | 10 | 21.5 | 22.5 | 46 (46) |
| 7-BR system | 5.5 | 18 | 24 | 52.5 (49) |
| 10-BR system | 2 | 5 | 9 | 84 (84) |
| 20-BR system | 1 | 7 | 8 | 84 (84) |

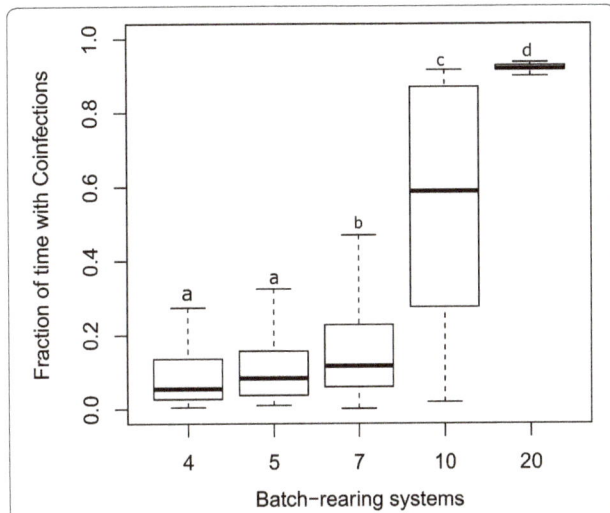

**Figure 5 Boxplots representing the occurrence of co-infections in growing pigs (number of days with co-infected pigs/number of days with infected pigs) according to the batch-rearing system (4-, 5-, 7-, 10- or 20-BR system) (Kruskal–Wallis test, $p < 0.001$).** Different letters indicate significant differences between BR systems (Wilcoxon rank sum test for pairwise comparisons).

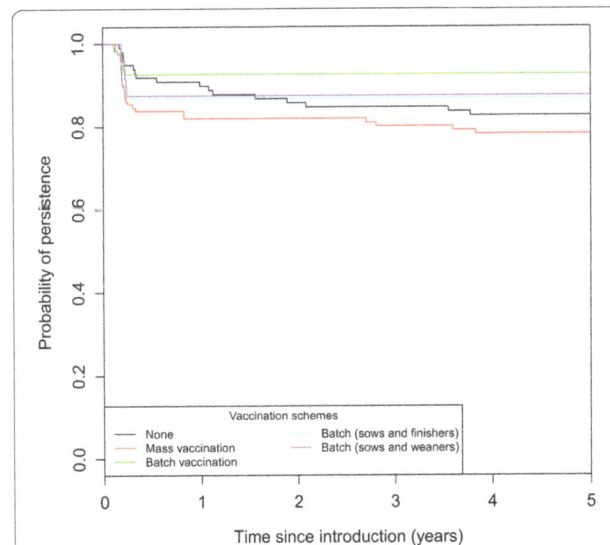

**Figure 6 Survival analysis of swIAV within-herd fade-out in pig herds reared in 5-BR system according to the vaccination scheme.** Batch-to-batch vaccination in sows, sows and five consecutive batches of weaned piglets, sows and five consecutive batches of finishing pigs, and mass vaccination. 200 simulations per scenario. χ2 Log rank test = 13.8, 4 df, $p < 0.05$.

fade-out compared to vaccination alone (Figure 7A). The concurrent export of two successive batches led to a higher probability of fade-out than the export of two batches 24 weeks apart, e.g. within the batch-to-batch

vaccination scheme: HR = 13.0 [7.6–22.0] vs. HR = 6.2 [3.65–10.5], respectively, taking the "No measure" scenario as the baseline (Cox proportional hazard model, $p$ values < 0.05). No significant difference was observed between the vaccination schemes when combined with export of weaned piglets (Figure 7A). In the 20-BR system, the simultaneous export of four consecutive batches was required to achieve a probability of swIAV within-herd fade-out of 14% (Figure 7B).

## Discussion

In this study, we extended a validated modeling framework to investigate swIAV transmission dynamics of two subtypes within a farrow-to-finish pig herd and to evaluate control strategies to prevent endemic persistence. Our model simulations showed an almost-mechanic repetition of swIAV outbreaks with infections in successive batches of piglets at a similar age. This pattern has also been shown in field conditions [4] by studying three endemically infected herds. Co-circulation of two distinct subtypes (H1$_{av}$N1 and H1$_{hu}$N2) was observed at the batch level and/or at the individual level, resulting in two distinct outbreaks or episodes with co-infections and reassortant viruses. They also identified a faster spread of the virus in pigs in finishing rooms compared to nursery rooms. Simulations from our model are consistent with this behaviour with a sharper epidemic peak in the three outbreaks occurring in older animals although the transmission characteristics between both subtypes were the same in our model. When two influenza outbreaks affect animals consecutively (slight overlap), the order of subtype infection changed from batch to batch. This phenomenon has not been shown in field conditions to date but could contribute to the understanding of repeated infections from batch to batch.

The present model highlighted the difficulty in containing transmission once a virus is introduced within the farm, consistently with White et al. [20]. Indeed, independently from the batch-rearing system, at least one of the two introduced viruses was still circulating 5 years after a unique introduction in 78% of the simulations. However, some differences were observed according to the BR systems. The 10- and 20-BR systems, characterized by short between-batch intervals and a large herd size (430 and 620 sows, respectively), inducing a huge number of animals in nursery and fattening facilities, showed a systematic persistence of swIAVs after introduction. However, both rearing systems displayed different occurrence of co-infections. Although both subtypes were circulating in the majority of the cases, a higher variability was associated with the 10-BR system due to an important number of simulations with a long persistence of a unique subtype. Moreover, the occurrence

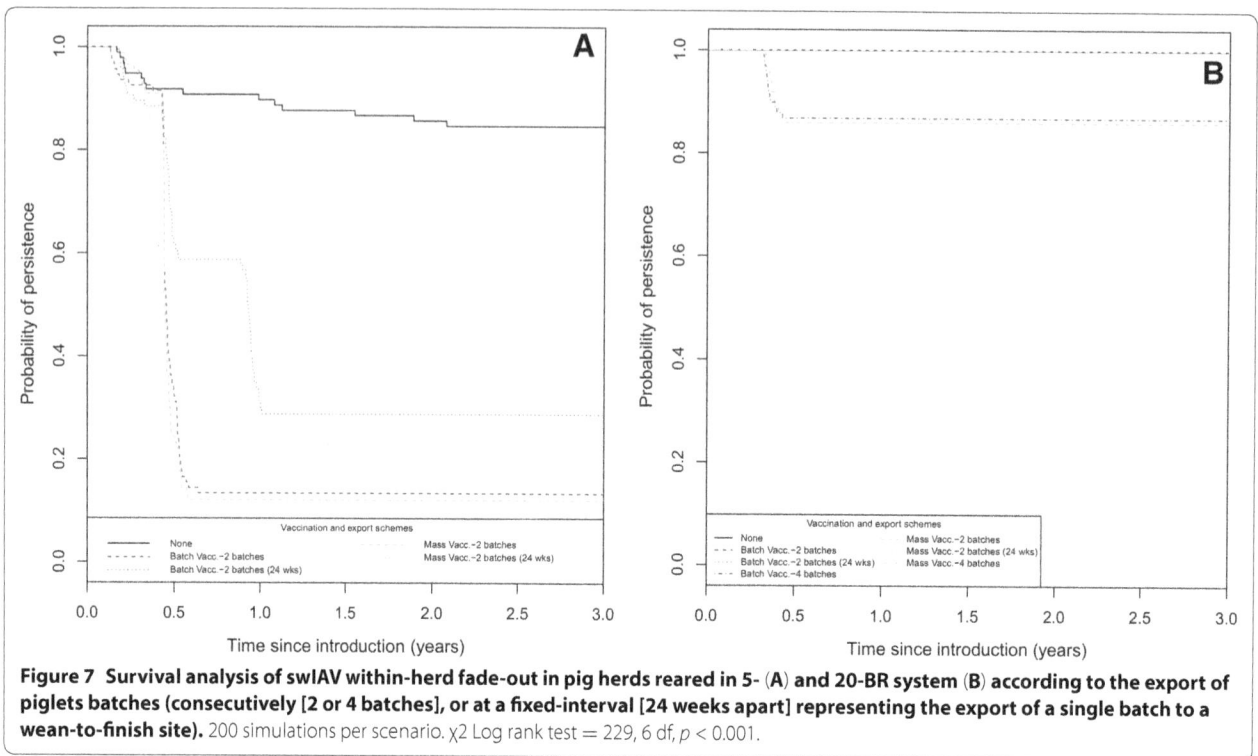

**Figure 7  Survival analysis of swIAV within-herd fade-out in pig herds reared in 5- (A) and 20-BR system (B) according to the export of piglets batches (consecutively [2 or 4 batches], or at a fixed-interval [24 weeks apart] representing the export of a single batch to a wean-to-finish site).** 200 simulations per scenario. χ2 Log rank test = 229, 6 df, $p < 0.001$.

of co-infection events appeared sporadic as compared to 20-BR system when both subtypes were circulating within the herd (median duration of the presence of both subtypes: 767 vs. 1831 days in the 20-BR system) with temporary switch between subtypes. However, because of the size of the population and the frequent introduction of susceptible animals (every 2 weeks) in this BR system, the persistence of a unique subtype for 5 years occurred more frequently than in BR systems with larger between-batch intervals.

The batch-rearing systems with the largest between-batch intervals (4 and 5 batches) have intrinsic specific characteristics that favour swIAV fade-out on top of the interval duration between batches. Fade-out of the virus in 10% of the simulations in the month following the introduction was due to the particular structure of the pig herds reared with the 4-BR system. Indeed, there is a unique batch in service room in herds reared with this system. Therefore, as sows are housed in this facility during 33 days and the virus was introduced at the entrance of the animals within the room, the epidemic outbreak could resume before the end of this period. Thus, recovered sows entering in gestating rooms couldn't initiate the infectious process in other batches. The fade-out of the virus in around 10% of the simulations 1 month later in pig herds reared in the 5-BR system was also likely due to the structure of the herd. Although two batches are housed in the service room at the same time helping the

transmission of the virus in the gestation room, the duration until the first entrance of pregnant sows in farrowing room is 23 days (only 9 days in the 4-BR system), yielding to the possible termination of the infectious process in the gestation room with a less likely spread to the farrowing rooms.

Once the virus introduced in growing pigs, a higher persistence was observed in the 4- and 5-BR compared to the 7-BR system probably due to the batch size (48 and 49 vs. 29 sows per batch respectively) and a different weaning age (21 vs. 28 days-old), which could favour fade-out in farrowing rooms before nursery entrance. The persistence could also be enhanced in the 5-BR system by the larger number of animals in the herd (245 total sows vs. 192 and 203 in the 4- and 7-BR systems). A modeling study focusing on the circulation of one influenza strain corroborates this effect of population size on swIAV persistence [18]. The choice was made to represent each BR system with the corresponding average herd size from statistics available at the country level [21]. Another option could have been to control for herd size and to evaluate only the impact of the herd organization and the time-interval between batches. However, this would have led to unrealistic situations as the choice of the BR system is governed partly by the herd size (large herds are generally reared using a 10- or 20-BR system). Moreover, representing realistic situations showed that the time-interval between batches is not the only determinant of swIAV persistence but the batch size and possibly the weaning-age also have an impact on infection dynamics.

The development of a model representing co-circulation of two swine influenza strains within pig herds had not been carried out before while models on the co-circulation of influenza A virus strains in humans exist [32, 33]. The model developed by Moghadas et al. [32] allowed consecutive infections of individuals assuming a partial cross-immunity after a first infection. In our model, no cross-immunity between subtypes was included as all the available experimental [34, 35] or field data [4] suggested an extremely limited cross-reactivity between the main subtypes known to endemically co-infect swine herds in the EU context ($H1_{av}N1$ and $H1_{hu}N2$). Zhang et al. [33] modelled the possibility of co-infections and the generation of a reassortant strain at a rate function of the days with co-infections. Only co-infection events were represented in our model as data were lacking to parameterize the likelihood of reassortant generation in case of co-infection in the swine context. Experimental in vitro, ex vivo and in vivo studies would be required to further parameterize this phenomenon. However, using our co-infections event as a proxy and combining the proportion of simulations with co-infections with the daily probability of occurrence, weighted by the relative proportion of each BR system in the population, the probability of co-infection events (16.8%) was found higher than the actual proportion of reassortant strains reported by the national surveillance system of swine influenza infections in French herds (3–5% according to years; [36]). The difference might be due to the probability of successful virus reassortment, which is not accounted in our analysis.

Control strategies were evaluated based on two BR systems selected among the five tested. According to the global spread of the virus, two subsets of BR systems were distinguished with similar behaviors obtained with the 4-, 7- and 5-BR systems, and with the 10- and 20-BR systems, respectively. To assess the impact of control measure, the 5- and 20-BR systems resulting in the longest swIAV persistence has been selected within each subset.

A key finding of this study was the selection of the export of piglet batches as the most effective measure favoring infection fade-out. The number of batches to export to obtain a significant effect depended on the BR system. Indeed, the export of four consecutive batches was required in the 20-BR system while the export of a single batch in the 5-BR system was sufficient to observe a significant decrease of swIAV persistence. The theoretical export of four consecutive batches appears difficult to set up in field conditions but highlights the necessity to insert "gaps" in the growing pigs facilities in order to block the swIAV infection dynamics. In this type of large

herds with short between-batch intervals, a solution could be to breed the minimum of batches on the main breeding site and to export, if possible, other batches to another wean-to-finish site. Indeed, lower swIAV persistence has been observed in specialized growing sites compared to farrow-to-finish pig herds [18, 37]. The consecutive export of piglet batches also led to an increased virus extinction compared to a regular export (24 weeks apart), suggesting a synergic effect on the infection disruption of consecutive exports. This is probably due to the longer period without introduction of a new cohort of potentially susceptible piglets in nursery.

Our model indicates that none of current vaccination strategies were sufficient to eliminate influenza in farrow-to-finish pig herds although it is a frequent measure implemented for swIAV control in pig herds [38]. Similarly to other modeling studies [19, 20], mass vaccination as well as batch-to-batch vaccination alone did not significantly reduce swIAV within-herd persistence. Although vaccination was found to favour swIAV fade-out in breeding sows in large between-batch interval BR systems, it had no impact on the global swIAV persistence. Indeed, even when sows were vaccinated, the viruses could still circulate and be maintained in the growing pig subpopulation and be further reintroduced in the breeding part of the herd when sows and piglets have contact (e.g. weaning stage). Usually carried out at the end of gestation, the aim of the batch-to-batch vaccination is to protect sows against reproductive disorders and to deliver maternal immunity to neonatal piglets. However, the adverse effect of maternal immunity previously highlighted [17] suggested thinking flu vaccination in swine operations differently. Incidentally, the batch-to-batch vaccination of sows, although allowing a 10% infection fade-out probability after implementation compared to the control scenario, did not affect the probability of fade-out afterwards, probably because the impact was counterbalanced by the adverse effect of maternal immunity in piglets. The mass vaccination was expected to confer a herd immunity to the sows [39] but the model showed a better efficiency of the batch-to-batch vaccination in breeding sows. This might be due to the systematic boost of immunity in sows a couple of weeks before farrowing preventing the relaunch of the infectious process in the breeding herd by growing pigs. White et al. [20] showed that early weaning of piglets after 0–7 days of age reduced endemic prevalence in farrow-to-wean units. Because such early-weaning is not allowed in Europe (Council Directive 91/630/EEC), we evaluated the export of 3-week-old piglets aiming at breaking the infectious process in growing pig population in combination with vaccination schemes. When the export of batches was implemented, the mass vaccination appeared more helpful to decrease swIAV within-herd persistence. Conversely, no differences between vaccination schemes were observed in the case of the concurrent export of consecutive batches, probably because of the limited effect of vaccination within the large impact of the export. The additional vaccination of five consecutive batches (deemed as the maximum affordable) of growing pigs or finishers did not significantly increase swIAV fade-out and could not mimic the effect of growing-pigs batches exports.

In the present model, the vaccination of the animals induced a tenfold lower transmission rate and a twofold reduction of the duration of the shedding period compared to fully-susceptible animals [29]. To the best of our knowledge, no quantitative data on the amount of virus shed by vaccinated animals have been published to date. Thus, this reduction of transmission could be due to a reduction of susceptibility in piglets having vaccine-induced immunity. A tenfold lower susceptibility has been tested with the present model but model outcomes as regards vaccine impact were not modified (data not shown). However, parameterization of the vaccine effect was made using the only data available and corresponding to a US vaccine evaluated in front of a US strain challenge. Further data should be collected on vaccine efficacy regarding the reduction in transmission and/or susceptibility to infection in the EU context to consolidate our conclusions.

swIAV endemic persistence in farrow-to-finish herds was shown in this study to be determined by multiple characteristics, which are not independent. Hence the choice of a BR system involves a specific herd structure, subpopulation sizes and between-batch time intervals. They all participate to a different degree to the persistence of the infectious process. As such, the advantage of long intervals between batches is possibly counterbalanced by large subpopulations. The observed chronic persistence of swIAVs at the herd level in field conditions and the difficulty to eradicate the infection once introduced even using different vaccination programs can be understood in the light of the present study. Control and progressive eradication of the infection requires combined vaccination programs adapted to the BR system in association with rearing practices aiming at introducing gaps in the growing part of the herd and an adequate separation between the breeding and the growing part of the herd to prevent reactivation.

## Competing interests
The authors declare that they have no competing interests.

## Authors' contributions
CC and MA developed the mathematical model and participated in data analyses and interpretations. CC drafted the manuscript; LW optimized the mathematical model; NR coordinated the study and participated in data

analyses and interpretations. All the co-authors revised the manuscript. All authors read and approved the final manuscript.

## Acknowledgements
LW is supported by the Research Foundation Flanders (FWO, G043815N) and the Antwerp Study Centre for Infectious Diseases (ASCID) at the University of Antwerp. The authors thank the CRP Regional Pig Committees for Bretagne, Pays de la Loire and Normandie, the INAPORC National Pork Council and the Brittany Region for their financial support. The funders had no role in study design, data collection and analysis, decision to publish, or preparation of the manuscript.

## Author details
[1] Swine Epidemiology and Welfare Research Unit, French Agency for Food, Environmental and Occupational Health & Safety (ANSES), BP 53, 22440 Ploufragan, France. [2] Centre for Health Economics & Modeling Infectious Diseases, Vaccine and Infectious Disease Institute, University of Antwerp Research, Antwerp, Belgium. [3] Université Bretagne Loire, Rennes, France.

## References
1.  Van Reeth K, Brown IH, Olsen CW (2012) Influenza virus. In: Zimmerman JJ, Karriker LA, Ramirez A, Schwartz KJ, Stevenson GW (eds) Diseases of Swine 10th. Wiley-Blackwell, Iowa, pp 557–571
2.  Deblanc C, Robert F, Pinard T, Gorin S, Quéguiner S, Gautier-Bouchardon AV, Ferré S, Garraud JM, Cariolet R, Brack M, Simon G (2013) Pre-infection of pigs with *Mycoplasma hyopneumoniae* induces oxidative stress that influences outcomes of a subsequent infection with a swine influenza virus of H1N1 subtype. Vet Microbiol 162:643–651
3.  Fablet C, Marois-Créhan C, Simon G, Grasland B, Jestin A, Kobisch M, Madec F, Rose N (2012) Infectious agents associated with respiratory diseases in 125 farrow-to-finish pig herds: a cross-sectional study. Vet Microbiol 157:152–163
4.  Rose N, Hervé S, Eveno E, Barbier N, Eono F, Dorenlor V, Andraud M, Camsusou C, Madec F, Simon G (2013) Dynamics of influenza a virus infections in permanently infected pig farms: evidence of recurrent infections, circulation of several swine influenza viruses and reassortment events. Vet Res 44:72
5.  Simon-Grifé M, Martin-Valls GE, Vilar MJ, Busquets N, Mora-Salvatierra M Bestebroer TM, Fouchier RA Martín M, Mateu E, Casal J (2012) Swine influenza virus infection dynamics in two pig farms; results of a longitudinal assessment. Vet Res 43:24
6.  Brown IH (2000) The epidemiology and evolution of influenza viruses in pigs. Vet Microbiol 74:29–46
7.  Kyriakis CS, Rose N, Foni E, Maldonado J, Loeffen WLA, Madec F, Simon G, Van Reeth K (2013) Influenza A virus infection dynamics in swine farms in Belgium, France, Italy and Spain, 2006–2008. Vet Microbiol 162:543–550
8.  Van Reeth K, Brown IH, Durrwald R, Foni E, Labarque G, Lenihan P, Maldonado J, Markowska-Daniel I, Pensaert M, Pospisil Z, Koch G (2008) Seroprevalence of H1N1, H3N2 and H1N2 influenza viruses in pigs in seven European countries in 2002–2003. Influenza Other Respir Viruses 2:99–105
9.  Simon-Grifé M, Martín-Valls GE, Vilar MJ, García-Bocanegra I, Mora M, Martín M, Mateu E, Casal J (2011) Seroprevalence and risk factors of swine influenza in Spain. Vet Microbiol 149:56–63
10. Hiromoto Y, Parchariyanon S, Ketusing N, Netrabukkana P, Hayashi T, Kobayashi T, Takemae N, Saito T (2012) Isolation of the pandemic (H1N1) 2009 virus and its reassortant with an H3N2 swine influenza virus from healthy weaning pigs in Thailand in 2011. Virus Res 169:175–181
11. Howard WA, Essen SC, Strugnell BW, Russell C, Barass L, Reid SM, Brown IH (2011) Reassortant pandemic (H1N1) 2009 virus in pigs, United Kingdom. Emerg Infect Dis 17:1049–1052
12. Ma W, Lager KM, Vincent AL, Janke BH, Gramer MR, Richt JA (2009) The role of swine in the generation of novel influenza viruses. Zoonoses Public Health 56:326–337
13. Kitikoon P, Vincent AL, Gauger PC, Schlink SN, Bayles DO, Gramer MR, Darnell D, Webby RJ, Lager KM, Swenson SL, Klimov A (2012) Pathogenicity

and transmission in pigs of the novel A (H3N2)v influenza virus isolated from humans and characterization of swine H3N2 viruses isolated in 2010–2011. J Virol 86:6804–6814

14. Liu Q, Ma J, Liu H, Qi W, Anderson J, Henry SC, Hesse RA, Richt JA, Ma W (2012) Emergence of novel reassortant H3N2 swine influenza viruses with the 2009 pandemic H1N1 genes in the United States. Arch Virol 157:555–562

15. Vincent A, Awada L, Brown I, Chen H, Claes F, Dauphin G, Donis R, Culhane M, Hamilton K, Lewis N, Mumford E, Nguyen T, Parchariyanon S, Pasick J, Pavade G, Pereda A, Peiris M, Saito T, Swenson S, Van Reeth K, Webby R, Wong F, Ciacci-Zanella J (2013) Review of influenza A virus in swine Worldwide: a call for increased surveillance and research. Zoonoses Public Health 61:4–17

16. Dorjee S, Revie CW, Poljak Z, McNab WB, Sanchez J (2016) One-health simulation modelling: a case study of influenza spread between human and swine populations using NAADSM. Transbound Emerg Dis 63:36–55

17. Cador C, Rose N, Willem L, Andraud M (2016) Maternally derived immunity extends swine influenza A virus persistence within farrow-to-finish pig farms: insights from a stochastic event-driven metapopulation model. PLoS One 11:e0163672

18. Pitzer VE, Aguas R, Riley S, Loeffen WLA, Wood JL, Grenfell BT (2016) High turnover drives prolonged persistence of influenza in managed pig herds. J R Soc Interface 13(119):20160138

19. Reynolds JJ, Torremorell M, Craft ME (2014) Mathematical modeling of influenza A virus dynamics within swine farms and the effects of vaccination. PLoS One 9:e106177

20. White LA, Torremorell M, Craft ME (2017) Influenza A virus in swine breeding herds: combination of vaccination and biosecurity practices can reduce likelihood of endemic piglet reservoir. Prev Vet Med 138:55–69

21. Agriculture chamber of Brittany Region (2017) Résultats des élevages de porcs en Bretagne–2014. Gestion Technique des Troupeaux de Truies-Chambre d'agriculture Bretagne. http://www.bretagne.synagri.com/ca1/PJ.nsf/TECHPJPARCLEF/25099/$File/RésultatsPorcs2014VF.pdf?OpenElement

22. Gillespie DT (1977) Exact stochastic simulation of coupled chemical reactions. J Phys Chem 81:2340–2361

23. Lloyd AL (2001) Realistic distributions of infectious periods in epidemic models: changing patterns of persistence and dynamics. Theor Popul Biol 60:59–71

24. Vergu E, Busson H, Ezanno P (2010) Impact of the infection period distribution on the epidemic spread in a metapopulation model. PLoS One 5:e9371

25. Wearing HJ, Rohani P, Keeling MJ (2005) Appropriate models for the management of infectious diseases. PLoS Med 2:e174

26. Cador C, Hervé S, Andraud M, Gorin S, Paboeuf F, Barbier N, Quèguiner S, Deblanc C, Simon G, Rose N (2016) Maternally-derived antibodies do not prevent transmission of swine influenza A virus between pigs. Vet Res 47:86

27. Simon G, Larsen LE, Dürrwald R, Foni E, Harder T, Van Reeth K, Markowska-Daniel I, Reid SM, Dan A, Maldonado J, Huovilainen A, Billinis C, Davidson I, Agüero M, Vila T, Herve S, Breum SØ, Chiapponi C, Urbaniak K, Kyriakis CS, Brown IH, Loeffen W (2014) European surveillance network for influenza in pigs: surveillance programs, diagnostic tools and Swine influenza virus subtypes identified in 14 European countries from 2010 to 2013. PLoS One 9:e115815

28. RESPIPORC FLU3 (2009) Annex 1. Summary of product characteristics. http://www.ema.europa.eu/docs/en_GB/document_library/EPAR_-_Product_Information/veterinary/000153/WC500067628.pdf. pp 1–21

29. Romagosa A, Allerson M, Gramer M, Joo H, Deen J, Detmer S, Torremorell M (2011) Vaccination of influenza a virus decreases transmission rates in pigs. Vet Res 42:120

30. Vincent AL, Ma W, Lager KM, Richt JA, Janke BH, Sandbulte MR, Gauger PC, Loving CL, Webby RJ, García-Sastre A (2012) Live attenuated influenza vaccine provides superior protection from heterologous infection in pigs with maternal antibodies without inducing vaccine-associated enhanced respiratory disease. J Virol 86:10597–10605

31. Van Reeth K, Labarque G, Pensaert M (2006) Serological profiles after consecutive experimental infections of pigs with European H1N1, H3N2, and H1N2 swine influenza viruses. Viral Immunol 19:373–382

32. Moghadas S, Bowman CS, Arino J (2009) Competitive interference between influenza viral strains. Can Appl Math Q 17:309–316

33. Zhang XS, De Angelis D, White PJ, Charlett A, Pebody RG, McCauley J (2013) Co-circulation of influenza A virus strains and emergence of pandemic via reassortment: the role of cross-immunity. Epidemics 5:20–33

34. Trebbien R, Bragstad K, Larsen LE, Nielsen J, Bøtner A, Heegaard PM, Fomsgaard A, Viuff B, Hjulsager CK (2013) Genetic and biological characterisation of an avian-like H1N2 swine influenza virus generated by reassortment of circulating avian-like H1N1 and H3N2 subtypes in Denmark. Virol J 10:290

35. Van Reeth K, Brown I, Essen S, Pensaert M (2004) Genetic relationships, serological cross-reaction and cross-protection between H1N2 and other influenza a virus subtypes endemic in European pigs. Virus Res 103:115–124

36. Simon G, Hervé S, Rose N (2013) Epidemiosurveillance of swine influenza in France from 2005 to 2012: programs, viruses and associated epidemiological data. Bull Epidémiol Santé Animale Aliment 56:17–22 **(in French)**

37. Loeffen WL, Hunneman WA, Quak J, Verheijden JH, Stegeman JA (2009) Population dynamics of swine influenza virus in farrow-to-finish and specialised finishing herds in the Netherlands. Vet Microbiol 137:45–50

38. Hervé S, Garin E, Rose N, Marcé C, Simon G (2014) French network for the surveillance of influenza viruses in pigs (Résavip). results of the first three years of operation. Bulletin Epidémiol Santé Animale Aliment Anses-DGAl 63:10–14

39. Corzo CA, Gramer M, Kuhn M et al (2012) Observations regarding influenza A virus shedding in a swine breeding farm after mass vaccination. J Swine Health Prod 20:283–289

# 12

# In vitro antibiotic susceptibility and biofilm production of *Staphylococcus aureus* isolates recovered from bovine intramammary infections that persisted or not following extended therapies with cephapirin, pirlimycin or ceftiofur

Céline Ster[1], Valérie Lebeau[1], Julia Leclerc[1], Alexandre Fugère[1], Koui A. Veh[1], Jean-Philippe Roy[2*] and François Malouin[1*]

## Abstract

*Staphylococcus aureus* intramammary infections (IMIs) have low cure rates using standard antibiotic treatment and increasing the duration of treatment usually improves therapeutic success. Chronic IMIs are thought to be caused by bacteria presenting a specific virulence phenotype that includes the capacity to produce greater amounts of biofilm. In this study, antibiotic susceptibility and biofilm production by *S. aureus* isolates recovered from IMIs that were cured or not following an extended therapy with cephapirin, pirlimycin or ceftiofur for 5, 8 and 8 days, respectively, were compared. An isolate was confirmed as from a persistent case (not cured) if the same *S. aureus* strain was isolated before and after treatment as revealed by the same VNTR profile (variable number of tandem repeats detected by multiplex PCR). The antibiotic minimal inhibitory concentrations (MICs) were determined for these isolates as well as the capacity of the isolates to produce biofilm. Isolates from persistent cases after extended therapy with cephapirin or ceftiofur had higher MICs for these drugs compared to isolates from non-persistent cases ($p < 0.05$) even though the antibiotic susceptibility breakpoints were not exceeded. Isolates of the ceftiofur study significantly increased their biofilm production in presence of a sub-MIC of ceftiofur ($p < 0.05$), whereas isolates from the pirlimycin group produced significantly less biofilm in presence of a sub-MIC of pirlimycin ($p < 0.001$). Relative antibiotic susceptibility of the isolates as well as biofilm production may play a role in the failure of extended therapies. On the other hand, some antibiotics may counteract biofilm formation and improve cure rates.

## Introduction

*Staphylococcus aureus* (*S. aureus*) is a major bacterial pathogen causing intramammary infections (IMIs) [1] and is most often responsible for a chronic and contagious mastitis that is difficult to treat with antibiotics [2]. Reported cure rates for *S. aureus* mastitis are usually low but vary from 4 to 92% and seem to depend on many host and bacterial factors such as cow parity, level of somatic cell counts or the genetic background of *S. aureus* isolates and their ability to produce biofilm [2, 3]. Biofilm is an extracellular matrix in which bacteria are more resistant to antibiotics, the immune system or disinfectants [4]. It is commonly believed that the discrepancy between the antimicrobial susceptibility in vitro and

*Correspondence: jean-philippe.roy@umontreal.ca;
francois.malouin@usherbrooke.ca
[1] Centre d'Étude et de Valorisation de la Diversité Microbienne (CEVDM), Département de Biologie, Faculté des Sciences, Université de Sherbrooke, Sherbrooke, QC J1K 2R1, Canada
[2] Département de Sciences Cliniques, Faculté de Médecine Vétérinaire, Université de Montréal, C.P. 5000, St-Hyacinthe, QC J2S 7C6, Canada

cure rate is related to the capacity of *S. aureus* to produce biofilm during IMIs [5].

Cephapirin, pirlimycin and ceftiofur are antibiotics available for the treatment of bovine mastitis in North America [6]. Cephapirin is a first generation cephalosporin antibiotic while ceftiofur is a third generation. Cephalosporins (part of the β-lactam class) inhibit bacterial transpeptidases, which are responsible for cell wall peptidoglycan biosynthesis [7]. Pirlimycin belongs to the lincosamide class of antibacterial agents [8]. It acts by inhibiting bacterial protein synthesis via binding to the 50S subunit of the ribosome.

Extending the duration of antibiotic treatment seems to improve therapeutic success [2, 6]. In a study evaluating the efficacy of a 5-day cephapirin treatment of chronic subclinical *S. aureus* IMIs, cow bacteriological cure rates were of 25.8 and 3.3% for the treated and untreated control groups, respectively [9]. In another study comparing 2-, 5- and 8-day therapies with pirlimycin, quarter bacteriological cure rates were of 13.3, 31.3 and 83.3%, respectively, while no cure (0%) for untreated controls was observed [10]. Several ceftiofur treatment durations for subclinical *S. aureus* IMIs were compared in a study by Oliver et al. [7]. Bacteriological cure rates were of 36, 17, 7 and 0% for the 8-, 5-, 2-day ceftiofur treatment and for the untreated control groups, respectively. A more recent study also assessed the impact of an extended therapy using ceftiofur for the treatment of clinical mastitis caused by *S. aureus* IMIs. A quarter bacteriological cure rate of 0% was observed for the group of cows treated for 2 days (conventional treatment) while a bacteriological cure rate of 47.4% was observed for cows treated for 8 days [11].

It is thus apparent that extended therapies increase cure rates for IMIs caused by *S. aureus*. However, not all *S. aureus* IMIs are cured and cure rates vary based on the type of antibiotic treatment used. This study aimed at making associations between *S. aureus* biofilm formation, antibiotic susceptibility and the success or failure of extended therapies with cephapirin, pirlimycin or ceftiofur.

## Materials and methods
### Extended antibiotic therapy
For the purpose of this study, we used *S. aureus* strains that were collected in three different field studies in which extended therapies were used for treatment of *S. aureus* IMIs. *S. aureus* isolates were identified from milk samples as Gram-positive cocci showing a positive catalase test, hemolysis on blood agar, and positive nuclease and coagulase tests.

An IMI was confirmed if at least one colony of *S. aureus* from a 10-μL milk sample (i.e., ≥ 100 cfu/mL) was found. Only one isolate was kept from each sample. Since only 10 μL milk samples were initially plated to assess the bacterial content, it was assumed that this isolate was predominant but IMI caused by multiple isolates each present in large numbers cannot be ruled out. Each of the three field studies are briefly described below.

### Extended therapy with cephapirin
The *S. aureus* isolates were collected during a study that assessed the efficacy of an extended therapy with cephapirin against chronic subclinical IMIs [9]. Briefly, 14 herds from a group of dairy herds in the Saint-Hyacinthe region of the Province of Quebec (Canada) were enrolled in this study. Milk samples were collected from dairy cows with a history of chronic IMIs caused by *S. aureus*. When *S. aureus* IMI was confirmed based on the presence of the bacterium in milk, cephapirin (200 mg/dose, Cefa-Lak®, Boehringer Ingelheim, Burlington, ON, Canada) was administered in all 4 quarters at each milking for 5 consecutive days and 3 milk samples were taken 10, 24 and 31 days after treatment for bacteriological analysis. The labelled treatment for cephapirin is 2 doses 12 h apart (2 consecutive milkings). Among the 29 cases analyzed in this study, 12 cases (41.4%) showed bacteriological cure, i.e., showed 3 consecutive negative milk samples after the end of the extended therapy (Table 1). For the other 17 cases, *S. aureus* was isolated from at least one of the 3 samplings collected after the end of the treatment, indicating a failure of the extended therapy (i.e., persistent cases based on bacteriology, Table 1).

### Extended therapy with pirlimycin
The bacterial isolates were collected from primiparous cows with *S. aureus* IMIs that were treated in the first week of lactation with pirlimycin (50 mg/dose, once a day, Pirsue®, Zoetis, Kirkland, QC, Canada) in the affected quarters for 8 consecutive days. The labelled treatment for pirlimycin in Canada is 2 or 8 doses 24 h apart. The cows were coming from 23 herds in the Drummondville region of the Province of Québec (Canada) and this treatment protocol was part of the usual udder health control program on these herds. Treatment success or failure was assessed by bacteriological milk cultures of quarter milk samples collected 3–8 weeks after treatment (average of 32 days). Forty quarters from 36 cows were subjected to this treatment regimen and 82.5% of *S. aureus* isolates (i.e., from 33 quarters) were from successful therapy based on bacteriology (Table 1). In 7 cases, *S. aureus* was isolated after treatment indicating therapeutic failure (i.e., 7 persistent cases based on bacteriology, Table 1). Due to the large number of isolates from cured cases, we only randomly included a total of 23 distinct isolates from cured cases (on a possibility of

**Table 1  Overview _S. aureus_ isolates collected in three different field studies in which extended therapies were used for treatment of IMIs**

|  | Extended therapy with | | |
|---|---|---|---|
|  | Cephapirin | Pirlimycin | Ceftiofur |
| Total number of cases[a] | 29 | 40 | 17 |
| Based on bacteriology |  |  |  |
|   Cases in which _S. aureus_ was eliminated | 12 | 33 | 9 |
|   Cases in which _S. aureus_ was isolated after therapy | 17 | 7 | 8 |
|   Proportion of isolates that were eliminated (%) | 41.3 | 82.5 | 52.9 |
| Based on VNTR analysis |  |  |  |
|   Isolates that were eliminated or that were distinct by VNTR before and after therapy | 19 | 34 | 9 |
|   Isolates from persistent cases (same VNTR before and after therapy) | 10 | 6 | 8 |
|   Proportion of isolates that were eliminated (%) | 65.5 | 85.0 | 52.9 |
| Number of isolates characterized in this study[b] |  |  |  |
|   Isolates from cured cases | 12 | 23[c] | 9 |
|   Isolates from persistent cases (VNTR-confirmed)[c] | 10 | 6 | 8 |

[a]  Cases are quarters infected with _S. aureus_. Isolates from cured cases are revealed when one _S. aureus_ isolate is found before treatment but no _S. aureus_ is detected after the end of treatment. Persistent cases are revealed when one _S. aureus_ isolate is found before treatment and at least one _S. aureus_ isolate is also found after the end of treatment.

[b]  Cases that were not validated as persistent (possible new infections by a different _S. aureus_ isolate) were excluded of the study. When multiple isolates were collected from the same cow (different quarters), only one isolate was selected for the study.

[c]  Only the isolates collected before treatment were used for the rest of the study.

33) for further characterization in this study (as indicated in Table 1).

### Extended therapy with ceftiofur

_Staphylococcus aureus_ isolates were collected during a study that assessed the efficacy of an extended therapy with ceftiofur for the treatment of mild to moderate clinical mastitis [11]. Labelled treatment in Canada is 2 doses 24 h apart. Briefly, 22 herds located in the Province of Quebec and Eastern Ontario (Canada) were enrolled in this study. A total of 17 _S. aureus_ isolates from 17 cases treated with an extended therapy with ceftiofur for 8 consecutive days (125 mg/dose, once a day, Spectramast® LC, Pfizer Animal Health, Kirkland, QC) were available for analysis. Milk samples were taken 7, 14 and 21 days after the end of the treatment to assess bacteriological cure. Based on bacteriological results, 8 cases responded to treatment (52.9%, Table 1), whereas in 9 cases, _S. aureus_ was isolated in at least one of the milk samples collected after the end of treatment, indicating therapeutic failure.

### VNTR analysis

VNTR analysis (variable number of tandem repeats) was used to validate bacterial persistence of the same _S. aureus_ strain before and after the extended therapy. First, genomic DNA of the different isolates was purified using the Gene Elute kit according to the recommendations of the manufacturer (Sigma Aldrich, Oakville, ON, Canada).

Then, VNTR analysis for five genes (_sdr_, _clfA_, _clfB_, _ssp_ and _spa_) was performed by multiplex PCR as previously described by Sabat et al. [12]. Isolates from each case were processed at the same time (same PCR mix) and their PCR products were migrated on the same electrophoresis agarose gel. Pattern of the isolates, recovered before and after treatment, from a same case were compared visually to assess their similarity. As described by Veh et al. [13], a control strain (SHY97-3906) was added to each multiplex PCR batch and electrophoresis gel to ensure the repeatability of the method.

This VNTR analysis aimed at excluding the possible cases of a cure followed by a new infection with a distinct _S. aureus_ isolate or also cases in which multiple strains could be involved. Isolates before and after extended therapy were considered as the same strain, from a persistent case, if their electrophoretic VNTR profiles were identical. If the isolates before and after extended therapy showed different VNTR profiles, this case was excluded from the study.

### Antibiotic minimal inhibitory concentration

The minimal inhibitory concentrations (MICs) of cephapirin, pirlimycin and ceftiofur for all isolates were determined by a 96-well plate broth microdilution technique, following the recommendations of the Clinical Laboratory Standards Institute (CLSI) [14]. Briefly, the antibiotics were serially diluted (doubling dilutions) in Mueller–Hinton broth (cation adjusted, CAMHB; BD,

Mississauga, ON) within a 96-well plate before the same volume of the bacterial inoculum was added to each well. The inoculum was prepared from an overnight culture in CAMHB, first diluted to a 0.5-McFarland standard ($\approx 1.5 \times 10^8$ CFU/mL) before adding $\approx 10^5$–$10^6$ CFU/mL to each well. The *S. aureus* strain ATCC29213 was used as a quality control as recommended by Clinical Laboratory Standards Institute (CLSI). The MIC was the lowest concentration of antibiotic preventing growth. Susceptibility thresholds used were 8, 2 and 2 µg/mL for cephapirin, pirlimycin and ceftiofur, respectively. Resistance breakpoints used were 32, 4 and 8 µg/mL for cephapirin, pirlimycin and ceftiofur, respectively.

## Biofilm production

Biofilm formation was evaluated by spectrophotometry using crystal violet staining, as previously described with few modifications [13, 15]. Briefly, isolates were cultured from frozen stocks onto tryptic soy agar plates and incubated at 35 °C overnight. Colonies were then inoculated into brain heart infusion containing 0.25% of glucose (Sigma Aldrich) to obtain a 0.5-McFarland standard ($\approx 1.5 \times 10^8$ CFU/mL). The suspension was then transferred into wells of a flat bottom polystyrene microtiter plates containing half the volume of the same medium. The plates were incubated at 35 °C for 24 h, without agitation and under aerobic conditions. The supernatant was then discarded and the wells were delicately washed three times with 200 µL of PBS. The plates were dried, and then stained for 30 min with crystal violet (Sigma Aldrich). Wells were then washed twice with 200 µL of water and allowed to dry again. A volume of 200 µL of 95% ethanol was added to each well and plates were incubated at room temperature for 1 h with frequent agitation. The absorbance of each well was then measured at 560 nm using a plate reader (Epoch, Bio-Tek instruments, Vinooski, VT). The *S. aureus* reference strain Newbould (ATCC 29740), initially isolated from a bovine mastitis case, was included into each plate to normalize for plate-to-plate variations. This strain is a moderate biofilm producer with an average OD 560 nn value of 0.15 in biofilm assays. Biofilm measurements were averages of three independent experiments performed on different days. Each independent experiment included four wells for each strain (four technical replicates). Average biofilm production for each isolate in each plate was calculated and normalized by dividing the average biofilm production of the isolates by the average production of the reference train. Then, the normalized measured biofilm enumeration of each isolate obtained from the three independent assays were combined.

To evaluate the effect of a subinhibitory concentration of cephapirin, pirlimycin or ceftiofur on biofilm production, measurements were also performed for each isolate grown in the presence of a sub-MIC ($0.25 \times$ MIC) of those antibiotics for the isolate. For example, if a strain had a MIC of 1 µg/mL for pirlimycin, biofilm assay was performed with 0.25 µg/mL of pirlimycin. The concentration was thus adjusted for each isolate and for each antibiotic.

## Statistical analysis

Statistical analyses were performed using the GraphPad Prism software (v5.00). The distribution of the isolates from cured cases vs the isolates from persistent cases according to their MIC for an antibiotic was compared using a Chi square trend test. Biofilm production for the different groups of isolates was compared with the Kruskal–Wallis test (nonparametric one way analysis of variance) followed by a Dunn's multiple comparisons test. The biofilm production of the isolates from cured cases vs the isolates from persistent cases and biofilm production in presence or absence of a sub-MIC of antibiotics were compared with the Mann–Whitney test (nonparametric *t* test). Statistical tests used for the analysis of each of the experiments are specified in the Figure legends. Differences were considered statistically significant when $p < 0.05$.

## Results

### VNTR analysis of the isolates and validation of persistent IMI cases

VNTR analysis was performed to validate IMI persistence despite extended therapy. A persistent case was validated when the *S. aureus* isolates collected before and after the extended therapy showed an identical VNTR electrophoretic profile (see Additional file 1 for examples). Among the IMIs that were classified as persistent based on the bacteriological analyses of the milk samples, 10/17, 6/7 and 8/8 of the IMIs from the extended therapy with cephapirin, pirlimycin and ceftiofur, respectively, were confirmed as persistent after VNTR analysis (see the number of isolates from persistent cases based on VNTR analysis, Table 1). For each pair of isolates from persistent cases (before and after therapy), only the results obtained for the "before therapy isolate" are presented here as no difference in VNTR, MICs or biofilm production among the pair members was observed (data not shown). Isolates from the non-validated cases of persistence (i.e., showing different VNTR profiles before and after therapy) were excluded for the rest of this study as these non-validated cases might represent cases where the quarter was successfully treated by the extended therapy but then re-infected by a new isolate having a different VNTR profile. The non-validated cases might also have represented cases in which multiple strains were involved. The data available about those cases did not permit to select the most likely hypothesis and these non-validated cases were thus excluded from the study.

### Antibiotic MICs among the study groups

Antibiotic resistance of bacterial isolates may cause failure of antibiotic therapy (standard or extended). Here, no difference in the antibiotic $MIC_{50}$ or $MIC_{90}$ (MIC that inhibits the growth of 50 or 90% of the tested strains, respectively) was observed between the isolates from cured and persistent cases for the three extended therapies. Cephapirin $MIC_{50}$ and $MIC_{90}$ values were of 0.12 and 0.25 µg/mL, respectively, for isolates of the cephapirin study, pirlimycin $MIC_{50}$ and $MIC_{90}$ were 0.25 and 0.25 µg/mL for isolates of the pirlimycin study, and ceftiofur $MIC_{50}$ and $MIC_{90}$ were 0.25 and 1 µg/mL for isolates of the ceftiofur study. Based on CLSI susceptibility thresholds of 8, 2 and 2 µg/mL for cephapirin, pirlimycin and ceftiofur, respectively (resistance breakpoints are 32, 4 and 8 µg/mL respectively), none of the isolates could be considered as resistant in vitro. However, the distribution of the antibiotic MICs for the isolates from cured and persistent cases was different within the three study groups (i.e., extended therapies to cephapirin, pirlimycin and ceftiofur) (Figure 1). This comparison demonstrates that the *S. aureus* isolate populations collected from those three studies were different. Noteworthy, cephapirin and ceftiofur generally had higher MICs for the isolates from the persistent cases in two of the three extended therapy studies, whereas the distribution of pirlimycin MICs for the isolates from cured and persistent cases did not differ in any of the three studies (Figure 1). Note that the isolates from the persistent cases tested were the "before therapy isolates" as mentioned in "Materials and methods" section and some of the observed differences in antibiotic susceptibility could therefore not have resulted from a selective pressure by the therapy under investigation.

### Biofilm production

The *S. aureus* isolates collected from the three different therapy studies were also distinct based on their in vitro biofilm production. The isolates from the ceftiofur study produced significantly less biofilm than isolates from the two other studies although for each of the study groups, there was no difference in biofilm production between isolates from cured or persistent cases (Figure 2).

Biofilm production by each isolate was also evaluated in presence of a sub-MIC (0.25 × MIC) of the different antibiotics previously determined against each of the isolates (Figure 3). No difference in biofilm production was observed in presence or absence of the sub-MIC of cephapirin for the entire set of isolates collected in

the cephapirin study (Figure 3A). Also, taken individually, each of the cephapirin-therapy isolates from cured or persistent cases showed the same ability to produce biofilm in presence or absence of the sub-MIC of cephapirin (Figure 3B). On the other hand, isolates from the extended therapy with pirlimycin produced significantly less biofilm in presence of a sub-MIC of pirlimycin ($p < 0.0001$, Figure 3C). Even though the group of isolates from the extended therapy with ceftiofur produced significantly less biofilm than the two other studied groups (Figure 2), the presence of a sub-MIC of ceftiofur significantly increased the biofilm production of these isolates ($p < 0.05$, Figure 3E). Finally, there was a tendency for the isolates from persistent cases from the pirlimycin study to produce more biofilm than isolates from the cured cases in presence of the sub-MIC of the antibiotic ($p = 0.07$, Figure 3D), but like for the isolates from the persistent cases of the ceftiofur study (Figure 3F), this difference was not statistically significant.

### Discussion

The incidence of new IMI may increase with duration of intramammary treatments [2]. Indeed, some studies that have evaluated the efficacy of extended antibiotherapies reported an increase in new IMI rates [10, 11, 16]. It was reported that new infections with *E. coli* or *Klebsiella* can occur during extended therapy. New IMIs can also occur between the end of a treatment and post-treatment samplings, which may appear as a therapeutic failure. In the present study, we used VNTR analysis to validate persistent cases. We found that some cases that were initially considered persistent IMIs based on the bacteriological analysis of milk samples needed to be re-classified as either potentially cured and followed by a new infection or cases in which multiple strains were involved since post-therapy samplings revealed *S. aureus* isolates having different VNTR profiles. VNTR analysis is therefore a useful tool to quickly discriminate between a persistent case and more complex cases where distinct strains are observed. VNTR analysis was also used to discriminate epidemic strains from sporadic strains in hospitals [17]. The effectiveness of VNTR as a molecular typing tool make VNTR analysis highly comparable to more complex methods such as PFGE and MLST [12, 18]. VNTR analysis can thus provide information on the diversity of isolates present in a herd, identify predominant clones and help management of IMIs [2].

Several differences other than the antibiotic treatment prevent a direct comparison of these therapies. First, case definitions and definition of cure were different. In the study using cephapirin [9], the *S. aureus* IMI cases were chronic subclinical infections and cure was defined using three milk cultures at 10, 24 and 31 days

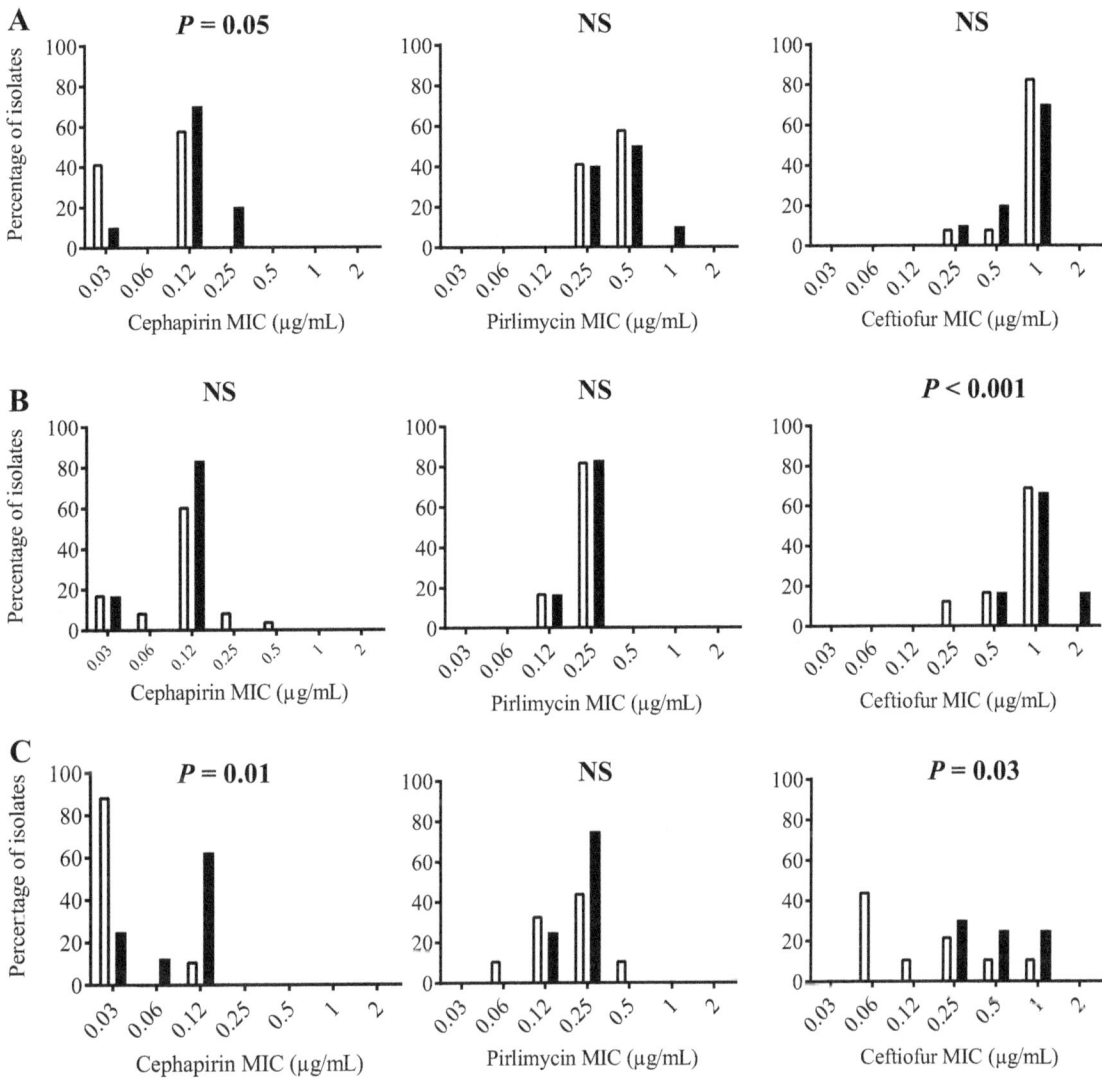

**Figure 1 Distribution of antibiotic MICs for isolates that were from cured or persistent cases.** Isolates from cured cases were represented with open bars while isolates from persistent cases are represented with closed bars. Isolates were collected from an extended therapy study with cephapirin (**A**), pirlimycin (**B**) or ceftiofur (**C**). The distribution of the isolates from cured vs the persistent cases according to their MIC for an antibiotic was compared using a Chi square trend test: NS, not statistically significant.

post-treatment. In the study using ceftiofur [11], *S. aureus* isolates were collected from clinical mastitis cases and cure was defined using three milk cultures at 7, 14 and 21 days post-treatment. Finally, the study with pirlimycin (unpublished) used first or second lactation cows at calving and only one milk culture between 3 and 8 weeks post-treatment was used for cure definition. Also, the three antibiotic treatments were not applied on the same population of cows and herd level factors may certainly affect cure rates. Finally, the bacterial isolate populations collected from the cephapirin, ceftiofur and pirlimycin studies also differed. The distribution of the

antibiotic MICs (Figure 1) and the overall differences in biofilm production for the three isolate populations (Figure 2) attest that bacterial factors may affect the outcome of the therapy.

The specific aim of the present study was indeed to examine some of the bacterial factors such as biofilm production that could influence or explain the relative success of extended therapies with cephapirin, pirlimycin or ceftiofur. By comparing biofilm formation and antibiotic susceptibility of the *S. aureus* isolates from cured and persistent cases we could suggest some explanations for failure or success of therapy as discussed below.

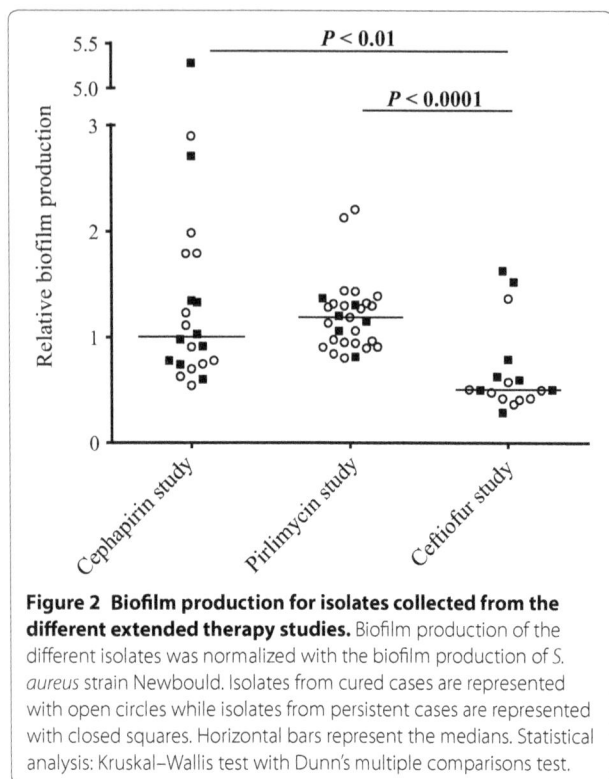

**Figure 2 Biofilm production for isolates collected from the different extended therapy studies.** Biofilm production of the different isolates was normalized with the biofilm production of *S. aureus* strain Newbould. Isolates from cured cases are represented with open circles while isolates from persistent cases are represented with closed squares. Horizontal bars represent the medians. Statistical analysis: Kruskal–Wallis test with Dunn's multiple comparisons test.

The cephapirin and ceftiofur MICs for the isolates from cases that persisted to the extended therapy with these antibiotics were generally higher than the MICs determined for the isolates from the cured cases. Although the isolates from persistent cases can still be considered as clinically susceptible to cephapirin (MIC $\leq$ 8 µg/mL) or ceftiofur (MIC $\leq$ 2 µg/mL), the higher MICs generally found for these isolates compared to the isolates from the cured cases (Figures 1A and 1C, respectively) may improve their capacity to persist in the mammary gland. The mammary gland is a large organ and intramammary antibiotic diffusion might not be homogenous [2]. A slight decrease in antibiotic activity (i.e., slightly higher MICs) against specific *S. aureus* strains and an unequal tissue distribution of the antibiotic may result in a persistent case. Then again, another study with cephapirin could not demonstrate a correlation between in vitro susceptibility test results (MICs) and the outcome of therapy [19], although this was a study on multiple Gram-positive pathogens and the standard prescribed cephapirin therapy was used.

Biofilms offer protection from antibiotic activity and host defenses and is one of the causes often proposed for therapeutic failure [2, 4, 20]. Interestingly, we report here that *S. aureus* isolates from both cured and persistent cases are producing significantly more biofilm in the presence of a sub-MIC of ceftiofur (Figure 3E).

Noteworthy however, there were at least 3 of the 17 strains that showed less biofilm production in presence of this antibiotic and this indicated that there were strain to strain variations in the response to this antibiotic (Figure 3E). This sub-MIC effect on biofilm production, combined to the higher MICs of the ceftiofur-persistent isolates mentioned above may both have contributed to treatment failure. The mechanism responsible for the increase biofilm production in the presence of a sub-MIC of ceftiofur is not known at this time but it is possible that the damage produced to the bacterial cell wall by this β-lactam antibiotic activates a sigma factor B-dependent stress response that helps biofilm formation [21]. On the other hand, as far as pirlimycin is concerned, we observed no difference in the degree of susceptibility of the *S. aureus* isolates collected from cases that persisted or that were cured by the extended therapy (Figure 1B), and remarkably, the presence of a sub-MIC of pirlimycin significantly reduced biofilm production (Figure 3C). The cure rates of pirlimycin may have been helped by such conditions. Extended pirlimycin treatments with cure rates up to 86% were also previously reported [7, 9, 10, 22, 23]. Pirlimycin is a lincosamide antibiotic that blocks proteins synthesis. Huang et al. [24] showed that clindamycin, another lincosamide, can also reduce the biofilm surface of *S. aureus*. Rachid et al. [25] showed that sub-inhibitory concentrations of clindamycin had no effect on the expression of the *ica* operon (involved in biofilm production) in *S. epidermidis* during biofilm formation. However, using *S. epidermidis* cells embedded in a biofilm, Gomes et al. [26], showed that the clindamycin–rifampicin combination reduces the expression of genes *icaA* and *rsbU* (two genes involved in biofilm formation) compared to that is observed with rifampicin alone.

Here, we have measured the impact of sub-inhibitory concentrations of antibiotics on the capacity of *S. aureus* to produce biofilm. Another interesting approach that may have facilitated the evaluation of the effect of biofilm production on antibiotic action and associations with treatment efficacy was proposed by Melchior et al. [27], i.e., the use of an antibiotic susceptibility assay for bacteria embedded in biofilms and the determination of the minimum concentration of biofilm eradication (MBEC) [5]. This would have provided information on the impact of antibiotics on an already formed biofilm. These in vitro methods address two different aspects of the possible action of antibiotics on biofilms and vice versa. It is still however very difficult to predict the success of treatment using in vitro tests.

Each antibiotic possesses different physical and biological properties (solubility, protein binding, absorption, tissue distribution, half-life, MIC, etc.) that certainly influence therapeutic efficacy. The host (cow) can also

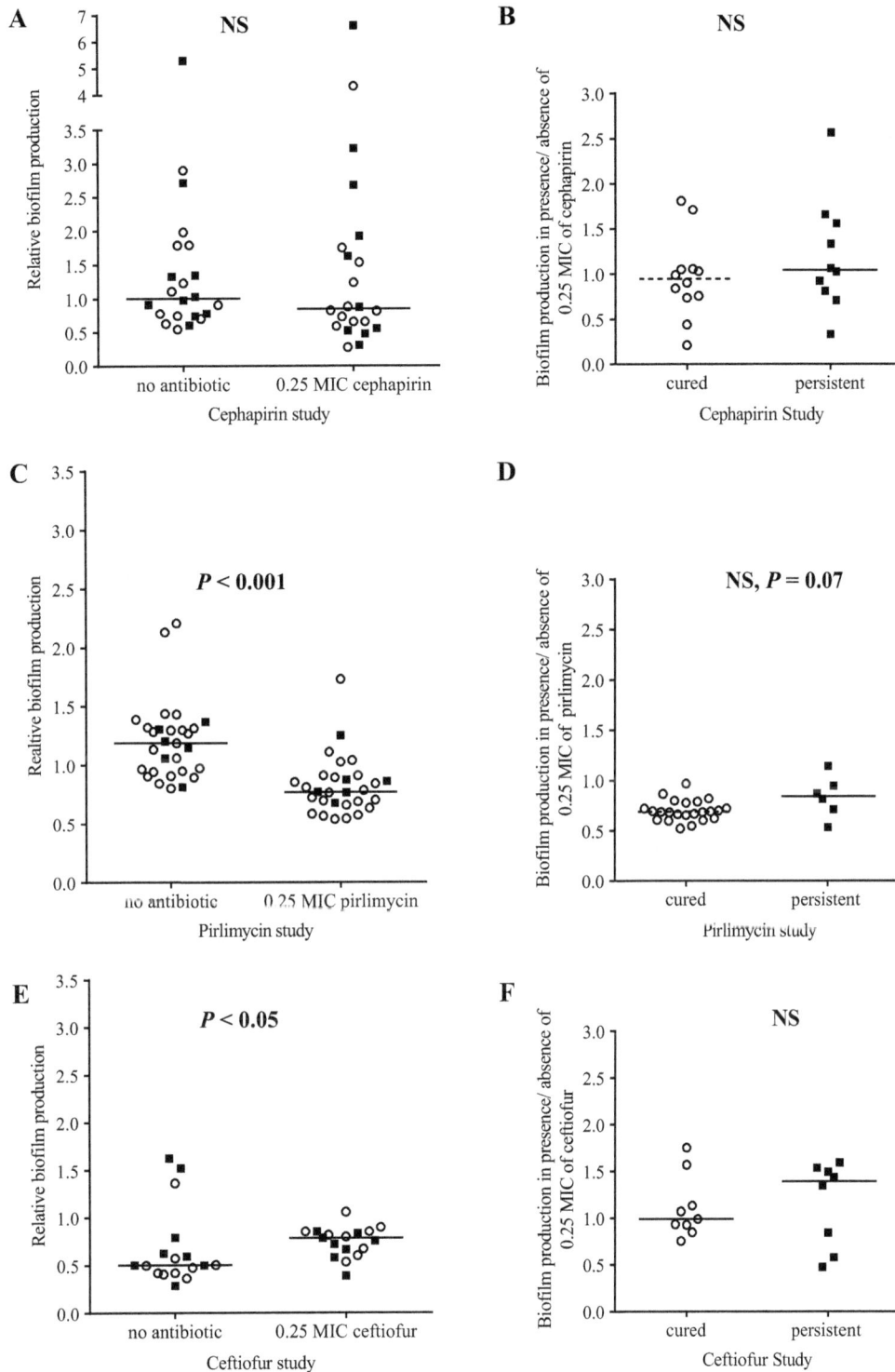

**Figure 3 Biofilm production in presence or absence of the sub-MIC of the different antibiotics. A, B** *S. aureus* isolates collected from the cephapirin study. **C, D** *S. aureus* isolates collected from the pirlimycin study; and **E, F** *S. aureus* isolates collected from the ceftiofur study. For all graphs, open circles represent data for isolates from cured cases and closed squares represent data for isolates from persistent cases. Horizontal bars represent the medians. **A**, **C**, and **E** present biofilm production (relative to the *S. aureus* strain Newbould) for each of the isolates grown in presence or absence of the sub-MIC (0.25 × MIC) of cephapirin, pirlimycin or ceftiofur for that isolate, respectively. **B, D, F** present the biofilm production of each of the isolates from cured or persistent cases as determined in the presence of the sub-MIC of cephapirin, pirlimycin or ceftiofur, respectively, relative to the biofilm production of the same isolate in absence of antibiotic. Statistical analysis: Mann–Whitney: NS, not statistically significant.

influence the outcome of treatment. For examples, cow parity and the position of the infected quarter (rear vs front) can affect cure rates [2]. Therefore, this study could not take in account all these factors but for each study group (i.e., each extended therapy taken individually), the study and comparison of both isolates from cured and persistent cases revealed some interesting bacterial factors and antibiotic effects that may influence the therapeutic outcome. The generic representation we made of the observed biological responses may however not be valid for a proportion of *S. aureus* isolates due to strain-to-strain variations. More work is needed to determine all host and bacterial factors, in addition to the pharmacological factors, involved in the success and failure of extended therapies for bovine *S. aureus* IMIs.

## Additional file

**Additional file 1. Examples of VNTR profiles for bacteriology-defined persistent cases from the cephapirin therapy study.** S1 represents the VNTR profile of the *S. aureus* isolate before treatment with cephapirin while S2 represents the VNTR profile of the *S. aureus* isolate recovered after treatment. The asterisk (*) shows identical VNTR profile, i.e., the VNTR-validated persistent cases that were investigated in this study. The arrows indicate some of the differences between two profiles, and as such, the isolate recovered after treatment was considered to be the result of a new infection; the case was considered neither cured or persistent and was therefore not evaluated in this work.

### Competing interests
The authors declare that they have no competing interests.

### Authors' contributions
VL and JL performed VNTR analysis and determined the biofilm production of the *S. aureus* isolates. AF and KV performed MICs determination and biofilm production in presence of antibiotics. JPR collected the isolates and the associated field study data and reviewed the manuscript. FM directed the project and reviewed the manuscript. CS supervised the experiments and wrote the manuscript. All authors read and approved the final manuscript.

### Acknowledgements
The authors thank Wyeth/Fort Dodge Animal Health and Zoetis for their financial support of initial field studies. We would like to recognize the contribution of the Canadian Bovine Mastitis and Milk Quality Research Network (CBMMQRN, St-Hyacinthe, QC, Canada) in the realization of this study. The CBMMQRN was supported by the Natural Sciences and Engineering Research Council (NSERC) of Canada, Alberta Milk, Dairy Farmers of New Brunswick, Nova Scotia, Ontario and Prince Edward Island, Novalait Inc., Dairy Farmers of Canada, Canadian Dairy Network, AAFC, PHAC, Technology PEI Inc., Université de Montréal, and University of Prince Edward Island. This work was also supported by Discovery Grant 89758-2010 from NSERC to FM. The authors want to thank all milk producers involved in the initial field studies, Drs. Jean-Yves Perreault and Line Simoneau for sharing bacterial strains and David Lalonde Séguin for his excellent technical and scientific advices on VNTR analyses. Additionally, we acknowledge the logistic support from Op + Lait, *le Regroupement de recherche pour un lait de qualité optimale* supported by the FRQNT, les *Fonds de Recherche du Québec, Nature et Technologies* (St-Hyacinthe, Québec, Canada).

## References

1. Reyher KK, Dufour S, Barkema HW, DesCôteaux L, Devries TJ, Dohoo IR, Keefe GP, Roy JP, Scholl DT (2011) The national cohort of dairy farms—a data collection platform for mastitis research in Canada. J Dairy Sci 94:1616–1626
2. Barkema HW, Schukken YH, Zadoks RN (2006) Invited review: the role of cow, pathogen, and treatment regimen in the therapeutic success of bovine *Staphylococcus aureus* mastitis. J Dairy Sci 89:1877–1895
3. Fox LK, Zadoks RN, Gaskins CT (2005) Biofilm production by *Staphylococcus aureus* associated with intramammary infection. Vet Microbiol 107:295–299
4. Hathroubi S, Mekni MA, Domenico P, Nguyen D, Jacques M (2017) Biofilms: microbial shelters against antibiotics. Microb Drug Resist 23:147–156
5. Melchior MB, Fink-Gremmels J, Gaastra W (2007) Extended antimicrobial susceptibility assay for *Staphylococcus aureus* isolates from bovine mastitis growing in biofilms. Vet Microbiol 125:141–149
6. Roy JP, Keefe G (2012) Systematic review: what is the best antibiotic treatment for *Staphylococcus aureus* intramammary infection of lactating cows in North America? Vet Clin N Am Food Anim Pract 28:39–50
7. Oliver SP, Gillespie BE, Headrick SJ, Moorehead H, Lunn P, Dowlen HH, Johnson DL, Lamar KC, Chester ST, Moseley WM (2004) Efficacy of extended ceftiofur intramammary therapy for treatment of subclinical mastitis in lactating dairy cows. J Dairy Sci 87:2393–2400
8. Thornsberry C, Marler JK, Watts JL, Yancey RJ Jr (1993) Activity of pirlimycin against pathogens from cows with mastitis and recommendations for disk diffusion tests. Antimicrob Agents Chemother 37:1122–1126
9. Roy JP, DesCôteaux L, DuTremblay D, Beaudry F, Elsener J (2009) Efficacy of a 5-day extended therapy program during lactation with cephapirin sodium in dairy cows chronically infected with *Staphylococcus aureus*. Can Vet J 50:1257–1262
10. Gillespie BE, Moorehead H, Lunn P, Dowlen HH, Johnson DL, Lamar KC, Lewis MJ, Ivey SJ, Hallberg JW, Chester ST, Oliver SP (2002) Efficacy of extended pirlimycin hydrochloride therapy for treatment of environmental *Streptococcus* spp. and *Staphylococcus aureus* intramammary infections in lactating dairy cows. Vet Ther 3:373–380
11. Truchetti G, Bouchard E, DesCôteaux L, Scholl D, Roy JP (2014) Efficacy of extended intramammary ceftiofur therapy against mild to moderate clinical mastitis in Holstein dairy cows: a randomized clinical trial. Can J Vet Res 78:31–37
12. Sabat A, Krzyszton-russjan J, Strzalka W, Filipek R, Kosowska K, Hryniewicz W, Travis J, Potempa J (2003) New method for typing *Staphylococcus aureus* strains: multiple-locus variable-number tandem repeat analysis of polymorphism and genetic relationships of clinical isolates. J Clin Microbiol 41:1801–1804
13. Veh KA, Klein RC, Ster C, Keefe G, Lacasse P, Scholl D, Roy JP, Haine D, Dufour S, Talbot BG, Ribon AO, Malouin F (2015) Genotypic and phenotypic characterization of *Staphylococcus aureus* causing persistent and nonpersistent subclinical bovine intramammary infections during lactation or the dry period. J Dairy Sci 98:155–168
14. CLSI (2011) Performance standards for antimicrobial susceptibility testing; twenty-first informational supplement. 31:M100-S21
15. Christensen GD, Simpson WA, Younger JJ, Baddour LM, Barrett FF, Melton DM, Beachey EH (1985) Adherence of coagulase-negative staphylococci to plastic tissue culture plates: a quantitative model for the adherence of staphylococci to medical devices. J Clin Microbiol 22:996–1006
16. Middleton JR, Luby CD (2008) *Escherichia coli* mastitis in cattle being treated for *Staphylococcus aureus* intramammary infection. Vet Rec 162:156–157
17. Luczak-Kadlubowska A, Sabat A, Tambic-Andrasevic A, Payerl-Pal M, Krzyszton-Russjan J, Hryniewicz W (2008) Usefulness of multiple-locus VNTR fingerprinting in detection of clonality of community- and hospital-acquired *Staphylococcus aureus* isolates. Antonie Van Leeuwenhoek 94:543–553
18. Malachowa N, Sabat A, Gniadkowski M, Krzyszton-Russjan J, Empel J, Miedzobrodzki J, Kosowska-Shick K, Appelbaum PC, Hryniewicz W (2005) Comparison of multiple-locus variable-number tandem-repeat analysis with pulsed-field gel electrophoresis, spa typing, and multilocus

sequence typing for clonal characterization of *Staphylococcus aureus* isolates. J Clin Microbiol 43:3095–3100

19. Apparao D, Oliveira L, Ruegg PL (2009) Relationship between results of in vitro susceptibility tests and outcomes following treatment with pirlimycin hydrochloride in cows with subclinical mastitis associated with gram-positive pathogens. J Am Vet Med Assoc 234:1437–1446

20. Melchior MB, Vaarkamp H, Fink-Gremmels J (2006) Biofilms: a role in recurrent mastitis infections? Vet J 171:398–407

21. Mitchell G, Brouillette E, Séguin DL, Asselin AE, Jacob CL, Malouin F (2010) A role for sigma factor B in the emergence of *Staphylococcus aureus* small-colony variants and elevated biofilm production resulting from an exposure to aminoglycosides. Microb Pathog 48:18–27

22. Roy JP, Du Tremblay D, DesCôteaux L, Messier S, Scholl D, Bouchard É (2007) Effect of precalving intramammary treatment with pirlimycin in nulliparous *Holstein heifers*. Can J Vet Res 71:283–291

23. Deluyker HA, Van Oye SN, Boucher JF (2005) Factors affecting cure and somatic cell count after pirlimycin treatment of subclinical mastitis in lactating cows. J Dairy Sci 88:604–614

24. Huang Q, Yu H-J, Liu G-D, Huang X-K, Zhang L-Y, Zhou Y-G, Chen J-Y, Lin F, Wang Y, Fei J (2012) Comparison of the effects of human β-defensin 3, vancomycin, and clindamycin on *Staphylococcus aureus* biofilm formation. Orthopedics 35:e53–60

25. Rachid S, Ohlsen K, Witte W, Hacker J, Ziebuhr W (2000) Effect of subinhibitory antibiotic concentrations on polysaccharide intercellular adhesin expression in biofilm-forming *Staphylococcus epidermidis*. Antimicrob Agents Chemother 44:3357–3363

26. Gomes F, Teixeira P, Cerca N, Ceri H, Oliveira R (2011) Virulence gene expression by *Staphylococcus epidermidis* biofilm cells exposed to antibiotics. Microb Drug Resist 17:191–196

27. Melchior MB, van Osch MH, Lam TJ, Vernooij JC, Gaastra W, Fink-Gremmels J (2011) Extended biofilm susceptibility assay for *Staphylococcus aureus* bovine mastitis isolates: evidence for association between genetic makeup and biofilm susceptibility. J Dairy Sci 94:5926–5937

# 13

# Identification of two mutation sites in spike and envelope proteins mediating optimal cellular infection of porcine epidemic diarrhea virus from different pathways

Min Sun, Jiale Ma, Zeyanqiu Yu, Zihao Pan, Chengping Lu and Huochun Yao[*] ⓘ

## Abstract

Entry of the α-coronavirus porcine epidemic diarrhea virus (PEDV) requires specific proteases to activate spike (S) protein for the membrane fusion of the virion to the host cell following receptor binding. Herein, PEDV isolate 85-7 could proliferate and induce cell–cell fusion in a trypsin independent manner on Vero cells, and eight homologous mutation strains were screened by continuous proliferation in the absence of trypsin on Vero cells. According to the whole genome sequence comparative analysis, we identified four major variations located in nonstructural protein 2, S, open reading frame 3, and envelope (E) genes, respectively. Comparative analyses of their genomic variations and proliferation characteristics identified a single mutation within the S2′ cleavage site between C30 and C40 mutants: the substitution of conserved arginine (R) by a glycine (G) (R895G). This change resulted in weaker cell–cell fusion, smaller plaque morphology, higher virus titer and serious microfilament condensation. Further analysis confirmed that this mutation was responsible for optimal cell-adaptation, but not the determinant for trypsin-dependent entry of PEDV. Otherwise, a novel variation (16–20 aa deletion and an L25P mutation) in the transmembrane domain of the E protein affected multiple infection processes, including up-regulation of the production of the ER stress indicator GRP78, improving the expression of pro-inflammatory cytokines IL-6 and IL-8, and promoting apoptosis. The results of this study provide a better understanding of the potential mechanisms of viral functional proteins in PEDV replication, infection, and fitness.

## Introduction

Porcine epidemic diarrhea (PED), characterized by watery diarrhea and dehydration, results in significant economic losses in the swine industry worldwide [1–3]. The causative agent, porcine epidemic diarrhea virus (PEDV), was identified as a member of the alphacoronavirus from the family *Coronaviridae* [1]. The PEDV genome is approximately 28 kb in length, comprising 7 open reading frames (ORF): ORF 1a/1b, spike (S), ORF3, envelope (E), membrane (M) and nucleocapsid (N), in that order [4]. In the process of cell culture and clinical spread of PEDV, several genomic sites show variation and

recombination, which are closely related with PEDV cell adaptation, pathogenicity, and evolution [5, 6].

The PEDV spike (S) glycoprotein was recognized as a class I fusion protein, and could be divided structurally into the S1 and S2 regions, mediating the receptor binding and membrane fusion, respectively [7]. Therein S2 contains the S2′ cleavage site, fusion peptide (FP), heptad repeat region 1 (HR1), HR2, and transmembrane domain (TM), in that order [8]. The propagation of PEDV isolates requires supplementation with trypsin in the cell culture supernatant in vitro [1]. Trypsin cleaves the S protein, allowing a conformational change and then mediating fusion activity [8, 9]. The S1/S2 junction and S2′ location have been identified as the important protease cleavage sites [10]. The S2′ cleavage site, FP position, and HR1 domain have been predicted as the determinants for

*Correspondence: yaohch@njau.edu.cn
College of Veterinary Medicine, Nanjing Agricultural University, Nanjing, Jiangsu, China

trypsin-dependent entry, and the trypsin-induced cell–cell fusion is weakened by mutation of the S2′ site [8].

The membrane vesicles for coronavirus' transcription, replication, and generation of new virus particles could be derived from the endoplasmic reticulum (ER) of infected cells [11]. The ER is likely to be overloaded by the extensive use of intracellular membranes, which would cause ER stress responses [11]. Subsequently, the unfolded protein response (UPR) would be triggered to restore the ER homeostasis via three ER-resident transmembrane proteins, otherwise cell apoptosis might be induced [12]. In fact, PEDV has been reported to induce ER stress, UPR, and caspase-independent apoptosis [12, 13].

The envelope (E) protein is a small membrane protein that shares low sequence homology among the coronavirus groups [14]. The E protein, especially the transmembrane domain, is involved in ion-conduction properties, and is highly associated with virus maturation, production, efficient release, and virus-host interactions, which are reflected in the cellular stress, UPR, apoptosis, inflammatory response and pathogenicity [11, 15–17]. Different coronaviruses have varied requirements for the E protein in morphogenesis and virus release. The E protein is absolutely essential for transmissible gastroenteritis virus (TGEV) and middle east respiratory syndrome (MERS-CoV), but not for the mouse hepatitis virus (MHV) and severe acute respiratory syndrome virus (SARS-CoV) [14, 18, 19]. In PEDV, the E protein is located in the ER or nucleus, and has been reported to induce ER stress alone in intestinal epithelial cells (IEC) expressing the PEDV E protein [20]. It remains poorly understood whether or how the E protein participates in PEDV production and infection, and what the critical region is.

In this study, PEDV strain 85-7, which could be cultured on Vero cells in a trypsin independent manner, was isolated successfully. We performed mutation screening by continuous proliferation on Vero cells, and used these strains to evaluate PEDV's genetic stability. We also identified the major variation regions that were active during cell culture, based on whole genome comparison. Furthermore, we compared the proliferation of these virus characteristics, and identified the functional sites involved in PEDV replication, infection, and fitness. The results were helpful in revealing the PEDV infection mechanism, and demonstrate how PEDV employs specific evolutionary strategies to adapt to the host microenvironment for better survival.

## Materials and methods
### Cell cultures and experimental reagents
Vero cells were cultured in Dulbecco modified Eagle medium (DMEM; Hyclone, USA) with 10% fetal bovine serum (FBS; TCB, USA) and maintained at 37 °C with 5% $CO_2$. Cyclosporin A (CsA), Z-VAD-FMK (caspase inhibitor), Dimethyl sulfoxide (DMSO), and Cy3-labeled Goat Anti-Mouse IgG (H+L) were purchased from Beyotime (Shanghai, China). The PEDV specific monoclonal antibody 5E2-C4 was made in our laboratory.

### RNA extraction, reverse transcription (RT)-PCR and quantitative real-time PCR (qPCR)
Viral RNA was extracted from homogenized samples or supernatants of PEDV-infected Vero cells using a Viral RNA Mini kit (Geneaid Biotech), according to the manufacturer's instructions. PEDV positivity was identified by RT-PCR using specific primers (Additional file 1) and determining its sequence (GENEWIZ, China). The virus cDNA synthesis and PCR amplification were performed according to previously published methods [21].

Total RNA of the PEDV-infected cells, or recombinant plasmid transfected-cells was extracted using the RNAiso Plus reagent (Takara, Japan), according to the manufacturer's protocols. The concentrations of the extracted RNA were measured using a Thermo Scientific NanoDrop 2000c (Thermo Scientific, USA). The gene-specific primers for qPCR are listed in Additional file 1 [20, 22, 23]. The qPCR was performed with SYBR® Premix Ex Taq™ II (Takara, Japan) and was conducted on an ABI 7300 Real-Time PCR System. The β-Actin gene served as the endogenous control [23]. The relative quantities of mRNA accumulation were evaluated based on the $2^{-\Delta\Delta Ct}$ method compared with mock-treated results [22]. Each sample was run in triplicate.

### Virus isolation and propagation
PEDV isolation from Vero cells was performed as previously described, with some modifications [1]. Intestinal homogenates or fecal samples were prepared as 30% (wt/vol) suspensions, vortexed, and centrifuged at 3000 × g for 10 min. The supernatant was then filtered through a 0.22-μm-pore-size syringe filter (Millipore, USA). Confluent Vero cells were then washed three times with DMEM, and inoculated with 1 mL of the above supernatant and 4 mL of post-inoculation medium [1] by adding trypsin (Gibco, USA) to a final concentration of 2.5, 10, 20, 30 ng/μL, respectively. The cells were incubated at 37 °C with 5% $CO_2$ for 3 days. Viral propagation was confirmed by daily observation of the cytopathic effects (CPE), and using RT-PCR, indirect immunofluorescence assay (IFA), and transmission electron microscopy (TEM). If no positive CPE, RT-PCR or IFA staining results was observed within continuously six blind passages, the result was then considered negative.

### Virus titration and growth characteristics
Confluent Vero cells were washed with DMEM three times, and then infected with the parent 85-7 strain

(Passage 5, P5) or the isolated mutants at a multiplicity of infection (MOI) of 0.1 in the presence (10 ng/μL) or absence of trypsin at 37 °C for 1 h, after which the incubation virus was discarded. The infected cells were washed three times with DMEM, cultured at 37 °C by adding the maintenance medium (DMEM supplied with 2% FBS), and the culture supernatants were collected at different time points [12, 24, 36, 48, and 60 h post infection (hpi)]. As to the trypsin-dependency assay, Vero cells were infected with parent 85-7 strain at an MOI of 0.1 within different concentrations trypsin or absence of trypsin, and the culture supernatants were collected at 48 hpi. Finally, titers of the culture supernatants at the indicated times were determined by plaque assay on Vero cells, and quantified as plaque-forming units (pfu) per milliliter (mL).

The viral binding or entry assays were performed as previously described [24], with some modifications. For the viral binding assay, cells were incubated with the same amount of parent 85-7 (P5), C30 or C40 viruses at 4 °C for 1 h in the presence (10 ng/μL) or absence of trypsin. After that the samples were washed three times with DMEM, then the binding efficiency was determined by plaque assay. The entry assay was performed following the viral attachment step. The samples were maintained in DMEM at 37 °C for 1 h in the presence (10 ng/μL) or absence of trypsin, and the cells were washed with cold acidic PBS (pH 3.0) to remove the virus binding to the cell membrane, then the entry efficiency was determined by plaque assay.

### Genome sequencing and genetic stability analysis
The culture supernatants of parent strain 85-7 (P5) and the corresponding variant strains were collected and then viral genomes were extracted. The whole genomes excluding the poly(A) tail, were amplified, sequenced, assembled, and analyzed as previously described [21]. The complete genome sequences of these strains were submitted to the GenBank database, with the accession numbers of KX839246 (parent strain 85-7), KY486713 (strain A40), KX839248 (strain B40), KX839249 (strain C30), KY486714 (strain C40), KX839250 (strain D40), and KX839251 (strain E40).

### Computational analysis and multiple sequence alignments
The transmembrane domain of the PEDV E protein was predicted by TMHMM 2.0 [25]. The schematic overview of the PEDV S2 domain was referred to as the SARS-CoV and then drawn to scale [26]. The nucleotides (S gene or the whole genome of PEDV) or amino acid sequence alignments (S or E protein) were performed using ClustalW with default parameters, using reference sequences of strain DR13 (PEDV, JQ023161.1),

cell-adapted DR13 (ca-DR13, JQ023162), strain CV777 (PEDV, AF353511), and strain Tor2 (SARS-CoV, NP828851.1).

### Annexin V and propidium iodide (PI) staining assay
Vero cells were mock- or PEDV-infected at an MOI of 0.1 in the absence of trypsin, and then collected at 36 hpi with 0.25% trypsin. The Annexin V and PI staining assays were measured using an Alexa Fluor 488 Annexin V/ Dead Cell Apoptosis kit (Vazyme, China), according to the manufacturer's protocols. A fluorescence-activated cell sorter (FACS) Accuri C6 flow cytometer (BD Accuri) detected the fluorescent signals of Annexin V and PI using channels FL-1 and FL-2 respectively, and the data was then analyzed by CFlow plus software (BD Accuri).

### Immunofluorescence assay (IFA) staining
IFA staining was performed as follows: first, the mock or PEDV-infected Vero cells were fixed with 4% methanal at 37 °C for 10 min, and then permeabilized with 0.1% Triton X-100 at 37 °C for 5 min. Second, the cells were blocked with 1% bovine serum albumin (BSA) at 37 °C for 1 h, and then stained with mouse anti-PEDV monoclonal antibody 5E2-C4 in 1% BSA (1:200, overnight, 4 °C). Third, the cells were incubated with the Cy3-labeled Goat Anti-Mouse IgG (H+L) (1:500, 37 °C, 1 h, in dark) and then stained with DAPI (37 °C, 10 min, in dark). Finally, the stained-cells were examined by fluorescence microscopy (Zeiss, Germany). All the above mentioned solutions were prepared in PBS, and the cells were washed with PBS containing 0.5% Tween-20 for five times between each step. Furthermore, the Vero cells infected with 85-7 parent, C30, or C40 mutant strains were stained with phalloidin to examine the effects on cytoskeletal organization, as described previously [27].

### Transmission electron microscopy
The mock or PEDV-infected Vero cells were collected gently with a rubber policeman, washed twice with cold PBS (with centrifugation at 2500 × g for 5 min between washing), and then fixed in 2.5% glutaraldehyde overnight at 4 °C. The cell pellet was used to prepare thin sections for observation under TEM, as described previously [28]. The final samples were visualized using a Hitachi-7650 transmission electron microscope (Hitachi Ltd., Japan).

### Virus competition assays
Vero cells were co-infected with PEDV 85-7 C30 and C40 mutant strains at an MOI of 0.1. The initial proportion of C30 and C40 was 1:1 or 4:1, respectively [17]. The co-infected supernatants were then collected at 36 hpi, and serially passaged three times. The relative abundance of

the C30 and C40 viruses at passage 3 was determined by comparing the plaque size and sequencing the genetic marker of the S2′ cleavage site. The isolation of viral genomes, gene sequencing, and virus titer determination were performed as described above.

## Western blotting assay

Vero cells were infected with PEDV 85-7 parent, C30, or C40 strains at an MOI of 0.1 for 24 h. The mock Vero cells served as the control. Total proteins were harvested with the RIPA Lysis and Extraction Buffer (ThermoFisher) with protease inhibitor (PMSF, 10%), and prepared for western blot as described previously [24]. The anti-GRP78 antibody (Beyotime, China) was used as the primary antibody, and β-Actin served as the loading control.

## Overexpression of PEDV parent and mutant E proteins

The parent or mutant E genes were amplified from the 85-7 parent or C40 strains by RT-PCR, then cloned into the pIRES2-EGFP expression vector to generate PI-E and PI-mE plasmids, respectively. The PCR primers are listed in Additional file 1, and both the parent and mutant E proteins were C-terminally labeled with HA-tag. The recombinant plasmids were transfected into Vero cells using Lipofectamine 3000 (Invitrogen, USA) according to the manufacturer's instructions. The overexpression of proteins was examined by dual-staining IFA with anti-HA-tag antibody.

## Statistical analysis

All data were analyzed with the GraphPad Prism 5 software. A $P$-value $< 0.05$ was considered as significant, and labeled with an asterisk in the figures (*).

# Results

## Virus isolation and characterization

Fourteen individual PEDV-positive samples were collected and prepared for virus isolation in Vero cells, however, only PEDV strain 85-7 was isolated successfully from the intestinal homogenate. Compared with the negative-control, the Vero cells infected by strain 85-7 (P5) showed a distinct CPE, characterized by cell fusion, and eventually flaking off the culture flask surface (Figure 1A). The CPE was observed at 12 hpi, and became remarkable by 48 hpi (Figure 1A). Each virus passage was assessed using PEDV M gene-based RT-PCR (Additional file 1), and confirmed by gene sequencing (data not shown). Virus propagation was further demonstrated by an IFA assay. The red-stained PEDV were distributed widely in the cytoplasm rather than in the nucleus (Figure 1B). As shown in Figure 1C, numerous virus particles were visible in the infected cells under TEM, which adhered to the cytoplasm membrane and replicated in cytoplasm at 24 hpi.

## Trypsin is not essential for the infection of PEDV strain 85-7 in Vero cells

To further study the proliferation characteristics of strain 85-7, Vero cells were infected with strain 85-7 at an MOI of 0.1 in the presence of trypsin (10 ng/μL). The results show that strain 85-7 proliferated effectively, and reached the peak viral titer (about $10^{5.5}$ pfu/mL) at 48 hpi (Figure 2A). The essential first step of virus infection is binding to the host cell receptor, and for PEDV, this is related closely to the release of the fusion peptide of the spike protein into target cellular membranes [7]. A large number of host proteases have been identified to activate the CoV-spike protein proteolytically, including the cell surface transmembrane type II serine protease 2 (TMPRSS2), furin, and trypsin [10, 29]. Supplementation with trypsin could assist the virion entry effectively and enhanced their release [8]. By contrast, some PEDV mutants infected Vero cells using a trypsin-independent process [8]. Therefore, the trypsin-dependency of strain 85-7 was further tested, indeed, the virus could infect Vero cells with or without the trypsin in the entry stage (Figure 2B). It should be noted that our results showed a gradual attenuation in the infection of strain 85-7 with increasing trypsin concentration (Figure 2B), as the highest virus titer was reached about $10^6$ pfu/mL in the absence of trypsin at 48 hpi (Figure 2B). These observations indicated that the release of infectious PEDV particles was more efficient without the assistance of trypsin activity, suggesting that strain 85-7 might employ a specific protease cleavage mechanism of the S protein for its infection process.

## Identification of PEDV variants with different infection characteristics by serial passaging in Vero cells

Previous reports showed that the PEDV genome might display frequent variation in the process of clinical evolution and cell culture, and some of the variant sites are closely related to PEDV pathogenicity and cell adaptation [5, 21], which provides useful clues to explore the molecular functions of viral proteins, and further clarify PEDV's infection mechanism. Herein, five repeats of strain 85-7 (purified from different virus plaques from the same generation and genetic background) were propagated serially for over 40 passages successfully in Vero cells. For subsequent research, the corresponding strains were designated as A40, B40, C40, D40, and E40 (Figure 3A). Growth kinetic analysis was performed on Vero cells at an MOI of 0.1 under the trypsin-free conditions. Strains A40, B40, and D40 showed a similar growth pattern to the parent virus, while C40 and E40 strains yielded significantly higher titers than other strains during the whole infection process (Figure 3B). The C40 and E40 strains induced CPE morphology of cell pycnosis and

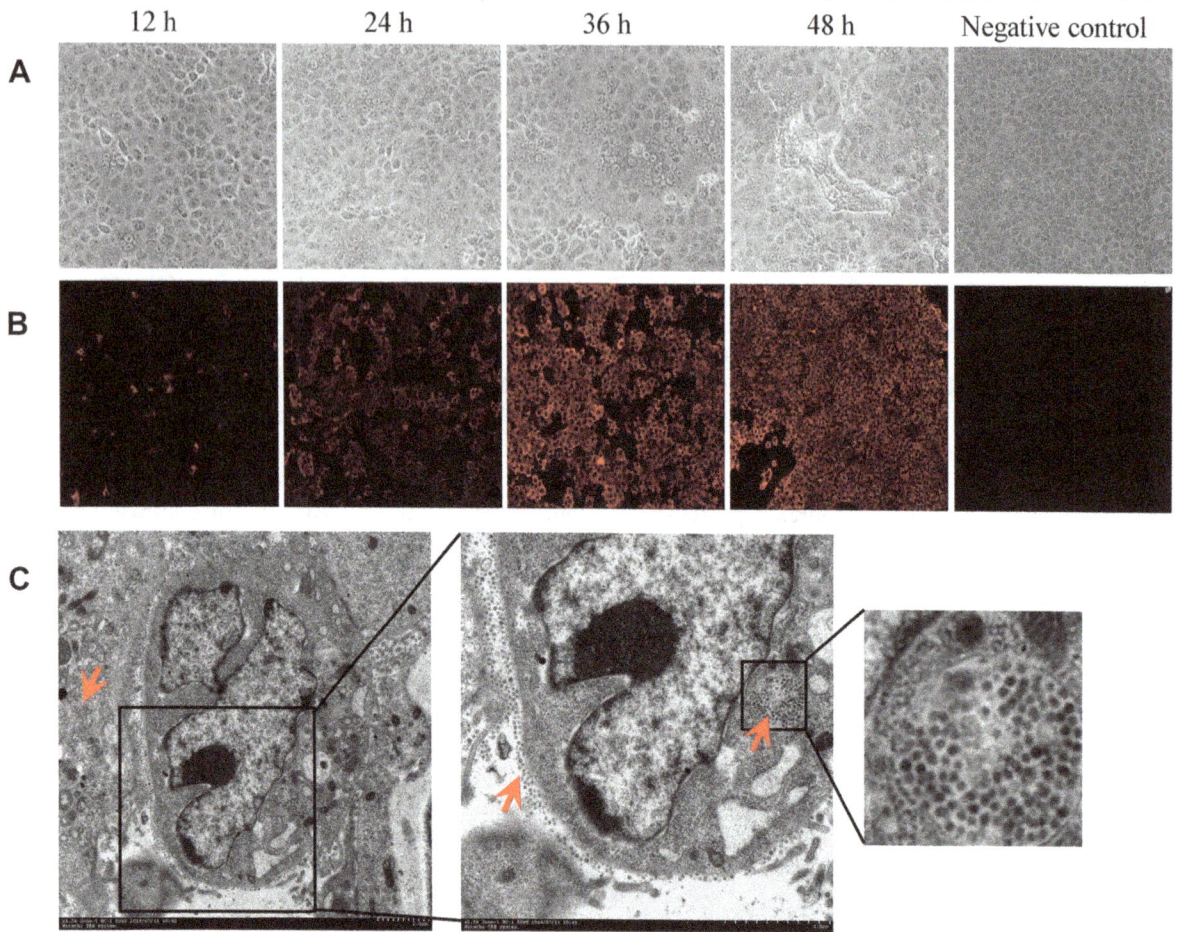

**Figure 1  Infection characteristics of the isolated PEDV strain 85-7. (A)** A distinct CPE (P5) was observed and photographed at 12, 24, 36, 48 hpi (magnification of 100×). **(B)** For IFA assay of P5, cells were fixed and incubated with PEDV-specific monoclonal antibody 5E2-C4, followed by Cy3-labeled Goat Anti-Mouse IgG (H+L) (secondary antibody), and then examined by fluorescence microscopy (magnification of 100×). **(C)** A thin section of infected cells (P5) at 24 hpi showing accumulation of virus particles in the cytoplasm membrane and cytoplasm (magnification 1200× and 2500×, Dai = 200 nm. Some virus particles are indicated by red arrows. An enlarged image of part of the cytoplasm is shown.

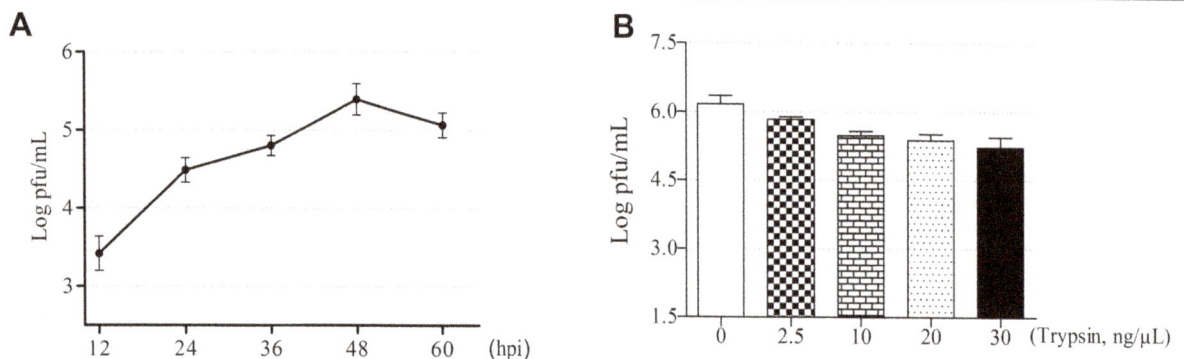

**Figure 2  PEDV strain 85-7 (P5) proliferated on Vero cells in a trypsin independent manner. (A)** Virus proliferation curve in the presence of 10 ng/μL trypsin at an MOI of 0.1. Plaque titrations from the indicated time points were carried out. Error bars indicate the standard deviation of the mean of three independent experiments. **(B)** The strain 85-7 could proliferate on Vero cells trypsin-independently. Vero cells were infected at an MOI of 0.1 in the indicated trypsin concentrations (0, 2.5, 10, 20, 30 ng/μL) and the viral titers at 48 hpi were measured and compared.

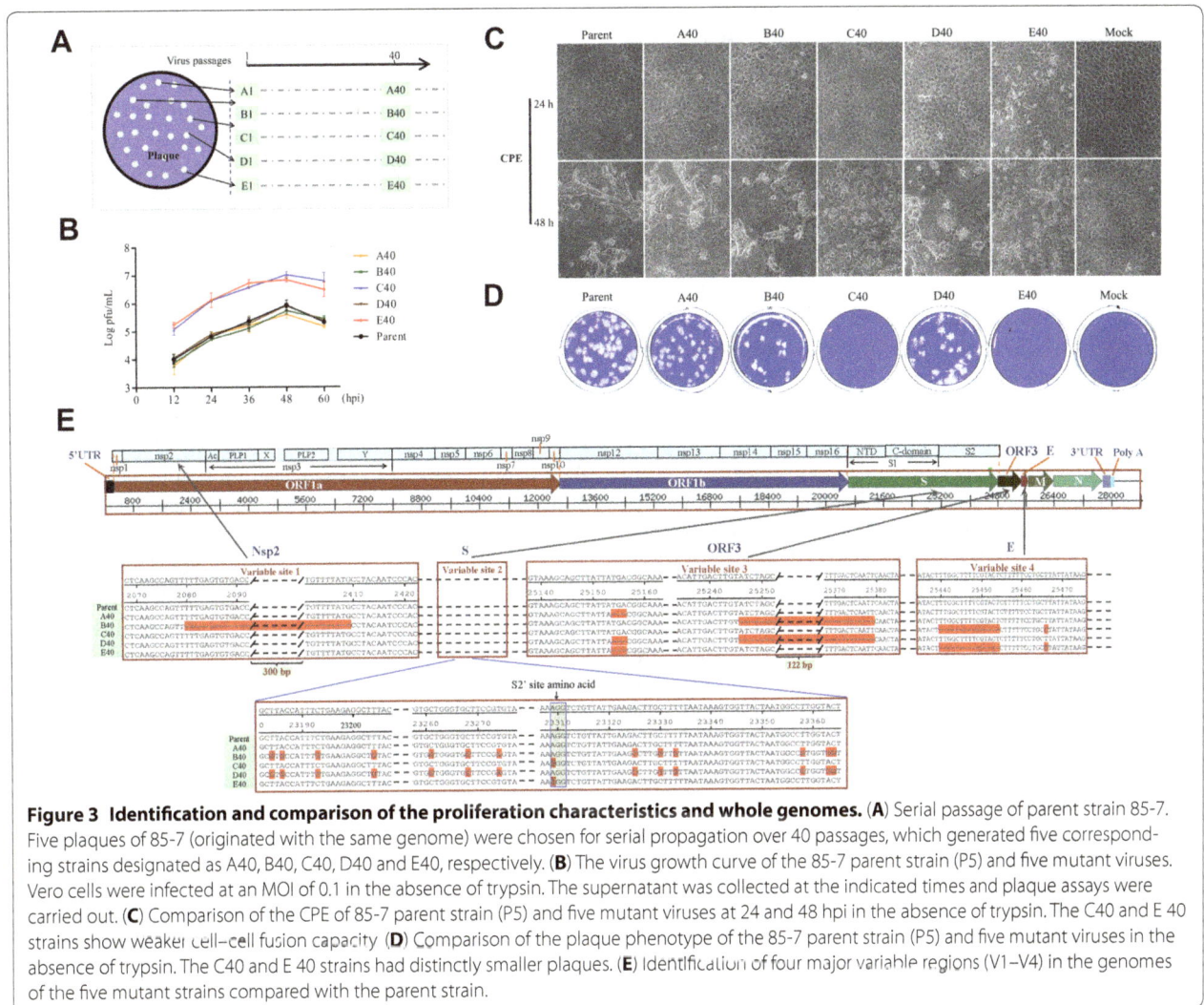

**Figure 3  Identification and comparison of the proliferation characteristics and whole genomes. (A)** Serial passage of parent strain 85-7. Five plaques of 85-7 (originated with the same genome) were chosen for serial propagation over 40 passages, which generated five corresponding strains designated as A40, B40, C40, D40 and E40, respectively. **(B)** The virus growth curve of the 85-7 parent strain (P5) and five mutant viruses. Vero cells were infected at an MOI of 0.1 in the absence of trypsin. The supernatant was collected at the indicated times and plaque assays were carried out. **(C)** Comparison of the CPE of 85-7 parent strain (P5) and five mutant viruses at 24 and 48 hpi in the absence of trypsin. The C40 and E 40 strains show weaker cell–cell fusion capacity **(D)** Comparison of the plaque phenotype of the 85-7 parent strain (P5) and five mutant viruses in the absence of trypsin. The C40 and E 40 strains had distinctly smaller plaques. **(E)** Identification of four major variable regions (V1–V4) in the genomes of the five mutant strains compared with the parent strain.

non-syncytium formation, which was completely different to that of the other strains (Figure 3C), being consistent with the above observations. Furthermore, the C40 and E40 viruses yielded smaller plaques, even at 5 days post-infection (Figure 3D). All of these observations suggest that C40 and E40 strains might contain some important mutations that contributed to the difference of infection characteristics.

## Mapping the potential genetic determinants for infection characteristics

To evaluate the PEDV genetic stability and explore the potential mechanism that caused the dissimilar infection characteristics in C40 and E40 strains, the whole genomes of the five variant strains and the parent 85-7 were sequenced. The whole genome of the parent 85-7 strain (P5), similar to the published PEDV genomes, was about 27 988 nucleotides (nt) excluding the poly(A) tail,

and had a PEDV characteristic gene order of 5′ untranslated region (UTR)-ORF1a/1b-S-ORF3-E-M–N-3′ UTR (Figure 3E).

Comparing the whole genome sequences of the 85-7 parent strain with the five variant strains (A40 to E40), we found that a total of 91 nucleotide sites were changed, leading to 84 amino acid (aa) variations (summarized in Additional files 2 and 3). The analysis of the variable regions of the five mutant strains show that the nucleotide sequences of the non-structural protein Nsp8, Nsp9, and Nsp15 were not subject to any variations during the Vero cell adaptation process of PEDV strain 85-7. Overall, we identified four major variable regions (V1–V4) that contained the most mutation sites (Figure 3E). V1 was located in Nsp2 and comprised a 330 nt deletion (at position 2080–2409) in the C-terminal coding region that led to 110 aa deletion. V2 was located in the S gene and comprised numerous point mutations that were dispersed in the S1 and S2 domains, but with no insertions or deletions. Compared with the parental S gene, there were 7 nt and 27 nt variation points in S1 and S2 regions that induced 6 and 24 aa mutations among the five stable passage strains, respectively. V3 was located in the ORF3 gene with a 3 nt (at position 25 148–25 150) and a 134 nt (at position 25 240–25 373) deletion, causing a 1 aa deletion and the early-termination of encoding mRNA, respectively. V4 was located in the E gene and comprised a 15 nt deletion (at position 25 432–25 446) and 1 nt mutation (T25460C), which caused a 5 aa deletion (16–20 aa) and 1 aa (L25P) mutation in the E protein, respectively (Additional files 2 and 3). The mutation regions of PEDV strain 85-7 varied with unfixed patterns: only two mutation sites were shared among the five variant strains, namely T24530C and G24572C in the S2 region.

To search for potential sites that contributed to the different infection characteristics, we focused on the identification of specific mutations in the C40 and E40 genomes. The shortened ORF3 with a deletion of 3 nt in A40, D40, and E40 strains; the early-terminated ORF3 with a 134 nt deletion in B40 and D40 strains; and the shortened Nsp2 with a deletion of 330 nt in B40 strains, were judged not to be involved in the infection characteristics of PEDV strain 85-7 (Figures 3, 5I and J). Given that the S protein plays a key role in the coronavirus infection process [26], we identified important sites in the S protein of the five variant strains. The fusion peptide (FP) residues located immediately on the C-terminus of the S2′ cleavage site are very highly conserved across all CoV [30]; however, strains B40 and D40 showed the mutations from 898IEDLLF903 to 898IEALVV903 in the FP domain (Additional file 4), which had no significant difference in infection characteristics between them and the parent strain (Figures 3, 5I and J). The only mutational position shared by strains C40 and E40 strains in S protein was the substitution of conserved arginine (R) by a glycine (G) in the S2′ cleavage site (R895G) (Figures 3E and 4B; Additional files 2 and 3). Notably, this site has been reported to be associated with trypsin-induced cell–cell fusion in the PEDV infection process [8], and also serves as the location of the putative cleavage site within the S2 subunit of SARS-CoV and infectious bronchitis virus (IBV) S protein [10, 31]. In addition, the C40 and E40 strains also shared a novel variation region in the E gene, namely V4 region with a 15 nt deletion and a 1 nt mutation (Figure 3E; Additional file 2).

### The R895G mutation of the S2′ site is crucial for virus replication and infection

To identify the decisive sites that mediated the change in infection characteristics of the C40 and E40 strains, we compared the infection characteristics of the precursor strains of C40 strain, namely the 10th (C10), 20th (C20), and 30th (C30) generation strains, with the parent strain. As shown in Figure 4A, the CPE and plaque morphologies of the C10, C20, and C30 strains were the same as the parent strain. Using the close strains C30 and C40 for comparative genomic analysis to avoid the occurrence of chaotic mutations, we managed to identify the sites involved in the above phenotypes. Over the whole genome of the C30 and C40 strains, there was just one mutation (R895G) located in the S2′ site (Figure 4B; Additional files 2 and 3).

In fact, a specific region (named as Part A), including putative S2′ cleavage site, fusion peptide and HR1 domain, has been confirmed as the determinant for PEDV trypsin-dependent entry [8]. The single mutation R895G in putative S2′ cleavage site was speculated to play a key role for this phenotype [8], addressing the difference of biological activities between C30 and C40 strains would define the real function of this novel site. Thus we managed to compare their virus titers on the entry step in the presence or absence of trypsin. The results show that the R895G mutation had no effect on viral binding and entry efficiency (Figures 4C and D), and the presence of trypsin could significantly reduce the infectivity of both C30 and C40 strains in the entry stage (Figures 4C and D), indicating that the S2′ site was not the determinant for trypsin-dependent entry.

We next asked why the R895G mutation caused the more significant cell pycnosis and non-syncytium formation in CPE morphology. To do so we tested the cell microfilament rearrangement after virus infection. As shown in Figure 4E, the control cells were filled with extending microfilaments that formed a complex network, while the parent- and C30-infected cells showed diffuse microfilaments in cytoplasm after 24 hpi, which disappeared significantly at 48 hpi. However, the microfilaments of the C40-infected cells were condensed throughout the cytoplasm and formed bright foci at 48 hpi, indicating that R895G mutation was involved in the microfilaments remodeling of PEDV infected cells.

As to the S2′ site mutant strains C40 and E40 showed higher virus titers than parent and other mutant strains, then we asked whether the S2′ site was involved in PEDV replication. Indeed, the growth curve of C30 was also consistent with the parent stain, and the virus titers were significantly lower than those of the C40 and E40 strains (Figure 4F). Although C40 showed higher virus production and dissimilar infection characteristics in cell culture, it remains unknown whether these differences could improve viral fitness. Thus, we performed a competition assay between the C30 and C40 strains at ratios of 1:1 or 4:1. Through serial subculture three times, the abundance of the C30 strain decreased significantly and was

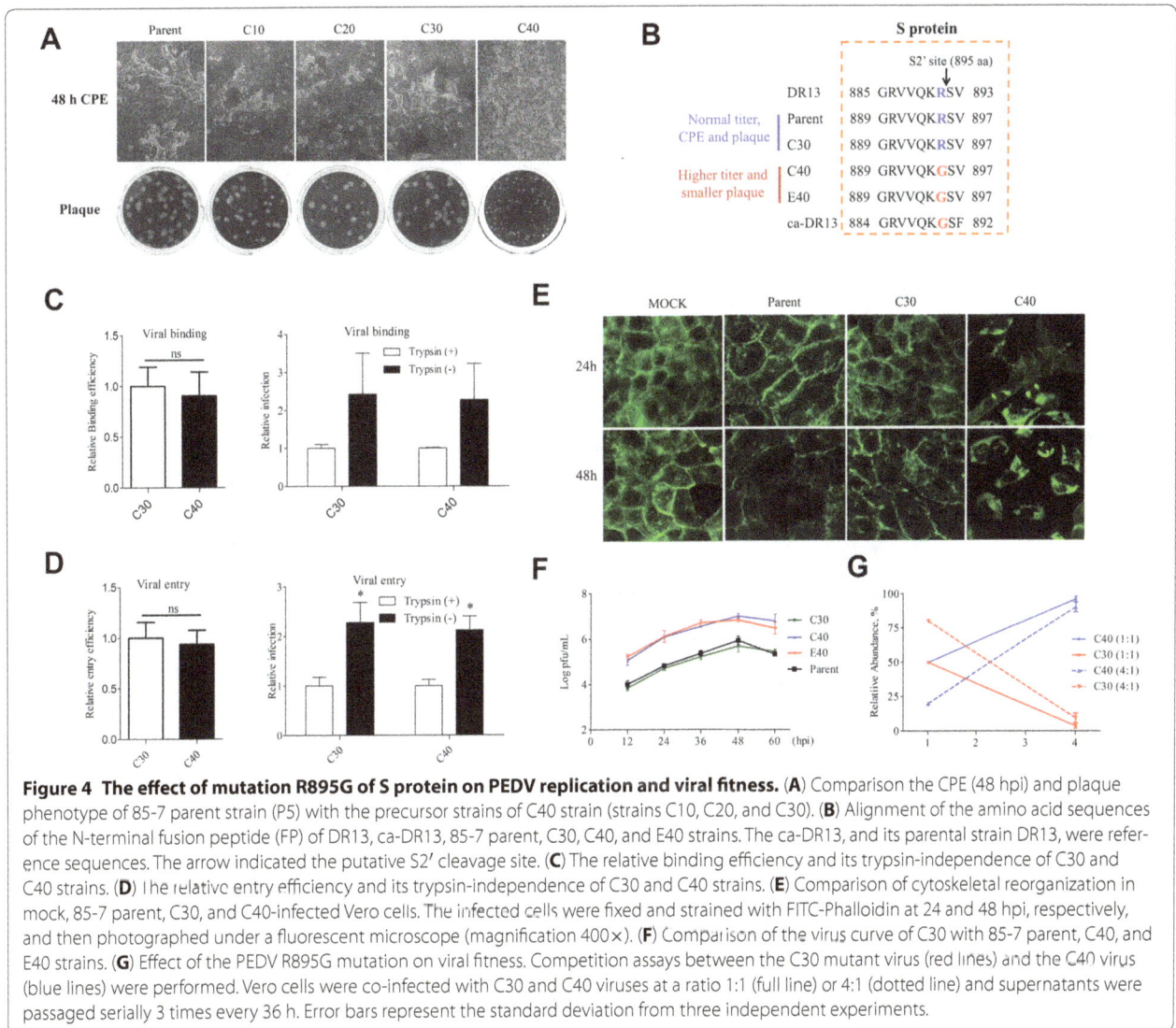

**Figure 4  The effect of mutation R895G of S protein on PEDV replication and viral fitness.** (**A**) Comparison the CPE (48 hpi) and plaque phenotype of 85-7 parent strain (P5) with the precursor strains of C40 strain (strains C10, C20, and C30). (**B**) Alignment of the amino acid sequences of the N-terminal fusion peptide (FP) of DR13, ca-DR13, 85-7 parent, C30, C40, and E40 strains. The ca-DR13, and its parental strain DR13, were reference sequences. The arrow indicated the putative S2′ cleavage site. (**C**) The relative binding efficiency and its trypsin-independence of C30 and C40 strains. (**D**) The relative entry efficiency and its trypsin-independence of C30 and C40 strains. (**E**) Comparison of cytoskeletal reorganization in mock, 85-7 parent, C30, and C40-infected Vero cells. The infected cells were fixed and strained with FITC-Phalloidin at 24 and 48 hpi, respectively, and then photographed under a fluorescent microscope (magnification 400×). (**F**) Comparison of the virus curve of C30 with 85-7 parent, C40, and E40 strains. (**G**) Effect of the PEDV R895G mutation on viral fitness. Competition assays between the C30 mutant virus (red lines) and the C40 virus (blue lines) were performed. Vero cells were co-infected with C30 and C40 viruses at a ratio 1:1 (full line) or 4:1 (dotted line) and supernatants were passaged serially 3 times every 36 h. Error bars represent the standard deviation from three independent experiments.

always outcompeted by the C40 strain (Figure 4G), which showed a distinct growth advantage, indicating that strain C40 had evolved for better adaptation to cell culture. All the above results suggest that the R895G mutation of the S2′ cleavage site was the genetic determinant mediating the difference of CPE characteristics, plaque size, growth capability, and cell adaptation between the C30 and C40 strains.

### The novel variation in transmembrane domain of E protein is responsible for stronger ER stress response, inflammatory effect, and higher apoptosis level

It should be noted that the strains C30, C40, and E40 also shared the same variation in E protein with a 5 aa deletion and a 1 aa mutation (Figures 3E and 5A). The PEDV parent E protein contains 76 aa and is predicted to be a

transmembrane protein. However, the variant E protein (C30, C40, and E40) was just 71 aa, and its predicted TM domain position was changed to $L_{10}$ to $L_{32}$ (23 aa) (Figure 5B). In fact, the TM domain structure was predicted to be more integral in the variant E protein, while its N-terminal domain was 5 aa shorter compared with the parent E protein (Figure 5B). The coronavirus E protein, especially the TM domain, is involved in many biological processes, including ion channel activity, stress response, and apoptosis [11, 17, 32, 33], thus its potential role in the cell-adaptation process of PEDV could not be overlooked.

A broad range of stresses, including virus infection, can perturb ER function seriously [12]. The intracellular stress response UPR was triggered to recover ER homeostasis and initiate inflammation through the release of

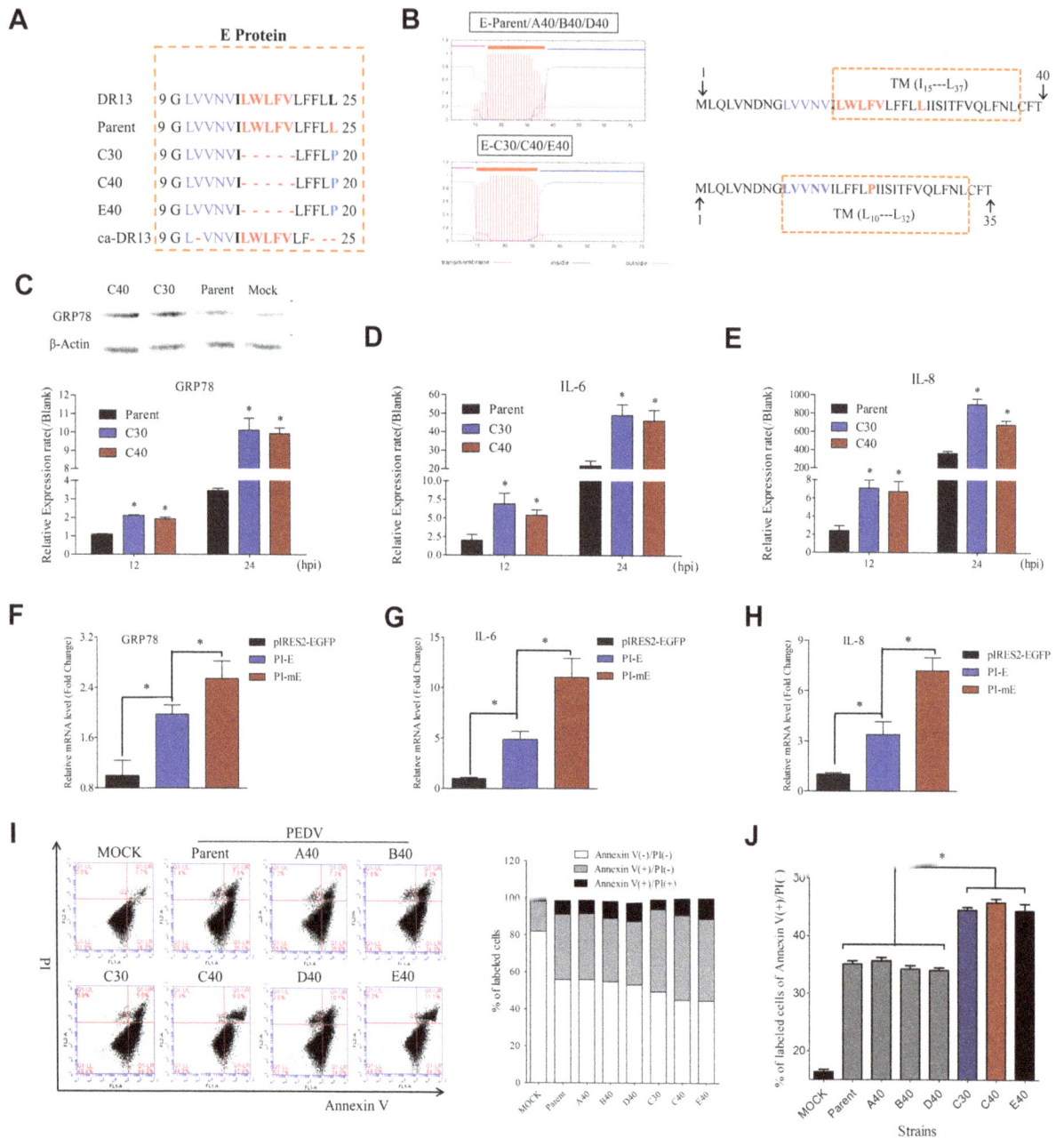

**Figure 5  The variation in the TM domain of E protein played a potential role in PEDV-host interaction.** (**A**) Alignment of the amino acid sequences of the V4 region in E protein from DR13, ca-DR13, 85-7 parent, C30, C40, and E40 strains. C30, C40, and E40 shared the same variation, with a deletion of [16]LWLFV[20] and the L25P mutation. (**B**) Analysis of the putative TM domain of the PEDV parent and variant E protein with TMHMM Server v.2.0 [25]. The TM domain was predicted as $I_{15}$ to $L_{37}$ and $I_{10}$ to $L_{32}$, respectively. (**C**) Comparative analysis of the mRNA levels of HSPA5 (encoding GRP78) and the protein production of GRP78 among the parent-, C30-, and C40-infected Vero cells. (**D**, **E**) Comparative analysis of the mRNA levels of the genes encoding IL-6 and IL-8 among the parent-, C30-, and C40-infected Vero cells by qPCR assay. The β-Actin gene served as an endogenous control. Error bars indicated the means of three independent experiments. (**F** and **G**) and (**H**) Comparative analysis of the mRNA levels of the genes encoding GRP78, IL-6, and IL-8 among the recombinant plasmids-transfected Vero cells by qPCR assay. The corresponding amount of empty plasmid (pIRES2-EGFP) was used as the mock control. (**I**) Comparison of the cell apoptosis level by flow cytometry with dual Annexin V-PI cell labeling. The infected cells were collected at 36 hpi, and the mock-infected cells were used as the control. Fluorescence-activated cell sorting was used to detect the fluorescent signals of Annexin V and PI, using channels FL-1 and FL-2, respectively. The figure was representative of two independent experiments. The graph representing the percentage of fluorescent signals of Annexin V and PI in each quadrant was shown on the left. (**J**) Comparative analysis of the levels of early apoptosis. C30, C40, and E40 showed higher early apoptosis levels than the 85-7 parent, A40, B40, and D40 strains.

inflammatory cytokines [12, 34]. GRP78 is a well-characterized ER chaperone protein and a marker of ER stress [12]. Our results show that C30 and C40 strains significantly activated *HSPA5* (the gene encoding GRP78) transcription and GRP78 production during the virus replication process compared with those of the parent strain (Figure 5C). Meanwhile, the transcriptions of pro-inflammatory cytokines IL-6 and IL-8 were also significantly up-regulated in C30 and C40 infected cells than parent virus infected cells (Figures 5D and E). Further study showed that overexpression of mutant E protein could induce significantly higher mRNA level of IL-6, IL-8, and GRP78 than parent E protein (Figures 5F–H; Additional file 6). These results indicate that the variation in the TM domain of the E protein caused a notable effect on its interaction with the host cells.

It should be noted that the continuous or too strong stimulation of ER stress can induce cell apoptosis [11]. Thus, we tested the apoptosis levels of the parent and mutant strains using flow cytometry. Compared with the mock-infected cells, the parent 85-7 strain triggered a positive result for caspase-independent apoptosis, with the percentage of early apoptotic cells (Annexin V positive/PI negative) increasing from 16.3 to 35.1% (Figure 5I; Additional file 5). Notably, the C30, C40, and E40 strains induced significantly higher apoptosis levels than the parent strain (Figures 5I and J). Furthermore, the similar apoptosis levels induced by the C30 and C40 strains indicated that the R895G mutation might not contribute to this pathogenic pathway (Figures 5I and J). The apoptosis levels induced by strains A40, B40, and D40 strains also showed no difference compared with the parent strain (Figures 5I and J), further confirming that the other mutations were not involved in this phenotype.

## Discussion

In recent years, PEDV has reemerged in Asia and Europe, and has spread into America and Australia, demonstrating a complex virulence situation, genetic recombination, and evolution [3, 4, 35, 36]. In this study, the infection of PEDV strain 85-7 could significantly up-regulate GRP78 production and the level of the mRNA encoding pro-inflammatory factors, and induced cell apoptosis and microfilament rearrangement on Vero cells, which provided clues to further explore PEDV's pathogenic mechanism. Furthermore, PEDV undergoes frequent variation in the process of clinical evolution and cell culture, which contributes to its fast adaptation to the host micro-environment [5, 21, 37, 38]. Indeed, genomic stability analysis of PEDV strain 85-7 identified four major variable regions, located in the Nsp2, S, ORF3, and E genes, respectively. Full understanding of the effects of these variations on infection characteristics was necessary to

reveal the PEDV infection mechanism and evolutionary trend.

Truncation of the C-terminus of Nsp2 had no distinct effects on PEDV replication (Figure 3). Similarly, mutations in Nsp2 did not affect viral replication but caused a modest reduction in titers and viral RNA synthesis in MHV and SARS-CoV [39]. The protein domains of Nsp1 to Nsp3 homologs showed minimal sequence identity among different coronavirus groups [39]. In fact, Nsp2 is one of the most variable regions, with diverse recombination events being identified in field strains of PEDV [4], but is not involved in the PEDV-induced IFN antagonistic effect [37], all of which suggest that Nsp2 might mediate virus evolution, rather than playing a role in viral replication. Similarly, the early termination of ORF3 gene studied here had no significant effects on PEDV replication, while the function of ORF3 in PEDV replication is controversial and requires further exploration [5, 37, 40–42].

More importantly, the C30 and C40 mutant strains, differing just with R895G mutation, showed significant difference in viral yields, cytoskeletal structure, CPE effects and plaque morphologies. A previous study has reported that the disordered microfilaments induced by PEDV infection in IPEC-J2 cells could suppress the replication and release of viruses [27], which implied that R895G mutation might contribute to higher viral titers via mediation of the cytoskeleton rearrangement. Furthermore, virus infection could also induce cellular conformational changes and cytopathic effect via rearranging host cell cytoskeletal and membrane compartments [43], suggesting that the R895G mutation might be the decisive site that allows the virus to evolve toward better survival in host cells.

Several protease cleavage sites in the S proteins of *coronavirus* have been identified, and most of them play key roles in the virus infection process [8, 10]. The R895 site of PEDV S protein forms the novel XXXR/S motif, and has been identified as a putative S2′ cleavage site, which was predicted as the determinant in trypsin-dependent entry of PEDV [8]. However, PEDV 85-7 parent and all the mutant strains (including the C30 and C40 strains differing single mutation R895G) could effectively proliferate in Vero cells in a trypsin-independent manner, and the entry or release of infectious PEDV particles was more efficiently without trypsin supplementation, indicating that the S2′ site was not the determinant for trypsin-dependent entry of PEDV. Coupled with the reports that R895G mutation in S protein could inhibit cell–cell fusion specifically in both PEDV and SARS-CoV [8, 10], suggesting that the PEDV induced cell–cell fusion capacity might be more closely related with the S2′ cleavage site than with trypsin supplementation.

Thus, supplementation with trypsin is required for the virus-cell fusion process of trypsin-dependent PEDV infection, while the cell–cell fusion process might be mediated by the S2' cleavage site via a completely different mechanism.

The specific region of S protein, including the putative S2' cleavage site, fusion peptide, and HR1 domain, has been confirmed as the determinant for trypsin-dependent entry of PEDV in the attenuated DR13 strain [8]. An amino acid sequence alignment of this region between trypsin-dependent strains (CV777 and DR13) and trypsin-independent strains (ca-DR13 and 85-7), revealed only one position difference, from Y977 (CV777 and DR13) to H977 (ca-DR13 and 85-7) (Additional file 7). These observations suggest that the Y977H mutation might be the determinant for PEDV trypsin-independent entry and served as a crucial proteolytic cleavage site.

Furthermore, the fusion peptides located close to the C-terminus of the S2' cleavage site are highly conserved across the *Coronaviridae*, particularly the [898]IEDLLF[903] motif, which contains four hydrophobic residues (I, Isoleucine; L, Leucine; F, Phenylalanine) and two negative-charged residues (E, Glutamic acid; D, Aspartic acid) [30]. Notably, the residues [901]LLF[903], but not the D[900], have been shown to have a crucial role in membrane fusion in SARS-CoV [30]. However, the B40 and D40 strains with point mutations comprising D900A (Alanine), L902 V (Valine), and F903 V showed similar infection characteristics to the parent strain (Figure 3; Additional file 4). Alanine (A) and Valine (V) are also hydrophobic residues, which suggests that the occasional conservative substitution in the [898]IEDLLF[903] motif caused only a minimal change in PEDV infection.

It is noteworthy that C30, C40, and E40 mutant strains sharing the same variation in TM domain of the E protein could up-regulate the transcription of GRP78, IL-6 and IL-8, and induce higher apoptosis levels compared with that of the parent strain. The SARS-CoV E protein alone was sufficient to reduce the expression of GRP78 and GRP94 (two ER stress inducible proteins) [11], whereas the PEDV E protein could be located in the ER, and then induced ER stress and up-regulated GRP78 alone [20], suggesting that the E proteins from diverse *Coronavirus* viruses might employ different mechanisms to mediate the stress response. Furthermore, SARS-CoV lacking the E gene (rSARS-CoV-ΔE) has been demonstrated to reduce the expression of pro-inflammatory cytokines [11]. In PEDV, the E protein also increased IL-8 expression in intestinal epithelial cells (IEC) [33] and Vero cells (Figures 5E and H), suggesting that the E protein is closely related to inflammation. These studies, coupled with the reports that TM domain alterations of CoV E

protein are involved in virus assembly, replication and release [15, 32], supported our speculation that the TM domain of PEDV E protein plays a potential role in interaction with host cells, including ER stress, pro-inflammatory cytokine production and apoptosis. Especially, it is the variation of the E protein, not the amount of virus production, that is responsible for the increase of the cell stress response. Some recent studies have reported that the ion channel (IC) activity of CoV E protein has important functions in immune response modulation via NLRP3 inflammasome, and the IC activity relies on its TM domain [17, 44]. However, it needs further study whether the variation of the TM domain in this study has an impact on the ion channel activity of PEDV E protein and the following immune response modulation.

In conclusion, we performed a comprehensive analysis of the viral proliferation characteristics and the alignment of whole genomes among the isolated PEDV strain 85-7 and several of its mutants screened from serial propagation on Vero cells. The results allowed us to hypothesize that the R895G mutation in S protein is the determinant of PEDV-induced cell–cell fusion, and also promotes PEDV replication and fitness. Furthermore, the E protein, especially the V4 region in the TM domain, is crucial for modulating the PEDV cell stress response and immune response. In short, continuous passage of PEDV strain 85-7 induces the above two variations to adapt the virus to the host microenvironment for better proliferation.

## Additional files

**Additional file 1. Primers designed for RT-PCR, qPCR and recombinant vector constructing.**

**Additional file 2. Summary of nucleotide changes of PEDV strain 85-7 during serial passages in cell culture.**

**Additional file 3. Summary of amino acid variations of PEDV strain 85-7 during serial passages in cell culture.**

**Additional file 4. The alignment of the amino acid sequences [898]IEDLLF[903] in the fusion peptide (FP).** Minimal divergence with occasional conservative substitutions in B40 and D40 strains were shown. The amino acids of I, Isoleucine; L, Leucine; F, Phenylalanine; V, Valine were hydrophobic amino acids. The E, Glutamic acid, and D, Aspartic acid were negative-charged amino acids.

**Additional file 5. PEDV strain 85-7 induced caspase-independent apoptosis on Vero cells.** (A) IFA of 85-7 parent strain in infected Vero cells with treatment of CsA (10 μM), V-ZAD-FMK (100 μM) and DMSO at 36 hpi. CsA treatment suppressed PEDV replication, while the V-ZAD-FMK had no significant effect on virus growth. Vero cells were pretreated with CsA, V-ZAD-FMK or DMSO for 1 h, and then infected with PEDV with the presence of CsA, V-ZAD-FMK or DMSO in the whole infected process. (B) Viral titers of the infected cells with CsA (1, 5, 10 μM) or DMSO treatment at 12, 24 and 36 hpi. Viral titers were determined as Log pfu/mL. Error bars indicate the average results of two independent experiments. (C) Viral titers of the infected cells with V-ZAD-FMK (100 μM) or DMSO treatment at 36 hpi.

**Additional file 6. The dual-staining IFA assay to verify the overexpression of PEDV parent E protein and mutant E proteins in Vero cells.** The recombinant plasmids (PI-E or PI-mE) were transfected into Vero cells for 24 h. The corresponding amount of empty plasmid (pIRES2-EGFP) was used as the mock control. The primary antibody was the anti-HA-tag antibody. The red staining (recombinant protein) was almost merged with the green staining (EGFP-tag protein).

**Additional file 7. Multiple amino acid sequence alignment of the determinant region for PEDV trypsin-dependent entry.** A schematic overview of the S2 domain is referred to as the SARS-CoV. FP, fusion peptide; HR1 and HR2, heptad repeat regions; S2′ site (R895), location of putative cleavage site within the S2 subunit; drawn to scale. Virus abbreviations (and GenBank accession numbers) were as follows: SARS-CoV (Tor2, NP_828851.1), DR13 (JQ023161.1), ca-DR13 (JQ023162.1), CV777 (AF353511.1). The Y977H was the only site that differed the trypsin-independent strains (ca-DR13 and 85-7 strain) from the trypsin-dependent strains (DR13 and CV777).

## Abbreviations

PEDV: porcine epidemic diarrhea virus; Nsp: nonstructural protein; ORF: open reading frame; PED: porcine epidemic diarrhea; FP: fusion peptide; HR: heptad repeat region; TM: transmembrane domain; ER: endoplasmic reticulum; UPR: unfolded protein response; TGEV: transmissible gastroenteritis virus; MERS-CoV: Middle East Respiratory Syndrome-coronavirus; MHV: mouse hepatitis virus; IBV: infectious bronchitis virus; SARS-CoV: severe acute respiratory syndrome-coronavirus; IEC: intestinal epithelial cells; DMEM: Dulbecco modified eagle medium; FBS: fetal bovine serum; CsA: cyclosporin A; DMSO: dimethyl sulfoxide; RT-PCR: reverse transcription-polymerase chain reaction; qPCR: quantitative real-time polymerase chain reaction; CPE: cytopathic effects; IFA: indirect immunofluorescence assay; MOI: multiplicity of infection; hpi: hours postinfection; pfu: plaque-forming units; PI: propidium iodide; FACS: fluorescence-activated cell sorter; BSA: bovine serum albumin; PBS: phosphate-buffered saline; TEM: transmission electron microscopy; TMPRSS2: transmembrane type II serine protease 2; UTR: untranslated region.

## Competing interests

The authors declared that they have no competing interests.

## Authors' contributions

HY and MS designed the study and drafted the paper; MS, JM, ZY and ZP performed the experiments; MS and HY analyzed the results; CL and HY contributed the materials and provided valuable suggestions. All authors read and approved the final manuscript.

## Acknowledgements

This work was supported by a grant from the Priority Academic Program Development of Jiangsu Higher Education Institutions (PAPD).

## References

1. Chen Q, Li G, Stasko J, Thomas JT, Stensland WR et al (2014) Isolation and characterization of porcine epidemic diarrhea viruses associated with the 2013 disease outbreak among swine in the United States. J Clin Microbiol 52:234–243
2. Trujillo-Ortega ME, Beltrán-Figueroa R, Garcia-Hernández ME, Juárez-Ramirez M, Sotomayor-González A et al (2016) Isolation and characterization of porcine epidemic diarrhea virus associated with the 2014 disease outbreak in Mexico: case report. BMC Vet Res 12:132
3. Steinrigl A, Fernández SR, Stoiber F, Pikalo J, Sattler T et al (2015) First detection, clinical presentation and phylogenetic characterization of porcine epidemic diarrhea virus in Austria. BMC Vet Res 11:310
4. Huang YW, Dickerman AW, Piñeyro P, Li L, Fang L et al (2013) Origin, evolution, and genotyping of emergent porcine epidemic diarrhea virus strains in the United States. MBio 4:e00737–e0073713
5. Chen F, Zhu Y, Wu M, Ku X, Ye S et al (2015) Comparative genomic analysis of classical and variant virulent parental/attenuated strains of porcine epidemic diarrhea virus. Viruses 7:5525–5538
6. Sato T, Takeyama N, Katsumata A, Tuchiya K, Kodama T et al (2011) Mutations in the spike gene of porcine epidemic diarrhea virus associated with growth adaptation in vitro and attenuation of virulence in vivo. Virus Genes 43:72–78
7. Li W, Wicht O, van Kuppeveld FJ, He Q, Rottier PJ et al (2015) A single point mutation creating a furin cleavage site in the spike protein renders porcine epidemic diarrhea coronavirus trypsin independent for cell entry and fusion. J Virol 89:8077–8081
8. Wicht O, Li W, Willems L, Meuleman TJ, Wubbolts RW et al (2014) Proteolytic activation of the porcine epidemic diarrhea coronavirus spike fusion protein by trypsin in cell culture. J Virol 88:7952–7961
9. Park JE, Cruz DJ, Shin HJ (2011) Receptor-bound porcine epidemic diarrhea virus spike protein cleaved by trypsin induces membrane fusion. Arch Virol 156:1749–1756
10. Belouzard S, Chu VC, Whittaker GR (2009) Activation of the SARS coronavirus spike protein via sequential proteolytic cleavage at two distinct sites. Proc Natl Acad Sci U S A 106:5871–5876
11. DeDiego ML, Nieto-Torres JL, Jiménez-Guardeño JM, Regla-Nava JA, Alvarez E et al (2011) Severe acute respiratory syndrome coronavirus envelope protein regulates cell stress response and apoptosis. PLoS Pathog 7:e1002315
12. Wang Y, Li JR, Sun MX, Ni B, Huan C et al (2014) Triggering unfolded protein response by 2-Deoxy-D-glucose inhibits porcine epidemic diarrhea virus propagation. Antiviral Res 106:33–41
13. Kim Y, Lee C (2014) Porcine epidemic diarrhea virus induces caspase-independent apoptosis through activation of mitochondrial apoptosis-inducing factor. Virology 460–461:180–193
14. Kuo L, Masters PS (2003) The small envelope protein E is not essential for murine coronavirus replication. J Virol 77:4597–4608
15. Ye Y, Hogue BG (2007) Role of the coronavirus E viroporin protein transmembrane domain in virus assembly. J Virol 81:3597–3607
16. Machamer CE, Youn S (2006) The transmembrane domain of the infectious bronchitis virus E protein is required for efficient virus release. Adv Exp Med Biol 581:193–198
17. Nieto-Torres JL, DeDiego ML, Verdiá-Báguena C, Jiménez-Guardeño JM, Regla-Nava JA et al (2014) Severe acute respiratory syndrome coronavirus envelope protein ion channel activity promotes virus fitness and pathogenesis. PLoS Pathog 10:e1004077
18. Ortego J, Ceriani JE, Patiño C, Plana J, Enjuanes L (2007) Absence of E protein arrests transmissible gastroenteritis coronavirus maturation in the secretory pathway. Virology 368:296–308
19. DeDiego ML, Alvarez E, Almazán F, Rejas MT, Lamirande E et al (2007) A severe acute respiratory syndrome coronavirus that lacks the E gene is attenuated in vitro and in vivo. J Virol 81:1701–1713
20. Xu X, Zhang H, Zhang Q, Dong J, Liang Y et al (2013) Porcine epidemic diarrhea virus E protein causes endoplasmic reticulum stress and up-regulates interleukin-8 expression. Virol J 10:26
21. Sun M, Ma J, Wang Y, Wang M, Song W et al (2015) Genomic and epidemiological characteristics provide new insights into the phylogeographical and spatiotemporal spread of porcine epidemic diarrhea virus in Asia. J Clin Microbiol 53:1484–1492
22. Jing H, Fang L, Wang D, Ding Z, Luo R et al (2014) Porcine reproductive and respiratory syndrome virus infection activates NOD2-RIP2 signal pathway in MARC-145 cells. Virology 458–459:162–171
23. Kim Y, Lee C (2013) Ribavirin efficiently suppresses porcine nidovirus replication. Virus Res 171:44–53
24. Hu W, Zhu L, Yang X, Lin J, Yang Q (2016) The epidermal growth factor receptor regulates cofilin activity and promotes transmissible gastroenteritis virus entry into intestinal epithelial cells. Oncotarget 7:12206–12221
25. Krogh A, Larsson B, von Heijne G, Sonnhammer EL (2001) Predicting transmembrane protein topology with a hidden Markov model: application to complete genomes. J Mol Biol 305:567–580

26. Bosch BJ, van der Zee R, de Haan CA, Rottier PJ (2003) The coronavirus spike protein is a class I virus fusion protein: structural and functional characterization of the fusion core complex. J Virol 77:8801–8811

27. Zhao S, Gao J, Zhu L, Yang Q (2014) Transmissible gastroenteritis virus and porcine epidemic diarrhoea virus infection induces dramatic changes in the tight junctions and microfilaments of polarized IPEC-J2 cells. Virus Res 192:34–45

28. Doane FW, Anderson N (1987) Electron microscopy in diagnostic virology a practical guide and atlas, vol XIV. Cambridge University Press, Cambridge, p 178

29. Shirato K, Matsuyama S, Ujike M, Taguchi F (2011) Role of proteases in the release of porcine epidemic diarrhea virus from infected cells. J Virol 85:7872–7880

30. Madu IG, Roth SL, Belouzard S, Whittaker GR (2009) Characterization of a highly conserved domain within the severe acute respiratory syndrome coronavirus spike protein S2 domain with characteristics of a viral fusion peptide. J Virol 83:7411–7421

31. Yamada Y, Liu DX (2009) Proteolytic activation of the spike protein at a novel RRRR/S motif is implicated in furin-dependent entry, syncytium formation, and infectivity of coronavirus infectious bronchitis virus in cultured cells. J Virol 83:8744–8758

32. Lopez LA, Riffle AJ, Pike SL, Gardner D, Hogue BG (2008) Importance of conserved cysteine residues in the coronavirus envelope protein. J Virol 82:3000–3010

33. DeDiego ML, Nieto-Torres JL, Jimenez-Guardeño JM, Regla-Nava JA, Castaño-Rodriguez C et al (2014) Coronavirus virulence genes with main focus on SARS-CoV envelope gene. Virus Res 194:124–137

34. Liu YP, Zeng L, Tian A, Bomkamp A, Rivera D et al (2012) Endoplasmic reticulum stress regulates the innate immunity critical transcription factor IRF3. J Immunol 189:4630–4639

35. Li W, Li H, Liu Y, Pan Y, Deng F et al (2012) New variants of porcine epidemic diarrhea virus, China, 2011. Emerg Infect Dis 18:1350–1353

36. Boniotti MB, Papetti A, Lavazza A, Alborali G, Sozzi E et al (2016) Porcine epidemic diarrhea virus and discovery of a recombinant swine enteric coronavirus, Italy. Emerg Infect Dis 22:83–87

37. Zhang Q, Shi K, Yoo D (2016) Suppression of type I interferon production by porcine epidemic diarrhea virus and degradation of CREB-binding protein by nsp1. Virology 489:252–268

38. Wang J, Zhao P, Guo L, Liu Y, Du Y et al (2013) Porcine epidemic diarrhea virus variants with high pathogenicity, China. Emerg Infect Dis 19:2048–2049

39. Graham RL, Sims AC, Brockway SM, Baric RS, Denison MR (2005) The nsp2 replicase proteins of murine hepatitis virus and severe acute respiratory syndrome coronavirus are dispensable for viral replication. J Virol 79:13399–13411

40. Li C, Li Z, Zou Y, Wicht O, van Kuppeveld FJ et al (2013) Manipulation of the porcine epidemic diarrhea virus genome using targeted RNA recombination. PLoS One 8:e69997

41. Ye S, Li Z, Chen F, Li W, Guo X et al (2015) Porcine epidemic diarrhea virus ORF3 gene prolongs S-phase, facilitates formation of vesicles and promotes the proliferation of attenuated PEDV. Virus Genes 51:385–392

42. Wang K, Lu W, Chen J, Xie S, Shi H et al (2012) PEDV ORF3 encodes an ion channel protein and regulates virus production. FEBS Lett 586:384–391

43. Foo KY, Chee HY (2015) Interaction between flavivirus and cytoskeleton during virus replication. Biomed Res Int 2015:427814

44. Nieto-Torres JL, Verdiá-Báguena C, Jiménez-Guardeño JM, Regla-Nava JA, Castaño-Rodriguez C et al (2015) Severe acute respiratory syndrome coronavirus E protein transports calcium ions and activates the NLRP3 inflammasome. Virology 485:330–339

# 14

# Serotype-specific role of antigen I/II in the initial steps of the pathogenesis of the infection caused by *Streptococcus suis*

Sarah Chuzeville[1,2†], Jean-Philippe Auger[1,2†], Audrey Dumesnil[1,2], David Roy[1,2], Sonia Lacouture[1,2], Nahuel Fittipaldi[3], Daniel Grenier[1,4] and Marcelo Gottschalk[1,2*] (iD)

## Abstract

*Streptococcus suis* is one of the most important post-weaning porcine bacterial pathogens worldwide. The serotypes 2 and 9 are often considered the most virulent and prevalent serotypes involved in swine infections, especially in Europe. However, knowledge of the bacterial factors involved in the first steps of the pathogenesis of the infection remains scarce. In several pathogenic streptococci, expression of multimodal adhesion proteins known as antigen I/ II (AgI/II) have been linked with persistence in the upper respiratory tract and the oral cavity, as well as with bacterial dissemination. Herein, we report expression of these immunostimulatory factors by *S. suis* serotype 2 and 9 strains and that AgI/II-encoding genes are carried by integrative and conjugative elements. Using mutagenesis and different in vitro assays, we demonstrate that the contribution of AgI/II to the virulence of the serotype 2 strain used herein appears to be modest. In contrast, data demonstrate that the serotype 9 AgI/II participates in self-aggregation, induces salivary glycoprotein 340-related aggregation, contributes to biofilm formation and increased strain resistance to low pH, as well as in bacterial adhesion to extracellular matrix proteins and epithelial cells. Moreover, the use of a porcine infection model revealed that AgI/II contributes to colonization of the upper respiratory tract of pigs. Taken together, these findings suggest that surface exposed AgI/II likely play a key role in the first steps of the pathogenesis of the *S. suis* serotype 9 infection.

## Introduction

*Streptococcus suis* is one of the most important post-weaning bacterial pathogens of pigs and a major economic problem for the porcine industry [1]. Septicemia with sudden death, meningitis, arthritis, and endocarditis are the most frequent clinical signs caused by *S. suis* in pigs [2]. *S. suis* is also a zoonotic agent responsible for numerous human cases of meningitis, septicemia, and streptococcal toxic shock-like syndrome [2]. In Western countries, human *S. suis* infections mostly occur in

individuals directly or indirectly linked with the porcine industry. In contrast, the general population is at risk of *S. suis* disease in certain Asian countries where this pathogen has been shown to be an important cause of adult meningitis [3]. Serotype 2 is, globally, considered the most virulent serotype and the one most frequently isolated from both porcine and human infections [4]. The use of multilocus sequence typing has revealed that serotype 2 strains belonging to certain sequence types (STs) are more virulent than others. ST1 strains (virulent) predominate in most Eurasian countries, whereas ST25 and ST28 strains (intermediate and low virulence, respectively) are mainly present in North America [4]. Meanwhile, highly virulent ST7 strains, responsible for at least two important human outbreaks in China, have only been reported in that country [5]. The serotype 9 has recently emerged in certain European countries, such as Spain, the Netherlands, and Germany [4]. Yet,

---

*Correspondence: marcelo.gottschalk@umontreal.ca
†Sarah Chuzeville and Jean-Philippe Auger contributed equally to this work
² Groupe de recherche sur les maladies infectieuses en production animale (GREMIP), Department of Pathology and Microbiology, Faculty of Veterinary Medicine, University of Montreal, 3200 Sicotte St., Saint-Hyacinthe, QC J2S 2M2, Canada
Full list of author information is available at the end of the article

very few studies have addressed the presence of virulence factors in this serotype, and putative virulence factors described for serotype 2 strains may not always be present in serotype 9 strains [6]. Moreover, the first *S. suis* serotype 9 human case of infection was reported in 2015 [7].

The early steps of the pathogenesis of the *S. suis* infection are not well understood [1, 8]. Currently, the most accepted hypothesis is that virulent strains reach the bloodstream after breaching the mucosal epithelium of either the upper respiratory or the gastrointestinal tracts of pigs [1]. Similarly, infection of humans occurs via skin wounds or at the intestinal interface following ingestion of raw or undercooked infected meat [1]. However, the precise mechanisms and virulence factors involved remain unknown. Of note, the upper respiratory tract of pigs, particularly the tonsils and nasal cavities, are important reservoirs of *S. suis* [1]. Furthermore, *S. suis* has also been shown to be present in nearly half of the submaxillary lymph node samples of clinically healthy pigs [9]. Bacterial loads in saliva swab and tonsillar brush samples are similar, indicating that *S. suis* is indeed a natural inhabitant of the oral cavity [10].

Antigens I/II (AgI/II) have been extensively described in oral as well as in invasive pathogenic streptococci, including *Streptococcus mutans*, *Streptococcus gordonii*, *Streptococcus pyogenes*, and *Streptococcus agalactiae* [11]. AgI/II are immunostimulatory components and multimodal adhesion proteins implicated in host upper respiratory tract and oral cavity persistence and dissemination [11]. Affinity of AgI/II-like proteins for binding salivary glycoproteins, especially the glycoprotein (gp) 340 (also called DMBT1 protein) is a common feature of this protein family [12]. Large quantities of gp340 are present in the saliva of mammals in either a surface-immobilized form or fluid phase form. It is also present at all mucosal surfaces, including the nasal and intestinal cavities [13, 14]. Interestingly, it has been shown that *S. suis* is able to adhere to gp340 and that this protein aggregates certain strains of *S. suis* [15]. However, the strains tested did not express AgI/II when using a heterologous monospecific antibody [15].

In this study, using in silico analyses, genes with homology to those coding for AgI/II were identified in *S. suis* serotype 2 and 9 strains. Using isogenic mutants deficient for the expression and production of AgI/II in both serotype 2 (S2Δ*agI/II*) and serotype 9 (S9Δ*agI/II*), the role of this protein in different aspects of the pathogenesis of the infection caused by *S. suis* was evaluated. We report for the first time that these proteins play a limited or important role in the pathogenesis of the infection caused by *S. suis* serotype 2 and 9, respectively.

## Materials and methods

### Bacterial strains and culture conditions

Bacterial strains and plasmids used in this study are listed in Table 1. The virulent serotype 2 ST7 strain SC84, responsible for the 2005 human outbreak in China [5], and the serotype 9 strain 1135776 (isolated from a diseased pig in Canada) were used herein as models to study the role of Ag I/II in the pathogenesis of the infection caused by *S. suis*. Twenty-five additional *S. suis* serotype 9 strains recovered from diseased pigs were also used to evaluate the prevalence of *agI/II* genes by PCR (Additional file 1). Seventeen of these strains originated from Canada, 3 from Brazil, 1 from Denmark (reference strain), and 4 from Germany. A strain isolated from a human case of infection was also included [7]. The *S. mutans* strain Ingbritt was used as a tool for collection of porcine salivary agglutinins (pSAGs) whereas the *Escherichia coli* TOP10 (Invitrogen, Carlsbad, CA, USA), MC1061 [16], and BL21(DE3) (Invitrogen) strains were used for DNA manipulations and/or AgI/II protein production. The different *Streptococcus* and *E. coli* strains were grown at 37 °C in Todd Hewitt (THB) under static conditions or in Luria-Bertani broth (Becton Dickinson, Franklin Lakes, NJ, USA) with shaking, respectively. Antibiotics (Sigma-Aldrich, St-Louis, MO, USA), where needed, were used at the following concentrations for *S. suis* and *E. coli*: spectinomycin at 500 and 50 µg/mL and erythromycin at 5 and 200 µg/mL, respectively. Ampicillin was also used at a concentration of 50 µg/mL for *E. coli*.

### Bioinformatics analyses

In silico analyses of AgI/II-coding DNA sequences (CDS) in *S. suis* genomes were performed using BLASTN (expected threshold $< 10^{-3}$) as previously described [17]. The *S. suis* nucleotide collection nr/nt database available in GenBank (taxid 1307) was queried for *S. suis* genomes. Alongside, a bank of *S. suis* serotype 2 North American ST25 and ST28 strains isolated from diseased pigs whose genomes were previously published [18, 19] were also queried. Moreover, BLASTN was used to detect homologies with genes coding for AgI/II or orthologues that have already been described in other bacterial species: *S. mutans* SpaP (accession number NC_004350.2), *S. gordonii* SspA and SspB (accession number CP000725.1), *S. pyogenes* (accession number NC_007296.1), *S. agalactiae* (accession number AAJP01000002.1), and *Enterococcus faecalis* (accession number AY855841.2). Examination of CDS carriage by putative integrative and conjugative elements (ICEs) was conducted using the ICEberg database [20], followed by BLASTN using the *S. suis* serotype 2 SC84 (accession number GCA_000026725.1) and serotype 9 D12 (accession number GCA_000231905.1)

**Table 1  Strains and plasmids used in the study**

| Strain or plasmid | Characteristics | References |
|---|---|---|
| *Streptococcus suis* | | |
| SC84 | Serotype 2 strain isolated from a patient with streptococcal toxic shock-like syndrome in China | [47] |
| 1135776 | Serotype 9 strain isolated from pig following sudden death in Canada | This study |
| S2Δ*agI/II* | SC84-derived strain carrying an in-frame deletion of the *agI/II* gene | This study |
| S9Δ*agI/II* | 1135776-derived strain carrying an in-frame deletion of the *agI/II* gene | This study |
| S2CΔ*agI/II* | SC84-derived strain carrying pOri23-S2*agI/II* | This study |
| S9CΔ*agI/II* | 1135776-derived strain carrying pOri23-S9*agI/II* | This study |
| *Escherichia coli* | | |
| TOP10 | Host for pCR2.1 and pSET4s derivatives | Invitrogen |
| MC1061 | Host for pOri23 derivatives | [16] |
| BL21(DE3) | Host for pET151 derivatives | Invitrogen |
| Plasmids | | |
| pET151 | Ap$^r$, pBR322 *ori*, T7 promotor | Invitrogen |
| pCR2.1 | Ap$^r$, Km$^r$, pUC *ori*, *lacZ*ΔM15 | Invitrogen |
| pSET4s | Spc$^r$, pUC *ori*, thermosensitive pG+host3 *ori*, *lacZ*ΔM15 | [37] |
| pOri23 | Erm$^r$, ColE1 *ori*, P23 | [28] |
| pET151–S2*agI/II* | pET151 carrying the S2 *agI/II* gene | This study |
| pSET4s–S2*agI/II* | pSET4s carrying regions upstream and downstream of the S2 *agI/II* gene | This study |
| pSET4s–S9*agI/II* | pSET4s carrying regions upstream and downstream of the S9 *agI/II* gene | This study |
| pOri23$_{spc}$–S2*agI/II* | pOri23 carrying the S2 *agI/II* gene as well as its promotor and terminator | This study |
| pOri23$_{spc}$–S9*agI/II* | pOri23 carrying the S9 *agI/II* gene as well as its promotor and terminator | This study |

genomes as queries. Protein domains were analyzed using the NCBI conserved domain database with the help of the BatchCD tool [21]. Cell wall anchored domains were predicted using CW-PRED [22], while transmembrane domains and signal peptide cleavage sites were detected using the TMHMM [23] and the SignalP [24] tools, respectively. The Expasy bioinformatics resource portal was used to determine the theoretical protein molecular weight [25].

## DNA manipulations

Chromosomal *S. suis* DNA was prepared using standard methods [26] or InstaGene matrix (Bio-Rad, Hercules, CA, USA) according to the manufacturer's instructions. Plasmid DNA preparations and purification of PCR amplicons were performed using the QIAprep Spin Miniprep Kit and the QIAquick PCR Purification Kit (Qiagen, Hilden, Germany), respectively, according to the manufacturer's instructions. Oligonucleotide primers (listed in Additional file 2) were purchased from Integrated DNA Technologies (Coralville, IA, USA). Primers were designed from the available *S. suis* serotype 2 (strain SC84) and serotype 9 (strain D12) genomes. DNA ligations and transformation of competent *E. coli* were performed as previously described [27]. Sequencing reactions were carried out using an ABI 3730xl Automated DNA Sequencer and the ABI PRISM Dye Terminator

Cycle Version 3.1 (Applied Biosystems, Foster City, CA, USA) and analyses of sequences performed using the BioEdit© software and/or BLASTN.

## Generation of the isogenic *agI/II*-deficient mutants and complemented strains

For precise in-frame deletions of the *agI/II* genes in the *S. suis* serotype 2 strain SC84 and serotype 9 strain 1135776, regions upstream and downstream of the genes were amplified and fused by overlap-extension PCR. The amplification products were subcloned into vector pCR2.1 (Invitrogen), excised using *Hin*dIII (Promega, Madison, WI, USA), and cloned into the thermosensitive gene replacement vector pSET4s as previously described [27]. The resulting serotype 2 and serotype 9 pSET4S-*agI/II* vectors were introduced into recipient serotype 2 and 9 strains, respectively. Allelic replacement and absence of AgI/II expression in resulting serotype 2 and serotype 9 *agI/II*-deficient mutants were confirmed by sequencing and Western blot, respectively.

The pOri23 plasmid [28], which carries a gene conferring resistance to erythromycin, was used for complementation assays. A DNA fragment composed of the full sequence of the *agI/II* genes, as well as their putative endogenous promotors and terminators was cloned into pOri23 using the *Eco*RI and *Pst*I restriction enzymes (two constructs, one for the serotype 2 *agI/II* and another for the serotype 9 *aglI/II*). Since the serotype 9 strain used is highly resistant to erythromycin (data not shown), and several reports have described increased resistance to this antimicrobial among serotype 2 strains [29, 30], a spectinomycin resistance cassette derived from pSET4s was introduced into the pOri23–S2*aglI/II* and pOri23–S9*aglI/II* plasmids. Following subcloning steps using *E. coli* MC1061, the generated pOri23$_{spc}$–S2*aglI/II* and pOri23$_{spc}$–S9*aglI/II* plasmids were then introduced into the S2Δ*aglI/II* and S9Δ*aglI/II* strains to generate the complemented S2CΔ*aglI/II* and S9CΔ*aglI/II* strains, respectively.

## Cloning, expression, and purification of the His-tagged recombinant AgI/II protein and production of polyclonal mono-specific antibodies

A 4430 bp fragment of the serotype 2 *aglI/II* gene, excluding the sequences coding for the cell wall anchorage and the LPXTG domains, was cloned into the pET151 expression vector (Invitrogen) according to the manufacturer's instructions (Figure 1). Protein synthesis was induced using 0.5 mM of isopropyl β-D-1-thiogalactopyranoside and cells lysed using lysozyme (Sigma-Aldrich) and sonication. The resulting recombinant His-tagged AgI/II, henceforth rAgI/II, was purified by affinity chromatography using the His-Bind Resin Chromatography Kit (Novagen, Madison, WI, USA,) according to manufacturer's instructions. Protein purity was evaluated by sodium dodecyl sulfate–polyacrylamide gel electrophoresis following dialysis. Protein concentration was determined using the Pierce Bicinchoninic Acid (BCA) Protein Assay Kit (Thermo Scientific, Waltham, MA, USA). Rabbits were inoculated with the purified rAgI/II to produce a mono-specific polyclonal serum as previously described [31]. This serum was then used to verify presence of the

protein in wild-type, isogenic *aglI/II*-deficient mutants, and complemented strains by Western blot as previously described [32].

## Cell surface hydrophobicity

The relative surface hydrophobicity of the *S. suis* wild-type strains and *aglI/II*-deficient mutants was determined by measuring their adsorption to *n*-hexadecane as previously described [33]. A serotype 2 non-encapsulated mutant strain showing a high percentage of hydrophobicity was used as a positive control [33].

## In vitro pathogenesis assays
### Self-aggregation and biofilm assays

For the self-aggregation assays, overnight cultures of *S. suis* were washed twice with phosphate-buffered saline (PBS), pH 7.3, and re-suspended in THB to obtain an optical density (OD) at 600 nm of 0.05. Samples were incubated at 37 °C for 24 h under static conditions and self-aggregation quantified as previously described [34]. Biofilm formation capacity was determined as previously described [35] in the absence or presence of 2 mg/mL of porcine fibrinogen (Sigma-Aldrich).

### *S. suis* aggregation to soluble porcine salivary agglutinins

Saliva was obtained from pigs as previously described [36] with a few modifications. Briefly, cotton ropes were suspended for 30 min to allow a total of 80 growing pigs from a high health status herd with no recent history of endemic *S. suis* disease to chew. No clinical signs of disease were present during collection. Whole saliva was decanted and impurities eliminated by centrifugation at 8000×*g* for 20 min at 4 °C. pSAGs were then purified from clarified saliva as previously described for human salivary agglutinins using *S. mutans* [37]. The pSAGs

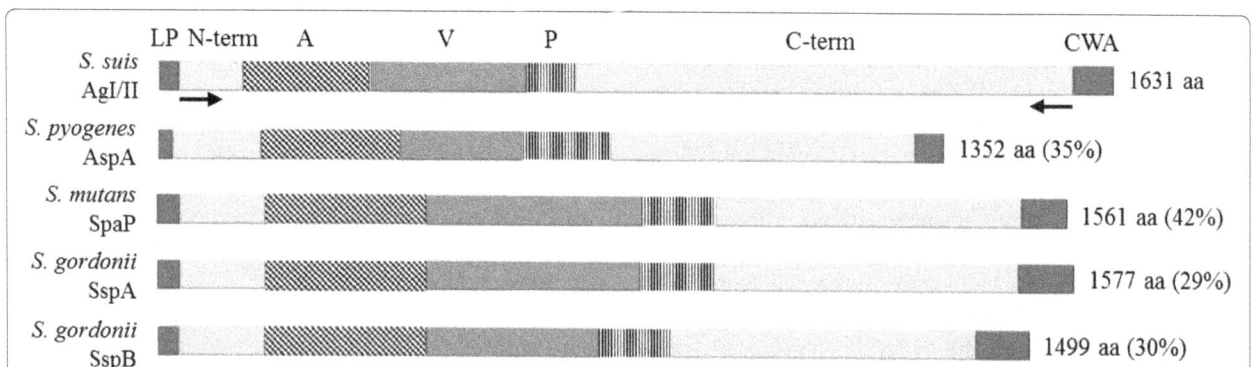

**Figure 1 Characteristics of AgI/II proteins present in different streptococci.** The leader peptide signal (LP), N-terminal domain (N-term), alanine-rich region (A), variable region (V), proline-rich region (P), and C-terminal domain, and the cell wall anchorage domain (CWA) containing the LPXTG domain are illustrated for the *S. suis* AgI/II, *S. pyogenes* AspA, *S. mutans* SpaP, and *S. gordonii* SspA and SspB. Amino acid (aa) size and percentage of *S. suis* AgI/II protein identity are also indicated. Black arrows indicate the location of primers pET151_S2*aglI/II*ΔCWA_F and pET151_S2*aglI/II*_ΔLPXTG_R, which were used to produce the his-tagged recombinant AgI/II protein, rAgI/II.

were dialyzed in PBS and the concentration determined using the Pierce BCA Protein Assay Kit. Bacterial aggregation was quantified every 20 min for 1 h in the absence or presence of pSAGs [37].

### Evaluation of *S. suis* adhesion to extracellular matrix proteins, porcine salivary agglutinins, and the gp340-derived SRCRP2 peptide by ELISA

Bacterial cultures were produced as previously described [38]. Formaldehyde-killed bacteria were washed using either PBS-T (PBS containing 0.05% Tween-20) for experiments involving extracellular matrix proteins (ECM), or TBS-T (10 mM Tris–HCl, 150 mM NaCl, pH 7.5 containing 0.1% Tween-20) supplemented with 1 mM $CaCl_2$, for experiments involving pSAGs and the gp340-derived SRCRP2 peptide [39]. Maxisorp flat-bottom microtiter plates (NUNC, Rochester, NY, USA) were coated with 12.5 µg/mL of human plasma fibronectin (Sigma-Aldrich), 15 µg/mL of human type I collagen (Corning, Corning, NY, USA), 1 mg/mL of porcine fibrinogen or 50 µg/mL of pSAGs, all diluted in carbonate coating buffer (0.1 M, pH 9.6), or with 200 µg/mL of the SRCRP2 peptide (Bio Basic Canada Inc., Markham, ON, Canada) diluted in water, overnight at 4 °C. After washing with PBS-T or TBS-T and blocking with non-fat dry milk, bacterial suspensions equivalent to $1 \times 10^8$ CFU/mL were added to the plates and incubated at 37 °C for 2 h. Subsequent steps were undertaken as previously described [38] using serotype 2 or 9 specific rabbit antisera and the OD at 450 nm determined.

### Acid stress killing assay

The ability of *S. suis* to withstand acid challenge was determined as previously described with some modifications [39]. Briefly, *S. suis* strains were grown in THB, washed twice with PBS, and adjusted to a concentration of $1 \times 10^8$ CFU/mL. Cells were then resuspended in 0.1 M glycine buffer adjusted to either pH 3.0 or 5.0 and incubated at 37 °C. Surviving bacteria were accurately determined using an Autoplate 4000 Spiral Plater (Spiral Biotech, Norwood, MA, USA).

### Cell adhesion and invasion assays

The newborn porcine tracheal epithelial cell line (NPTr) was cultured until confluent as previously described [40]. Cells were infected with *S. suis* as previously described with minor modifications [41]. Briefly, PBS-washed NPTr cells were incubated at 37 °C with 5% $CO_2$ and infected with *S. suis* at a multiplicity of infection of 10. After 2 h of incubation, wells were washed with PBS to remove non-associated bacteria. For adhesion assays, cells were lysed with 1 mL of cold water, while the invasion assay was performed using the antibiotic protection method as

previously described [40], and associated or intracellular bacteria enumerated as described above.

### Intranasal colonization in a porcine model of infection

All experiments involving animals were conducted in accordance with the guidelines and policies of the Canadian Council on Animal Care and the principles set forth in the Guide for the Care and the Use of Laboratory Animals by the Animal Welfare Committee of the University of Montreal, which approved the protocols and procedures used herein (permit number RECH-1570). Four-week old pigs (providing from the same high health status herd mentioned above) were used. The 10 pigs were randomly separated into two rooms upon arrival and their nasal cavities, saliva, and tonsils swabbed to confirm absence of serotype 9. The *S. suis* serotype 9 wild-type strain 1135776 and *agI/II*-deficient mutant were cultured as previously described [42] to obtain a final concentration of $2 \times 10^9$ CFU/mL. Intranasal infections were carried out as previously described with some modifications [43]. Pigs were inoculated with 1 mL of 2% acetic acid per nostril 1 h prior to infection with 1 mL per nostril of either the wild-type or the S9Δ*agI/II* mutant strain.

Nasal cavities were swabbed using sterile cotton-tipped applicators. Swabs were placed in sterile tubes containing PBS supplemented with 0.1% bovine serum albumin and immediately cultured. Serial dilutions of swab samples ($10^0$–$10^{-6}$) were plated on Colombia agar supplemented with 5% defibrinated sheep blood (Cedarlane, Burlington, ON, Canada), *Streptococcus* selective reagent SR0126 (Oxoid, Hampshire, UK), and selected antibiotics to which the serotype 9 strain is resistant at the concentrations used (50 µg/mL spectinomycin, 5 µg/mL erythromycin, 0.2 µg/mL penicillin G, and 1 µg/mL tetracycline). After incubation for 24 h at 37 °C with 5% $CO_2$, plates containing 30–300 colonies were selected. Suspected alpha-hemolytic colonies were enumerated and 10 *S. suis*-like colonies per plate were sub-cultured and tested by coagglutination assay using anti-*S. suis* serotype 9 rabbit serum as previously described [44]. Three weeks post-infection, pigs were euthanized and tonsils recovered. Tonsil samples were processed as previously described [45] and *S. suis* serotype 9 carriage evaluated as described above.

### Statistical analyses

At least three independent biological replicates were performed for each experiment and results expressed as mean ± standard error of the mean (SEM). Raw data were analyzed using the non-parametric statistical Mann–Whitney test. Statistical differences are defined as being greater than $p < 0.05$.

## Results

### Prevalence and molecular characteristics of the *S. suis* AgI/II

Bioinformatics analyses using the *S. suis* (taxid 1307) genome database available in GenBank revealed the presence of genes coding for AgI/II-like proteins in the genomes of serotype 2 strains, including the ST7 strain SC84, ST1 strain BM407, ST25 strain 89–1591, and in a bank of North American *S. suis* serotype 2 ST25 and ST28 strain genomes [18, 19]. However, they were absent from the genome of the reference ST1 strain P1/7. The gene was also present in the genome of the serotype 9 strain D12. Given the low number of published *S. suis* serotype 9 genomes, PCR analyses were undertaken using field strains, which confirmed the presence of the gene in the 25 strains tested (Additional file 1), including strains from Canada, Germany, and Brazil, as well as in the *S. suis* serotype 9 reference strain from Denmark and a human isolate from Thailand. *S. suis* serotype 2 and 9 genes coding for AgI/II share approximately 95% of nucleotide identity. In addition, the promotors share 92% of nucleotide identity with the −35 and −10 boxes and the ribosome binding site for *agI/II* genes being present in all available genomes. Moreover, the terminators of *agI/II* genes are conserved in all strains (100% of nucleotide identity). The percentage of identity between the AgI/II proteins of serotypes 2 and 9 is 95%, being both highly similar. Alignment of the amino acid sequence of both proteins is presented in Additional file 3. Bioinformatics analyses revealed that the *S. suis* AgI/II has a theoretical molecular weight of 180 kDa, which is slightly larger than that of other described AgI/II, probably due to the SspB-like isopeptide-forming domain being repeated thrice in the C-terminal part of the *S. suis* AgI/II (Figure 1) [11]. The *S. suis* AgI/II shares between 29 and 42% of protein sequence identity with other streptococcal AgI/II, such as AspA (*S. pyogenes*), SpaP (*S. mutans*), SspA (*S. gordonii*), and SspB (*S. gordonii*) (Figure 1). Alongside, the *S. suis* AgI/II also shares 32% of protein identity with the aggregation substance PrgB (also called Asc10) of *E. faecalis* [46]. The *S. suis* AgI/II has similar characteristic domains to those described in oral streptococci (Figure 1) [11].

Further bioinformatics investigations, including the use of the ICEberg database, revealed that the gene encoding for the AgI/II protein in the serotype 2 strain SC84 is carried by the 89 K ICE (89 Kbp) [47], while that of the serotype 2 ST1 strain BM407 is carried by two putative ICEs annotated as ICE*Ssu*(BM407)1 and ICE*Ssu*(BM407)2 (75 and 80 Kbp, respectively). Moreover, the gene coding for AgI/II in the serotype 9 strain D12 is also carried by an element sharing 95% of nucleotide identity with the whole sequence of ICE*Ssu*(BM407)1. Altogether, these analyses suggest that the *S. suis* AgI/II are mainly carried by ICEs.

### Confirmation of AgI/II-deficient mutants in both *S. suis* serotypes 2 and 9

Production of AgI/II by the serotype 2 and 9 strains SC84 and 1135776, respectively, was confirmed by immunoblotting using mono-specific antisera produced with the recombinant protein, rAgI/II (Figure 2). The proteins had a molecular weight of approximately 180 kDa, as predicted by bioinformatics analyses. Deletion of the *agI/II* gene resulted in absence of detectable signal while complementation of the mutant strains restored detection with a band at the expected molecular weight (Figure 2). Growth of the S2Δ*agI/II* and S9Δ*agI/II* mutants as well as that of the complemented strains was similar to their respective wild-type strains (data not shown).

It was previously described that AgI/II positively impacts surface hydrophobicity of oral streptococci. However, we did not observe significant differences in hydrophobicity between the *S. suis* serotype 2 or 9 wild-type strains and their AgI/II-deficient mutants (S2Δ*agI/II* and S9Δ*agI/II*) (Additional file 4). Interestingly, the serotype 2 wild-type strain was significantly more hydrophobic than that of serotype 9 ($p < 0.05$).

### In vitro pathogenesis assays

#### Serotype-dependent role of the *S. suis* AgI/II in self-aggregation and biofilm formation

*S. suis* serotype 2 self-aggregation was not modified by the absence of AgI/II (Figure 3A). However, deletion of AgI/II significantly reduced self-aggregation of *S. suis* serotype 9 by 80% ($p < 0.01$) (Figure 3A). On the other hand, self-aggregation was completely restored when using the complemented S9CΔ*agI/II* strain (Figure 3A).

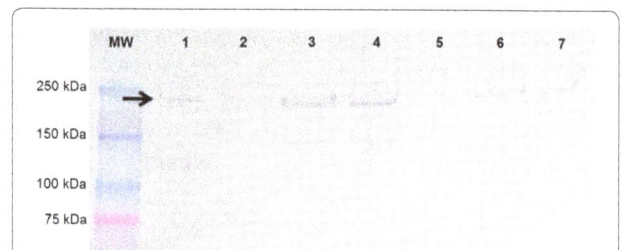

**Figure 2 The AgI/II protein is expressed in the *S. suis* serotype 2 and 9 wild-type strains but is absent in S2Δ*agI/II* and S9Δ*agI/II* mutant strains.** Western blot using cell wall extracts from *S. suis* serotype 2 (wells 1–3) and serotype 9 (wells 4–6): serotype 2 wild-type strain SC84 (well 1) and serotype 9 wild-type strain 1135776 (well 4); mutant strains S2Δ*agI/II* (well 2) and S9Δ*agI/II* (well 5); and complemented strains S2CΔ*agI/II* (well 3) and S9CΔ*agI/II* (well 6). Expected bands at approximately 180 kDa, shown by the black arrow, were observed for the serotype 2 and 9 wild-type and complemented strains, similar to that obtained with the purified AgI/II protein, rAgI/II (well 7), used as a positive control. MW: molecular weight marker.

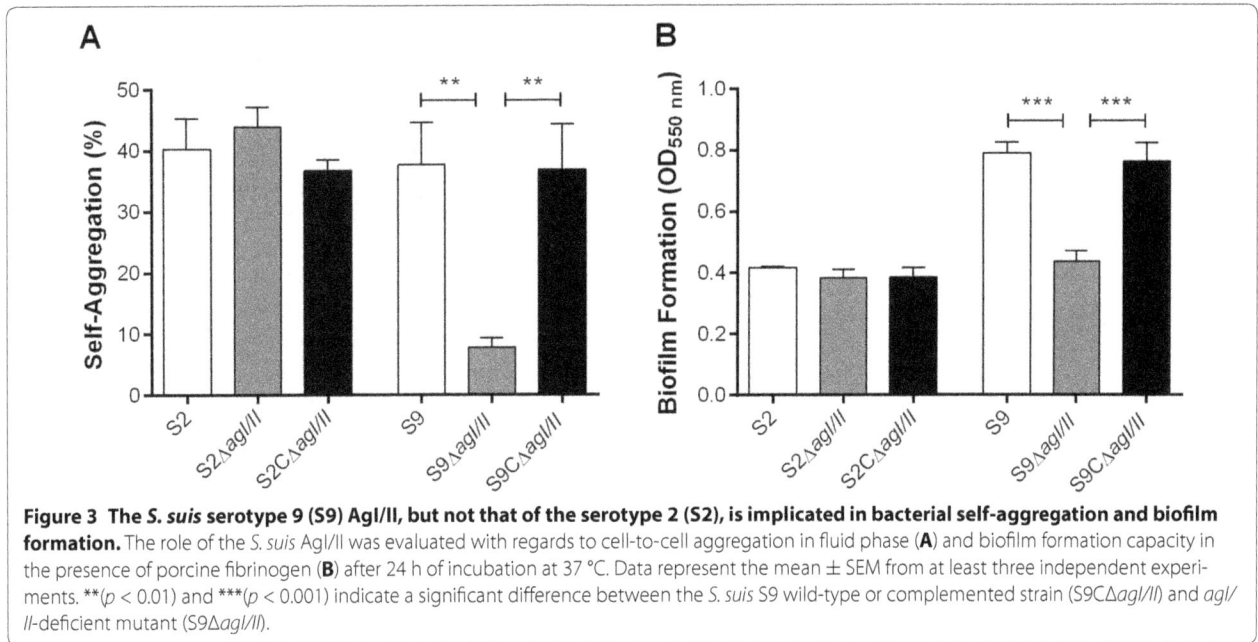

**Figure 3 The *S. suis* serotype 9 (S9) AgI/II, but not that of the serotype 2 (S2), is implicated in bacterial self-aggregation and biofilm formation.** The role of the *S. suis* AgI/II was evaluated with regards to cell-to-cell aggregation in fluid phase (**A**) and biofilm formation capacity in the presence of porcine fibrinogen (**B**) after 24 h of incubation at 37 °C. Data represent the mean ± SEM from at least three independent experiments. **($p < 0.01$) and ***($p < 0.001$) indicate a significant difference between the *S. suis* S9 wild-type or complemented strain (S9CΔ*agI/II*) and *agI/II*-deficient mutant (S9Δ*agI/II*).

Thus, the serotype 9 AgI/II, but not that of serotype 2, is involved in bacterial self-aggregation.

The role of AgI/II in biofilm formation was evaluated for both serotype 2 and 9 in the presence of porcine fibrinogen. The capacity of the serotype 2 strain to form biofilm was relatively low, and no difference was observed in the absence of AgI/II (Figure 3B). On the other hand, the serotype 9 wild-type strain showed a significantly greater capacity to form biofilm than the wild-type serotype 2 strain in the presence of porcine fibrinogen ($p < 0.01$). Furthermore, the serotype 9 AgI/II was significantly involved in this bacterial function ($p < 0.001$) (Figure 3B). The capacity to form biofilm was restored in the complemented S9CΔ*agI/II* strain (Figure 3B). Minimal biofilm formation was observed in the absence of porcine fibrinogen for both the serotype 2 and 9 strains (Additional file 5). Consequently, the serotype 9 AgI/II, but not that of serotype 2, plays an important role in the capacity to form biofilm.

### The *S. suis* AgI/II increases both porcine salivary agglutinin induced-aggregation and adhesion to salivary agglutinins
Salivary agglutinins are major receptors of streptococcal AgI/II [12]. Thus, we investigated the interactions of the *S. suis* serotype 2 and 9 AgI/II with fluid phase (miming the conditions in saliva) and surface-immobilized (miming mucosa such as in the oral cavity) pSAGs. pSAGs collected from pig saliva was obtained at a concentration of 50 µg/mL, which is similar to that usually obtained for human salivary agglutinins [37].

Results showed a significantly more rapid and greater aggregation of both *S. suis* serotype 2 or serotype 9 strains in the presence of pSAGs ($p < 0.05$) (Figure 4). Moreover, this fluid phase pSAG-induced aggregation significantly increased with time ($p < 0.05$) (Figure 4). However, the pSAG-mediated aggregation induced by the serotype 9 strain was significantly higher than that induced by the serotype 2 strain, but only after 60 min of incubation ($p < 0.05$) (Figure 4). AgI/II-deficiency significantly reduced fluid phase pSAG-induced aggregation for both serotypes ($p < 0.05$) (Figures 5A and B), and complementation of AgI/II-deficient mutants restored fluid phase pSAG-induced aggregation ($p < 0.01$) (Figures 5A and B).

The adhesion of *S. suis* to surface-immobilized pSAGs was then evaluated using ELISA. Since background obtained with crude pSAGs was very elevated (data not shown), the gp340-derived peptide SRCRP2, described as the major binding sequence for AgI/II [37], was used. Results showed that deletion of the *S. suis* serotype 2 *agI/II* had no effect on adhesion to SRCRP2 (Figure 5C), while that of serotype 9 significantly reduced adhesion to SRCRP2 ($p < 0.05$), but only at a concentration of 200 µg/mL (Figure 5D). As expected, complementation of the *S. suis* serotype 9 AgI/II-deficient mutant restored adhesion to SRCRP2 (Figure 5D).

Taken together, these results demonstrate that AgI/II promotes pSAG-induced aggregation when in fluid phase for both serotypes, and adhesion to the gp340-derived peptide SRCRP2 at a high concentration for serotype 9 only.

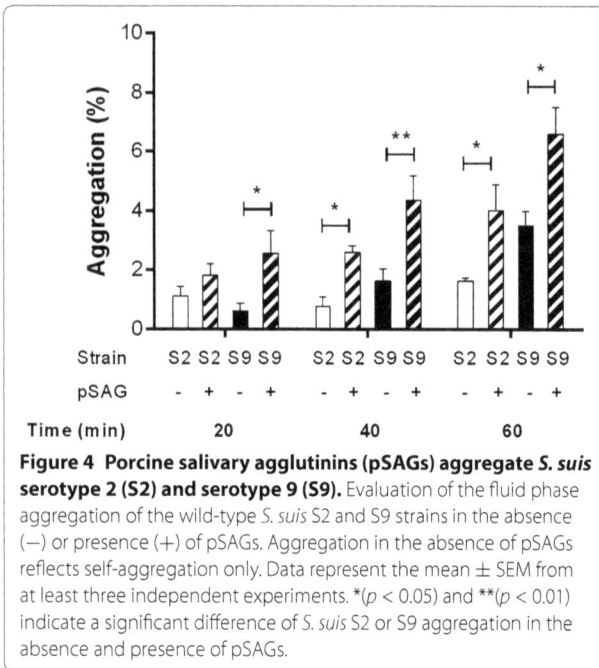

**Figure 4  Porcine salivary agglutinins (pSAGs) aggregate *S. suis* serotype 2 (S2) and serotype 9 (S9).** Evaluation of the fluid phase aggregation of the wild-type *S. suis* S2 and S9 strains in the absence (−) or presence (+) of pSAGs. Aggregation in the absence of pSAGs reflects self-aggregation only. Data represent the mean ± SEM from at least three independent experiments. *($p < 0.05$) and **($p < 0.01$) indicate a significant difference of *S. suis* S2 or S9 aggregation in the absence and presence of pSAGs.

### The *S. suis* AgI/II confers protection to acid stress

Once swallowed, *S. suis* will reach the stomach, in which it must overcome hostile environmental conditions such as low pH. We thus investigated the role of AgI/II and aggregation in resistance to low pH. Acid stress killing assays revealed that the *S. suis* serotype 2 AgI/II was not involved in acid resistance at pH 3 (Figure 6A) nor at pH 5 (Figure 6C). On the other hand, results showed that the S9Δ*agI/II* mutant strain survived significantly less than its wild-type strain ($p < 0.05$) at both pH 3 (Figure 6B) and pH 5 (Figure 6D). Thus, AgI/II confers partial protection to *S. suis* serotype 9, but not to serotype 2, against acidic environments.

### The *S. suis* serotype 9 AgI/II contributes to adhesion to extracellular matrix proteins and to porcine epithelial cells

AgI/II was previously described in other streptococci as binding ECM proteins and contributing to adhesion to and invasion of epithelial cells. Our results showed that while the serotype 2 AgI/II was not involved in adhesion to collagen I, that of the serotype 9 played a significant role ($p < 0.01$) (Figures 7A and B). In accordance, complementation of the S9Δ*agI/II* mutant restored the wild-type phenotype (Figure 7B). Moreover, as previously described with other serotype 2 strains [38], the serotype 2 wild-type strain used in this study (SC84) did not bind porcine fibrinogen (Figure 7C). On the other hand, the serotype 9 wild-type strain did bind to porcine fibrinogen, with absence of AgI/II significantly reducing this ability ($p < 0.05$) (Figure 7D). Once again, complementation of

the S9Δ*agI/II* mutant strain restored this adhesion capacity (Figure 7D). Finally, the deletion of the *S. suis* serotype 9 *agI/II* gene and, to a lesser extent, that of the serotype 2, significantly decreased adhesion to plasma fibronectin ($p < 0.05$) (Figures 7E and F). Consequently, these results demonstrate the importance of AgI/II as a multimodal adhesin for *S. suis* serotype 9 while only playing a minor role for serotype 2.

The role of AgI/II in adhesion to and invasion of porcine tracheal epithelial cells was subsequently investigated. Interestingly, the serotype 9 wild-type strain adhered significantly more to epithelial cells than did the serotype 2 ($p < 0.05$) (Figure 8). Adhesion assays revealed a significant decrease in adhesion to epithelial cells in the absence of AgI/II for the serotype 9 ($p < 0.05$), equivalent to 30% of wild-type strain adhesion, with complementation restoring adhesion (Figure 8). On the other hand, no differences were observed between the *S. suis* serotype 2 wild-type strain and its AgI/II-deficient mutant (Figure 8). Low levels of epithelial cell invasion were observed for both serotypes, with no role of AgI/II being evident (data not shown). Taken together, these results reveal that AgI/II is implicated in adhesion to host proteins and epithelial cells for serotype 9 and, to a lesser extent, for serotype 2.

### Role of AgI/II in colonization of the oral and nasal cavities of pigs

Given that in vitro results demonstrated an important role of AgI/II for *S. suis* serotype 9, we next evaluated the contribution of this protein in colonization using a porcine infection model. Animals were divided into two groups and infected with either the serotype 9 wild-type strain or the AgI/II-deficient mutant by intranasal inoculation. Evaluation of serotype 9 colonization revealed that the number of wild-type strain recovered from the nasal cavities significantly increased over time until day 12 post-infection (p.i.) ($p < 0.05$), whereas the number of S9Δ*agI/II* remained stable throughout the experiment (Figure 9A). Moreover, AgI/II-deficient mutants were recovered in significantly lower numbers from the nasal cavities of pigs on days 5, 8, and 12 p.i. ($p < 0.05$) (Figure 9A). Although the number of serotype 9 wild-type strain and AgI/II-deficient mutant in the nasal cavities of pigs was similar 21 days p.i. (Figure 9A), AgI/II-deficiency resulted in significantly reduced colonization of tonsils ($p < 0.05$) (Figure 9B). Together, these results strongly suggest that the serotype 9 AgI/II contributes to colonization of the porcine respiratory tract.

### Discussion

AgI/II proteins have been extensively described in oral pathogenic streptococci as multimodal adhesion proteins and immunostimulatory components implicated in host

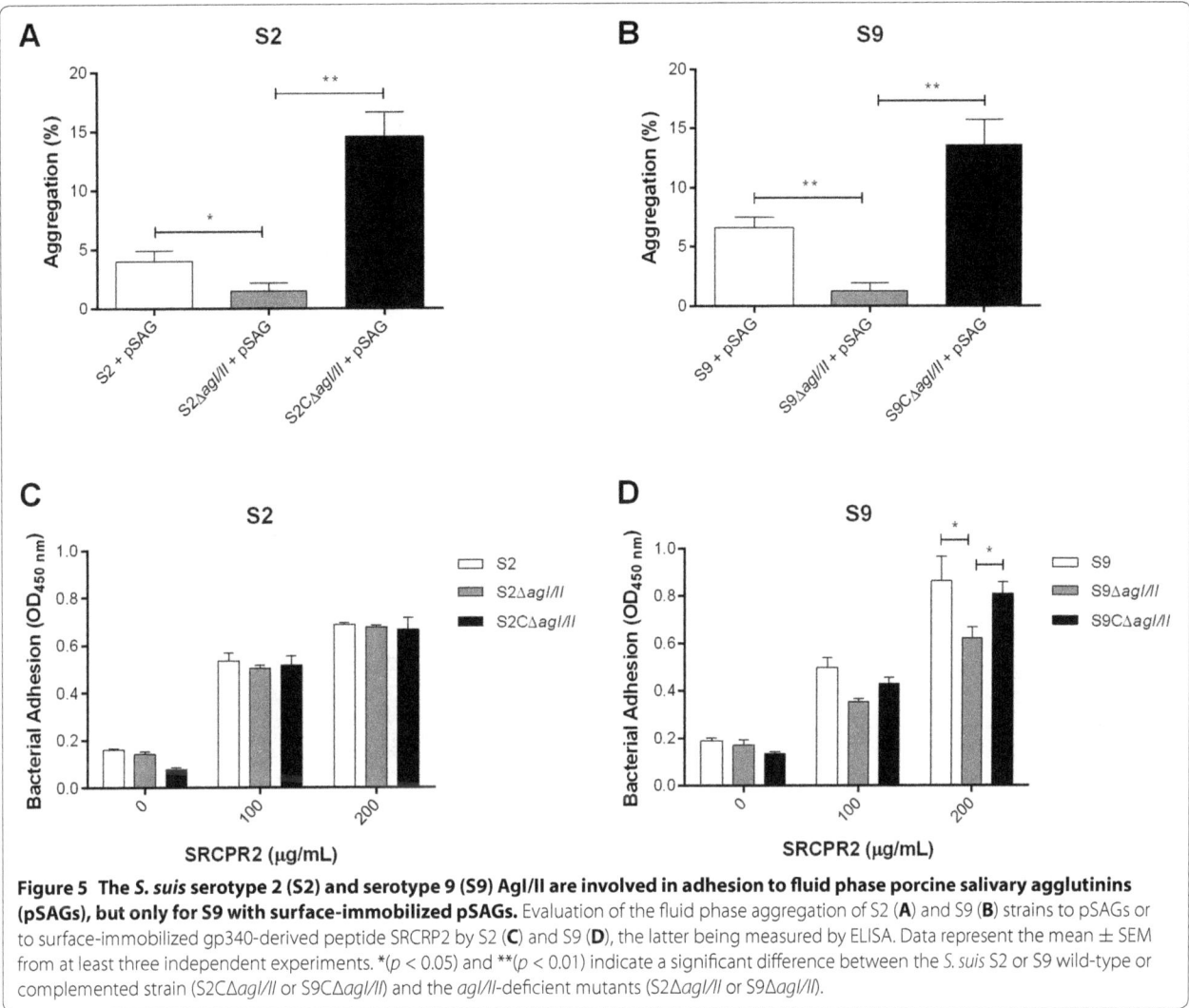

**Figure 5 The S. suis serotype 2 (S2) and serotype 9 (S9) AgI/II are involved in adhesion to fluid phase porcine salivary agglutinins (pSAGs), but only for S9 with surface-immobilized pSAGs.** Evaluation of the fluid phase aggregation of S2 (**A**) and S9 (**B**) strains to pSAGs or to surface-immobilized gp340-derived peptide SRCRP2 by S2 (**C**) and S9 (**D**), the latter being measured by ELISA. Data represent the mean ± SEM from at least three independent experiments. *($p < 0.05$) and **($p < 0.01$) indicate a significant difference between the S. suis S2 or S9 wild-type or complemented strain (S2CΔagI/II or S9CΔagI/II) and the agI/II-deficient mutants (S2ΔagI/II or S9ΔagI/II).

upper respiratory tract and oral cavity persistence and dissemination [11]. In addition, it has been shown that AgI/II proteins potentially play multiple roles in *Streptococcus* adherence, colonization, and microbial community development [11]. These proteins have also been described in pyogenic streptococci, such as *S. pyogenes* and *S. agalactiae*, but they have never been identified in *Streptococcus pneumoniae* [11]. An initial goal of this study was to determine whether *S. suis* possesses these putative virulence factors. We showed that most of the *S. suis* serotype 2 available genomes, including from different STs, possess genes encoding AgI/II. Interestingly, the gene was absent from the ST1 strain P1/7, which is commonly used as a reference for investigation of virulence [6]. We also identified AgI/II-encoding genes in the genome of the Chinese serotype 9 strain D12, in the serotype 9 reference strain 22083, as well as in a collection of 25 serotype 9 field strains (added herein given the limited

number of serotype 9 genomes available), alongside a human isolate, tested by PCR.

It is widely recognized that mobile genetic elements such as insertion sequences, transposons, bacteriophages, plasmids, and genomic islands are key drivers of genomic evolution and bacterial adaptation. Among them, ICEs are chromosomal genetic elements that play an important role in horizontal gene transfer [48]. In both *S. pyogenes* and *S. agalactiae*, AgI/II are encoded by genes carried by ICEs, which can spread not only to other *S. pyogenes* and *S. agalactiae* strains, but also to other streptococci [49, 50]. Meanwhile, different ICEs have been described in *S. suis* [51], of which the 89 K ICE carried by the *S. suis* serotype 2 strain SC84 has been suggested to be responsible, at least in part, for the higher virulence of this strain [52]. Interestingly, results obtained in this study showed that the *S. suis agI/II* genes are mainly carried by ICEs. As such, it may be suggested

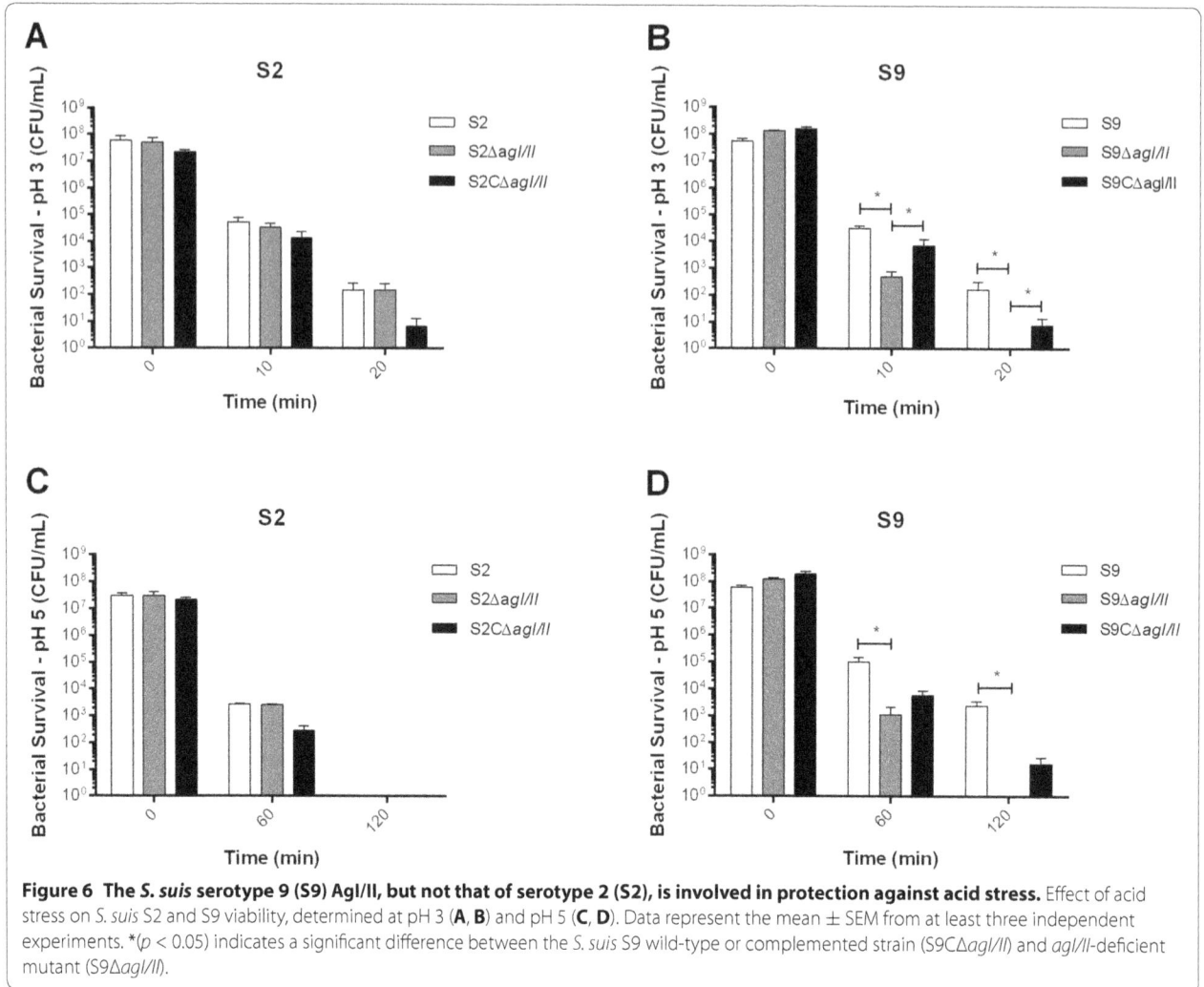

**Figure 6 The _S. suis_ serotype 9 (S9) AgI/II, but not that of serotype 2 (S2), is involved in protection against acid stress.** Effect of acid stress on _S. suis_ S2 and S9 viability, determined at pH 3 (**A**, **B**) and pH 5 (**C**, **D**). Data represent the mean ± SEM from at least three independent experiments. *($p < 0.05$) indicates a significant difference between the _S. suis_ S9 wild-type or complemented strain (S9C$\Delta$agI/II) and agI/II-deficient mutant (S9$\Delta$agI/II).

that acquisition of AgI/II by _S. suis_ occurred via horizontal transfer following acquisition of ICEs.

Persistence of _S. suis_ in the oral cavity may contribute to the pathogenesis of the infection. Our data showed that AgI/II plays an important role in self-aggregation for _S. suis_ serotype 9. This role was even more important in the presence of salivary glycoproteins, such as gp340. It has been previously shown that human salivary gp340 was able to aggregate an untypeable, a serotype 1, and a serotype 2 _S. suis_ strain [15]. However, these strains were negative for the expression of AgI/II as evaluated by immunoblot using a polyclonal antibody raised against the _S. mutans_ proteins [15]. In the present study, we showed that purified soluble pSAGs increase the ability of _S. suis_ to aggregate and that AgI/II played an important role in such interactions for serotype 9 and, to a lesser extent, serotype 2. Fluid phase and surface-immobilized gp340 expose different binding properties and, consequently, differentially recognize adhesive phenotypes of

diverse bacterial species. Herein, we showed that AgI/II also played a role in the _S. suis_ serotype 9 adhesion to the surface-immobilized gp340-derived peptide SRCRP2. Similarly, the AgI/II from _S. suis_ serotype 9 also played an important role in biofilm formation.

The relationship between the saliva-dependent aggregation, attachment to salivary glycoproteins, and biofilm formation in the oral cavity and pathogenesis of the infection caused by pathogenic streptococci is not very clear. On the one hand, aggregation (clumping) may presumably allow "bacterial clearance" from the oral cavity via swallowing [53]. It is usually accepted that the main route of infection for pigs is through the respiratory tract. However, more recently, the oral route (as clearly described in humans) has also been suggested as a portal of entry in pigs [54]. Although a recent report showed that disease could not be induced in an experimental infection by the oral route in post-weaned animals [55], a role of early colonization of the intestine of pre-weaned piglets followed

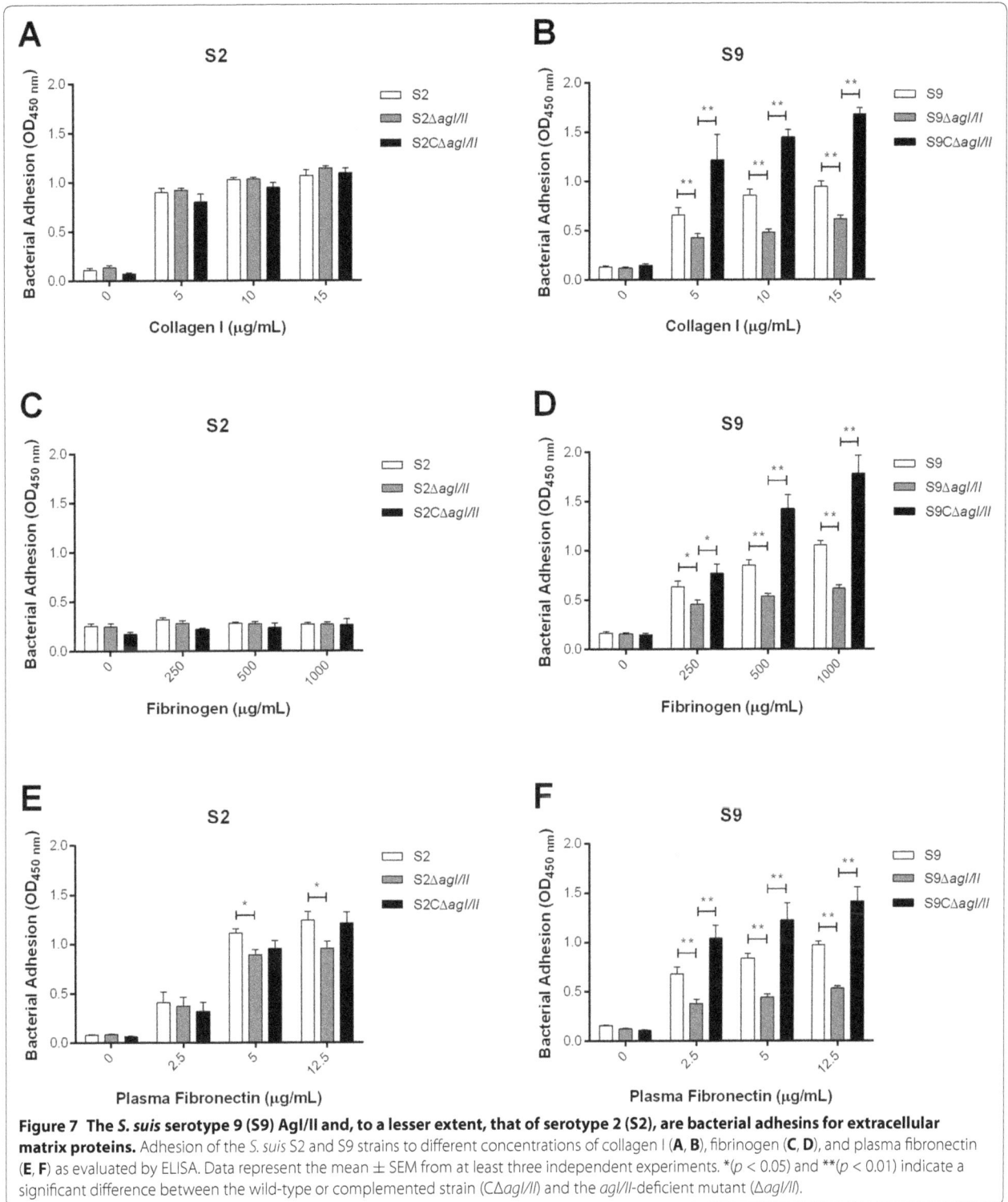

**Figure 7  The *S. suis* serotype 9 (S9) AgI/II and, to a lesser extent, that of serotype 2 (S2), are bacterial adhesins for extracellular matrix proteins.** Adhesion of the *S. suis* S2 and S9 strains to different concentrations of collagen I (**A**, **B**), fibrinogen (**C**, **D**), and plasma fibronectin (**E**, **F**) as evaluated by ELISA. Data represent the mean ± SEM from at least three independent experiments. *($p < 0.05$) and **($p < 0.01$) indicate a significant difference between the wild-type or complemented strain (C$\Delta agI/II$) and the *agI/II*-deficient mutant ($\Delta agI/II$).

by direct invasion through intestinal epithelial cells in animals under post-weaned stress could not be completely ruled out [1]. In the present study, an increased susceptibility to low pH (usually found in the stomach) was observed for *S. suis* serotype 9 in the absence of the *agI/II* gene. As such, it may be hypothesized that AgI/II induces bacterial self-mediated and salivary agglutinin-mediated aggregation and biofilm formation for serotype 9, which would increase, at certain moments, the swallowing of large amounts of bacteria. AgI/II would subsequently

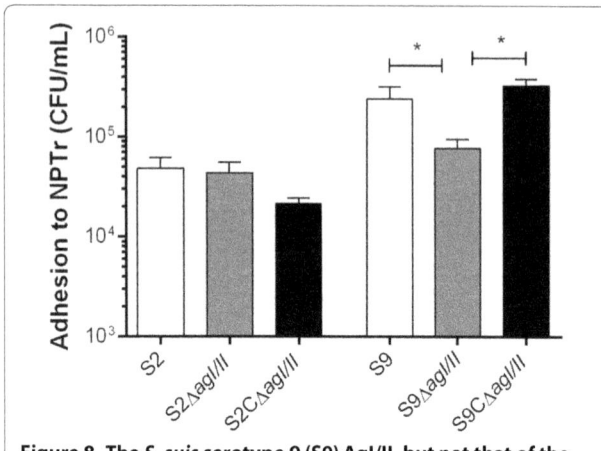

**Figure 8 The *S. suis* serotype 9 (S9) AgI/II, but not that of the serotype 2 (S2), is involved in adhesion to porcine tracheal epithelial cells.** Adhesion of the *S. suis* S2 and S9 strains to NPTr cells after 2 h of incubation with a multiplicity of infection of 10. Data represent the mean ± SEM from at least three independent experiments. *($p < 0.05$) indicates a significant difference between the *S. suis* S9 wild-type or complemented strain (S9C∆*agI/II*) and the *agI/II*-deficient mutant (S9∆*agI/II*).

increase bacterial protection against the low pH of the stomach, thus allowing colonization of the intestine. However, this hypothesis remains to be confirmed.

It has been proposed that adhesion to epithelial cells is one of the most important initial steps of the pathogenesis of the infection caused by *S. suis* [1]. Similarly to other pathogens, *S. suis* is also able to bind ECM components, which have been suggested to be implicated as cell receptors [1]. At least 28 different *S. suis* components have been described to be involved in such interactions

so far [1, 6]. In the present study, it was clearly shown that the AgI/II plays an important role in the adhesion of *S. suis* serotype 9 to collagen I, fibrinogen, and fibronectin. In the case of serotype 2, this protein plays a minimal role in adhesion to fibronectin and none to collagen I. As previously described, the serotype 2 strain was unable to bind fibrinogen [38]. The lack of binding to the latter may also explain differences observed in biofilm formation (in the presence of this protein) between serotype 2 and serotype 9 strains and the important role played by the serotype 9 AgI/II.

The implication of AgI/II in the adhesion to epithelial cells was further evaluated using porcine tracheal epithelial cells as a model [40]. Firstly, it was interesting to note that the serotype 9 wild-type strain presented higher adhesion levels than the serotype 2 strain, a fact that has been previously reported with other porcine cells [54]. A role was attributed to AgI/II in the adhesion of serotype 9 since a significant reduction of adhesion to these cells was observed using the S9∆*agI/II* mutant. This reduction of adhesion could be explained by a reduction in the interactions with ECM components (as described above) or through a direct effect of the AgI/II as an adhesin. In fact, this protein has been described to be directly involved in epithelial cell adhesion and invasion by *S. gordonii* through β1 integrin recognition [56]. Using a different mechanism, this protein was also involved in adhesion/invasion of *S. pyogenes* to these cells [56].

Previous studies showed that the *S. pyogenes* AgI/II is implicated in upper respiratory tract colonization [57]. Since results showed that AgI/II plays important roles in vitro for serotype 9, its implication in colonization of

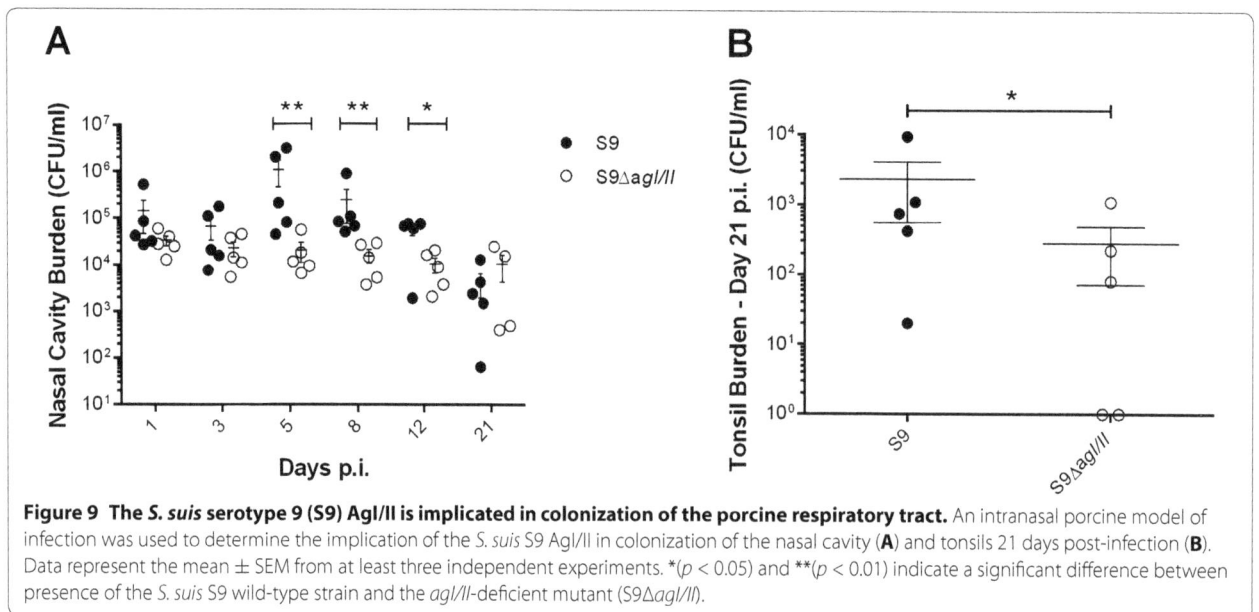

**Figure 9 The *S. suis* serotype 9 (S9) AgI/II is implicated in colonization of the porcine respiratory tract.** An intranasal porcine model of infection was used to determine the implication of the *S. suis* S9 AgI/II in colonization of the nasal cavity (**A**) and tonsils 21 days post-infection (**B**). Data represent the mean ± SEM from at least three independent experiments. *($p < 0.05$) and **($p < 0.01$) indicate a significant difference between presence of the *S. suis* S9 wild-type strain and the *agI/II*-deficient mutant (S9∆*agI/II*).

the upper respiratory tract was investigated in pigs. As previously described, pigs infected by the serotype 9 wild-type strain and its isogenic S9Δ*agI/II* mutant via the intra-nasal route did not develop clinical signs of infection [43]. However, a slight, yet significantly lower colonization of the upper respiratory tract by the mutant strain, and, subsequently at the tonsillar level, was observed, suggesting that this protein may collaborate in bacterial colonization during the first steps of the infection. However, additional studies should be carried out to confirm this hypothesis.

In conclusion, the presence of AgI/II is herein reported for the first time in *S. suis*. This protein appears to play important or limited roles during the first steps of the pathogenesis of the infection caused by serotypes 9 and 2, respectively. Since the gene and protein sequences are highly similar between both serotypes, the observed differences are more difficult to explain than anticipated, and several hypotheses may be proposed. Firstly, a particular motif specific to the gene coding for the serotype 9 AgI/II might be responsible for the phenotypic differences highlighted in this study. Secondly, the *S. suis* serotype 2 and 9 *agI/II* genes are both carried by ICEs, which vary, creating differing genetic contexts and, consequently, differential gene regulation. Thirdly, critical *S. suis* virulence factors still remain poorly known [6]; the lack of a dominant role of the serotype 2 AgI/II observed herein might also be due to compensation by other virulence factors that result in bacterial redundancy [6]. Further studies are presently underway to explore these avenues. Overall, AgI/II may contribute to the colonization of the upper respiratory tract of pigs and could represent important surface bacterial components implicated in the first steps of the pathogenesis of the infection caused by *S. suis*.

## Additional files

**Additional file 1. List of *S. suis* serotype 9 strains used in this study and their characteristics.**

**Additional file 2. List of primers used in this study.** Restriction sites are underlined and in bold.

**Additional file 3. *S. suis* serotype 2 (S2) and serotype 9 (S9) AgI/II amino acid sequence alignment.** Alignment was performed using Vector NTI 11.5. Conserved amino acids appear in light gray and identical amino acids in dark gray.

**Additional file 4. Percent hydrophobicity of the *S. suis* serotype 2 (S2) and serotype 9 (S9) wild-type and *agI/II*-deficient mutant strains.** Hydrophobicity was determined using *n*-hexadecane and the non-encapsulated *S. suis* serotype 2 strain, S2Δ*cpsF*, included as a positive control. Data represent the mean ± SEM from at least three independent experiments.

**Additional file 5. Biofilm formation by the *S. suis* serotype 2 (S2) and serotype 9 (S9) wild-type and *agI/II*-deficient mutant strains in the absence of porcine fibrinogen.** Biofilm formation capacity was quantified after 24 h of incubation at 37 °C in the absence of porcine fibrinogen. Data represent the mean ± SEM from at least three independent experiments.

## Abbreviations
AgI/II: antigen I/II; BCA: bicinchoninic acid; CDS: coding DNA sequence; ECM: extracellular matrix protein; gp340: glycoprotein 340; ICE: integrative and conjugative element; NPTr: newborn porcine tracheal epithelial cell; OD: optical density; PBS: phosphate-buffered saline; p.i.: post-infection; pSAG: porcine salivary agglutinin; SEM: standard error of the mean; ST: sequence type; THB: Todd Hewitt broth.

## Competing interests
The authors declare that they have no competing interests.

## Authors' contributions
Conception of the work: SC, JPA, NF, DG, MG; laboratory techniques: SC, JPA, AD, DR, SL; acquisition, analysis and interpretation of data: SC, JPA, AD, NF, DG, MG; preparation of the manuscript: SC, JPA, MG. All authors read and approved the final manuscript.

## Acknowledgements
The authors would like to thank Prof. Jianguo Xu (Chinese Center for Disease Control and Prevention, Beijing, China), Prof. Christoph Baums (Leipzig University, Germany), and Dr. Anusak Kerdsin (Lampang Province, Thailand) for providing certain of the *S. suis* strains used in this study. The authors would also like to thank Dr. Paula J. Crowley (University of Florida, USA) for providing the human gp340 used herein as a control for pSAG, as well as Dr. Marisa Haenni and Dr. Pierre Châtre (Anses, France) for providing the pOri23 plasmid. The authors would also like to thank Annabelle Mathieu-Denoncourt, Léa Martelet, and Corinne Letendre for technical support.

## Author details
[1] Swine and Poultry Infectious Diseases Research Center (CRIPA), Saint-Hyacinthe, QC, Canada. [2] Groupe de recherche sur les maladies infectieuses en production animale (GREMIP), Department of Pathology and Microbiology, Faculty of Veterinary Medicine, University of Montreal, 3200 Sicotte St., Saint-Hyacinthe, QC J2S 2M2, Canada. [3] Public Health Ontario Laboratory Toronto and Department of Laboratory Medicine and Pathobiology, University of Toronto, Toronto, ON, Canada. [4] Oral Ecology Research Group, Faculty of Dentistry, Laval University, Quebec City, QC, Canada.

## Funding
This study was funded by the Natural Sciences and Engineering Research Council of Canada (NSERC) to MG (Grant #154280).

## References
1. Segura M, Calzas C, Grenier D, Gottschalk M (2016) Initial steps of the pathogenesis of the infection caused by *Streptococcus suis*: fighting against nonspecific defenses. FEBS Lett 590:3772–3799
2. Gottschalk M, Xu J, Calzas C, Segura M (2010) *Streptococcus suis*: a new emerging or an old neglected zoonotic pathogen? Future Microbiol 5:371–391
3. Wertheim HF, Nghia HD, Taylor W, Schultsz C (2009) *Streptococcus suis*: an emerging human pathogen. Clin Infect Dis 48:617–625
4. Goyette-Desjardins G, Auger JP, Xu J, Segura M, Gottschalk M (2014) *Streptococcus suis*, an important pig pathogen and emerging zoonotic agent-an update on the worldwide distribution based on serotyping and sequence typing. Emerg Microbes Infect 3:e45
5. Ye C, Zhu X, Jing H, Du H, Segura M, Zheng H, Kan B, Wang L, Bai X, Zhou Y, Cui Z, Zhang S, Jin D, Sun N, Luo X, Zhang J, Gong Z, Wang X, Wang L, Sun H, Li Z, Sun Q, Liu H, Dong B, Ke C, Yuan H, Wang H, Tian K, Wang Y, Gottschalk M, Xu J (2006) *Streptococcus suis* sequence type 7 outbreak, Sichuan, China. Emerg Infect Dis 12:1203–1208

6.  Segura M, Fittipaldi N, Calzas C, Gottschalk M (2017) Critical *Streptococcus suis* virulence factors: are they all really critical? Trends Microbiol. doi:10.1016/j.tim.2017.02.005

7.  Kerdsin A, Hatrongjit R, Gottschalk M, Takeuchi D, Hamada S, Akeda Y, Oishi K (2015) Emergence of *Streptococcus suis* serotype 9 infection in humans. J Microbiol Immunol Infect. doi:10.1016/j.jmii.2015.06.011

8.  Fittipaldi N, Segura M, Grenier D, Gottschalk M (2012) Virulence factors involved in the pathogenesis of the infection caused by the swine pathogen and zoonotic agent *Streptococcus suis*. Future Microbiol 7:259–279

9.  Tharavichitkul P, Wongsawan K, Takenami N, Pruksakorn S, Fongcom A, Gottschalk M, Khanthawa B, Supajatura V, Takai S (2014) Correlation between PFGE groups and *mrp/epf/sly* genotypes of human *Streptococcus suis* serotype 2 in Northern Thailand. J Pathog 2014:350416

10. Dekker N, Bouma A, Daemen I, Klinkenberg D, van Leengoed L, Wagenaar JA, Stegeman A (2013) Effect of spatial separation of pigs on spread of *Streptococcus suis* serotype 9. PLoS One 8:e61339

11. Brady LJ, Maddocks SE, Larson MR, Forsgren N, Persson K, Deivanayagam CC, Jenkinson HF (2010) The changing faces of *Streptococcus* antigen I/II polypeptide family adhesins. Mol Microbiol 77:276–286

12. Jakubovics NS, Stromberg N, van Dolleweerd CJ, Kelly CG, Jenkinson HF (2005) Differential binding specificities of oral streptococcal antigen I/II family adhesins for human or bacterial ligands. Mol Microbiol 55:1591–1605

13. Madsen J, Mollenhauer J, Holmskov U (2010) Review: Gp-340/DMBT1 in mucosal innate immunity. Innate Immun 16:160–167

14. Kaemmerer E, Schneider U, Klaus C, Plum P, Reinartz A, Adolf M, Renner M, Wolfs TG, Kramer BW, Wagner N, Mollenhauer J, Gassler N (2012) Increased levels of deleted in malignant brain tumours 1 (DMBT1) in active bacteria-related appendicitis. Histopathology 60:561–569

15. Loimaranta V, Jakubovics NS, Hytönen J, Finne J, Jenkinson HF, Strömberg N (2005) Fluid- or surface-phase human salivary scavenger protein gp340 exposes different bacterial recognition properties. Infect Immun 73:2245–2252

16. Casadaban MJ, Cohen SN (1980) Analysis of gene control signals by DNA fusion and cloning in *Escherichia coli*. J Mol Biol 138:179–207

17. Chuzeville S, Dramsi S, Madec JY, Haenni M, Payot S (2015) Antigen I/II encoded by integrative and conjugative elements of *Streptococcus agalactiae* and role in biofilm formation. Microb Pathog 88:1–9

18. Athey TB, Auger JP, Teatero S, Dumesnil A, Takamatsu D, Wasserscheid J, Dewar K, Gottschalk M, Fittipaldi N (2015) Complex population structure and virulence differences among serotype 2 *Streptococcus suis* strains belonging to sequence type 28. PLoS One 10:e0137760

19. Athey TB, Teatero S, Takamatsu D, Wasserscheid J, Dewar K, Gottschalk M, Fittipaldi N (2016) Population structure and antimicrobial resistance profiles of *Streptococcus suis* serotype 2 sequence type 25 strains. PLoS One 11:e0150908

20. Bi D, Xu Z, Harrison EM, Tai C, Wei Y, He X, Jia S, Deng Z, Rajakumar K, Ou HY (2012) ICEberg: a web-based resource for integrative and conjugative elements found in bacteria. Nucleic Acids Res 40:D621–D626

21. Marchler-Bauer A, Derbyshire MK, Gonzales NR, Lu S, Chitsaz F, Geer LY, Geer RC, He J, Gwadz M, Hurwitz DI, Lanczycki CJ, Lu F, Marchler GH, Song JS, Thanki N, Wang Z, Yamashita RA, Zhang D, Zheng C, Bryant SH (2015) CDD: NCBI's conserved domain database. Nucleic Acids Res 43:D222–D226

22. Fimereli DK, Tsirigos KD, Litou ZI, Liakopoulos TD, Bagos PG, Hamodrakas SJ (2012) CW-PRED: a HMM-based method for the classification of cell wall-anchored proteins of Gram-positive bacteria. Artificial intelligence: theories and applications. Springer, Berlin, pp 285–290

23. Krogh A, Larsson B, von Heijne G, Sonnhammer EL (2001) Predicting transmembrane protein topology with a hidden Markov model: application to complete genomes. J Mol Biol 305:567–580

24. Petersen TN, Brunak S, von Heijne G, Nielsen H (2011) SignalP 4.0: discriminating signal peptides from transmembrane regions. Nat Methods 8:785–786

25. Artimo P, Jonnalagedda M, Arnold K, Baratin D, Csardi G, de Castro E, Duvaud S, Flegel V, Fortier A, Gasteiger E, Grosdidier A, Hernandez C, Ioannidis V, Kuznetsov D, Liechti R, Moretti S, Mostaguir K, Redaschi N, Rossier G, Xenarios I, Stockinger H (2012) ExPASy: SIB bioinformatics resource portal. Nucleic Acids Res 40:W597–W603

26. Wilson K (2001) Preparation of genomic DNA from bacteria. Curr Protoc Mol Biol. doi:10.1002/0471142727.mb0204s56

27. Takamatsu D, Osaki M, Sekizaki T (2001) Thermosensitive suicide vectors for gene replacement in *Streptococcus suis*. Plasmid 46:140–148

28. Que YA, Haefliger JA, Francioli P, Moreillon P (2000) Expression of *Staphylococcus aureus* clumping factor A in *Lactococcus lactis* subsp. *cremoris* using a new shuttle vector. Infect Immun 68:3516–3522

29. Chu YW, Cheung TK, Chu MY, Tsang VY, Fung JT, Kam KM, Lo JY (2009) Resistance to tetracycline, erythromycin and clindamycin in *Streptococcus suis* serotype 2 in Hong Kong. Int J Antimicrob Agents 34:181–182

30. Ngo TH, Tran TB, Tran TT, Nguyen VD, Campbell J, Pham HA, Huynh HT, Nguyen VV, Bryant JE, Tran TH, Farrar J, Schultsz C (2011) Slaughterhouse pigs are a major reservoir of *Streptococcus suis* serotype 2 capable of causing human infection in southern Vietnam. PLoS One 6:e17943

31. Li Y, Martinez G, Gottschalk M, Lacouture S, Willson P, Dubreuil JD, Jacques M, Harel J (2006) Identification of a surface protein of *Streptococcus suis* and evaluation of its immunogenic and protective capacity in pigs. Infect Immun 74:305–312

32. Maddocks SE, Wright CJ, Nobbs AH, Brittan JL, Franklin L, Stromberg N, Kadioglu A, Jepson MA, Jenkinson HF (2011) *Streptococcus pyogenes* antigen I/II-family polypeptide AspA shows differential ligand-binding properties and mediates biofilm formation. Mol Microbiol 81:1034–1049

33. Roy D, Grenier D, Segura M, Mathieu-Denoncourt A, Gottschalk M (2016) Recruitment of factor H to the *Streptococcus suis* cell surface is multifactorial. Pathogens 5:E47

34. Bordeleau E, Purcell EB, Lafontaine DA, Fortier LC, Tamayo R, Burrus V (2015) Cyclic di-GMP riboswitch-regulated type IV pili contribute to aggregation of *Clostridium difficile*. J Bacteriol 197:819–832

35. Bonifait L, Grignon L, Grenier D (2008) Fibrinogen induces biofilm formation by *Streptococcus suis* and enhances its antibiotic resistance. Appl Environ Microbiol 74:4969–4972

36. Cook NJ, Hayne SM, Rioja-Lang FC, Schaefer AL, Gonyou HW (2013) The collection of multiple saliva samples from pigs and the effect on adrenocortical activity. Can J Anim Sci 93:329–333

37. Brady LJ, Piacentini DA, Crowley PJ, Oyston PC, Bleiweis AS (1992) Differentiation of salivary agglutinin-mediated adherence and aggregation of mutans streptococci by use of monoclonal antibodies against the major surface adhesin P1. Infect Immun 60:1008–1017

38. Esgleas M, Lacouture S, Gottschalk M (2005) *Streptococcus suis* serotype 2 binding to extracellular matrix proteins. FEMS Microbiol Lett 244:33–40

39. Bikker FJ, Ligtenberg AJ, Nazmi K, Veerman EC, van't Hof W, Bolscher JG, Poustka A, Nieuw Amerongen AV, Mollenhauer J (2002) Identification of the bacteria-binding peptide domain on salivary agglutinin (gp-340/DMBT1), a member of the scavenger receptor cysteine-rich superfamily. J Biol Chem 277:32109–32115

40. Wang Y, Gagnon CA, Savard C, Music N, Srednik M, Segura M, Lachance C, Bellehumeur C, Gottschalk M (2013) Capsular sialic acid of *Streptococcus suis* serotype 2 binds to swine influenza virus and enhances bacterial interactions with virus-infected tracheal epithelial cells. Infect Immun 81:4498–4508

41. Roy D, Fittipaldi N, Dumesnil A, Lacouture S, Gottschalk M (2014) The protective protein Sao (surface antigen one) is not a critical virulence factor for *Streptococcus suis* serotype 2. Microb Pathog 67–68:31–35

42. Auger JP, Fittipaldi N, Benoit-Biancamano MO, Segura M, Gottschalk M (2016) Virulence studies of different sequence types and geographical origins of *Streptococcus suis* serotype 2 in a mouse model of infection. Pathogens 5:E48

43. Pallarés FJ, Halbur PG, Schmitt CS, Roth JA, Opriessnig T, Thomas PJ, Kinyon JM, Murphy D, Frank DE, Hoffman LJ (2003) Comparison of experimental models for *Streptococcus suis* infection of conventional pigs. Can J Vet Res 67:225–228

44. Gottschalk M, Higgins R, Boudreau M (1993) Use of polyvalent coagglutination reagents for serotyping of *Streptococcus suis*. J Clin Microbiol 31:2192–2194

45. Fittipaldi N, Broes A, Harel J, Kobisch M, Gottschalk M (2003) Evaluation and field validation of PCR tests for detection of *Actinobacillus pleuropneumoniae* in subclinically infected pigs. J Clin Microbiol 41:5085–5093

46. Hedberg PJ, Leonard BA, Ruhfel RE, Dunny GM (1996) Identification and characterization of the genes of *Enterococcus faecalis* plasmid pCF10 involved in replication and in negative control of pheromone-inducible conjugation. Plasmid 35:46–57

47. Chen C, Tang J, Dong W, Wang C, Feng Y, Wang J, Zheng F, Pan X, Liu D, Li M, Song Y, Zhu X, Sun H, Feng T, Guo Z, Ju A, Ge J, Dong Y, Sun W, Jiang Y, Wang J, Yan J, Yang H, Wang X, Gao GF, Yang R, Wang J, Yu J (2007)

A glimpse of streptococcal toxic shock syndrome from comparative genomics of *Streptococcus suis* 2 Chinese isolates. PLoS One 2:e315

48. Wozniak RA, Waldor MK (2010) Integrative and conjugative elements: mosaic mobile genetic elements enabling dynamic lateral gene flow. Nat Rev Microbiol 8:552–563

49. Puymège A, Bertin S, Chuzeville S, Guédon G, Payot S (2013) Conjugative transfer and cis-mobilization of a genomic island by an integrative and conjugative element of *Streptococcus agalactiae*. J Bacteriol 195:1142–1151

50. Sitkiewicz I, Green NM, Guo N, Mereghetti L, Musser JM (2011) Lateral gene transfer of streptococcal ICE element RD2 (region of difference 2) encoding secreted proteins. BMC Microbiol 11:65

51. Palmieri C, Princivalli MS, Brenciani A, Varaldo PE, Facinelli B (2011) Different genetic elements carrying the *tet(W)* gene in two human clinical isolates of *Streptococcus suis*. Antimicrob Agents Chemother 55:631–636

52. Zhang A, Yang M, Hu P, Wu J, Chen B, Hua Y, Yu J, Chen H, Xiao J, Jin M (2011) Comparative genomic analysis of *Streptococcus suis* reveals significant genomic diversity among different serotypes. BMC Genom 12:523

53. Scannapieco FA (1994) Saliva-bacterium interactions in oral microbial ecology. Crit Rev Oral Biol Med 5:203–248

54. Ferrando ML, de Greeff A, van Rooijen WJ, Stockhofe-Zurwieden N, Nielsen J, Wichgers Schreur PJ, Pannekoek Y, Heuvelink A, van der Ende A, Smith H, Schultsz C (2015) Host-pathogen interaction at the intestinal mucosa correlates with zoonotic potential of *Streptococcus suis*. J Infect Dis 212:95–105

55. Warneboldt F, Sander SJ, Beineke A, Valentin-Weigand P, Kamphues J, Baums CG (2016) Clearance of *Streptococcus suis* in stomach contents of differently fed growing pigs. Pathogens 5:E56

56. Nobbs AH, Shearer BH, Drobni M, Jepson MA, Jenkinson HF (2007) Adherence and internalization of *Streptococcus gordonii* by epithelial cells involves beta1 integrin recognition by SspA and SspB (antigen I/II family) polypeptides. Cell Microbiol 9:65–83

57. Franklin L, Nobbs AH, Bricio-Moreno L, Wright CJ, Maddocks SE, Sahota JS, Ralph J, O'Connor M, Jenkinson HF, Kadioglu A (2013) The AgI/II family adhesin AspA is required for respiratory infection by *Streptococcus pyogenes*. PLoS One 8:e62433

# 15

# Recall T cell responses to bluetongue virus produce a narrowing of the T cell repertoire

José-Manuel Rojas[1], Teresa Rodríguez-Calvo[1,2] and Noemí Sevilla[1*] (ID)

## Abstract

In most viral infections, recall T cell responses are critical for protection. The magnitude of these secondary responses can also affect the CD8 and CD4 epitope repertoire diversity. Bluetongue virus (BTV) infection in sheep elicits a T cell response that contributes to viremia control and could be relevant for cross-protection between BTV serotypes. Here, we characterized CD4$^+$ and CD8$^+$ T cell responses during primary and recall responses. During primary immune responses, both CD4$^+$ and CD8$^+$ T cell populations expanded by 14 days post-infection (dpi). CD4$^+$ T cell populations showed a lower peak of expansion and prolonged contraction phase compared to CD8$^+$ T cell populations. Recall responses to BTV challenge led to BTV-specific expansion and activation of CD8$^+$ but not of CD4$^+$ T cells. The evolution of the BTV-specific TCR repertoire was also characterized in response to VP7 peptide stimulation. Striking differences in repertoire development were noted over the time-course of infection. During primary responses, a broader repertoire was induced for MHC-I and MHC-II epitopes. However, during memory responses, a narrowed repertoire was activated towards a dominant motif in VP7 comprising amino acids 139–291. Monocytes were also examined, and expanded during acute infection resolution. In addition, pro-inflammatory cytokine levels increased after BTV inoculation and persisted throughout the experiment, indicative of a prolonged inflammatory state during BTV infections. These findings could have implications for vaccine design as the narrowing memory T cell repertoire induced after BTV re-infection could lead to the development of protective immunodominant TCR repertoires that differs between individual sheep.

## Introduction

The role of memory T cells is to help protect the host during secondary antigen encounters. These secondary responses can reinforce the quantity and quality of the immune response against the challenging pathogen [1]. This is reflected by the increased frequency of antigen-specific T cells able to mount accelerated responses, with shorter antigenic stimulation leading to efficient and quicker antigen clearance. However, T cell exhaustion can also occur in the presence of saturated levels of antigen or even after repetitive natural or vaccination exposures.

In particular, an understanding of T cell recruitment/expansion process during the recall response may have significant implications for effective control strategies. Different mechanisms of memory recruitment have been postulated. A memory population in which highly effective clones predominate may occur as a stochastic expansion, more likely maintaining the T cell diversity, which was shown to be beneficial for virus control [2]. Alternatively, by deterministic selection, high quality clones in the memory population may be expanded by antigen-driven mechanisms [3], narrowing the T cell repertoire [4].

Bluetongue virus (BTV) is the prototype member of the genus *Orbivirus* within the *Reoviridae* family, transmitted by *Culicoides* midges [5]. BTV infects ruminants, causing an acute disease with high morbidity and mortality [6]. The BTV genome is composed of 10 segments

*Correspondence: sevilla@inia.es
[1] Centro de Investigación en Sanidad Animal (CISA-INIA), Instituto Nacional de Investigación Agraria y Alimentaria, Ctra Algete a El Casar km 8, Valdeolmos, 28130 Madrid, Spain
Full list of author information is available at the end of the article

of double-stranded RNA encoding 4 non-structural and 7 structural proteins that is enclosed by a complex capsid structure [7, 8]. There are at least 27 serotypes circulating based on the specific neutralizing antibodies raised against VP2 [9–11]. The immune response against BTV is characterized by the induction of humoral responses, neutralizing antibodies, and cellular immunity that contributes significantly to protection in vaccinated animals [12–15]. Virus-specific $CD8^+$ cytotoxic T lymphocytes (CTL) are key components of the immune response, inducing cross-protection among different serotypes [16, 17]. In nature, high frequency of repeated BTV infections due to successive bites by biting midges may occur, meaning successive challenges with other BTV serotypes (heterologous virus) or with the same serotype (homologous virus).

Immune responses to viral infections are not mounted in immunological isolation, as the immune response to one virus may condition the host to elicit an altered immune response against a homologous or heterologous virus. Using successive challenge with BTV-8, we investigated the expansion of VP7-specific $CD8^+$ and $CD4^+$ T cells [18]. Furthermore, we studied the inflammatory response during recall responses. Here, we show that recall responses with BTV led to BTV-specific expansion and activation of $CD8^+$ but not of $CD4^+$ T cells. Interestingly, during primary responses, a broader repertoire of T cell epitopes was induced. However, during memory responses, a narrowed repertoire was activated towards a dominant epitope in VP7.

## Materials and methods

### Virus

A BTV-8 isolate (Belgium/06) from an infected calf in the 2006 Belgium outbreak was used in this study [19]. BTV-8 was expanded in baby hamster kidney (BHK) cells (ATCC CCL-10) and titered in semi-solid agar medium in Vero cells (ATCC CCL-81) as described [20]. BTV-8 inactivation with binary ethylenimine (BEI) was performed as described [21].

### Animals and experimental design

Three-month old BTV naive female Mallorquina sheep were kept in a disease-secure isolation facility (BSL3) at the Centro de Investigación en Salud Animal (CISA), in strict accordance with the recommendations in the guidelines of the Code for Methods and Welfare Considerations in Behavioural Research with Animals (Directive 86/609EC; RD1201/2005) and all efforts were made to minimize suffering. Experiments were approved by the Committee on the Ethics of Animal Experiments (CEEA) (Permit Number: 10/142792.9/12) of the Spanish Instituto Nacional de Investigación y Tecnología Agraria

y Alimentaria (INIA) and the "Comisión de ética estatal de bienestar animal" (Permit Numbers: CBS2012/06 and PROEX 228/14). An acclimatization period of 2 weeks was observed, during which the animals were monitored daily for general health status prior to the experiment.

Animals ($n = 8$) were inoculated subcutaneously with $1 \times 10^5$ pfu BTV-8 three times at 28 day intervals. Two naive controls were inoculated with PBS at the same time points as the control group.

### Peripheral blood mononuclear cell isolation

Venous blood from BTV-8 infected sheep was collected on days 0, 7, 14, 28, 35, 56, 63 and 70, and PBMC were isolated by standard centrifugation methods on Ficoll [18]. Flow cytometry studies were performed on freshly isolated PBMC. Remaining PBMC were frozen and stored in liquid nitrogen until use.

### Peptides and antibodies

Peptides from BTV-8 VP7 protein (ACJ06230) were selected as described in [18] and synthesized by Altabiosciences (Birmingham, UK) (Table 1 corresponds to oligonucleotide sequences). All peptides were resuspended in DMSO and stored at $-80$ °C. The following directly conjugated antibodies were used in this study: anti-sheep CD4 (44.38); anti-sheep CD8 (38.65); anti-human (cross-reactive with sheep) CD14 (TÜK4) (all from Biorad); anti-BTV-VP7 (CF-J-BTV-MAB-10ML).

### Flow cytometry

Surface flow cytometry stainings were performed using staining buffer (PBS + 2% FBS + 0.05% sodium azide). PBMC were washed twice, stained with antibodies for 20 min on ice, and finally washed twice in staining buffer. For BTV-VP7 intracellular staining, PBMC were fixed in 4% paraformaldehyde for 10 min, permeabilized and washed 3 times in staining buffer containing 0.2% saponin and incubated for 30 min on ice with antibody diluted in staining buffer supplemented with 0.2% saponin. For all stainings appropriate isotype and fluorescence minus one controls were included. Acquisitions were performed on a BD FACScalibur flow cytometer and analysis using FlowJo software (Tree Star Inc, USA).

**Table 1  Primer sequences for real-time RT-PCR**

| Gene | Forward (5′–3′) | Reverse (5′–3′) |
| --- | --- | --- |
| IL-6 | CCTCCAGGAACCCAGCTATG | GGAGACAGCGAGTGGACTGAA |
| IL-1β | CGAACATGTCTTCCGTGATG | TCTCTGTCCTGGGAGTTTGCAT |
| IL-12 | CGTGATGGAAGCTGTGCAC | CTTTCCTGGACCTGAACAC |
| CXCL10 | GCTCATCACCCTGAGCTGTT | AGCTGTCAGTAGCAAGGCTA |

## RNA isolation, reverse transcription and quantitative real-time PCR to determine viral load

RNA from total blood was obtained using Trizol Reagent Solution (Thermo Fisher Scientific) and following the manufacturer's protocol. Viral RNA loads were determined by amplification of segment 5 as described [12, 22] using the QIAGEN OneStep RT-PCR kit (QIAGEN) or the Ambion AgPath-ID One-Step RT-PCR (Thermo Fisher Scientific).

## Expression of immune genes by real time PCR

Total RNA was extracted from PBMC isolated at different times post-infection using Trizol Reagent Solution (Thermo Fisher Scientific). Isolated RNA was treated with DNase I (BioLabs New England) according to the manufacturer's protocol. 1 μg of RNA was used to obtain cDNA using the SuperScript™ II reverse Transcriptase (Thermo Fisher Scientific) and oligo $(dT)_{12-18}$ (0.5 μg/mL). To evaluate the levels of transcription of IL-12, IL-6, CXCL10 and IL-1β, real time was performed in a LightCycler 480 System instrument (Roche) using SYBR Green PCR core Reagents (Applied Biosystems) and specific primers (Table 1). Each sample was measured under the following conditions: 10 min at 95 °C followed by 45 amplification cycles (15 s at 95 °C and 1 min at 60 °C). The expression of individual genes was normalized to relative expression of ovine GPDH gene and the expression levels were calculated using $2^{-\Delta Ct}$ method, where $\Delta Ct$ is determined by subtracting the GPDH value from the target Ct. A melting curve for each PCR fluorescence reading, every degree between 60 and 95 °C, was determined to ensure that only a single product had been amplified.

## ELISA for sheep IFN-γ

PBMC ($2 \times 10^5$ per well) were stimulated for 24 h in U-bottom 96 well plates with BEI-BTV-8 (equivalent to $1 \times 10^5$ pfu prior to inactivation), concanavalin-A (2.5 μg/mL) as the positive control, VP7 peptide (10 μg/mL), or an equivalent volume of DMSO as the negative control. IFN-γ production in culture supernatants was then tested using a commercially available IFN-γ ELISA kit (Mabtech, Sweden). The ELISA detection limit was 20 pg/mL. Data were normalized to $1 \times 10^6$ PBMC.

## Statistical analysis

Statistical analysis was performed using Prism 5.0 software (Graphpad Software Inc, USA). Levels of significance were *$p < 0.05$; **$p < 0.01$; ***$p < 0.001$.

## Results
### Clinical responses

In order to evaluate and compare the expansion of the immune response after primary and secondary BTV infections, one in vivo experiment with 10 animals was done, in which 8 sheep were inoculated sc with BTV-8 three times at 28-day intervals (see "Materials and methods"). All animals inoculated with BTV-8 developed clinical signs and fever (> 40 °C during four successive days) at days 5–8 post-infection (Figure 1). The first sign of the disease was a slight to moderate increase in respiratory rate, accompanied by inflammation of the oral mucosa. After day 9, temperature declined to normal levels and disease signs were detectable up to day 15, achieving full recovery afterwards. BTV-8 inoculation at day 28 and 56 did not increase rectal temperature nor produce clinical signs, suggesting that an efficient BTV-specific immune response had been elicited in BTV-infected sheep. Control PBS-inoculated sheep did not show any clinical signs or fever during the experiment.

## Expansion of PBMC after challenge with BTV in primary and secondary responses

To evaluate the immune response after primary and secondary BTV infections, and according to the scheme indicated above, total PBMC were isolated from peripheral blood and quantified at different times post-inoculation. During primary response, a significant decrease in the number of PBMC was detected at day 7 post-infection (D7pi) returning to basal levels by D14pi (Figure 2A). Twenty-eight days later, sheep were inoculated with the same amount of BTV-8 sc (secondary BTV infection) and the number of PBMC was determined. In contrast to the primary infection, PBMC levels did not decrease 7 days after the second infection (D35pi) and significantly increased 14 days after this second infection (D42pi), followed by a contraction period. Similar results were obtained after the third challenge. Because BTV may infect lymphocytes causing cell death [23], we next asked whether BTV infection of PBMC would result

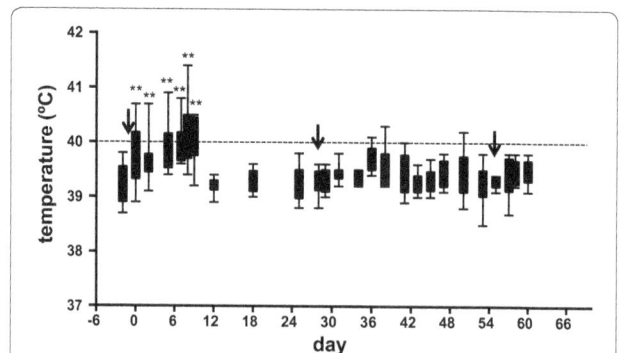

**Figure 1 Temperature measurements after primary and recall BTV-8 infections in sheep.** Sheep rectal temperatures were measured prior to BTV-8 sc inoculation and after primary and recall infections (indicated by red arrows). ** $p < 0.01$; one-way ANOVA test with Bonferroni's post-test (timepoints vs day −2).

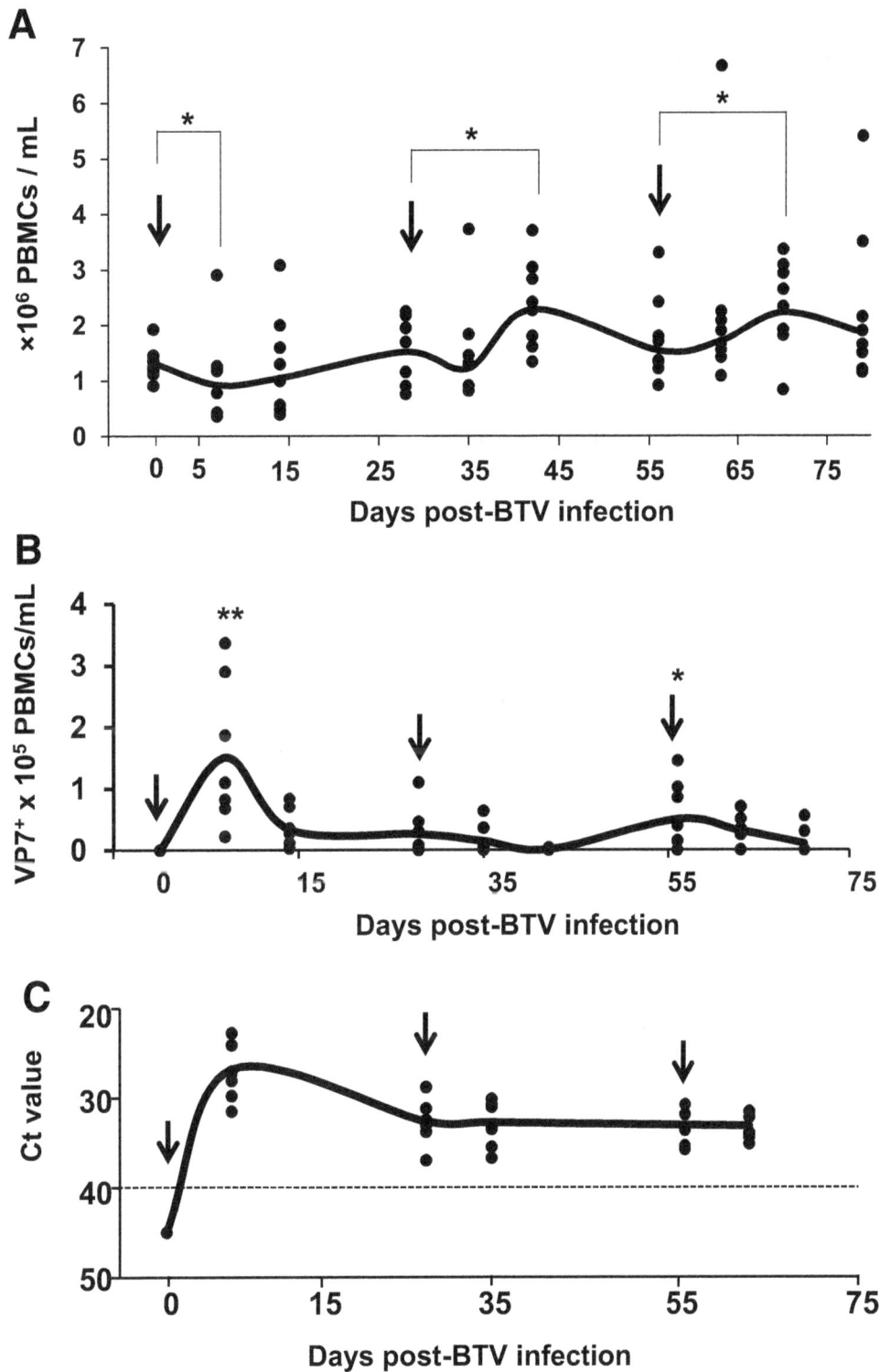

**Figure 2 Expansion of PBMC and viral load during acute and recall BTV infection.** Sheep were inoculated with BTV-8 three times at 28 day intervals (see "Materials and methods" section) and bled at different times post-inoculation. **A** Average count of PBMC relative to pre-BTV infection at different days post-inoculation. The arrow indicates the inoculation day. * $p < 0.05$; Mann-Whitney test (timepoint vs inoculation time). **B** Number of PBMC/mL of blood that were positive for VP7 by flow cytometry staining at different days post-BTV infection. Arrows indicate inoculation days. * $p < 0.05$, ** $p < 0.01$; Mann–Whitney test (timepoint vs day 0). **C** Whole blood was collected at different days post-BTV infection. Total RNA was extracted and RT-qPCR for BTV segment 5 was performed as indicated in the "Materials and methods". The results are expressed as Ct. The cut-off is indicated with a dotted lined (Ct $= 40$ according to [22]).

in PBMC depletion after primary infection. PBMC were labeled with a specific monoclonal antibody against the VP7 protein and directly coupled to a fluorochrome probe. A significant amount of PBMC were positive for VP7 protein by flow cytometry analysis (average of $1.51 \times 10^5 \pm 0.2$ PBMCs/mL from 8 sheep infected with BTV-8) by D7pi (Figure 2B), suggesting that the D7pi decrease in PBMC numbers might be due to BTV-induced cell death. The number of VP7 positive cells did not increase after secondary infection but it was maintained until at least D45pi. After the third infection, a significant increase of VP7 positive PBMC was observed, suggesting that a brief round of BTV infection occurred shortly after inoculation (D3pi). This contrasts with primary infection where the peak of VP7 positive cells was obtained at D7pi. To assess virus replication, blood samples for each sheep were examined for viral genome by RT-qPCR. A peak in viremia was found at D7pi (average Ct value of $26.82 \pm 3$) followed by a slow reduction in circulating virus. Importantly, the infection was not completely cleared by the end of the experiment (average Ct value $33.1 \pm 1.4$ at D63pi) (Figure 2C). New viremia peaks were nonetheless never detected after secondary or tertiary challenge. Taken together these data suggest that during secondary BTV infections PBMC expanded but BTV infection was not completely controlled.

### Re-exposure to virus controls the magnitude of the CD4 and CD8 T cell responses

Given that total PBMC numbers expanded 14 days after acute (D14pi vs D7pi) and secondary infections with BTV (D42pi vs D28pi and D56pi vs D70pi), we examined whether an increase in $CD4^+$ or $CD8^+$ T cell populations could explain this expansion. $CD4^+$ T cell numbers started to increase significantly at D7pi, maintaining this trend up to D28pi (Figure 3A). Surprisingly, the population of $CD4^+$ T cells slightly declined 7 days after the second infection (D35pi) but increased 15 days later (D42pi). After the third BTV challenge, the $CD4^+$ T cell population did not show any significant changes in numbers although at D15 post-third infection (D70pi) $CD4^+$ T cell numbers slightly increased. In general, $CD8^+$ T cell responses peak at about 1 week post-infection in most viral infections, and soon thereafter, virus-specific T cells eliminate the virus [24, 25]. Interestingly, $CD8^+$ T cell responses peaked at D14 post-BTV challenge both in acute (D14pi) and secondary responses (D42pi and D70pi) (Figure 3B). $CD8^+$ T cells thus proliferated in response to the virus, independently of primary or secondary infections. The decrease in $CD8^+$ T cell numbers following D15pi expansion led to a subsequent significant decrease in the CD8:CD4 T cell ratio (Figure 3C). Although repeated infections slightly increased $CD8^+$

T cell numbers (D42pi and D70pi), CD4:CD8 T cell ratios were unchanged as $CD4^+$ T cell numbers slightly increased concomitantly. This unchanged CD8:CD4 T cell ratio indicated that $CD8^+$ T cells did not significantly proliferate after antigen re-exposure. Thus, our findings indicate that levels of central $CD8^+$ memory T cells did not stabilize after primary infection, suggesting that in the absence of further infections the memory level of $CD8^+$ T cells would continually decline.

### Characterization of T cell responses after primary and secondary infections

We next sought to analyze the BTV-specific $CD4^+$ and $CD8^+$ T cell responses. The global T cell responses were first evaluated to determine differences in the overall magnitude of the responses to primary and secondary BTV infections. To this end, PBMC from BTV-infected sheep were isolated at different times post-infection, stimulated in vitro with inactivated-BTV-8, and IFN-γ production was evaluated by ELISA. A significant production of IFN-γ was found at D15pi after primary infection (D0) (Figure 4). Recall infections also induced significant IFN-γ responses 7 and 15 days after the second or third challenge (D35pi, D63pi and D70pi). In addition, the amplitude of these T cell responses increased over time, suggesting that there was a prolonged activation of T cell responses during the observed period, probably due to inefficient virus clearance that might continuously activate $CD8^+$ T cells responses.

T cell recognition of infected cells is accomplished by the interaction of clonally distributed TCR on effector cells with the complex of viral peptide/MHC class I-II on infected cells [26, 27]. The specificity of T cells for a particular MHC/peptide combination determines, at least in part, the TCR repertoires within an antigen-specific population. In order to determine the spectrum of the TCR repertoire against VP7 during primary and recall responses, PBMC from BTV-infected sheep were stimulated in vitro with peptides that comprise the main T cell epitopes in VP7 protein (Figure 5A) [18], and the production of IFN-γ was measured by ELISA. During acute infection, most T cells synthesized IFN-γ in response to most of the epitopes (D7pi and D14pi) (Figure 5B), showing a broad distribution of TCR diversity. This was also observed after secondary response, in which T cell responses to all the epitopes were detected. However, by D70pi, after the third BTV challenge, a T cell response bias towards 3 MHC-I epitopes [VP(175), VP(245) and VP(283)] and 2 MHC-II epitope [VP(139) and VP(181)] became apparent. All these epitopes were grouped in a cluster of 100 amino acids of VP7, indicating a restriction in the TCR diversity that responds to BTV after repeated infections and thereby a narrowing of the TCR repertoire during memory responses.

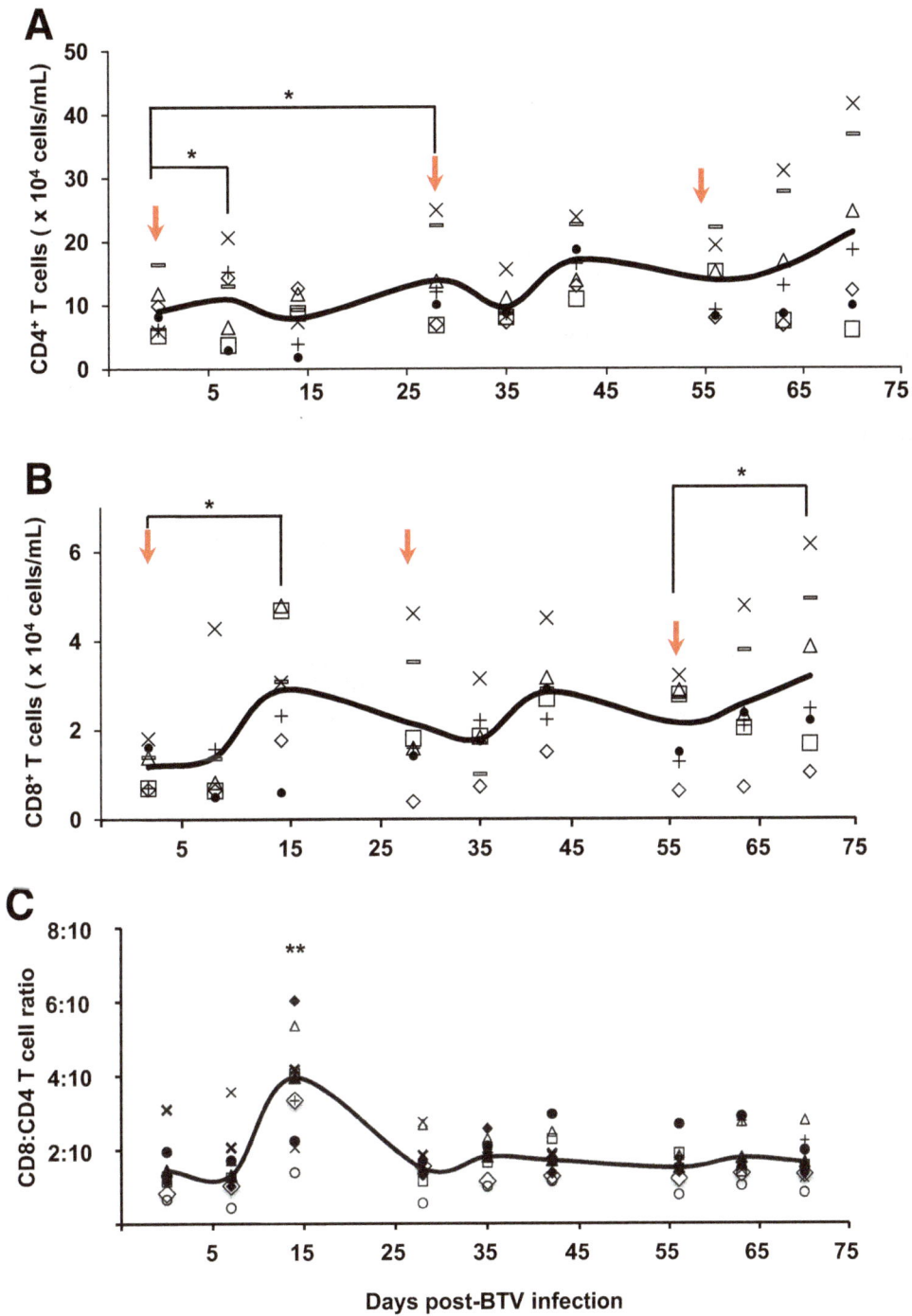

**Figure 3  CD4$^+$ and CD8$^+$ T cell expansion during acute and recall BTV infection.** PBMC were obtained at the indicated time points after primary, secondary or tertiary BTV infection (indicated by an arrow) and staining for CD4 and CD8-T cell was done by flow cytometry (see "Materials and methods"). **A** Number of CD4$^+$-T cells over time in PBMC of individual sheep. * $p < 0.05$; Mann-Whitney test (timepoints vs inoculation time). **B** Number of CD8$^+$-T cells in PBMC over time of individual sheep. * $p < 0.05$; Mann-Whitney test (time points vs inoculation time). **C** Kinetics of specific CD8:CD4 T-cell ratio. The number of CD8$^+$ T cells was divided by the number of CD4$^+$ T-cells during the time course of infection. ** $p < 0.01$; Mann-Whitney test (day 14 vs all timepoints).

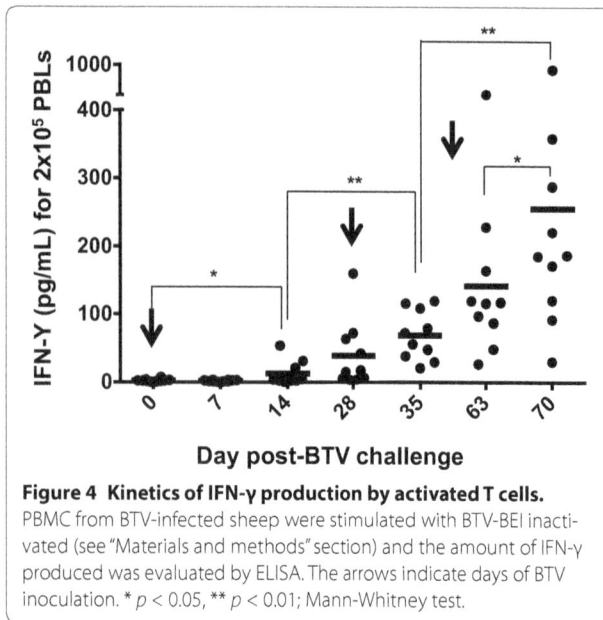

**Figure 4 Kinetics of IFN-γ production by activated T cells.**
PBMC from BTV-infected sheep were stimulated with BTV-BEI inactivated (see "Materials and methods" section) and the amount of IFN-γ produced was evaluated by ELISA. The arrows indicate days of BTV inoculation. * $p < 0.05$, ** $p < 0.01$; Mann-Whitney test.

### Persistent inflammation during acute and secondary responses

Upon virus infection, monocytes play a role in initiating the adaptive immune response, and affect Th1/Th2 polarization by producing proinflammatory and immune-modulatory cytokines [28]. Therefore, we studied the magnitude of the monocyte response during primary and secondary BTV responses by flow cytometry in PBMC from sheep infected with BTV. Analysis of CD14-expressing cells (Figure 6A) revealed a steady increase in CD14$^+$ monocytes during infection. This increase was transient and started to decline by D28pi, right after the second challenge with BTV. By day 15 after the second BTV challenge (D42pi), CD14$^+$ cell numbers increased followed by a progressive decline by D56pi. After the third BTV challenge (D56pi), the population of CD14-expressing cells increased until the experiment ended. To study the cytokine/chemokine response during BTV infection, we determined the amount of mRNA expressed by PBMC of BTV-infected sheep at different time points by RT-qPCR. IL-6 and IL-1β were chosen as representative pro-inflammatory cytokines [29, 30]. IL-6 transcription was significantly up-regulated during primary infection, starting at D7pi (Figure 6B) and during the course of the second BTV challenge. However, after D56pi, IL-6 mRNA transcripts declined to levels similar to prior BTV infection. In contrast, IL-1β mRNA levels showed an opposite transcription pattern to IL-6. IL-1β mRNA was not up-regulated until the third challenge, by D56pi (Figure 6B). In addition to these pro-inflammatory cytokines, transcript levels of IL-12, a classical

Th1 cytokine [31] and CXCL10, a chemokine that mediates leukocyte trafficking and activates Th1 responses (reviewed in [32]) were evaluated. Both cytokines showed a significant up-regulation of transcription during infection until D56pi (Figure 6B). Thus, IL-6, IL-12 and CXCL10 were significantly up-regulated after primary and secondary responses while IL-1β was up-regulated only after D56pi, suggesting that an active inflammatory response was induced during primary and secondary BTV infection that did not involve IL-1β.

### Discussion

In this report we analyzed the T cell immune response elicited in sheep after repetitive infections with BTV-8, mimicking several peaks of vector activity during the course of the year [33]. Our results show that although an expansion of PBMC occurs after serial BTV inoculations, the infection is not completely controlled, resulting in detectable BTV RNA by RT-qPCR. Similarly, in BTV-8-immunized calves BTV1/15 replication still occurred after heterologous challenge [34]. In our study, the characterization of the expansion of CD4$^+$ and CD8$^+$ T cell responses during primary and secondary responses demonstrated a burst in size of the CD8$^+$ but not the CD4$^+$ population 15 days after each challenge. Moreover, IFN-γ production was also detected 15 days after primary and secondary challenge, although the TCR repertoires present within primary responses and secondary recall responses were different. These findings indicate that during BTV reinfections there is a bias of T cell responses towards a more specialized T cell pool that results in the narrowing of the T cell repertoire.

The study of the fluctuation of the PBMC population during primary and secondary BTV infections revealed that after primary infection the number of PBMC declined significantly, whereas those numbers increased after secondary and tertiary infections. The early decline of PBMC during primary BTV infection support previous results where a high proportion of apoptosis in PBMC was observed during the peak of viremia [23]. In fact, our data show that a high number of PBMC are BTV-infected, which presumably triggers apoptosis in these cells [35]. When the virus is no longer detected in PBMC, the population expands after secondary and tertiary recall responses, supporting the hypothesis that BTV might induce PBMC apoptosis at early stages during infection. This becomes especially relevant during acute infections in which a potent T cell response is needed to mediate viral clearance. PBMC infection leading to cell death could thus dampen the immune response and promote BTV survival.

We have outlined differences between CD8$^+$ and CD4$^+$ T cell expansion after primary and secondary

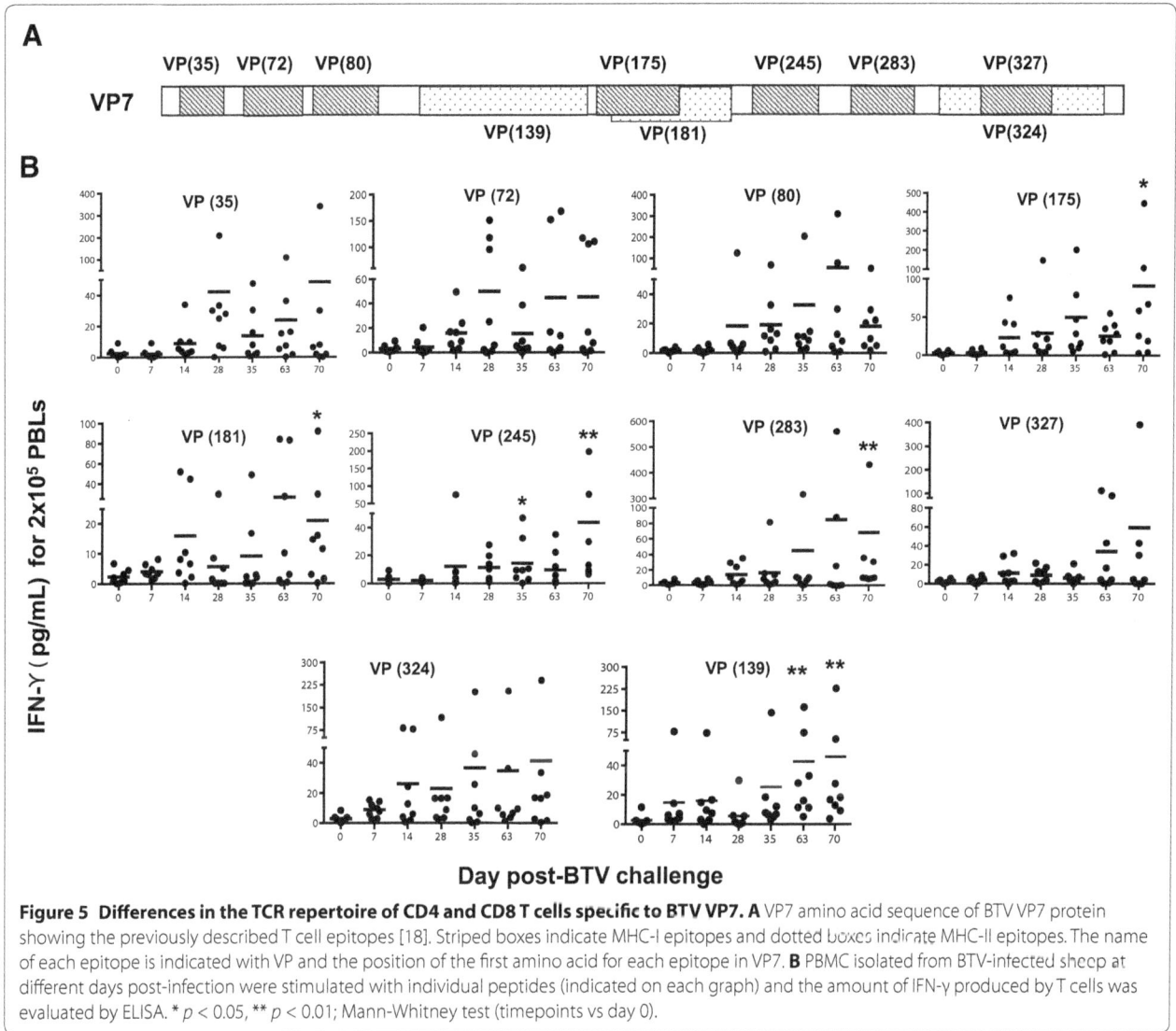

**Figure 5 Differences in the TCR repertoire of CD4 and CD8 T cells specific to BTV VP7. A** VP7 amino acid sequence of BTV VP7 protein showing the previously described T cell epitopes [18]. Striped boxes indicate MHC-I epitopes and dotted boxes indicate MHC-II epitopes. The name of each epitope is indicated with VP and the position of the first amino acid for each epitope in VP7. **B** PBMC isolated from BTV-infected sheep at different days post-infection were stimulated with individual peptides (indicated on each graph) and the amount of IFN-γ produced by T cells was evaluated by ELISA. * $p < 0.05$, ** $p < 0.01$; Mann-Whitney test (timepoints vs day 0).

responses. CD4$^+$ T cells, which help to promote B cell antibody production and are required for the generation of cytotoxic and memory CD8$^+$ T cells (reviewed in [36, 37]), did not significantly increase in numbers during the time course studied here, although they displayed a trend towards an increase. This lack of significant CD4$^+$ T cell expansion may be the consequence of a slowly controlled infection, or even a lack of control due to serial infections. This possible scenario in which high viral loads impair virus-specific CD4$^+$ T cell responses has been reported for other viral infections [38, 39]. For BTV, the viral load at the peak of primary infection (D7pi) is very high (*Ct* values < 25), and is kept low or medium (*Ct* value > 30–40) after recall responses and until the end of the experiment. Thus, we speculate that although the viral load may not be high enough to completely impair virus-specific CD4$^+$ T cell responses, our

data suggest that this low/medium viral load (antigen load) is affecting the expansion of CD4$^+$ T cells. The typical contraction phase of CD4$^+$ T responses after acute viral infection was not detected in our experiment, in which the CD8:CD4 T cell ratio was stabilized after primary infection and never decreased. Nevertheless, it is also plausible that these data reflect a rapid contraction phase combined with ongoing CD4$^+$ T cell recruitment to lymph nodes. By contrast, the kinetic of CD8$^+$ T cells displays an expansion by D15pi followed by a contraction phase and expansions after secondary infections. Our results support previous work in which the rate of proliferation was similar for naïve and memory CD8$^+$ T cells [3, 40]. In addition, our data show that CD8$^+$ T cell responses in acute infection reached their highest responses by D15pi, which indicates that optimal CD8$^+$ T cell expansion could require the presence of antigen

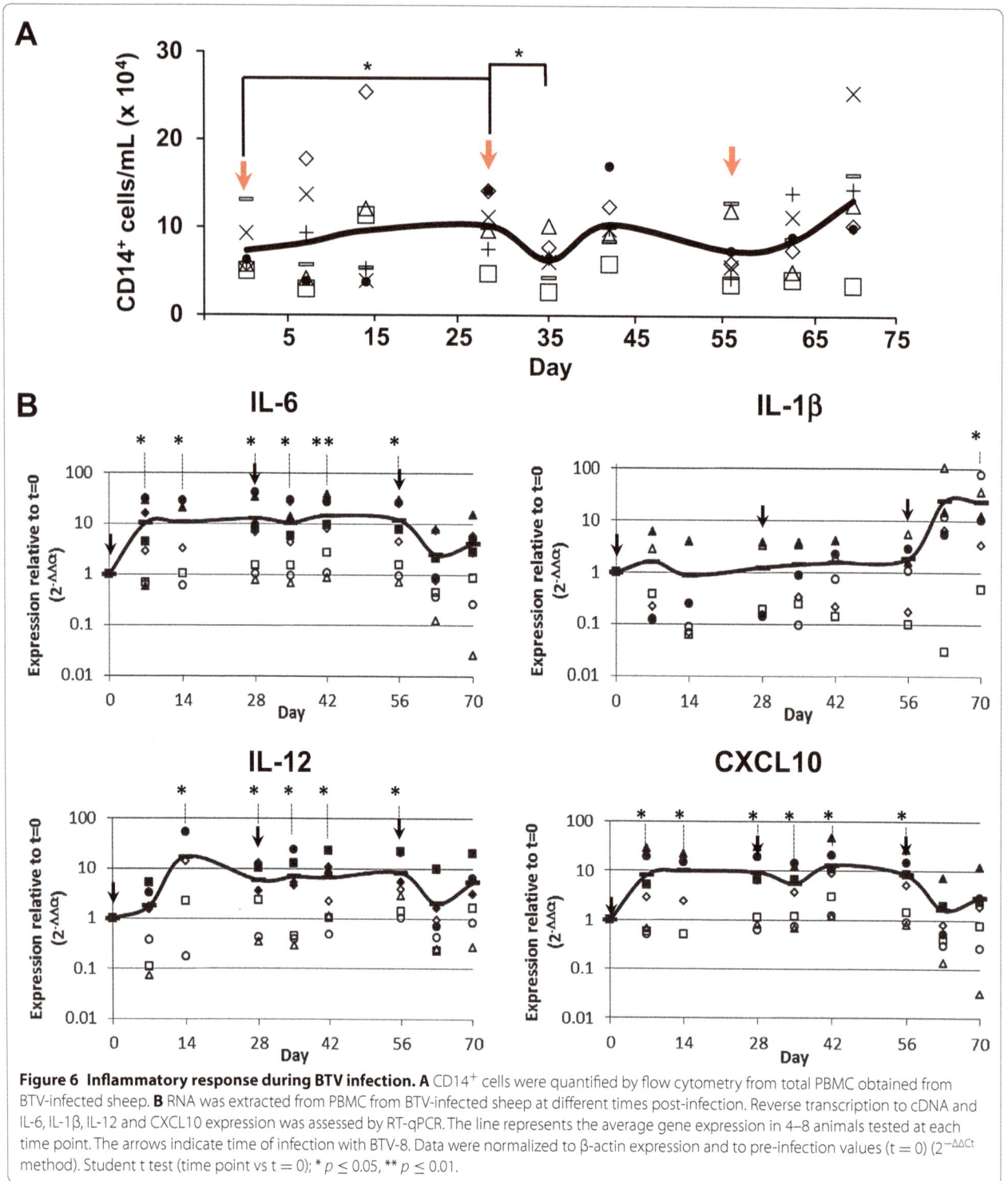

**Figure 6 Inflammatory response during BTV infection. A** CD14$^+$ cells were quantified by flow cytometry from total PBMC obtained from BTV-infected sheep. **B** RNA was extracted from PBMC from BTV-infected sheep at different times post-infection. Reverse transcription to cDNA and IL-6, IL-1β, IL-12 and CXCL10 expression was assessed by RT-qPCR. The line represents the average gene expression in 4–8 animals tested at each time point. The arrows indicate time of infection with BTV-8. Data were normalized to β-actin expression and to pre-infection values (t = 0) ($2^{-\Delta\Delta Ct}$ method). Student t test (time point vs t = 0); * $p \leq 0.05$, ** $p \leq 0.01$.

for at least 12 days following BTV infection. For memory response upon challenge, CD8$^+$ T cells initiate division and IFN-γ production with a significantly reduced duration of antigen exposure when compared to naïve T cells [41]. By D7 post-secondary infection CD8$^+$ T cells already expand and produce IFN-γ. Our data thus indicate a clear activation of CD8$^+$ T cells upon secondary challenge with BTV, due to the activation of memory CD8$^+$ T cells that may, ideally, cross-react [21] between previously and newly encountered BTV strains.

In many viral infections, bulk T cell responses correlate weakly with the control of virus replication, whereas T cell responses to subdominant epitopes can play an important role in limiting infection [42, 43]. Moreover, antigen dose can also modify the immunodominance hierarchy of T cell epitopes [44], and thus repeated infections (and thereby increased antigen exposure) could alter the antiviral T cell response. We have characterized the evolution of the TCR repertoires specific for the VP7 protein from acute to secondary homologous BTV infection. Acute and secondary infection with BTV induces very broad repertoires in which T cell responses target a relatively high number of epitopes in VP7 (Figure 4). By contrast, after a third BTV challenge, a profound narrowing of the TCR repertoire was observed, in which 3 MHC-I and 2 MHC-II epitopes were detected. The possibility of clonotyping and/or determining the TCRβ chain usage [45] of the narrowing anti-BTV T cell repertoire could prove useful to further understand T cell responses to BTV infections in future work. In conventional vaccine design, the most immunogenic epitopes have been chosen to generate a high number of T cells directed against these dominant epitopes, and thus the T cell repertoire tends to be focused on a few epitopes [42, 46]. However, our data show that a broader T cell repertoire is initially raised to fight the incoming virus but that after recurrent infection the virus is now more likely to select and drive the activation of a more focused T cell repertoire. These findings raise the interesting possibility that a broad anti-BTV T cell repertoire may induce a faster clearance of BTV infection than a narrowly focused T cell response.

Recombinant vaccines expressing BTV subunits could therefore prove useful to trigger a broad T cell repertoire against BTV. For instance, vaccination with a recombinant adenovirus vaccine expressing VP7 partially protected sheep from a virulent challenge [12]. Adenoviral vectors can induce CD4+ T cell mucosal immunity and strong memory CD8+ T cell responses to the transgene they express [47–50]. The recombinant vaccine expressing VP7 induced a CD4+ T cell response and a robust CD8+ T cell response which was likely responsible for the control of BTV after virulent challenge. These recombinant vaccine platforms that express BTV subunits and adequately activate T cells could therefore be ideal to broaden and induce long-term memory T cell responses.

The study of the inflammatory response after sequential BTV infections revealed interesting data. IL-6, a cytokine mainly produced by activated monocytes, with pleiotropic action affecting the functions of a variety of immune cells (reviewed in [29]), is up-regulated during primary and secondary responses, and declines after the third infection. IL-6 synthesis is triggered by pathogen-recognition receptor engagement [29], and probably induced by BTV dsRNA recognition by the cell. IL-6 induces the production of the cytokine VEGF (vascular endothelial growth factor), among others, leading to angiogenesis and increased vascular permeability [51]. BTV infection is characterized by increased vascular permeability and endothelial cell dysfunction, leading to hemorrhages and edema [52]. Therefore, the high levels of IL-6 found during primary and secondary BTV infections might contribute to BTV-induced vasoactive disease. IL-6 is nonetheless also important for the development of adaptive immunity and its upregulation could help combat the infection. IL-6 promotes T follicular cell help and thus favors antibody production [53]. Moreover, it has been linked to the differentiation of activated B cells into antibody-producing plasma cells and the differentiation of CD8+ T cells into cytotoxic T lymphocytes [29].

Intriguingly, BTV-8 infection only induced IL-1β expression after the third viral challenge. Our results are in accordance with others, which have reported that BTV-1 primary infection triggered IL-1β expression but BTV-8 inoculation failed to induce the production of this cytokine [54]. The pro-inflammatory cytokine IL-1β is produced mostly by monocytes, macrophages and dendritic cells after pattern recognition receptor engagement and inflammasome activation [55, 56]. IL-1β promotes the recruitment of inflammatory and immune competent cells to the inflamed tissue. It is also essential for T cell-dependent antibody production [57], a pathway that BTV disrupts during infection [58]. Blockade of IL-1β activation could thus facilitate BTV survival. The increase in IL-6 detected during the first and second challenge could also contribute to impaired IL-1β activity. IL-6 triggers the production of the IL-1 receptor antagonist IL-1Ra that blocks IL-1β and IL-1α signaling [56, 59]. IL-1Ra induction by IL-6 can protect mice from autoimmune disease [59]. Whether the high IL-6 levels detected after BTV-8 infection impairs IL-1β activity will nonetheless require further investigation.

IL-12 is also a pro-inflammatory cytokine produced by B cells, macrophages and dendritic cells in response to infection (reviewed in [31, 60]). IL-12 induces IFN-γ production by T cells and drives Th1 differentiation. CXCL10 is a chemoattractant for monocytes, T cells and NK cells towards inflamed areas (review in [32]). Our data were consistent with a positive feedback loop between IFN-γ-producing Th1 cells that induce CXCL10 production on resident cells, which in turn enables CXCL10 to attract and recruit more Th1 cells.

In conclusion, BTV-8 infection induces an inflammatory response in the host characterized by increased IL-6, IL-12 and CXCL10 levels, but IL-1β levels only increased after the third infection. Our data indicate that BTV-8 infection induces a memory T cell response to subsequent homologous BTV challenges. BTV-8 re-infection also produced a narrowing of the T cell repertoire to VP7. This narrowing T cell repertoire that responds better and faster to homologous BTV challenge is, however, not sufficient to eradicate viral load. The induction and maintenance of a diverse anti-BTV T cell repertoire may therefore be more beneficial for BTV control. These findings could have implications for the design of serotype-cross-reactive BTV vaccines.

## Competing interests

The authors declare that they have no competing interests.

## Authors' contributions

JMR carried out most of the experiments described in the manuscript and contributed to writing the article; TR carried out some of the experiments; NS, conceived the study, its design, coordination and wrote the article. All authors read and approved the final manuscript.

## Acknowledgements

This work was funded by Grants AGL2012-33289 and AGL2015-64290-R from the Spanish Ministry of Economy and Competitiveness and S2013/ABI-2906-PLATESA from Comunidad de Madrid and the European Union (European Regional development's Funds, FEDER).

## Author details

[1] Centro de Investigación en Sanidad Animal (CISA-INIA), Instituto Nacional de Investigación Agraria y Alimentaria, Ctra Algete a El Casar km 8, Valdeolmos, 28130 Madrid, Spain. [2] Present Address: Institute of Diabetes Research, Helmholtz Zentrum München, Deutsches Forschungszentrum für Gesundheit und Umwelt (GmbH), Neuherberg, Germany.

## References

1. Ahmed R, Gray D (1996) Immunological memory and protective immunity: understanding their relation. Science 272:54–60
2. Cukalac T, Chadderton J, Handel A, Doherty PC, Turner SJ, Thomas PG, La Gruta NL (2014) Reproducible selection of high avidity CD8+ T-cell clones following secondary acute virus infection. Proc Natl Acad Sci U S A 111:1485–1490
3. Blair DA, Turner DL, Bose TO, Pham QM, Bouchard KR, Williams KJ, McAleer JP, Cauley LS, Vella AT, Lefrancois L (2011) Duration of antigen availability influences the expansion and memory differentiation of T cells. J Immunol 187:2310–2321
4. Cornberg M, Chen AT, Wilkinson LA, Brehm MA, Kim SK, Calcagno C, Ghersi D, Puzone R, Celada F, Welsh RM et al (2006) Narrowed TCR repertoire and viral escape as a consequence of heterologous immunity. J Clin Invest 116:1443–1456
5. Mellor PS, Baylis M, Mertens PP (2009) Bluetongue. Academic Press, London
6. Schwartz-Cornil I, Mertens PP, Contreras V, Hemati B, Pascale F, Breard E, Mellor PS, MacLachlan NJ, Zientara S (2008) Bluetongue virus: virology, pathogenesis and immunity. Vet Res 39:46
7. Roy P (2005) Bluetongue virus proteins and particles and their role in virus entry, assembly, and release. Adv Virus Res 64:69–123
8. Ratinier M, Caporale M, Golder M, Franzoni G, Allan K, Nunes SF, Armezzani A, Bayoumy A, Rixon F, Shaw A et al (2011) Identification and characterization of a novel non-structural protein of bluetongue virus. PLoS Pathog 7:e1002477
9. Maan S, Maan NS, Belaganahalli MN, Potgieter AC, Kumar V, Batra K, Wright IM, Kirkland PD, Mertens PP (2016) Development and evaluation of real time RT-PCR assays for detection and typing of bluetongue virus. PLoS One 11:e0163014
10. Maan S, Maan NS, Belaganahalli MN, Rao PP, Singh KP, Hemadri D, Putty K, Kumar A, Batra K, Krishnajyothi Y et al (2015) Full-genome sequencing as a basis for molecular epidemiology studies of bluetongue virus in India. PLoS One 10:e0131257
11. Zientara S, Sanchez-Vizcaino JM (2013) Control of bluetongue in Europe. Vet Microbiol 165:33–37
12. Martin V, Pascual E, Avia M, Peña L, Valcarcel F, Sevilla N (2015) Protective efficacy in sheep of adenovirus-vectored vaccines against bluetongue virus is associated with specific T cell responses. PLoS One 10:e0143273
13. Stott JL, Osburn BI, Barber TL (1979) The current status of research on an experimental inactivated bluetongue virus vaccine. Proc Annu Meet U S Anim Health Assoc 83:55–62
14. Stott JL, Barber TL, Osburn BI (1985) Immunologic response of sheep to inactivated and virulent bluetongue virus. Am J Vet Res 46:1043–1049
15. Bouet-Cararo C, Contreras V, Caruso A, Top S, Szelechowski M, Bergeron C, Viarouge C, Desprat A, Relmy A, Guibert JM et al (2014) Expression of VP7, a bluetongue virus group specific antigen by viral vectors: analysis of the induced immune responses and evaluation of protective potential in sheep. PLoS One 9:e111605
16. Takamatsu H, Jeggo MH (1989) Cultivation of bluetongue virus-specific ovine T cells and their cross-reactivity with different serotype viruses. Immunology 66:258–263
17. Andrew M, Whiteley P, Janardhana V, Lobato Z, Gould A, Coupar B (1995) Antigen specificity of the ovine cytotoxic T lymphocyte response to bluetongue virus. Vet Immunol Immunopathol 47:311–322
18. Rojas JM, Rodriguez-Calvo T, Peña L, Sevilla N (2011) T cell responses to bluetongue virus are directed against multiple and identical CD4+ and CD8+ T cell epitopes from the VP7 core protein in mouse and sheep. Vaccine 29:6848–6857
19. Elbers AR, Backx A, Meroc E, Gerbier G, Staubach C, Hendrickx G, van der Spek A, Mintiens K (2008) Field observations during the bluetongue serotype 8 epidemic in 2006. I. Detection of first outbreaks and clinical signs in sheep and cattle in Belgium, France and the Netherlands. Prev Vet Med 87:21–30
20. Calvo-Pinilla E, Rodríguez-Calvo T, Anguita J, Sevilla N, Ortego J (2009) Establishment of a bluetongue virus infection model in mice that are deficient in the alpha/beta interferon receptor. PLoS One 4:e5171
21. Rojas JM, Peña L, Martin V, Sevilla N (2014) Ovine and murine T cell epitopes from the non-structural protein 1 (NS1) of bluetongue virus serotype 8 (BTV-8) are shared among viral serotypes. Vet Res 45:30
22. Toussaint JF, Sailleau C, Breard E, Zientara S, De Clercq K (2007) Bluetongue virus detection by two real-time RT-qPCRs targeting two different genomic segments. J Virol Methods 140:115–123
23. Umeshappa CS, Singh KP, Nanjundappa RH, Pandey AB (2010) Apoptosis and immuno-suppression in sheep infected with bluetongue virus serotype-23. Vet Microbiol 144:310–318
24. Davenport MP, Price DA, McMichael AJ (2007) The T cell repertoire in infection and vaccination: implications for control of persistent viruses. Curr Opin Immunol 19:294–300
25. Stipp SR, Iniguez A, Wan F, Wodarz D (2016) Timing of CD8 T cell effector responses in viral infections. R Soc Open Sci 3:150661
26. Chien YH, Davis MM (1993) How alpha beta T-cell receptors "see" peptide/MHC complexes. Immunol Today 14:597–602
27. Zinkernagel RM, Doherty PC (1976) The role of major histocompatibility antigens in cell-mediated immunity to virus infection. In: Baltimore D, Huang AS, Fox CF (eds) Animal virology. Academic Press, New York, pp 735–750
28. Ziegler-Heitbrock L (2007) The CD14+ CD16+ blood monocytes: their role in infection and inflammation. J Leukoc Biol 81:584–592
29. Tanaka T, Narazaki M, Kishimoto T (2014) IL-6 in inflammation, immunity, and disease. Cold Spring Harb Perspect Biol 6:a016295
30. Keyel PA (2014) How is inflammation initiated? Individual influences of IL-1, IL-18 and HMGB1. Cytokine 69:136–145
31. Vignali DA, Kuchroo VK (2012) IL-12 family cytokines: immunological playmakers. Nat Immunol 13:722–728

32. Liu M, Guo S, Hibbert JM, Jain V, Singh N, Wilson NO, Stiles JK (2011) CXCL10/IP-10 in infectious diseases pathogenesis and potential therapeutic implications. Cytokine Growth Factor Rev 22:121–130

33. Brugger K, Rubel F (2013) Bluetongue disease risk assessment based on observed and projected *Culicoides obsoletus* spp. vector densities. PLoS One 8:e60330

34. Martinelle L, Dal Pozzo F, Sarradin P, Van Campe W, De Leeuw I, De Clercq K, Thys C, Thiry E, Saegerman C (2016) Experimental bluetongue virus superinfection in calves previously immunized with bluetongue virus serotype 8. Vet Res 47:73

35. Barratt-Boyes SM, Rossitto PV, Stott JL, MacLachlan NJ (1992) Flow cytometric analysis of in vitro bluetongue virus infection of bovine blood mononuclear cells. J Gen Virol 73:1953–1960

36. Sant AJ, McMichael A (2012) Revealing the role of CD4(+) T cells in viral immunity. J Exp Med 209:1391–1395

37. Swain SL, McKinstry KK, Strutt TM (2012) Expanding roles for CD4(+) T cells in immunity to viruses. Nat Rev Immunol 12:136–148

38. Fuller MJ, Zajac AJ (2003) Ablation of CD8 and CD4 T cell responses by high viral loads. J Immunol 170:477–486

39. Schulze Zur Wiesch J, Ciuffreda D, Lewis-Ximenez L, Kasprowicz V, Nolan BE, Streeck H, Aneja J, Reyor LL, Allen TM, Lohse AW et al (2012) Broadly directed virus-specific CD4+ T cell responses are primed during acute hepatitis C infection, but rapidly disappear from human blood with viral persistence. J Exp Med 209:61–75

40. Stock AT, Jones CM, Heath WR, Carbone FR (2011) Rapid recruitment and activation of CD8+ T cells after herpes simplex virus type 1 skin infection. Immunol Cell Biol 89:143–148

41. Lauvau G, Boutet M, Williams TM, Chin SS, Chorro L (2016) Memory CD8(+) T cells: innate-like sensors and orchestrators of protection. Trends Immunol 37:375–385

42. Frahm N, Kiepiela P, Adams S, Linde CH, Hewitt HS, Sango K, Feeney ME, Addo MM, Lichterfeld M, Lahaie MP et al (2006) Control of human immunodeficiency virus replication by cytotoxic T lymphocytes targeting subdominant epitopes. Nat Immunol 7:173–178

43. Gallimore A, Dumrese T, Hengartner H, Zinkernagel RM, Rammensee HG (1998) Protective immunity does not correlate with the hierarchy of virus-specific cytotoxic T cell responses to naturally processed peptides. J Exp Med 187:1647–1657

44. Luciani F, Sanders MT, Oveissi S, Pang KC, Chen W (2013) Increasing viral dose causes a reversal in CD8+ T cell immunodominance during primary influenza infection due to differences in antigen presentation, T cell avidity, and precursor numbers. J Immunol 190:36–47

45. Lythe G, Callard RE, Hoare RL, Molina-París C (2016) How many TCR clonotypes does a body maintain? J Theor Biol 389:214–224

46. Borrow P, Lewicki H, Wei X, Horwitz MS, Peffer N, Meyers H, Nelson JA, Gairin JE, Hahn BH, Oldstone MB et al (1997) Antiviral pressure exerted by HIV-1-specific cytotoxic T lymphocytes (CTLs) during primary infection demonstrated by rapid selection of CTL escape virus. Nat Med 3:205–211

47. Benlahrech A, Harris J, Meiser A, Papagatsias T, Hornig J, Hayes P, Lieber A, Athanasopoulos T, Bachy V, Csomor E et al (2009) Adenovirus vector vaccination induces expansion of memory CD4 T cells with a mucosal homing phenotype that are readily susceptible to HIV-1. Proc Natl Acad Sci U S A 106:19940–19945

48. Holst PJ, Ørskov C, Thomsen AR, Christensen JP (2010) Quality of the transgene-specific CD8+ T cell response induced by adenoviral vector immunization is critically influenced by virus dose and route of vaccination. J Immunol 184:4431–4439

49. Zhou D, Wu TL, Emmer KL, Kurupati R, Tuyishime S, Li Y, Giles-Davis W, Zhou X, Xiang Z, Liu Q et al (2013) Hexon-modified recombinant E1-deleted adenovirus vectors as dual specificity vaccine carriers for influenza virus. Mol Ther 21:696–706

50. Suleman M, Galea S, Gavard F, Merillon N, Klonjkowski B, Tartour E, Richardson J (2011) Antigen encoded by vaccine vectors derived from human adenovirus serotype 5 is preferentially presented to CD8+ T lymphocytes by the CD8α+ dendritic cell subset. Vaccine 29:5892–5903

51. Nakahara H, Song J, Sugimoto M, Hagihara K, Kishimoto T, Yoshizaki K, Nishimoto N (2003) Anti-interleukin-6 receptor antibody therapy reduces vascular endothelial growth factor production in rheumatoid arthritis. Arthritis Rheum 48:1521–1529

52. Howerth EW (2015) Cytokine release and endothelial dysfunction: a perfect storm in orbivirus pathogenesis. Vet Ital 51:275–281

53. Ma CS, Deenick EK, Batten M, Tangye SG (2012) The origins, function, and regulation of T follicular helper cells. J Exp Med 209:1241–1253

54. Sánchez-Cordón PJ, Pérez de Diego AC, Gómez-Villamandos JC, Sánchez-Vizcaíno JM, Pleguezuelos FJ, Garfia B, del Carmen P, Pedrera M (2015) Comparative analysis of cellular immune responses and cytokine levels in sheep experimentally infected with bluetongue virus serotype 1 and 8. Vet Microbiol 177:95–105

55. Latz E, Xiao TS, Stutz A (2013) Activation and regulation of the inflammasomes. Nat Rev Immunol 13:397–411

56. Dinarello CA (2009) Immunological and inflammatory functions of the interleukin-1 family. Annu Rev Immunol 27:519–550

57. Nakae S, Asano M, Horai R, Iwakura Y (2001) Interleukin-1 beta, but not interleukin-1 alpha, is required for T-cell-dependent antibody production. Immunology 104:402–409

58. Melzi E, Caporale M, Rocchi M, Martin V, Gamino V, di Provvido A, Marruchella G, Entrican G, Sevilla N, Palmarini M (2016) Follicular dendritic cell disruption as a novel mechanism of virus-induced immunosuppression. Proc Natl Acad Sci U S A 113:E6238–E6247

59. Samavedam UK, Kalies K, Scheller J, Sadeghi H, Gupta Y, Jonkman MF, Schmidt E, Westermann J, Zillikens D, Rose-John S et al (2013) Recombinant IL-6 treatment protects mice from organ specific autoimmune disease by IL-6 classical signalling-dependent IL-1ra induction. J Autoimmun 40:74–85

60. Ma X, Trinchieri G (2001) Regulation of interleukin-12 production in antigen-presenting cells. Adv Immun 79:55–92

# 16

# Intracellular delivery of HA1 subunit antigen through attenuated *Salmonella* Gallinarum act as a bivalent vaccine against fowl typhoid and low pathogenic H5N3 virus

Nitin Machindra Kamble, Kim Je Hyoung and John Hwa Lee[*]

## Abstract

Introduction of novel inactivated oil-emulsion vaccines against different strains of prevailing and emerging low pathogenic avian influenza (LPAI) viruses is not an economically viable option for poultry. Engineering attenuated *Salmonella* Gallinarum (S. Gallinarum) vaccine delivering H5 LPAI antigens can be employed as a bivalent vaccine against fowl typhoid and LPAI viruses, while still offering economic viability and sero-surveillance capacity. In this study, we developed a JOL1814 bivalent vaccine candidate against LPAI virus infection and fowl typhoid by engineering the attenuated S. Gallinarum to deliver the globular head (HA1) domain of hemagglutinin protein from H5 LPAI virus through pMMP65 constitutive expression plasmid. The important feature of the developed JOL1814 was the delivery of the HA1 antigen to cytosol of peritoneal macrophages. Immunization of chickens with JOL1814 produced significant level of humoral, mucosal, cellular and IL-2, IL-4, IL-17 and IFN-γ cytokine immune response against H5 HA1 and S. Gallinarum antigens in the immunized chickens. Post-challenge, only the JOL1814 immunized chicken showed significantly faster clearance of H5N3 virus in oropharyngeal and cloacal swabs, and 90% survival rate against lethal challenge with a wild type S. Gallinarum. Furthermore, the JOL1814 immunized were differentiated from the H5N3 LPAI virus infected chickens by matrix (M2) gene-specific real-time PCR. In conclusion, the data from the present showed that the JOL1814 can be an effective bivalent vaccine candidate against H5N3 LPAI and fowl typhoid infection in poultry while still offering sero-surveillance property against H5 avian influenza virus.

## Introduction

*Salmonella enterica serovar* Gallinarum (*S.* Gallinarum) and avian influenza virus (AIV) are two contagious and infectious pathogens that are responsible for severe economic distress in poultry production [1, 2]. *S.* Gallinarum, an etiological agent of fowl typhoid (FT), causes a severe systemic disease with a high mortality rate in chickens. Similarly, infection of chickens with AIV causes either a mortality or respiratory distress with serious complications depending on the pathogenicity of the infecting virus [1, 2]. AIV is categorized as high-pathogenicity avian influenza (HPAI) or low-pathogenicity

avian influenza (LPAI) based on the pathogenicity and virulence in chickens [3]. The HPAI and LPAI viruses cause acute systemic disease with high flock mortality and mild respiratory disease, respectively [3]. The LPAI viruses are widespread around the globe since mid-nineties. According to OIE, from 2006 to 2014, the LPAI H9N2 virus incidences in domestic poultry were notified regularly from the Republic of Korea [4]. Since 2007, the Korean veterinary authority has permitted the use of inactivated H9N2 LPAI vaccine to control the disease [5]. Apart from LPAI H9N2 infection, during 2007–2010, the Republic of Korea has notified four H5 and twenty H7 LPAI subtype virus outbreaks with subclinical infection to the OIE. These regular outbreaks of LPAI viruses in poultry with detection of the H5 and H7 subtypes have raised the concerns about the possibility of emergence of

*Correspondence: johnhlee@jbnu.ac.kr
College of Veterinary Medicine, Chonbuk National University, Iksan Campus, Jeonju 570-752, Republic of Korea

HPAI viruses from pre-circulating LPAI virus in the poultry [6, 7]. Therefore, the implementation of the vaccination strategy for control and prevention of LPAI H5 and H7 subtype viruses infection in poultry are warranted.

Routine vaccination of chickens against *S.* Gallinarum and influenza viruses are the principle means to control the infection and subsequent outbreak of FT and AIV infection [4, 8]. We previously developed an attenuated *S.* Gallinarum vaccine candidate, JOL967 (Δ*lon* Δ*cpxR*), that effectively protected chickens against FT infection [9]. However, stamping out is the preferred method to control HPAI infection, whereas vaccination is principally directed against LPAI virus control. Vaccination programs to control LPAI virus outbreaks are specifically directed against a particular subtype prevalent in a particular area. Moreover, the possibility of HPAI emerging from LPAI increases the importance of vaccinating against LPAI [3, 7, 10]. The prophylactic use of traditional inactivated oil-emulsion vaccines to prevent infection with different LPAI subtypes is efficient but should possess capacity to differentiate between vaccinated and infected birds (DIVA) [11]. Moreover, developing and introducing a vaccine candidate against each LPAI virus subtype is not an economically viable option for poultry production. Therefore, a cost-effective vaccine candidate to control different subtypes of the LPAI virus without interfering with HPAI virus sero-surveillance is needed.

Among the new vaccine platforms, live bacterial vaccine vectors (LBVs) are a promising approach to express and deliver immunogenic heterologous proteins of AIV [12]. LBV-based vaccine development is highly cost effective and allows for a quick development of strain-matched vaccine against the novel circulating influenza viruses, as it circumvents the need for a constant supply of eggs [12]. Recently, an attenuated *Salmonella*-based LBV vaccine system has generated a new perspective

for delivering heterologous antigenic proteins [13]. Further, using routine vaccination with *S.* Gallinarum to deliver an LPAI vaccine can reduce the cost and facilitate mass-scale vaccine production [12, 14]. In addition, engineering an *S.* Gallinarum-based LBV system to control LPAI virus infection in poultry has an added advantage in simultaneously protecting chickens against FT. Another characteristic of bacterial vaccine vectors is ease of administration, along with humoral immunity generation of the mucosal and innate immune response against invading pathogens [15].

Hence, we hypothesized that immunization with a bivalent vaccine is a novel approach to simultaneously control bacterial origin FT and H5N3 LPAI virus infection in poultry. A bivalent vaccine candidate was constructed by engineering the *S.* Gallinarum vaccine to carry the globular head (HA1) domain of hemagglutinin from H5 LPAI virus. The candidate was evaluated for its potential to induce immunogenicity and protect against fowl typhoid and LPAI H5 virus infection in a chicken model. Further, as only HA1 gene were used to construct the LBV, the DIVA capability of the LBV was validated by matrix (M2) gene specific real-time PCR.

## Materials and methods
### Construction of *S.* Gallinarum strain JOL967 expressing HA1 from the H5N3 virus

The bacterial and viral strains used in this study are listed in Table 1. An attenuated auxotrophic mutant strain of *S.* Gallinarum, JOL967, was used as a delivery vehicle for the HA1 protein of the influenza A virus H5 subtype. JOL967 was constructed by deleting the *lon*, *cpxR*, and *asd* genes from wild-type *S.* Gallinarum JOL394, as previously described [16]. A computational, *codon-optimized*, *synthetic* HA1 gene fragment from the H5N1 and H5N8 subtype of influenza A virus was cloned in pMMP65,

**Table 1  List of plasmid, bacterial and viral strains used**

| Strains/plasmid | Description | Reference |
|---|---|---|
| *S.* Gallinarum | | |
| JOL967 | Δ*lon*, Δ*cpxR*, Δ*asd* mutant of *S.* Gallinarum | [16] |
| JOL394 | Wild-type *S.* Gallinarum from chicken with fowl typhoid | |
| JOL-1814 | JOL967 with pMMP65-HA1 plasmid | This study |
| JOL1820 | JOL967 with pMMP65 plasmid | This study |
| BL21 | *E. coli* cells for protein expression | |
| H5N3 virus | Influenza A/spot-billed duck/Korea/KNU SYG06/2006 LPAI | |
| Plasmids | | |
| pMMP65 | Asd+, pBR *ori*, -lactamase signal sequence-based periplasmic secretion plasmid, 6 His tag | |
| pMMP65-HA1 | pMMP65 harboring HA1 gene of H5N3 virus | This study |
| pET28a(+) HA1 | pET28(+) harborunf HA1 gene of H5N3 virus | |

The strains were maintained as frozen glycerol cultures in LB broth at −70 °C.

an Asd$^+$ constitutive expression vector (Figure 1A). The pMMMP65-HA1 plasmid was introduced into JOL967 by electroporation, designated JOL1814, and used for the chicken immunization study. The pMMP65 plasmid was electroporated into JOL967. A positive clone was coined JOL1820 and used as a vector control. The HA1 protein used for ELISA were prepared by cloning codon-optimized, synthetic HA1 gene fragment from the H5N1 and H5N8 subtype of influenza A virus in pET28a (+) plasmid and expressed in BL21 cells as 6× histidine (His)

tagged HA1 protein. The BL21 expressed 6× His tagged HA1 protein were purified by affinity chromatography with Ni–NTA agarose column as per manufacturer's instruction (Quigen, USA).

## Western blot analysis

Periplasmic expression of the H5 HA1 gene in JOL1814 was confirmed by Western blot assay. To express H5 HA1 protein, JOL1814 was cultured in Luria–Bertani (LB) broth (Becton, Dickinson and Company, USA) until the $OD_{600}$ reached 0.8, after which the pellet was harvested by centrifugation at 3400g for 20 min. The periplasmic protein fraction was prepared from harvested cell pellets by the lysozyme-osmotic shock method, as described elsewhere [17, 18]. Boiled protein samples from the pellet and periplasmic fraction were separated by 12% sodium dodecyl sulfate–polyacrylamide gel electrophoresis and transferred to polyvinylidene fluoride membranes (Millipore, USA). The membranes were blocked with 3% bovine serum albumin. Mouse influenza A avian H5N1 hemagglutinin (HA) (bird flu) polyclonal antibody (Cat. No. MBS396043; MyBioSource, USA) and horseradish peroxidase (HRP)-conjugated goat anti-mouse IgY antibodies (Cat. No. NB730-H; Novus Biologicals, USA) were used as primary and secondary antibodies, respectively. The Western blots were developed by adding 3,3′-diaminobenzidine and 4-chloro-1-naphthol (Sigma) in the presence of $H_2O_2$.

## Internalization of JOL1814 into avian peritoneal macrophages

Avian peritoneal exudate or macrophage cells were isolated for gentamicin protection assay, as described elsewhere [19, 20]. The 6-weeks-old chicken was injected intraperitoneally with Sephadex particles. Four days later, the peritoneal macrophages were collected, washed and incubated in six-well plates at 40 °C for 30 min. The non-adherent cells were washed away with Hanks solution and adherent cell monolayer were harvested for internalization assay. The live dead percentage in the scraped adherent peritoneal macrophages were estimated by trypan blue dye exclusion technique. The adherent peritoneal macrophages were seeded on gelatin-coated coverslips at a density of $5 \times 10^5$ cells per well in a six-well plate and were infected with JOL1814 and JOL1820 at a multiplicity of infection (MOI) of 100 for 20 min. Then, the infected peritoneal macrophages were washed three times with PBS and incubated with RPMI-1640 supplemented with 50 µg/mL gentamicin for 24 h. After incubation, the cells were fixed with 4% paraformaldehyde and permeabilized with 0.2% Triton-x. The infected cells were incubated with chicken anti-S. Gallinarum polyclonal antibody and mice anti-hemagglutinin (HA) H5N1 (Bird

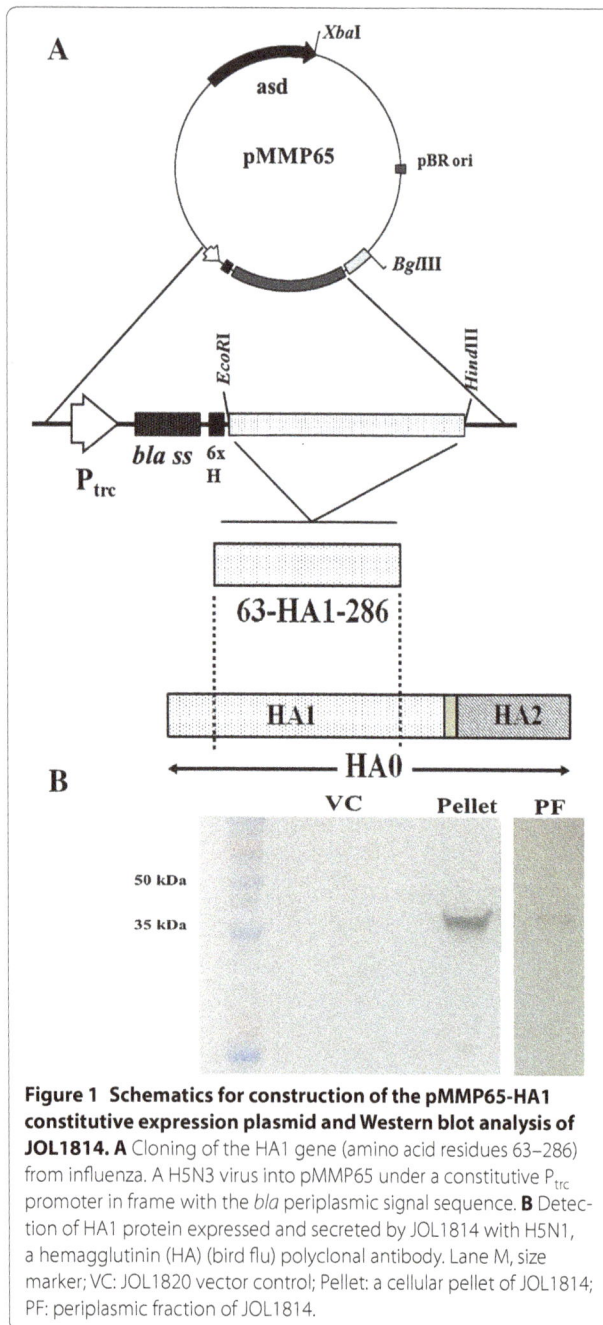

**Figure 1 Schematics for construction of the pMMP65-HA1 constitutive expression plasmid and Western blot analysis of JOL1814. A** Cloning of the HA1 gene (amino acid residues 63–286) from influenza. A H5N3 virus into pMMP65 under a constitutive P$_{trc}$ promoter in frame with the bla periplasmic signal sequence. **B** Detection of HA1 protein expressed and secreted by JOL1814 with H5N1, a hemagglutinin (HA) (bird flu) polyclonal antibody. Lane M, size marker; VC: JOL1820 vector control; Pellet: a cellular pellet of JOL1814; PF: periplasmic fraction of JOL1814.

Flu) Polyclonal Antibody (Cat. No. MBS396043; MyBio-Source, USA). Post-washing, the infected peritoneal macrophages were stained with anti-chicken-fluorescein isothiocyanate and anti-mice alexa-fluor monoclonal secondary antibodies. Finally, the cells were incubated for 10 min with 4 s, 6-diamidino-2-phenylindole nuclear stain and observed under a fluorescence microscope.

### Chicken experiments
The chicken experiments were approved by the Chonbuk National University Animal Ethics Committee (CBU 2014-1-0038) and were performed according to the guidelines of the Korean Council on Animal Care. Female, 1-day-old layer chickens (Brown Nick) were procured and provided antibiotic-free food and water ad libitum. Prior to immunizing the chickens with JOL1814, they were evaluated for the presence of pre-existing $S.$ Gallinarum-specific antibodies by ELISA. JOL1814 was cultured in LB broth at 37 °C to an $OD_{600}$ of 0.6 and adjusted to an appropriate concentration in sterile PBS (pH 7.4) before being administered to chickens. The chickens were immunized with JOL1814 and JOL1820 with a prime-boost immunization strategy. The chickens were primed at 4 weeks of age and boosted at 8 weeks of age. The chickens ($n = 60$) were divided into four equal groups ($n = 20$). One group was immunized orally (oral) with $10^8$ colony forming units (CFU) of JOL1814, and another group was immunized intramuscularly (IM) with $10^6$ CFU of JOL1814. The other two groups were inoculated intramuscularly with JOL1820 or sterile phosphate-buffered saline (PBS) and designated as vector and PBS controls, respectively.

### Indirect enzyme-linked immunosorbent assay (ELISA)
Plasma and intestinal lavage samples were collected as described elsewhere [21]. An indirect ELISA was performed to determine the concentrations of plasma IgY and secretory IgA (sIgA) specific for $S.$ Gallinarum and H5 HA1 protein. An antigenic outer membrane protein (OMP) extracted from JOL394 $S.$ Gallinarum and BL21 expressed 6× His tagged H5 HA1 protein were used separately to coat 96-well MICROLON® ELISA plates (Greiner Bio-One GmbH, Germany). Plasma and intestinal lavage samples were diluted to 1:100 and 1:3 to examine the IgY and sIgA titers, respectively. Goat anti-chicken IgY HRP-conjugate (Southern Biotech, USA) and goat anti-chicken IgA HRP-conjugate (ThermoFisher Scientific, USA) at 1:100 000 dilutions were used as secondary antibodies. The HRP activity of bound secondary antibody was determined with $o$-phenylenediamine dihydrochloride substrate (Sigma-Aldrich, USA). All assays were performed in triplicate. The plasma IgY and

intestinal sIgA responses against $S.$ Gallinarum were quantified by plotting a standard curve of ODs against a reference antibody concentration using a chicken IgY and IgA ELISA quantitation kit (Bethyl Laboratories, Montgomery, TX, USA), as per the manufacturer's instruction and described elsewhere [22].

### Lymphocyte proliferation assay (LPA)
Peripheral blood mononuclear cells (PBMCs) were isolated as described previously [23]. Harvested PBMCs were incubated in 96-well tissue culture plates at a concentration of $1 \times 10^6$ cells/mL in the RPMI-1640 medium. PBMCs were stimulated with a sonicated bacterial cell protein (sbcp) suspension prepared from JOL394 and purified H5 HA1 protein antigen in a separate PBMC culture for 72 h at 40 °C [24]. Proliferation of stimulated PBMCs was measured with thiazolyl blue tetrazolium bromide dye (Sigma-Aldrich, USA) according to the manufacturer's protocol. The blastogenic response was expressed as the mean stimulation index (SI), as described elsewhere [25].

### Quantitative analysis of cytokine mRNA level by real-time PCR (qRT-PCR)
PBMCs were harvested from blood samples collected from the JOL1814, JOL1820-inoculated, and PBS control groups at 7 weeks of age following primary inoculation. A total of $1 \times 10^6$ viable PBMCs were cultured in six-well tissue culture plates. The cultured PBMCs were stimulated with 4 µg/mL of H5 HA1 protein. The stimulated PBMCs cultures were incubated at 40 °C for 72 h. Total RNA isolated from the stimulated PBMCs were reverse transcribed into cDNA with a QuantiTect Reverse Transcription Kit (Qiagen, USA). The change in cytokine mRNA level was calculated by the $2^{-\Delta\Delta Ct}$ method [26]. The change in mRNA level in immunized chickens was calculated as a fold difference over the PBS control group after normalizing ct value against endogenous control β-actin.

### Hemagglutinin inhibition assay
The haemagglutination inhibition (HI) assay was performed to evaluate functional antibodies in the sera of immunized and control chickens. Heat-inactivated (56 °C for 30 min) serum samples were serially diluted and incubated with 4 HA units of H5N3 virus for 30 min in a V-bottom microtiter plate. Further, chicken red blood cells (RBCs) were added to each well and incubated for 30 min at room temperature. The HAI titer was calculated as the reciprocal of the highest serum dilution that completely inhibited haemagglutination in chicken RBCs. Individual HAI antibody titers were transformed to $\log_2$ values, and average GMTs were calculated.

## DIVA and determination of protective efficacy

An influenza A/spot-billed duck/Korea/KNU SYG06/2006(H5N3) LPAI virus isolated previously from fecal samples of the spot-billed duck (*Anas poecilorhyncha*) were used as a challenge virus. The 50% egg infective dose ($EID_{50}$) of the H5N3 virus was calculated as described elsewhere [27]. Oropharyngeal swabs were collected form the immunized and control group chickens before and after the H5N3 virus challenge. An M2-gene specific real time PCR method was used to differentiate infected chickens from vaccinated 1 at 0 and 4 dpi, as described elsewhere [28]. At 12 weeks of age following booster immunization, chickens were challenged intra-nasally with $1 \times 10^7$ $EID_{50}$ of H5N3 virus. Chicken infection with H5N3 were monitored via oropharyngeal and cloacal swabs for 14 days after the challenge. Swabs positive for H5N3 virus were determined by qRT-PCR for the viral HA gene. After the H5N3 challenge, chickens from all groups were challenged orally with $5 \times 10^6$ CFU/0.1 mL of virulent JOL394 *S*. Gallinarum. The mortality was observed daily for 2 weeks post-challenge.

## Statistical analysis

ELISA, lymphocyte proliferation assay, and viral shedding data are expressed as mean ± standard error of the mean (SEM). HAI titers are expressed as GMT ± SD. Statistical analyses were performed with SPSS 16.0 software (SPSS Inc., USA). All analyses were one-tailed, and statistical significance was identified at $p$ values less than 0.05 or less than 0.005. A one-way ANOVA with post hoc Tuckey adjustments was used to analyze statistical differences in ELISA, CMI immune responses between the immunized and control groups.

## Results

### Construction and expression of HA1 protein from JOL1814

The codon-optimized synthetic HA1 gene from the H5 subtype of the influenza A virus was cloned into pMMP65, an Asd$^+$ constitutive expression vector (Figure 1A). The pMMP65-HA1 gene construct was electroporated into an auxotrophic mutant of *S*. Gallinarum, JOL967 ($\Delta cpxR$, $\Delta lon$, and $\Delta asd$). Colonies harboring the pMMP65-HA1 plasmid were confirmed by restriction enzyme analysis of isolated plasmids, and the strain was designated JOL1814. JOL1814 constitutively expressed a 36-kDa band corresponding to the HA1 protein of the H5 AIV subtype in precipitated cultures and periplasmic fractions, as shown by Western blot analysis (Figure 1B).

### In vitro delivery of HA1 antigen through JOL1814 to peritoneal macrophages

The in vitro macrophage invasion assay was performed to assess the delivery of the expressed HA1 proteins by JOL1814. We infected harvested chicken peritoneal macrophages with JOL1814 and a vector control strain, JOL1820. Direct plating of the lysate from infected PBMCs on BGA plates showed colonies and the JOL1814 and JOL1820 were recovered. The JOL1814 and JOL1820 colonies were confirmed by HA1 gene specific PCR. The fluorescence microscopy observation showed green fluorescence surrounding blue stained nuclei indicating uptake of JOL1814 and JOL1820 by peritoneal macrophages. Only the JOL1814-infected showed red fluorescence surrounding blue stained nuclei, suggesting the delivery of the HA1 antigen to the cytosol of the macrophage, in vitro (Figure 2).

### Specific humoral and mucosal immune responses against *S*. Gallinarum and H5 HA1 protein

Plasma and intestinal wash samples from JOL1814-immunized and control chickens were collected and analyzed by indirect ELISA using purified HA1 and OMP proteins from H5N3 virus and *S*. Gallinarum, respectively. The plasma IgY (μg/mL) and intestinal sIgA (ng/mL) immune responses to the *Salmonella* and HA1 antigens were quantified with a standard curve plotted against a reference antibody concentration (Figure 3). The HA1-specific IgY and sIgA concentrations in chickens from all JOL1814-immunized groups were significantly higher than in the vector and PBS control groups after primary and booster immunizations ($p < 0.05$) (Figures 3A and B). The additional booster immunizations primarily maintained the plasma IgY and intestinal sIgA concentrations at a significantly high level until 12 weeks of age relative to the PBS and vector control groups (Figures 3A and B).

A bivalent immune response to the HA1 and SG antigens was present only in the JOL1814 group. Along with the HA1-specific humoral and mucosal immune response, *S*. Gallinarum-specific IgY and sIgA concentrations were also significantly elevated in the JOL1814 group after primary and booster immunizations ($p < 0.05$) (Figures 3C and D). The OMP-specific plasma IgY and intestinal sIgA immune responses again peaked compared to the primary immunization at 11 and 12 weeks of age after the booster immunization, indicating a booster effect (Figures 3C and D). The vector control group had a significant ($p < 0.05$) humoral immune response to *S*. Gallinarum that was equivalent to that of JOL181, but failed to show any response to HA1. In summary, only the bivalent vaccines elicited high plasma IgY and intestinal sIgA titers specific to H5N3 and *S*. Gallinarum, whereas the vector control elicited a specific immune response to only *S*. Gallinarum, indicating that JOL1814 is a specific bivalent vaccine.

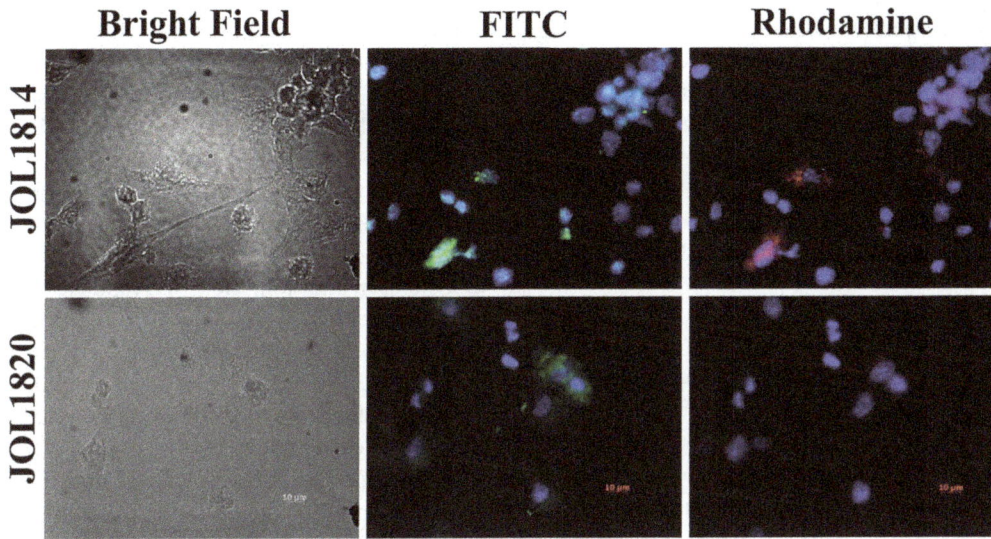

**Figure 2  In vitro delivery of HA1 antigen to peritoneal macrophages via JOL1814.** Harvested and cultured peritoneal macrophages were infected with JOL1814 and JOL1820 at an MOI of 100. The cells were fixed at 24 hpi and analysed for immunofluorescence by fluorescence microscopy (total magnification, 10 × 100). The JOL1814 infected peritoneal macrophages showed green and red fluorescence surrounding the blue fluorescence nuclei. The vector control JOL1820 showed only green fluorescence surrounding the blue fluorescence nuclei. DAPI: blue coloured nuclear stain; Rhodamine: tagged antibodies for localization of the HA1 antigen and FITC: tagged antibodies for localization of S. Gallinarum.

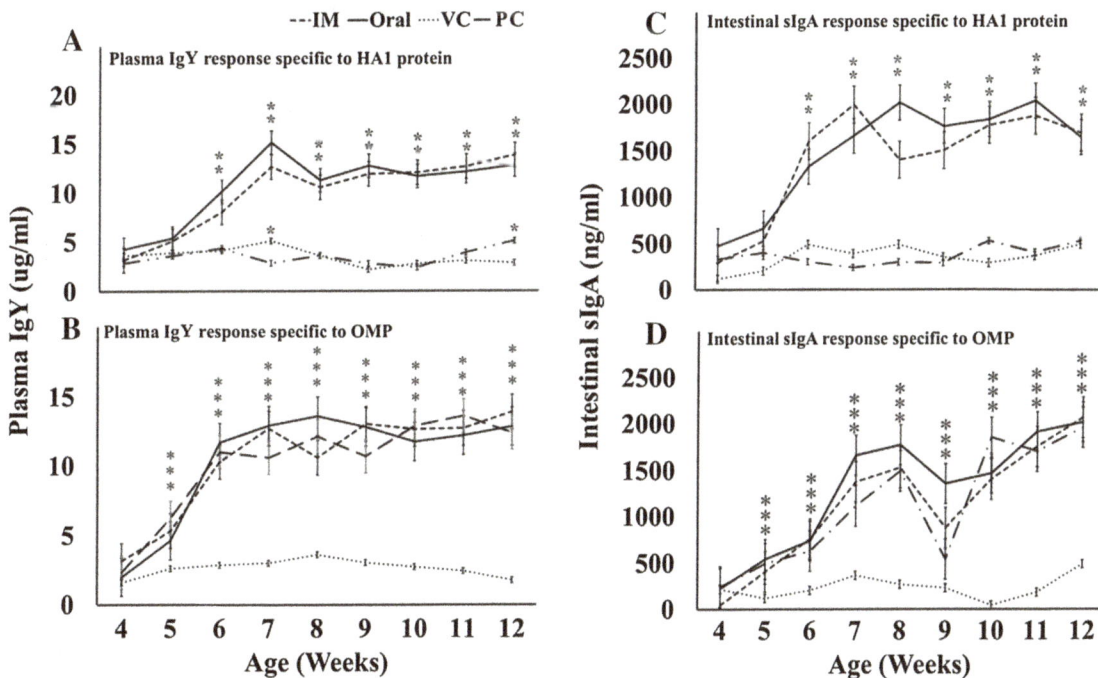

**Figure 3  Humoral and mucosal immune responses to LPAI H5 HA1-specific antigens and S. Gallinarum-specific antigens. A** The systemic IgY immune response to LPAI H5 HA1 purified protein antigen in plasma. **B** The mucosal sIgA immune response to LPAI H5 HA1 purified protein antigen in intestinal lavage. **C** The systemic IgY immune response to S. Gallinarum OMP protein in plasma. **D** The mucosal sIgA immune response to S. Gallinarum OMP protein in intestinal lavage. Oral: JOL1814 orally immunized group; IM: JOL1814 intramuscularly immunized group; VC: JOL1820 intramuscularly immunized group and PC: PBS inoculated group. *$p < 0.05$ when compared with PBS negative control group.

## Cell-mediated immune (CMI) response

The LPA assay was performed at 7 and 11 weeks of age to assess the CMI response in immunized and control chickens. HA1 and SG antigens specifically induced simultaneous and significant induction of PBMC proliferation only in the JOL1814 group (Figure 4A). The lymphocyte proliferation responses to the HA1 antigen in the JOL1814 group revealed 2.2- and 2.4-fold increases in the stimulation indices (SI) at 7 and 11 weeks of age,

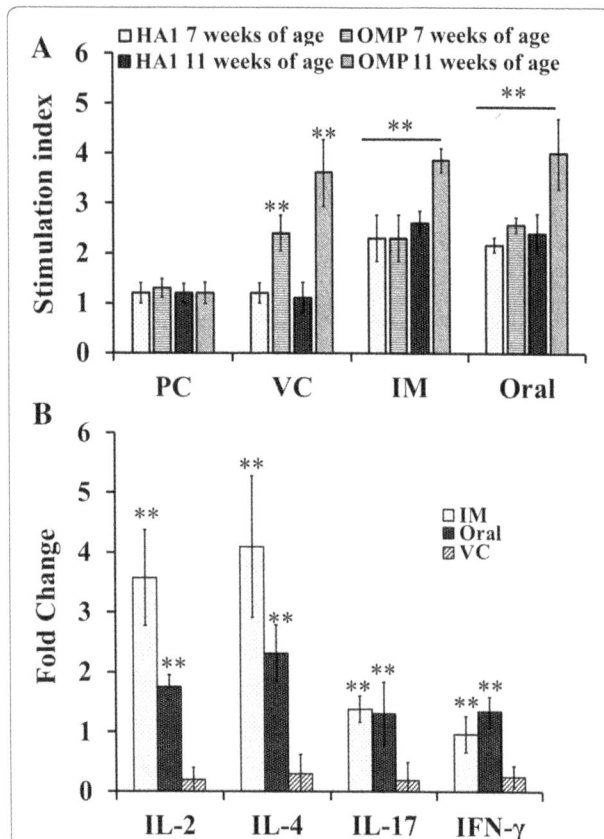

**Figure 4 Cytokine- and cell-mediated immune responses to LPAI H5N3 virus and soluble _S. Gallinarum_ antigen. A** The stimulation index (SI) in chicken PBMC samples stimulated with (1) H5N3 HA1 purified protein antigen and (2) soluble antigen from _S. Gallinarum_. The SI was calculated by dividing the mean OD value of antigen-stimulated wells by the mean OD of media-stimulated wells. **B** Cytokine levels in stimulated PBMCs from JOL1814 immunized and PBS control chickens. PBMCs from the 1814 oral, 1814 IM, vector and PBS control groups were collected at 11 weeks of age following booster immunization and stimulated with H5N3 HA1 purified protein antigen. Cytokine levels were assessed by qPCR with gene-specific primers, and the change was calculated using $2^{-\Delta\Delta Ct}$. The fold change was calculated by taking the ct value for PBS control group as baseline. Each column represents the mean ± SD of six individual values. Oral: JOL1814 orally immunized group; IM: JOL1814 intramuscularly immunized group; VC: JOL1820 intramuscularly immunized group and PC: PBS inoculated group *$p < 0.05$; **$p < 0.001$ when compared with the PBS control group.

respectively, over the vector and PBS controls ($p < 0.05$) (Figure 4A). In addition to the HA1-specific CMI response, JOL1814-immunized chickens also showed a specific CMI response to _S. Gallinarum_ antigens ($p < 0.05$) (Figure 4A). The vector control group showed a CMI response only to _S. Gallinarum_ (Figure 4A). The booster only affected the _S. Gallinarum_-specific immune response, as the SI value increased significantly by up to fourfold over the primary immunization (twofold) ($p < 0.05$). In addition, the CMI response to _S. Gallinarum_ was significantly higher ($p < 0.05$) than the response to HA1 after booster immunization.

## Cytokine gene expression following stimulation of PBMCs with HA1 protein

The expression of IL-2, IL-4, IL-17 and IFN-γ in PBMCs was determined by quantitative real-time PCR following recall antigenic stimulation with the HA1 antigen. Stimulated PBMCs from the JOL1814 group exhibited significantly higher expression levels of the Th1 cytokine IFN-γ ($p < 0.05$), IL-2 ($p = 0.05$), Th2 cytokine IL-4 ($p < 0.05$), and IL-17 cytokine genes than did those from the vector and PBS control groups (Figure 4B). Within immunized group, the JOL1814 IM group showed significantly higher ($p < 0.05$) production of IL-2 and IL-4 cytokine than oral group, indicating effective stimulation of Th1 as well as Th2 arm of immunity (Figure 4B).

## Induction of functional antibody response in chickens following immunization with JOL1814

Sera collected from chickens after primary and booster immunizations were assayed for the presence of H5N3-specific functional antibodies by HI assays. As shown in Figure 5, at 7 and 11 weeks of age, chickens that were immunized orally and IM with JOL1814 developed significantly higher ($p < 0.01$) HAI antibody titers against the LPAI H5N3 influenza virus. The HAI titers expressed as a geometric mean of the virus neutralization antibody titers (GMTs) in the JOL1814-immunized oral and IM groups were 6.45 ± 0.28 and 6.78 ± 0.29, respectively, at 7 weeks of age ($p < 0.01$) (Figure 5A). After booster immunization, the HAI titer in the JOL1814 oral and IM groups increased significantly over primary immunization ($p < 0.05$) (Figure 5B). The increases in the GMT for HAI following booster immunization in the oral and IM groups were 7.43 ± 0.30 and 8.45 ± 0.29, respectively ($p < 0.01$) (Figure 5B). The HAI titers in the PBS and vector control groups did not change significantly: 4.2 ± 0.28 and 4.15 ± 0.23 at 7 and 11 weeks of age, respectively (Figure 5).

## Protective efficacy against H5N3 LPAI virus and DIVA

The chickens were challenged intranasally with LPAI virus to evaluate protection conferred to chickens by

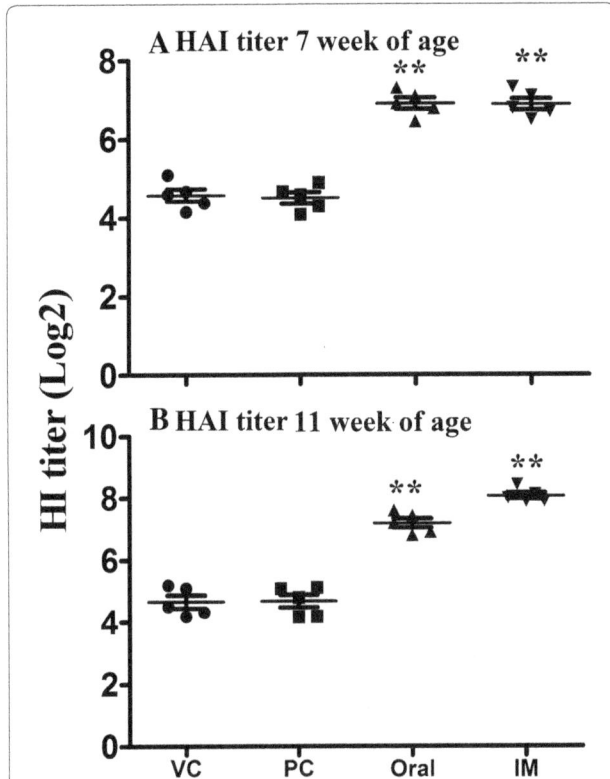

**Figure 5  The HAI titer in JOL1814-immunized and control groups.** HAI titers are expressed as $\log_2$ values of the highest dilution of serum that completely inhibited chicken RBC haemagglutination. **A** HAI titer at 7 weeks of age following post primary immunization; **B** HAI titer 11 weeks of age following post booster immunization. The SI values are presented as the mean ± SEM of each group. Significant differences in HAI titer value were estimated by calculating the GMT ± SD for each group. Oral: JOL1814 orally immunized group; IM: JOL1814 intramuscularly immunized group; VC: JOL1820 intramuscularly immunized group, and PC: PBS inoculated group. *$p < 0.05$ when compared with the PBS control group.

**Table 2  DIVA potential of the *S.* Gallinarum LBVs**

| Groups | No. of chickens positive for H5N3 virus | |
|---|---|---|
| | Before challenge (0 dpi) | Post challenge (4 dpi) |
| JOL1914 Oral | 0 | 7 |
| JOL1814 IM | 0 | 8 |
| JOL1820 VC | 0 | 9 |
| PBS control | 0 | 9 |

The M2e gene based qRT-PCR test were used to detect presence of H5N3 virus in the Oropharyngeal swabs collected from inoculated and challenged chickens at 0 dpi (before challenge) and 2 dpi, respectively.

that H5N3 virus was isolated from oropharyngeal and cloacal swabs at 2 dpi. The JOL1814 oral and IM groups completely cleared the H5N3 LPAI virus at 7 and 4 dpi, respectively, as determined by oropharyngeal and cloacal swabs (Figure 6). Contrary to the JOL1814 group, control chickens remained infected and shed H5N3 LPAI virus in oropharyngeal and cloacal swabs until 11 and 14 dpi, respectively (Figure 6).

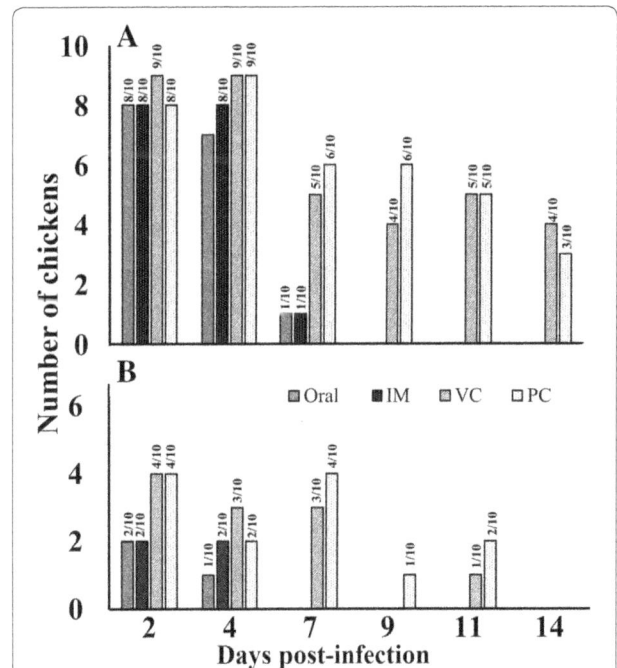

**Figure 6  Protective efficacy against LPAI H5N3 virus challenge in JOL1814-immunized and control group chickens.** Ten chickens from each group were infected with LPAI H5N3 virus. Oropharyngeal and cloacal swabs were collected at the indicated time points after infection (dpi). The swabs were evaluated for presence of H5N3 challenge virus by qRT-PCR. **A** Number of birds positive for LPAI H5N3 infection in oropharyngeal swabs. **B** Number of birds positive for LPAI H5N3 infection in cloacal swabs. The number above each column indicates the number of positive samples per total number of analyzed swab samples.

JOL1814 immunization. Despite intranasal challenge with $10^7$ EID$_{50}$ of H5N3 virus, no adverse clinical signs were observed in the JOL1814 or control chickens. In the absence of any adverse clinical signs, at 2 days post-infection (dpi) more than 80% of chickens from the immunized and control groups shown presence of H5N3 duck isolate virus in the oropharyngeal swab indicating infection of chickens. All the oropharyngeal swab samples collected before challenge at 0 dpi from JOL1814 immunized as well as control group chickens were found to be negative for amplification of M2 gene, whereas, post-challenge at 4 dpi 70, 80 and 90% swabs from JOL814 oral, JOL1814 IM, JOL1820 vector control and PBS control were tested positive for M2 gene amplification (Table 2). The successful infection of chickens with H5N3 LPAI virus was supported by the observation

### Evaluation of protective efficacy against lethal *S. Gallinarum* challenge in immunized and control chickens

The survival rate following lethal challenge with wild-type (WT) *S.* Gallinarum, JOL394, was evaluated to assess protection in JOL1814-immunized, vector, and control chickens until 14 days after the challenge. After the challenge, a few chickens from the JOL1814 and vector groups were depressed until 5 dpi, but recovered thereafter. The PBS control chickens had decreased feed intake, severe depression and subsequent mortality. The JOL1814 immunized and vector control groups showed significantly higher protection against the *S.* Gallinarum challenge. The oral and IM immunized groups had 10% mortality compared to 30 and 80% mortality in the vector and PBS control groups, respectively (Figure 7). All chickens were euthanized at 14 days after the challenge, and pathognomonic legions specific to *S.* Gallinarum infection were assessed on the liver and spleen. The livers and spleens from the PBS control chickens were hemorrhagic and enlarged, whereas JOL1814 chickens had normal livers and spleens.

### Discussion

A strain matched and cost-effective vaccine against different H5 subtypes of LPAI viruses with DIVA capacity is needed to control LPAI virus outbreaks and thus prevent emergence of HPAI viruses [3, 7]. Recently, attenuated *Salmonella*-based LBV systems that can be engineered to deliver a DNA vaccine for AIV have shown promising results [12]. A potential limitation of DNA vaccine delivery through *Salmonella* is the inability to stably maintain

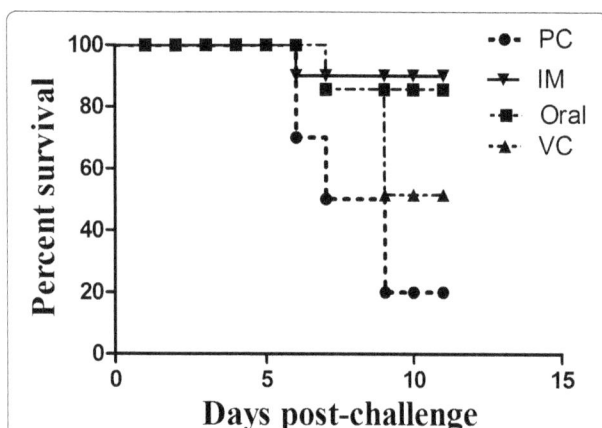

**Figure 7 Mortality rates of JOL1814-immunized and control group chickens post *S.* Gallinarum challenge.** The x-axis depicts the days for which the mortality rate was observed in chickens after challenge with virulent *S.* Gallinarum JOL394. The y-axis represents the percent survival rate. Until day 6 after challenge, no death was reported. Oral: JOL1814 orally immunized group; IM: JOL1814 intramuscularly immunized group; VC: JOL1820 intramuscularly immunized group; and PC: PBS inoculated group.

the plasmid inside the delivery vehicle. To overcome this limitation of a DNA vaccine, we constructed JOL1814, an attenuated auxotrophic mutant of *S.* Gallinarum expressing the HA1 antigen of the AIV H5 subtype virus on an Asd$^+$ plasmid, and used it to immunize chickens. The auxotrophic *S.* Gallinarum mutant, a balanced-lethal host-vector system was previously constructed by deletion of the aspartate-semialdehyde dehydrogenase (asd) from wild-type strain and which can be functionally complemented with Asd$^+$ plasmid [29]. The ability to infect and multiply inside macrophages makes *S.* Gallinarum an effective LBV for expressing and delivering heterologous antigens into APC [30, 31]. In a previous study have shown the invasion potential of attenuated *S.* Gallinarum (Δ*lon* and Δ*cpxR*) in peritoneal macrophages and quantified the results as colony forming unit per mL (CFU/mL), the attenuated *S.* Gallinarum (3.81 ± 0.03 CFU/mL) showed significantly higher viable cell counts than wild type (3.32 ± 0.03 CFU/mL), indicating more invasion potential of *S.* Gallinarum vaccine strain [32]. Further, the results of fluorescent microscopy showed that JOL1814 effectively delivered the HA1 antigen to the cytoplasm of infected peritoneal macrophages in vitro, suggesting that *S.* Gallinarum based JOL1814 LBVs was able to deliver the expressed HA1 antigenic protein to the APCs for further MHC presentation (Figure 2). Previously, we demonstrated that an attenuated *Salmonella typhimurium* vector-based influenza vaccine had efficacy for pandemic preparedness against H1N1 influenza viruses. Here, we further extend this approach by engineering attenuated *S.* Gallinarum to provide bivalent protection against fowl typhoid and LPAI H5N3 viruses.

Chickens immunized with JOL1814 by oral and IM routes had significantly induced levels of plasma IgY and intestinal sIgA antibodies specific to H5 and *S.* Gallinarum antigens. JOL1814 immunized chickens had highest HA1 specific ($p < 0.05$) plasma IgY and intestinal sIgA responses at 7 and 8 weeks of age, respectively, after primary immunization. Immunizing chickens with a JOL1814 booster dose failed to significantly increase the HA1 specific plasma IgY and intestinal sIgA concentrations compared to primary immunization. Furthermore, JOL1814 also induced a significant level of HAI titer against LPAI H5N3 virus. Live *Salmonella* vaccines can colonize the lymphoid organs and Peyer's patches at high concentrations and stimulate both mucosal and humoral immune responses [18]. Mucosal sIgA and systemic IgY antibodies specific to H5 HA1 and *S.* Gallinarum antigens provide immediate, early, and neutralizing immunity against invading *S.* Gallinarum and influenza viruses, respectively [33, 34]. Systemic plasma IgY antibodies clear *Salmonella* infections from the blood by opsonizing the *Salmonella* and promoting its phagocytosis by antigen-presenting cells [35]. Plasma IgY and neutralizing antibody-based immunity are sufficient to prevent systemic infection, but were inadequate to protect against upper respiratory tract infection in mice and ferrets [36, 37]. To protect chickens against both S. Gallinarum and H5N3 influenza virus infection, sIgA antibodies act as an immunological barrier at mucosal level, thus limiting the spread to internal organs [38, 39]. Collectively, these results indicate that JOL1814 can induce humoral and mucosal immunity via oral and IM immunization. In addition to humoral and mucosal immunity, cell-mediated immunity is required for chickens to completely recover from S. Gallinarum and influenza infections. The cellular immune responses induced by influenza viruses are necessary for viral clearance from the lungs and, therefore, are critical for chickens to recover from influenza virus infections [40]. Although the HA1-specific SI value at 11 weeks of age for the JOL1814 group did not increase significantly over 7 weeks of age ($p < 0.05$) (Figure 4A), a booster immunization maintained the HA1-specific CMI response at a level equivalent to primary immunization. In present study, it was observed the booster immunization was able to maintain and significantly elevate the cell mediated immunity against influenza and S. Gallinarum, respectively. Further, enhanced cellular immunity contributes significantly to both protecting chickens from primary Salmonella infection and clearing S. Gallinarum infection from macrophages [41]. Our results show that JOL1814 immunization significantly increased cellular immunity to S. Gallinarum and LPAI H5N3 virus.

Oral and IM JOL1814-immunized chickens had significantly higher levels of IL-2, IL-4, IL-17, and IFN-γ mRNA in stimulated PBMCs. The IFN-γ and IL-2 cytokines which is produced by stimulated natural killer cells, macrophages, CD4+ and CD8+ T cells, controls the generation of antigen-specific CMI, whereas IL-4 cytokines are generally produced by Th2 cells and mediate the generation of an antigen-specific antibody response [42]. Recent findings have shown that IL-17 cytokines are important for inducing innate and adaptive host responses and contribute to maintaining barrier function against pathogens in the host mucosa [43]. The PBMCs isolated from the immunized and control group chickens were stimulated only with purified HA1 antigen, hence the significant increase in fold change in IL-2, IL-4, IL17 and IFN-γ were observed only in JOL1814 immunized group, whereas, the JOL1820 vector control showed cytokine response equivalent to PBS control, indicating generation of HA1 antigen specific cytokine response. In previous reports, the PBMC pulsed with soluble antigen fraction of S. Gallinarum resulted in significant increase in IL-6 cytokine in the immunized chickens [24]. Overall, the cytokine analysis of the stimulated PBMC culture correlates with augmented immunogenicity specific to JOL1814 immunization in chickens.

The protective efficacy of the JOL1814 bivalent vaccine was evaluated by viral challenge with S. Gallinarum and LPAI H5N3. The LPAI H5N3 virus infected chickens and was continuously shed into the environment through the nasal and cloacal routes [44]. In this study, JOL1814-immunized chickens were protected against LPAI H5N3 virus infection. Both oral and IM JOL1814-immunized chickens cleared H5N3 virus infection by day 7 pi. Compared to the immunized group at 14 dpi, 30 and 40% challenged chickens from PBS control and vector control group were positive for presence of LPAI H5N3 virus in oropharyngeal swabs (Figure 6A). In a previous study, the efficacy of an LBV vaccine against LPAI viruses was evaluated in a mouse model [37]. Oral inoculation of BALB/c mice with Lactobacillus plantarum expressing the HA gene of LPAI H9N2 completely protected against lethal challenge with mouse-adapted H9N2 virus [45]. Further, after challenging H5N3-infected chickens with a virulent dose of S. Gallinarum (WT), PBS control chickens had 80% mortality with profound liver and spleen lesions. On the other hand, the JOL1814 group and JOL1820 (VC) chickens were well protected against virulent S. Gallinarum challenge, with only 10–30% mortality. Taken together, our results suggest that chickens in the JOL1814 group were significantly protected from LPAI H5N3 infection and shedding and survived virulent challenge with S. Gallinarum.

In conclusion, for the first time, we showed that an attenuated S. Gallinarum-based LBV for influenza virus is an efficient bivalent vaccine candidate against fowl typhoid and LPAI H5N3 virus in chickens. Immunizing chickens with JOL1814 significantly induced humoral, mucosal, and cell-mediated immunities against H5N3 HA1 and S. Gallinarum antigens, and this induced immunogenicity significantly reduced H5N3 viral infection and S. Gallinarum-induced mortality in chickens. Future studies are needed to determine the protective effect of JOL1814 against heterologous LPAI H5 subtype virus challenge.

**Abbreviations**

AIV: avian influenza virus; LPAI: low pathogenic avian influenza; HPAI: high Pathogenicity avian influenza; FT: fowl typhoid; LBVs: live bacterial vaccine vectors; DIVA: differentiate infected from vaccinated animals; LB: Luria–Bertani; ELISA: indirect enzyme-linked immunosorbent assay; PBMC: peripheral blood mononuclear cells; HI: haemagglutination inhibition; CMI: cell mediated immunity.

**Competing interests**

The authors declare that they have no competing interests.

**Authors' contributions**

JHL carried out conceptualization and design of the experiment. NMK carried out the cloning and expression of HA1 gene. NMK and KJH did chicken experimentation and analysed data. NMK and JHL co-drafted the manuscript.

All authors have significantly contributed to the manuscript preparation and editing of the manuscript. All authors read and approved the final manuscript.

## Funding

This work was supported by the National Research Foundation of Korea (NRF) Grant funded by the Korea government (MISP) (No. 2015R1A2A1A14001011).

## References

1. França MS, Brown JD (2014) Influenza pathobiology and pathogenesis in avian species. Curr Top Microbiol Immunol 385:221–242
2. Barrow PA, Freitas Neto OC (2011) Pullorum disease and fowl typhoid—new thoughts on old diseases: a review. Avian Pathol 40:1–13
3. Röhm C, Horimoto T, Kawaoka Y et al (1995) Do hemagglutinin genes of highly pathogenic avian influenza viruses constitute unique phylogenetic lineages? Virology 209:664–670
4. Lee D-H, Song CS (2013) H9N2 avian influenza virus in Korea: evolution and vaccination. Clin Exp Vaccine Res 2:26–33
5. Choi JG, Lee YJ, Kim YJ et al (2008) An inactivated vaccine to control the current H9N2 low pathogenic avian influenza in Korea. J Vet Sci 9:67–74
6. Kang HM, Kim MC, Choi JG et al (2011) Genetic analyses of avian influenza viruses in Mongolia, 2007 to 2009, and their relationships with Korean isolates from domestic poultry and wild birds. Poult Sci 90:2229–2242
7. Banks J, Speidel ES, Moore E et al (2001) Changes in the haemagglutinin and the neuraminidase genes prior to the emergence of highly pathogenic H7N1 avian influenza viruses in Italy. Arch Virol 146:963–973
8. de Paiva J, Penha Filho R, Argüello Y et al (2009) Efficacy of several Salmonella vaccination programs against experimental challenge with Salmonella gallinarum in commercial brown layer and broiler breeder hens. Rev Bras Ciência Avícola 11:65–72
9. Nandre RM, Lee JH (2014) Generation of a safe Salmonella Gallinarum vaccine candidate that secretes an adjuvant protein with immunogenicity and protective efficacy against fowl typhoid. Avian Pathol 43:164–171
10. Fouchier RAM, Schneeberger PM, Rozendaal FW et al (2004) Avian influenza A virus (H7N7) associated with human conjunctivitis and a fatal case of acute respiratory distress syndrome. Proc Natl Acad Sci U S A 101:1356–1361
11. Capua I, Terregino C, Cattoli G et al (2003) Development of a DIVA (differentiating infected from vaccinated animals) strategy using a vaccine containing a heterologous neuraminidase for the control of avian influenza. Avian Pathol 32:47–55
12. Medina E, Guzmán CA (2001) Use of live bacterial vaccine vectors for antigen delivery: potential and limitations. Vaccine 19:1573–1580
13. da Silva AJ, Zangirolami TC, Novo-Mansur MTM et al (2014) Live bacterial vaccine vectors: an overview. Braz J Microbiol 45:1117–1129
14. Wigley P, Hulme S, Powers C et al (2005) Oral infection with the Salmonella enterica serovar Gallinarum 9R attenuated live vaccine as a model to characterise immunity to fowl typhoid in the chicken. BMC Vet Res 1:2
15. Medaglini D, Pozzi G, King TP, Fischetti VA (1995) Mucosal and systemic immune responses to a recombinant protein expressed on the surface of the oral commensal bacterium Streptococcus gordonii after oral colonization. Proc Natl Acad Sci U S A 92:6868–6872
16. Byeon H, Hur J, Kim BR, Lee JH (2014) Generation of an attenuated Salmonella-delivery strains expressing adhesin and toxin antigens for progressive atrophic rhinitis, and evaluation of its immune responses in a murine model. Vaccine 32:5057–5064
17. Hur J, Lee JH (2011) Enhancement of immune responses by an attenuated Salmonella enterica serovar yyphimurium strain secreting an Escherichia coli heat-labile enterotoxin B subunit protein as an adjuvant for a live Salmonella vaccine candidate. Clin Vaccine Immunol 18:203–209
18. Kang HY, Srinivasan J, Curtiss R (2002) Immune responses to recombinant pneumococcal PspA antigen delivered by live attenuated Salmonella enterica serovar typhimurium vaccine. Infect Immun 70:1739–1749
19. Rosenberger CM, Finlay BB (2002) Macrophages inhibit Salmonella typhimurium replication through MEK/ERK kinase and phagocyte NADPH oxidase activities. J Biol Chem 277:18753–18762
20. Sabet T, Hsia W-C, Stanisz M et al (1977) A simple method for obtaining peritoneal macrophages from chickens. J Immunol Methods 14:103–110
21. Nandre RM, Matsuda K, Chaudhari AA et al (2012) A genetically engineered derivative of Salmonella Enteritidis as a novel live vaccine

candidate for salmonellosis in chickens. Res Vet Sci 93:596–603
22. Jawale CV, Lee JH (2013) Development of a biosafety enhanced and immunogenic Salmonella enteritidis ghost using an antibiotic resistance gene free plasmid carrying a bacteriophage lysis system. PLoS One 8:e78193
23. Kamble NM, Jawale CV, Lee JH (2016) Interaction of a live attenuated Salmonella Gallinarum vaccine candidate with chicken bone marrow-derived dendritic cells. Avian Pathol 45(2):235–243. doi:10.1080/03079457.2016.1144919
24. Jeon BW, Jawale CV, Kim SH, Lee JH (2012) Attenuated Salmonella Gallinarum secreting an Escherichia coli heat-labile enterotoxin B subunit protein as an adjuvant for oral vaccination against fowl typhoid. Vet Immunol Immunopathol 150:149–160
25. Rana N, Kulshreshtha RC (2006) Cell-mediated and humoral immune responses to a virulent plasmid-cured mutant strain of Salmonella enterica serotype gallinarum in broiler chickens. Vet Microbiol 115:156–162
26. Livak KJ, Schmittgen TD (2001) Analysis of relative gene expression data using real-time quantitative PCR and the 2(-Delta Delta C(T)) Method. Methods 25:402–408
27. Reed LJ, Muench H (1938) A simple method of estimating fifty percent endpoints. Am J Epidemiol 27:493–497
28. Karlsson M, Wallensten A, Lundkvist Å et al (2007) A real-time PCR assay for the monitoring of influenza a virus in wild birds. J Virol Methods 144:27–31
29. Matsuda K, Chaudhari AA, Lee JH (2011) Comparison of the safety and efficacy of a new live Salmonella Gallinarum vaccine candidate, JOL916, with the SG9R vaccine in chickens. Avian Dis 55:407–412
30. Lindgren SW, Stojiljkovic I, Heffron F (1996) Macrophage killing is an essential virulence mechanism of Salmonella typhimurium. Proc Natl Acad Sci U S A 93:4197–4201
31. Panthel K, Meinel KM, Sevil Domènech VE et al (2008) Salmonella type III-mediated heterologous antigen delivery: a versatile oral vaccination strategy to induce cellular immunity against infectious agents and tumors. Int J Med Microbiol 298:99–103
32. Matsuda K, Chaudhari AA, Kim SW et al (2010) Physiology, pathogenicity and immunogenicity of lon and/or cpxR deleted mutants of Salmonella Gallinarum as vaccine candidates for fowl typhoid. Vet Res 41:59
33. Barrow PA (2007) Salmonella infections: immune and non-immune protection with vaccines. Avian Pathol 36(1):1–13
34. Eggink D, Goff PH, Palese P (2014) Guiding the immune response against influenza virus hemagglutinin toward the conserved stalk domain by hyperglycosylation of the globular head domain. J Virol 88:699–704
35. Goh YS, Grant AJ, Restif O et al (2011) Human IgG isotypes and activating Fcγ receptors in the interaction of Salmonella enterica serovar typhimurium with phagocytic cells. Immunology 133:74–83
36. Epstein SL, Lo CY, Misplon JA et al (1997) Mechanisms of heterosubtypic immunity to lethal influenza A virus infection in fully immunocompetent, T cell-depleted, beta2-microglobulin-deficient, and J chain-deficient mice. J Immunol 158:1222–1230
37. Kris RM, Yetter RA, Cogliano R et al (1988) Passive serum antibody causes temporary recovery from influenza virus infection of the nose, trachea and lung of nude mice. Immunology 63:349–353
38. Griffin AJ, McSorley SJ (2011) Development of protective immunity to Salmonella, a mucosal pathogen with a systemic agenda. Mucosal Immunol 4:371–382
39. Rose MA, Zielen S, Baumann U (2012) Mucosal immunity and nasal influenza vaccination. Expert Rev Vaccines 11:595–607
40. Moss P (2003) Cellular immune responses to influenza. Dev Biol (Basel) 115:31–37
41. Penha Filho RAC, Moura BS, de Almeida AM et al (2012) Humoral and cellular immune response generated by different vaccine programs before and after Salmonella Enteritidis challenge in chickens. Vaccine 30:7637–7643
42. Or R, Renz H, Terada N, Gelfand EW (1992) IL-4 and IL-2 promote human T-cell proliferation through symmetrical but independent pathways. Clin Immunol Immunopathol 64:210–217
43. Guglani L, Khader SA (2010) Th17 cytokines in mucosal immunity and inflammation. Curr Opin HIV AIDS 5:120–127
44. Mundt E, Gay L, Jones L et al (2009) Replication and pathogenesis associated with H5N1, H5N2, and H5N3 low-pathogenic avian influenza virus infection in chickens and ducks. Arch Virol 154:1241–1248

# 17

# Phylodynamics of foot-and-mouth disease virus O/PanAsia in Vietnam 2010–2014

Barbara Brito[1,2], Steven J. Pauszek[1], Michael Eschbaumer[1,2,7], Carolina Stenfeldt[1,2], Helena C. de Carvalho Ferreira[1,2], Le T. Vu[3], Nguyen T. Phuong[3], Bui H. Hoang[3], Nguyen D. Tho[4], Pham V. Dong[5], Phan Q. Minh[5], Ngo T. Long[3], Donald P. King[6], Nick J. Knowles[6], Do H. Dung[5], Luis L. Rodriguez[1] and Jonathan Arzt[1*]

## Abstract

Foot-and-mouth disease virus (FMDV) is endemic in Vietnam, a country that plays an important role in livestock trade within Southeast Asia. The large populations of FMDV-susceptible species in Vietnam are important components of food production and of the national livelihood. In this study, we investigated the phylogeny of FMDV O/PanAsia in Vietnam, reconstructing the virus' ancestral host species (pig, cattle or buffalo), clinical stage (subclinical carrier or clinically affected) and geographical location. Phylogenetic divergence time estimation and character state reconstruction analyses suggest that movement of viruses between species differ. While inferred transmissions from cattle to buffalo and pigs and from pigs to cattle are well supported, transmission from buffalo to other species, and from pigs to buffalo may be less frequent. Geographical movements of FMDV O/PanAsia virus appears to occur in all directions within the country, with the South Central Coast and the Northeast regions playing a more important role in FMDV O/PanAsia spread. Genetic selection of variants with changes at specific sites within FMDV VP1 coding region was different depending on host groups analyzed. The overall ratio of non-synonymous to synonymous nucleotide changes was greater in pigs compared to cattle and buffalo, whereas a higher number of individual amino acid sites under positive selection were detected in persistently infected, subclinical animals compared to viruses collected from clinically diseased animals. These results provide novel insights to understand FMDV evolution and its association with viral spread within endemic countries. These findings may support animal health organizations in their endeavor to design animal disease control strategies in response to outbreaks.

## Introduction

Foot-and-mouth disease (FMD) is a highly transmissible viral disease of cloven hooved animals and is considered one of the most important diseases of livestock. Countries in Southeast and East Asia have varying levels of FMD endemicity, with Cambodia, Thailand, Laos, China and Vietnam having relatively high FMD incidence throughout the year [1]. Vietnam is the largest pig trader in Southeast Asia, so FMD control in this country is critical for the entire region [2]. The economic burden of FMD is substantial for large and small-scale pig producers and pig owners [3]. Cattle and water buffalo (*Bubalus bubalis*) have similar and important roles in agricultural practice in Vietnam [2, 4]. Both species are kept in varying degrees of intensity for dairy and meat production and are additionally used for draught purposes. Both species are often allowed to range freely for variable periods of time, and are frequently moved across country borders [5].

A study carried out in Vietnam, targeting areas with recent history of FMDV, found 22.3% seropositivity (to non-structural proteins) amongst subclinical buffalo and cattle sampled [6]. FMDV serotypes A and O currently circulate in Vietnam, while serotype Asia 1 has not been reported in Vietnam since 2008 [7–9]. FMDV serotype O is the most prevalent in the country; a recent study sequenced 71 serotype O viruses from samples collected

*Correspondence: Jonathan.Arzt@ars.usda.gov
[1] Foreign Animal Disease Research Unit, Plum Island Animal Disease Center, ARS, USDA, Orient Point, NY, USA
Full list of author information is available at the end of the article

between 2009 and 2013 in Vietnam, 65 of these viruses belonged to O/ME-SA/PanAsia lineage, while only 6 were classified as O/SEA/Mya-98 [6, 8]. However, in Vietnam from 2014–2016 it is believed that there has been a resurgence of O/SEA/Mya-98 (Dung and Long, unpublished data). Additionally, an incursion of O/ME-SA/Ind2001d lineage was reported for the first time in the country in 2016 [10].

Ruminants infected with FMDV may either clear the virus within 1–2 weeks after initial infection or develop a subclinical, persistent infection [11–13]. The World Organization for Animal Health (OIE) defines persistent FMDV infection as the recovery of FMDV from oropharyngeal fluids >28 days post-infection (dpi). However, recent work has demonstrated that, under experimental conditions, cattle that clear the infection can be differentiated from those that develop persistent infection at 14 dpi for vaccinated animals and 21 dpi amongst non-vaccinated animals [14, 15]. These persistently infected animals are referred to as FMDV carriers [13, 16] and earlier studies have estimated that the proportion of infected cattle that become carriers range from 50 to 65% [14, 17]. The role of carriers in disease transmission amongst cattle has been extensively debated [17–19]. Researchers have conducted numerous experimental studies, but have failed to detect transmission from carrier cattle to susceptible animals, while others have concluded that transmission from persistently infected cattle may occur to a very limited extent [20, 21].

There are intrinsic challenges to investigating FMDV transmission between herds and between different host species under field conditions in areas where animal movements and husbandry practices are variable and inconsistently regulated. Molecular techniques used to study the evolution of a pathogen through phylogenetic reconstruction can help understand the geographical spread, transmission between species and transmission from carrier and acutely infected animals, respectively when records about animal movements and contacts are not available [22, 23].

The objective of this study was to reconstruct the phylogeny, inferred inter-species transmission, and geographic spread of FMDV using VP1 coding sequences obtained from different host species, clinical stages, and locations in Vietnam. These analyses can help identify characteristics of the host species, geographic location, and disease status that are associated with specific changes in the viral genome and selection pressures.

## Materials and methods
### Data source
This investigation of FMDV phylodynamics in Vietnam was based on 125 FMDV VP1 coding region sequences

[639 nucleotides (nt) total length]. The VP1 capsid protein comprises approximately 7.6% of the FMDV genome, and is commonly used for first-line phylogenetic analyses because it is known to be the most variable region of FMDV due to selective pressure on the immunogenic epitopes contained therein [24]. These sequences were obtained from three sources: (1) previous studies conducted by our group wherein 77 FMDVs collected in Vietnam were sequenced at the Plum Island Animal Disease Center, United States and identified as FMDV O/ME-SA topotype, PanAsia lineage as described in previous publications [6, 25], (2) eleven sequences generated by the OIE/FAO World Reference Laboratory for Foot-and-mouth disease (WRLFMD, The Pirbright Institute, UK), delivered directly to the Vietnam Department of Animal Health and deposited in GenBank for this study, and (3) 37 recently described, genetically related sequences that were retrieved from GenBank, 34 of which are from Vietnam, two from Kazakhstan and one from China. All sequences used in the study are currently available (see Additional file 1; Table 1). No animal experimentation or euthanasia was performed for the sake of completing this study. Because several VP1 sequences were shorter than complete length of the protein-coding segment (639 nt), we trimmed the alignment to the first 621 nt, to have consistent data for phylogenetic reconstruction.

### Phylogenetic reconstruction using divergence time estimation
We reconstructed the phylogeny of FMDV and estimated divergence times. Sequences were aligned using the MUSCLE algorithm [26]. To estimate the best codon partition and best substitution model, we analyzed the sequences using Partition Finder [27] and selected the best partition scheme based on the Bayesian Information Criterion (BIC). The purpose of this selection is to identify the best codon partition scheme and the best nt substitution model for each partition.

**Table 1 Bayesian stochastic search variable selection analysis results**

| Discrete character | Bayes factor |
| --- | --- |
| Species | |
|   Cattle to pig | 5900 |
|   Cattle to buffalo | 5900 |
|   Pig to cattle | 1179 |
| Persistent and outbreak | |
|   Carrier to clinical | 871 |
|   Clinical to carrier | 871 |

Significant (Bayes factor > 3) non-zero transmission rates between species and between outbreak and persistent animals are shown.

Using the best partition scheme and corresponding substitution model, we reconstructed the phylogeny of O/ME-SA/PanAsia FMD virus using a Bayesian statistical approach (Bayesian Evolutionary Analysis by Sampling Trees), implemented in BEAST 1.8.2 [28]. The sampling dates were specified to estimate times of divergence. We used the lognormal uncorrelated relaxed clock model, and the Coalescent Bayesian Skyline tree prior. The analysis was run for $2 \times 10^8$ iterations within a web-based platform with access to computational resources available in CIPRES [29]. Convergence of the chain was assessed using Tracer 1.6, by visualizing traces of parameters of trees sampled and confirming that mixing of the chain had been achieved so that the effective sample size of all parameters was >200 [30]. From all trees sampled, the maximum clade credibility tree (MCC) was annotated and depicted using FigTree 1.4.2 [31]. The initial 10% sampled trees were discarded as burn-in. Time to most recent common ancestor (tMRCA) of all nodes and 95% highest posterior densities (95% HPD) were obtained from the MCC tree.

### Phylogeographic analysis and ancestral character state reconstruction

We used discrete ancestral character state reconstruction to estimate the viral history, specifying traits according to 3 different characteristics: the host species, the clinical status, and the location. To reconstruct the host species, we defined three discrete characters: cattle, pig or buffalo. For the clinical status, we used two characters: sequences described as "Clinical" were obtained from samples derived from vesicular lesions of animals during outbreaks of clinical FMD in Vietnam, whereas "Carrier" sequences were obtained from oropharyngeal fluid (probang) from subclinical cattle and buffalo identified through active surveillance as previously described [6]. To infer ancestral states with respect to geographical location we categorized each viral sequence assigning one of the 8 different geographical regions defined within Vietnam: Northeast, Northwest, Red River Delta, North Central Coast, South Central Coast, Central Highlands, Southeast, and the Mekong River Delta.

For each host species, clinical disease and geographic location traits, we reconstructed the inferred character state for each node within the phylogenetic tree. We analyzed the inferred transmission rates between character states using an asymmetric model for the discrete traits and estimated the significance of the network with Bayesian stochastic search variable selection (BSSVS), which tests the hypothesis of non-zero transmission rates between discrete characters [22]. Statistical support was assessed using Bayes Factor (BF) for discrete traits

implemented in SPREAD1.0.6 [32], we considered BF > 3 as significant non-zero transmission. The analysis was carried out in BEAST 1.8.2 and the number of iterations and assessment of chains were performed as described above. Additionally, we obtained the count of character transitions ("jumps") from all trees (excluding initial burning). The 95% high-density interval (95% HDI) of the values collected for each character state change that had a non-zero rate BF > 3.0 was computed using HDInterval package in R [33].

### Evolutionary selection of nucleotide sites across different species and between clinically versus persistently infected animals

The VP1 coding region of the 122 FMDV O/ME-SA/PanAsia sequences described above and the additional related sequences ($n = 3$) from Kazakhstan and China were analyzed for positive and negative selection. Sequence groups from different species (cattle, pigs and buffalo-excluding samples from persistently infected animals) as well as clinical or persistent status were analyzed independently to study differences in viral selection by nt site and overall selection. The mean ratio of non-synonymous (dN) and synonymous changes (dS) (global $\omega = dN/dS$ ratio) was computed using the single-likelihood ancestor counting (SLAC) method, and 95% confidence intervals estimated from the data and the likelihood profile [34]. Individual site selection was also computed by the fixed effects likelihood (FEL) method and by the random effects likelihood (REL; which was used for the species groups but not for the clinical/carrier groups due to the size restriction -number of sequences- of the analysis) [34]. Only unique sequences were used in this analysis (i.e. identical sequences were removed). The HKY85 nt substitution model was used. A site was considered positively or negatively selected if identified by at least one of the methods described (dN-dS > 0 with a $p$ value cutoff 0.1 for SLAC, 0.1 for FEL and 50 BF for REL). We displayed the dN-dS values computed for each codon position and indicated the statistically significant positively selected sites. The analyses were performed in the HyPhy2.2.1 software package [34, 35].

## Results

### Divergence time estimation and ancestral character reconstruction

The partition scheme and substitution models selected were the K80 + I for codon positions 1 + 2, and the HKY + G substitution model, for codon position 3. The mean substitution/site/year for VP1 coding segment the O/ME-SA/PanAsia phylogeny reconstructed was $1.66 \times 10^{-2}$ (95% HPD 1.21–2.11 $\times 10^{-2}$).

## Ancestral state character reconstruction
### Host species
The MCC tree depicting the reconstruction based on FMDV host species is presented in Figure 1. The current FMD O/ME-SA/PanAsia viruses circulating in Vietnam diverged into two different clades in June 2010 (95% HPD March 2010 to September 2010). One of these lineages (Figure 1, branch A), initially found in all three hosts species, diverged into a cluster of viruses that subsequently were found predominantly in pigs. Transitions between host species character state inferred from the MCC tree (and 95% HDI) occurred from cattle to pigs (7 events 95% HDI 5–10), pigs to cattle (2 events 95% HDI 1–3), and from cattle to buffalo (8 events 95% HDI 7–11). Results

of the analysis to estimate significant transmission rates between species, BSSVS, are shown in Table 1. With respect to host species, non-zero inferred transmission rates were detected from cattle to pig, from cattle to buffalo and from pig to cattle.

### Clinical status
The MCC tree showing the ancestral reconstruction of clinically affected animals ("Clinical") and subclinically infected animals ("Carriers") is shown in Figure 2. In the upper main branch of the tree (Figure 2, branch A), there are two viruses from persistently infected animals (KT153098-O/VIT/12/2012pro and KT153128-O/VIT/25/2012pro) likely originating from previous

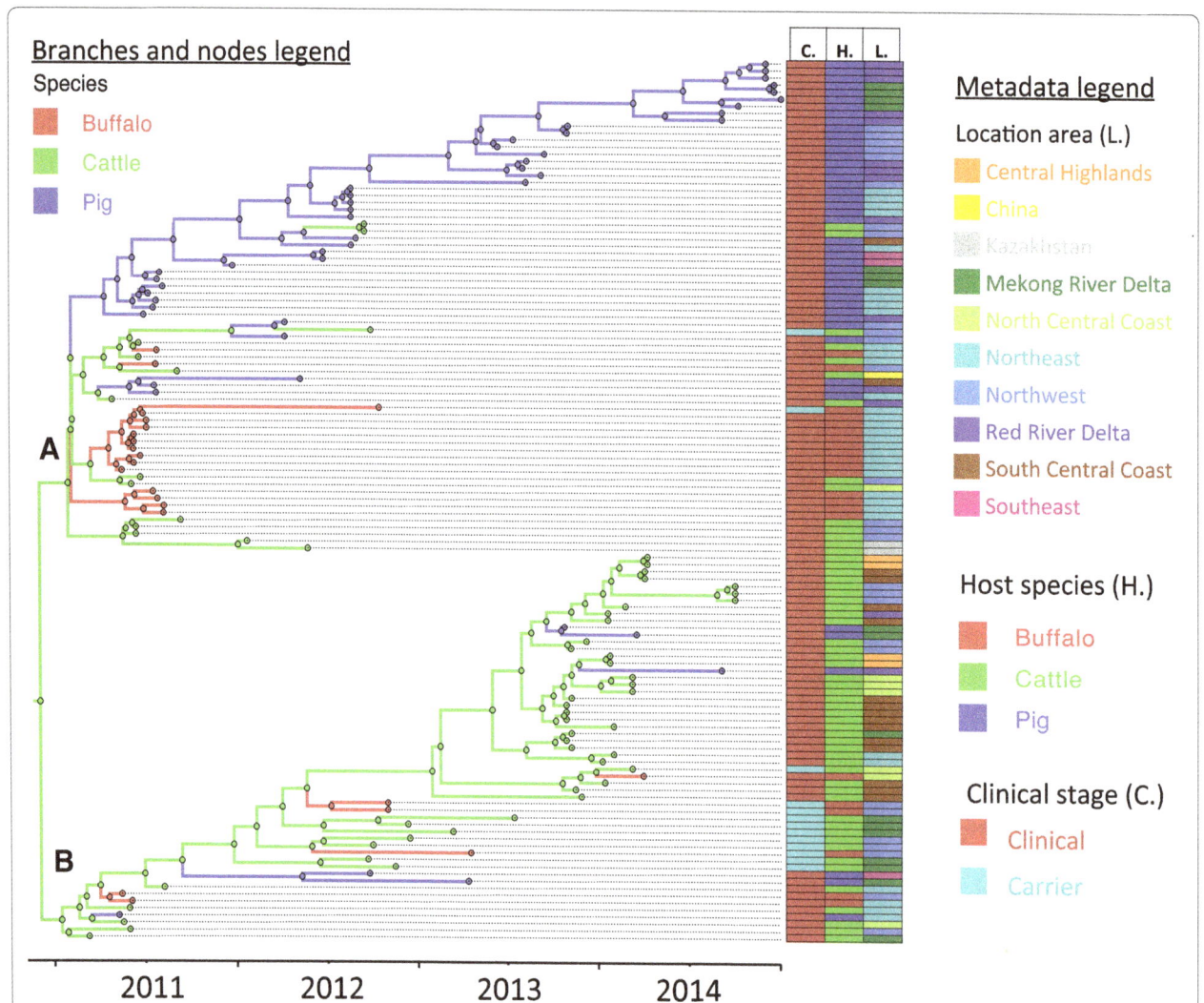

**Figure 1  Maximum clade credibility tree of FMDVs in Vietnam and related viruses from China and Kazakhstan between 2010 and 2014.** The color of tree branches and nodes indicates the ancestral host species for the reconstructed phylogeny. Clades **A** and **B** represent the two main O/ME-SA/PanAsia sublineages that have diverged recently in Vietnam. Characteristics of the sampled viruses (clinical stage: C., host species: H., and location: L.) are indicated in colored columns aligned to the right of the tree, color coding is indicated in the metadata legend.

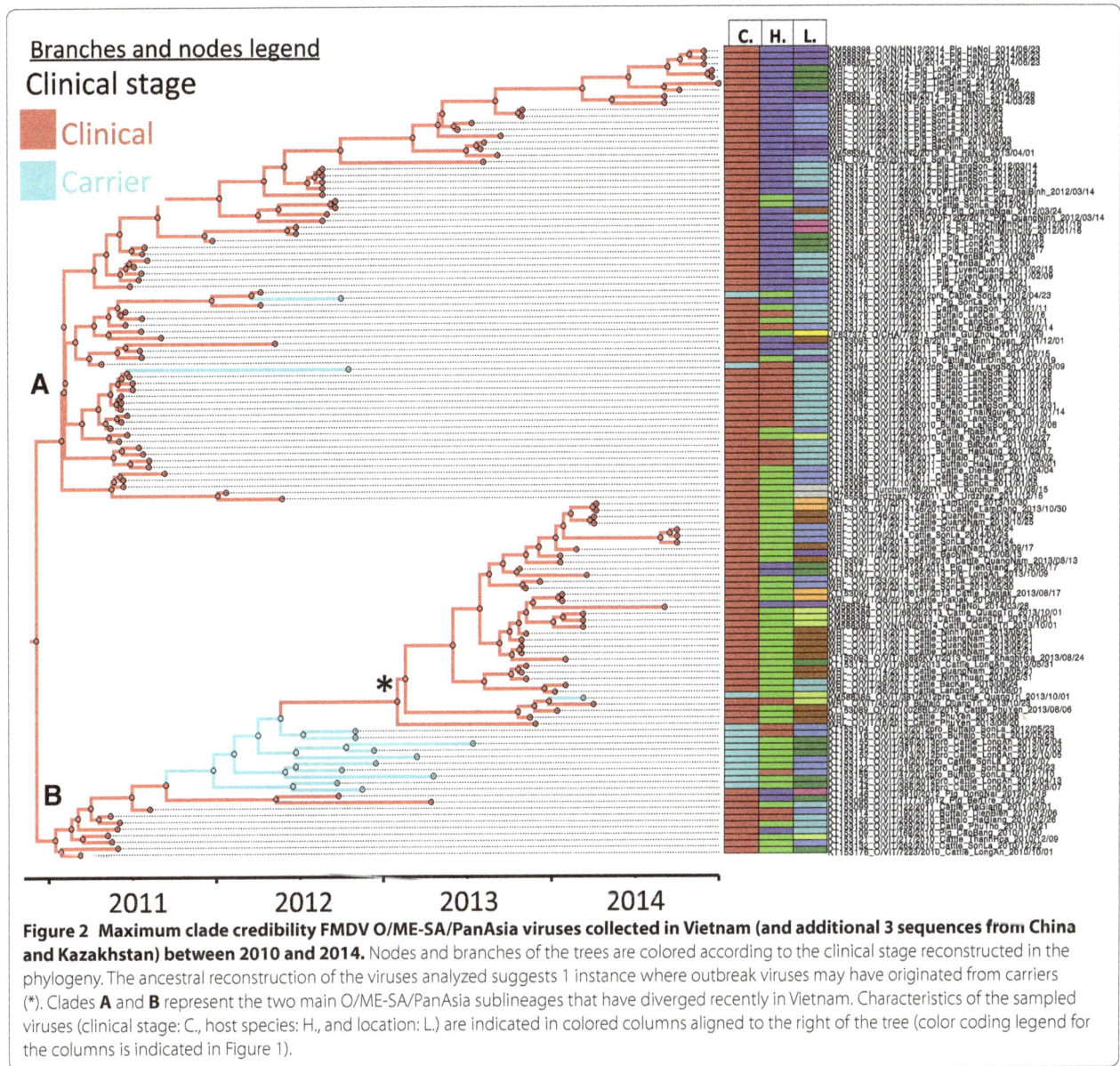

**Figure 2  Maximum clade credibility FMDV O/ME-SA/PanAsia viruses collected in Vietnam (and additional 3 sequences from China and Kazakhstan) between 2010 and 2014.** Nodes and branches of the trees are colored according to the clinical stage reconstructed in the phylogeny. The ancestral reconstruction of the viruses analyzed suggests 1 instance where outbreak viruses may have originated from carriers (*). Clades **A** and **B** represent the two main O/ME-SA/PanAsia sublineages that have diverged recently in Vietnam. Characteristics of the sampled viruses (clinical stage: C., host species: H., and location: L.) are indicated in colored columns aligned to the right of the tree (color coding legend for the columns is indicated in Figure 1).

outbreaks. However the tMRCA with the most closely genetically related 'clinical' viruses was relatively long (compared to tMRCA of related viruses), suggesting that they had already diverged approximately one year (1.32 and 0.53 years for viruses O/VIT/12/2012pro and O/VIT/25/2012pro respectively) from their ancestral "clinical" sample sequences. The lower branch of the tree (Figure 2, branch B) includes closely related viruses from 9 different persistently infected animals. The ancestral reconstruction of the set of viruses analyzed suggests that these viruses may have initiated an outbreak with clinical disease, which includes several closely related viruses (Figure 2, *).

Inferred non-zero transmission rates estimated by BSSVS analysis (Table 1), which is used to detect significant non-zero transmission from carrier to clinical and from clinical to carrier categories.

**Phylogeographic analysis**

The phylogeographic reconstruction of the viruses is shown in Figure 3. The common ancestor of all O/ME-SA/PanAsia sequences included in this study was located in the northeast region. Putative movements of this lineage from the Northeast of Vietnam into China and from the Northwest Region of Vietnam into Kazakhstan can be observed in Figure 3—branch A and

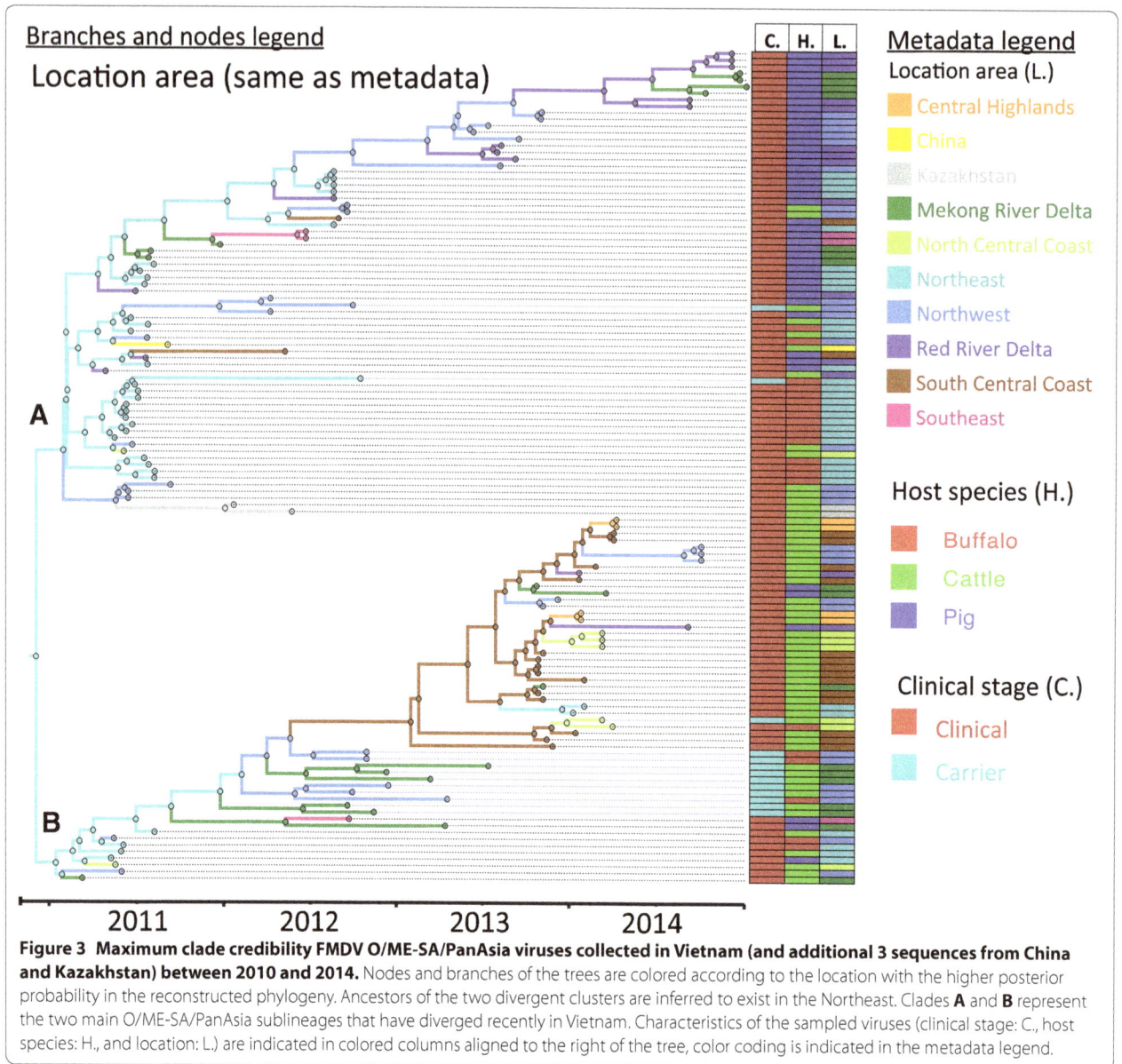

**Figure 3  Maximum clade credibility FMDV O/ME-SA/PanAsia viruses collected in Vietnam (and additional 3 sequences from China and Kazakhstan) between 2010 and 2014.** Nodes and branches of the trees are colored according to the location with the higher posterior probability in the reconstructed phylogeny. Ancestors of the two divergent clusters are inferred to exist in the Northeast. Clades **A** and **B** represent the two main O/ME-SA/PanAsia sublineages that have diverged recently in Vietnam. Characteristics of the sampled viruses (clinical stage: C., host species: H., and location: L.) are indicated in colored columns aligned to the right of the tree, color coding is indicated in the metadata legend.

may have occurred in December of 2010. The phylogeographic analysis demonstrates that the upper part of Figure 3—branch A, which contains a cluster of pig-derived viruses (Figure 2, branch A), may have initially originated from the Northeast and then spread into the Northwest, and the Red River Delta Regions.

To visualize the significant inferred transmission rates (BF > 3) between the geographical regions we overlaid these results on a map of Vietnam (Figure 4). The most significant inferred transmissions were detected from Northeast and South Central Coast to their corresponding adjacent regions, as well as transmission from Mekong River Delta into Southeast region. Inferred disease spread occurred in northern and southern directions, however there was a general trend of higher BF for southbound transfer of viruses. BF-inferred transmission is also shown in the heatmap displayed in Figure 4, and it further evidences that the South Central Coast and the Northeast are the regions from where the viruses are more frequently spread into other regions.

**Evolutionary selection of sites in different species and clinically versus persistently infected animals**
Results of the global dN/dS ratio (ratio of non-synonymous to synonymous changes) estimated by category are shown in Table 2. Considering only viruses from clinical outbreaks, pig-derived viruses had a higher overall positive selection ratio (dN/dS) compared to buffalo and

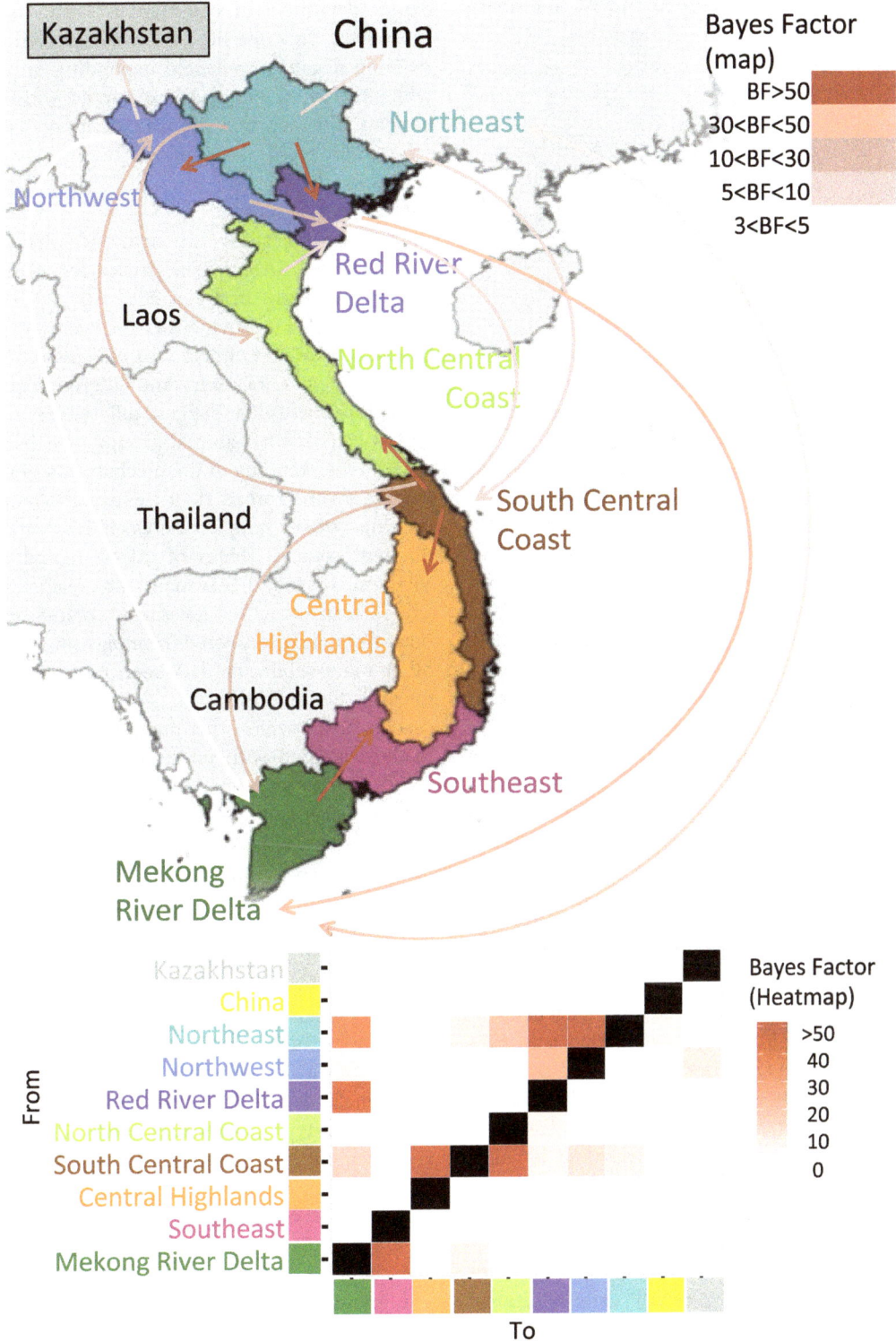

**Figure 4  Results from the Bayesian stochastic search variable selection of the Phylogeographic reconstruction of O/ME-SA/PanAsia in Vietnam regions, and related sequences from Kazakhstan and China.** Only Bayes factor > 3 are represented as arrows as significant non-zero transmission of O/ME-SA/PanAsia. Most significant transmissions were inferred for some adjacent regions, although inferred transmission between some distant regions was also statistically supported. The heatmap in the lower area of the figure depicts the magnitude of the statistical support (Bayes factor) for transmission rate between geographic regions in Vietnam. This heatmap allows visualizing that more transmission occurred from South Central Coast and the Northeast regions into other areas, whereas the Red River Delta and Mekong Delta were the ones with more incoming transmission from other regions.

**Table 2 Results of the global dN/dS ratio estimated for each of the categories and corresponding 95% confidence interval**

| Category | ω = dN/dS ratio | Lower 95% CI | Upper 95% CI |
| --- | --- | --- | --- |
| Cattle[a] | 0.161 | 0.107 | 0.23 |
| Pig[a] | 0.272 | 0.205 | 0.351 |
| Buffalo[a] | 0.181 | 0.094 | 0.312 |
| Carrier[b] | 0.160 | 0.112 | 0.222 |
| Outbreak[b] | 0.160 | 0.11 | 0.224 |
| All | 0.209 | 0.173 | 0.249 |

[a] Sequence from virus collected from clinical samples.

[b] Sequences from viruses collected from cattle and buffalo only.

cattle; however, only the difference with cattle was statistically significant at $p < 0.05$ (based on non-overlapping 95% confidence intervals). The extent of positive selection was similar in buffalo and cattle. Similarly, viruses collected from persistently infected animals and from clinically affected ones had almost the same dN/dS values (Table 2).

Results of the specific site selection for every codon (dN-dS) in all categories are shown in Figures 5A and B. No specific sites under positive selection were found to be statistically significant when analyzing viral sequences collected from cattle and buffalo, whereas few sites were detected when analyzing viral sequences from pig (site numbers: 1, 152, 153 and 172). Several statistically significant negatively selected sites were found for cattle (23 sites), pigs (28 sites), and buffalo (7 sites). Overall positive selection was mainly found within the known antigenic sites (GH loop, BC loop). Two statistically significant positively selected sites were found in the GH loop in pigs, compared to none in buffalo and cattle groups.

Although the global positive selection ratio was the same in carrier and clinically diseased animals, when dissecting the specific positively selected amino acid sites in the antigenic domains, carrier animals had a higher number of statistically significant positively selected sites compared to selection in viruses from clinical samples: Four statistically significant positively selected sites in the GH loop (near the RGD motif) and one in the BC loop were found in carriers, whereas two positively sites in the GH loop and two sites in the BC loop without statistical significance were found in clinical samples from cattle and buffalo (Figure 5B). Three additional sites of significant positive selection were also identified in viruses from carriers, but in non-antigenic regions. When analyzing all viral sequences together, several positively selected (non significant) sites were found within the GH-loop and the BC loop, whereas numerous significantly negatively selected sites were found throughout

VP1. Site 73 was consistently negatively selected (higher expected number of synonymous changes) in all group categories. Only one site (154) was detected as both positive and negatively selected depending on the category; while positive selection was detected within the carrier animals category, this site was identified as a negatively selected for pig viral sequences.

## Discussion

In the current study, we analyzed phylodynamics of FMDV O/ME-SA/PanAsia viruses recovered from livestock in Vietnam between 2010 and 2014. The results presented herein provide a novel overview of comparative viral evolution of field samples collected from different host species, locations, and different clinical stages of infection. These data suggest differences in viral evolution within distinct animal groups, which may contribute to understanding of the mechanisms of maintenance, emergence and spread of viruses across Vietnam.

Using viruses sampled between 2010 and 2014 from different species, stages of infection and provinces of Vietnam, we found two main sublineages of FMDV O/ME-SA/PanAsia. One of these sublineages has been most frequently recovered from pigs since 2011 while the other main sublineage has been most frequently found in cattle. Some FMDV strains may have a predilection to certain host species; this phenomenon has been extensively described with porcinophilic FMDV serotype O of the Cathay topotype [36, 37]. However, the data presented herein is not sufficient to determine limited host range of the mostly pig-derived FMDV subclade found in this study. This is because several other factors, including sampling bias, could have determined the apparent species-specificity. The hypothesis of limited host range could be confirmed by follow up studies in tissue culture or in vivo to determine if these viruses have evolved to a specific pig host predilection.

The substitution rate calculated herein for VP1 of FMDV O/ME-SA/PanAsia circulating in Vietnam between 2009 and 2014 was similar to a previous estimate of serotype O Cathay topotype ($1.06 \times 10^{-2}$) [38]. However, the rate estimated for this study was higher than those computed across other serotype O viruses estimated at $6.65 \times 10^{-3}$ [39], $6.34 \times 10^{-3}$ [40], or $4.81 \times 10^{-3}$ (serotype O collected globally between 1939 and 2010) [41] substitutions/site/year. The high mutation rate found in our analyses may be a result of capturing mutations that do not become fixed in a population, as a consequence of sampling a high number of outbreaks in a relatively short period of time. In contrast, isolated sequences from different regions sampled over longer periods may reflect fixed mutations, which may result in computing a different substitution rate. However, the

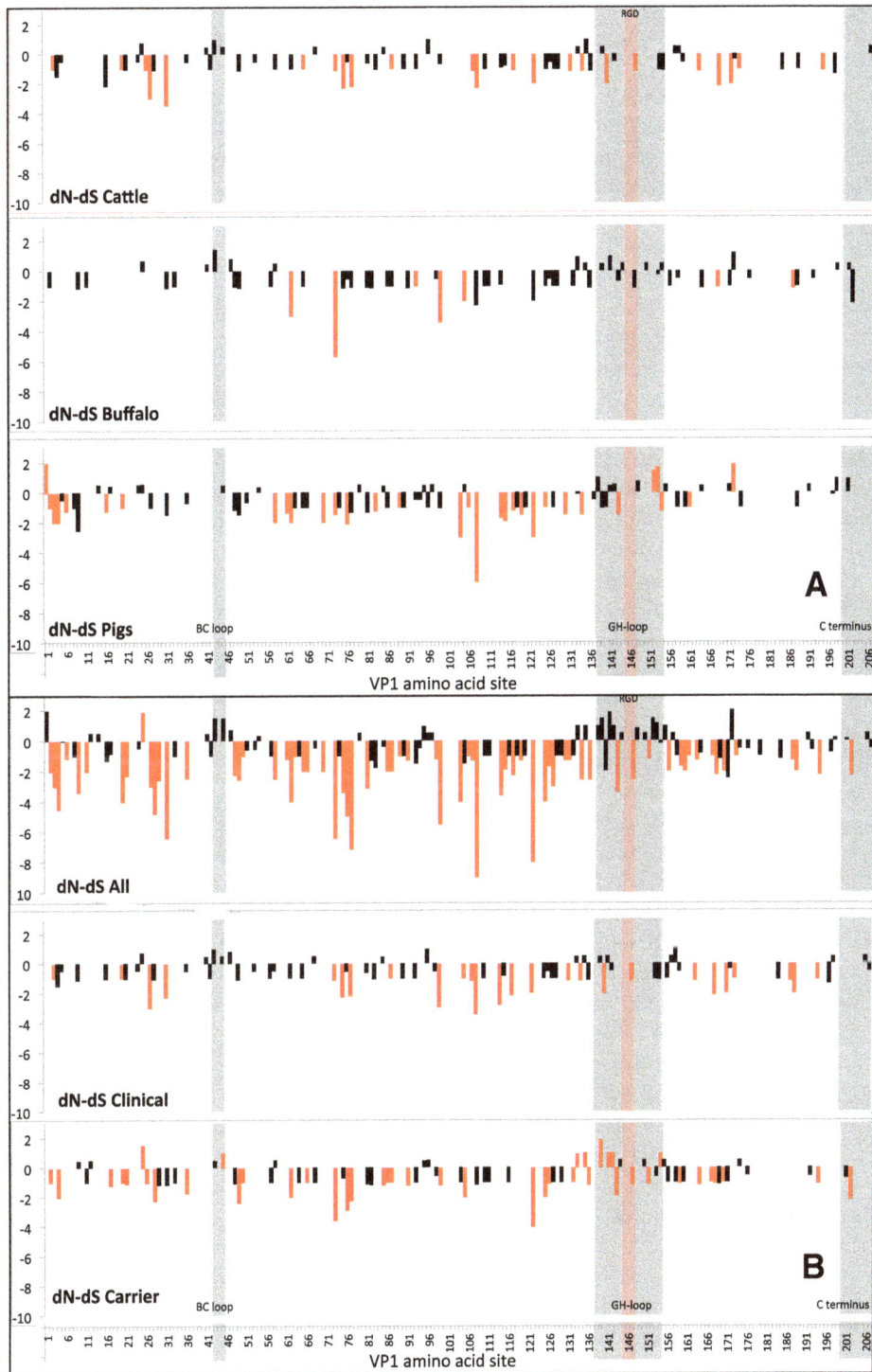

**Figure 5 Site selection (dN-dS) by VP1 coding region in alignments of FMDV sequences. A** Site selection (dN-dS) results per VP1 coding region in alignments of cattle viral sequences (excluding persistently infected), buffalo (excluding persistently infected) and pigs. Values >0 represent positive selection. Bars colored in red indicate sites where selection is statistically significant. Grey shaded areas correspond to known antigenic sites within VP1: BC loop (sites 43–45), GH loop (sites 238–254), and C terminus (sites 200–207). Pink-shaded sites correspond to the RGD integrin-binding motif. **B** Site selection (dN-dS) results per VP1 coding region in alignments including of all viral sequences, "clinical" (cattle and buffalo) viral sequences and "carrier" (cattle and buffalo) infected animals.

specific underlying mechanisms driving these differences across studies using different geotemporal conditions remain undetermined.

Inferred transmission as deduced by ancestral character reconstruction suggests that cattle have a relevant role in inter-species dissemination. Various factors may contribute to this phenomenon including subclinical infection in vaccinated cattle and a longer duration of FMDV infectiousness in cattle compared to other species [12, 13]. Similarly, our study also provides evidence of inferred transmission of viruses from pigs to cattle. This may be explained by the large pig population in the country, and husbandry practices including the highly common practice of co-mingling pigs with other species in rural households and villages. In contrast, based on the sequences obtained, we did not identify putative transmission from buffalo to either cattle or pigs. Although transmission from cattle to buffalo, and buffalo to cattle is known to occur [42, 43], to our knowledge, comparative quantitative estimates of transmission rates of these two species have not been estimated. We detected several instances of transfer of viruses from cattle to buffalo, but none from buffalo to cattle. The lack of detection may either represent lesser ability of buffalo to transmit the disease to cattle, differential ranging and transport of buffalo and cattle within and between different areas in Vietnam, or it may be an effect of sampling bias.

Phylogenetic analyses in this study, suggest that there are instances in which viruses found in carrier animals may have been the ancestors of viruses that later caused outbreaks. However, it is also possible that undersampling of outbreak sequences around the period of the apparent carrier-to-clinical transfer may have created sampling bias which influenced these results (Figure 2). Transmission from carriers to susceptible animals has been either low or inexistent in controlled experiments. However, the potential epidemiological role of the FMDV carrier state in maintaining FMDV and being the source of new outbreaks is still highly controversial [13, 17, 44]. Quantitatively, it has been estimated that the transmission rate from acutely (clinically) infected animals is more than 500 times that of the carrier [20]. However even though the probability is exceedingly low, it would only require one successful transmission event within the thousands of contacts to start an outbreak and thus have a substantial impact.

Overall, the number of outbreaks and potential infected animals included herein is low compared to the actual number of outbreaks and infections that occurred in the field. Thus, such findings must be interpreted conservatively. Because of the inability to obtain every relevant virus from the field, analyses derived from studies such as this, contain intrinsic sampling bias and must be interpreted as generating, rather than confirming hypotheses. Similarly, these phylogenetic analyses were carried out using only VP1 coding sequence of FMDV, which is 639 nt long of the ~7000 nt ORF length. This genetic segment is the most variable within FMDV genome and contains the most relevant antigenic sites. Full genome sequences in sufficient quantities to enable these studies of phylodynamics of Vietnam, were not available at the time of this work.

Geographic spread of FMD within Vietnam inferred by viral sequence suggests that transmission occurs between several different regions of the country. However transmission seems to be more frequent from South Central Coast and Northeast into other parts of the country. As expected, the greatest extent of transmission was to immediately adjacent regions, but also to distant parts of the country. These findings are partially consistent with previous studies conducted by the OIE, which assessed the livestock movement in Vietnam and neighboring countries [5]. That report describes that substantial ruminant movement occurs from central areas of the country into northern and southern regions. Within the northern regions, this flow tends to be towards northeastern region, whereas in the south, animal movement converges into northern areas of the Mekong River Delta region. In contrast, pig movement occurs mostly from northern into southern areas of Vietnam and from northern areas into China. Transmission occurring in different geographic directions inferred by our analysis reflects the combination of these reported pig and ruminant species movement. The movement of large ruminants and pigs into China, however, is supported by our current inferred viral transmission data. Additionally, animal movement from Thailand, Cambodia and Laos into Vietnam occurs frequently [5].

Selection pressure may be an important driver of viral evolution [45]. It is biologically plausible that selection pressures differ in different host species, or through different phases of infection within the same host (e.g. acute clinical infection in contrast to persistent infection). Viral evolution comparing different groups of infected animals has not been extensively explored previously. Potential specific molecular changes in the FMDV genome that establish persistent infection have been reported in few controlled studies [17, 21, 46]. Here, we found that the global positive selection of VP1 tended to be similar in carrier animals compared to viruses recovered from clinical outbreaks. Although the value of the global positive selection rate was almost equal in carrier and outbreak groups, the quantity of individual (statistically significant) positive selected codon sites was higher in carrier animals compared with those with acute clinical infection, especially in the antigenic regions.

Because animal movement and mixing animals from different origins is a common practice in Vietnam, persistently infected animals may play an important role in disease spread. Understanding specific molecular (genomic and/or antigenic) changes can eventually help to understand the mechanisms through which FMDV persistence is established and maintained. Although analyses of our data demonstrate potentially relevant trends, results should be interpreted carefully with mindfulness of the relatively low quantity of samples from carrier animals ($n = 12$).

Additionally, we found that statistically significant positive selection was greatest in pigs compared to buffalo and cattle, and that these sites were found mostly in regions that code for the known antigenic domains. This suggests that the viral evolution in the pig population may provide an important contribution to antigenic diversity and strain emergence compared to other species. Previous work has shown that most of the genomic variation occurs early in the course of infection, when there is greater viral replication [47].

In conclusion, the current study suggests that inferred virus transmission patterns in Vietnam may differ depending on the host species and clinical status of infected hosts. This may be related to differences in viral selection between species and in the persistently infected animals compared to clinically affected individuals. These differences can help to elucidate viral evolution within-host, across host species, and within populations. Application and combination of the methodologies described herein to study specific aspects of FMDV evolution may help to gain new knowledge in our understanding of FMDV, ultimately contributing to disease control and eradication in endemic countries.

### Abbreviations

BF: Bayes factor; BSSVS: Bayesian stochastic search variable selection; dN: substitution rates at non-synonymous sites; dpi: days post-infection; dS: substitution rates at synonymous sites; FMD: foot-and-mouth disease; FMDV: foot-and-mouth disease virus; MCC: maximum clade credibility; Nt: nucleotide; OIE: World Organization for Animal Health; tMRCA: time to most recent common ancestor.

### Competing interests

The authors declare that they have no competing interests.

### Authors' contributions

JA, LR, BB, NTL, DHD, PVD, and SP conceived the study. SP, HF, PQM, LTV, NTP, BHH, NDT, ME, DK and NK performed the laboratory analysis, BB performed the sequence and statistical analyses, LTV, NDT, BHH, NTP, DK and NK coordinated and performed the sample collection. BB, JA, CS and SP wrote the manuscript. All authors read and approved the manuscript.

### Acknowledgements

This research was funded in part by ARS-CRIS Project 1940-32000-057-00D and through an interagency agreement with the Science and Technology Directorate of the U.S. Department of Homeland Security under Award Number HSHQDC-12-X-0060. Additional funding was provided by the U.S. Department of State, Biosecurity Engagement Program through the USDA, ARS Office of International Research Programs and the Cooperative Biological Engagement Program of the U.S. Department of Defense, Defense Threat Reduction Agency. We acknowledge Ethan J. Hartwig and George R. Smoliga for expert technical support. Barbara Brito, Carolina Stenfeldt, Michael Eschbaumer, and Helena C. de Carvalho Ferreira are the recipients of a Plum Island Animal Disease Center Research Participation Program fellowship, administered by the Oak Ridge Institute for Science and Education (ORISE) through an interagency agreement between the U.S. Department of Energy (DOE) and the U.S. Department of Agriculture (USDA). All opinions expressed in this paper are the author's and do not necessarily reflect the policies and views of the USDA-ARS FADRU, Vietnam DAH or ORAU/ORISE. The Vietnam DAH and USDA-ARS FADRU are members of the Global Foot-and-Mouth Disease Research Alliance (GFRA). The work contributed by the WRLFMD was supported by the Department for Environment, Food and Rural Affairs (Project SE2943: Defra, UK), and funding provided to the EuFMD from the European Union.

### Author details

[1] Foreign Animal Disease Research Unit, Plum Island Animal Disease Center, ARS, USDA, Orient Point, NY, USA. [2] Oak Ridge Institute for Science and Education, PIADC Research Participation Program, Oak Ridge, TN, USA. [3] Regional Animal Health Office No. 6, Department of Animal Health, Ministry of Agriculture and Rural Development, Ho Chi Minh City, Vietnam. [4] National Centre for Veterinary Diagnostics, Hanoi, Vietnam. [5] Department of Animal Health, Ministry of Agriculture and Rural Development, Hanoi, Vietnam. [6] The Pirbright Institute, Pirbright, UK. [7] Present Address: Friedrich-Loeffler-Institut, Federal Research Institute for Animal Health, Insel Riems, Germany.

### References

1. Sumption K, Rweyemamu M, Wint W (2008) Incidence and distribution of foot-and-mouth disease in Asia, Africa and South America; combining expert opinion, official disease information and livestock populations to assist risk assessment. Transbound Emerg Dis 55:5–13
2. Di Nardo A, Knowles NJ, Paton DJ (2011) Combining livestock trade patterns with phylogenetics to help understand the spread of foot and mouth disease in sub-Saharan Africa, the Middle East and Southeast Asia. Rev Sci Tech 30:63–85
3. Pham HT, Antoine-Moussiaux N, Grosbois V, Moula N, Truong BD, Phan TD, Vu TD, Trinh TQ, Vu CC, Rukkwamsuk T, Peyre M (2016) Financial impacts of priority swine diseases to pig farmers in Red River and Mekong River Delta, Vietnam. Transbound Emerg Dis. doi:10.1111/tbed.12482
4. Gleeson LJ (2002) A review of the status of foot and mouth disease in South-East Asia and approaches to control and eradication. Rev Sci Tech 21:465–475
5. Smith P, Bourgeois Lüthi N, Huachun L, Naing Oo K, Phonvisay A, Premashthira S, Abila R, Widders P, Kukreja K, Miller C (2015) Movement pathways and market chains of large ruminants in the Greater Mekong Sub-region. Report of the World Organisation for Animal Health (OIE). Sub-regional representation for South-East Asia, Thailand. http://www.rr-asia.oie.int/fileadmin/SRR_Activities/documents/movement.pdf. Accessed Jan 2017
6. de Carvalho Ferreira HC, Pauszek SJ, Ludi A, Huston CL, Pacheco JM, Le VT, Nguyen PT, Bui HH, Nguyen TD, Nguyen T, Nguyen TT, Ngo LT, Do DH, Rodriguez L, Arzt J (2017) An integrative analysis of foot-and-mouth disease virus carriers in Vietnam achieved through targeted surveillance and molecular epidemiology. Transbound Emerg Dis 64:547–563
7. Brito BP, Rodriguez LL, Hammond JM, Pinto J, Perez AM (2015) Review of the global distribution of foot-and-mouth disease virus from 2007 to 2014. Transbound Emerg Dis 64:316–332
8. Le VP, Nguyen T, Park JH, Kim SM, Ko YJ, Lee HS, Nguyen VC, Mai TD, Do TH, Cho IS, Lee KN (2010) Heterogeneity and genetic variations of serotypes O and Asia 1 foot-and-mouth disease viruses isolated in Vietnam. Vet Microbiol 145:220–229
9. Le PV, Vu TTH, Duong HQ, Than VT, Song D (2016) Evolutionary phylodynamics of foot-and-mouth disease virus serotypes O and A circulating in Vietnam. BMC Vet Res 12:269

10. WRLFMD (2015) Reference laboratory reports. In: The Fao World Reference Laboratory for Foot-and-mouth Disease. http://www.wrlfmd.org/ref_labs/fmd_ref_lab_reports.htm. Accessed 15 Sept 2016

11. Mardones F, Perez A, Sanchez J, Alkhamis M, Carpenter T (2010) Parameterization of the duration of infection stages of serotype O foot-and-mouth disease virus: an analytical review and meta-analysis with application to simulation models. Vet Res 41:45

12. Alexandersen S, Zhang Z, Donaldson AI, Garland AJ (2003) The pathogenesis and diagnosis of foot-and-mouth disease. J Comp Pathol 129:1–36

13. Arzt J, Juleff N, Zhang Z, Rodriguez LL (2011) The pathogenesis of foot-and-mouth disease I: viral pathways in cattle. Transbound Emerg Dis 58:291–304

14. Stenfeldt C, Eschbaumer M, Rekant SI, Pacheco JM, Smoliga GR, Hartwig EJ, Rodriguez LL, Arzt J (2016) The foot-and-mouth disease carrier state divergence in cattle. J Virol 90:6344–6364

15. Stenfeldt C, Belsham GJ (2012) Detection of foot-and-mouth disease virus RNA in pharyngeal epithelium biopsy samples obtained from infected cattle: investigation of possible sites of virus replication and persistence. Vet Microbiol 154:230–239

16. Sutmoller P, McVicar JW, Cottral GE (1968) The epizootiological importance of foot-and-mouth disease carriers. I. Experimentally produced foot-and-mouth disease carriers in susceptible and immune cattle. Arch Gesamte Virusforsch 23:227–235

17. Salt J (2004) Persistence of Foot-and-mouth Disease Virus. In: Sobrino F, Domingo E (eds) Foot-and-mouth disease current perspectives. Horizon Bioscience, Wymondham, pp 103–144

18. Kitching RP (2002) Identification of foot and mouth disease virus carrier and subclinically infected animals and differentiation from vaccinated animals. Rev Sci Tech 21:531–538

19. Garland AJ, de Clercq K (2011) Cattle, sheep and pigs vaccinated against foot and mouth disease: does trade in these animals and their products present a risk of transmitting the disease? Rev Sci Tech 30:189–206

20. Tenzin Dekker A, Vernooij H, Bouma A, Stegeman A (2008) Rate of foot-and-mouth disease virus transmission by carriers quantified from experimental data. Risk Anal 28:303–309

21. Parthiban AB, Mahapatra M, Gubbins S, Parida S (2015) Virus excretion from foot-and-mouth disease virus carrier cattle and their potential role in causing new outbreaks. PLoS One 10:e0128815

22. Lemey P, Rambaut A, Drummond AJ, Suchard MA (2009) Bayesian phylogeography finds its roots. PLoS Comput Biol 5:e1000520

23. Baele G, Suchard MA, Rambaut A, Lemey P (2017) Emerging concepts of data integration in pathogen phylodynamics. Syst Biol 66:e47–e65

24. Jackson T, King AM, Stuart DI, Fry E (2003) Structure and receptor binding. Virus Res 91:33–46

25. Pauszek SJ, Eschbaumer M, Brito B, de Carvalho Ferreira HC, Vu LT, Phuong NT, Hoang BH, Tho ND, Dong PV, Tung N, Long NT, Dung DH, Rodriguez LL, Arzt J (2016) Site-specific substitution (Q172R) in the VP1 protein of FMDV isolates collected from subclinical field cases in Vietnam. Virol Rep 6:90–96

26. Edgar RC (2004) MUSCLE: multiple sequence alignment with high accuracy and high throughput. Nucleic Acids Res 32:1792–1797

27. Lanfear R, Calcott B, Ho SY, Guindon S (2012) Partitionfinder: combined selection of partitioning schemes and substitution models for phylogenetic analyses. Mol Biol Evol 29:1695–1701

28. Drummond AJ, Rambaut A (2007) BEAST: Bayesian evolutionary analysis by sampling trees. BMC Evol Biol 7:214

29. Miller MA, Pfeiffer W, Schwartz T (2010) Creating the CIPRES Science Gateway for inference of large phylogenetic trees. Gateway Computing Environments Workshop (GCE), New Orleans

30. Rambaut A, Drummond A (2007) Tracer version 1.4, Computer program and documentation distributed by the author. http://tree.bio.ed.ac.uk/software/tracer/. Accessed 15 Sept 2016

31. Rambault A (2006–2009) Fig Tree Tree Figure Drawing Tool, Version 13.1. http://tree.bio.ed.ac.uk/software/figtree/. Accessed 15 Sept 2016

32. Bielejec F, Rambaut A, Suchard MA, Lemey P (2011) SPREAD: spatial phylogenetic reconstruction of evolutionary dynamics. Bioinformatics 27:2910–2912

33. Meredith M, Kruschke J (2016) HDInterval: highest (posterior) density intervals. R package version 0.1.3. https://CRAN.R-project.org/package=HDInterval. Accessed 3 Mar 2017

34. Kosakovsky Pond SL, Frost SDW (2005) Not so different after all: a comparison of methods for detecting amino acid sites under selection. Mol Biol Evol 22:1208–1222

35. Kosakovsky Pond SL, Frost SDW, Muse SV (2005) HyPhy: hypothesis testing using phylogenies. Bioinformatics 21:676–679

36. Oem JK, Yeh MT, McKenna TS, Hayes JR, Rieder E, Giuffre AC, Robida JM, Lee KN, Cho IS, Fang X, Joo YS, Park JH (2008) Pathogenic characteristics of the Korean 2002 isolate of foot-and-mouth disease virus serotype O in pigs and cattle. J Comp Pathol 138:204–214

37. Beard CW, Mason PW (2000) Genetic determinants of altered virulence of Taiwanese foot-and-mouth disease virus. J Virol 74:987–991

38. Di Nardo A, Knowles NJ, Wadsworth J, Haydon DT, King DP (2014) Phylodynamic reconstruction of O CATHAY topotype foot-and-mouth disease virus epidemics in the Philippines. Vet Res 45:90

39. Jamal SM, Ferrari G, Ahmed S, Normann P, Belsham G (2011) Genetic diversity of foot-and-mouth disease virus serotype O in Pakistan and Afghanistan, 1997-2009. Infect Genet Evol 11:1229–1238

40. Subramaniam S, Mohapatra JK, Sharma GK, Biswal JK, Ranjan R, Rout M, Das B, Dash BB, Sanyal A, Pattnaik B (2015) Evolutionary dynamics of foot-and-mouth disease virus O/ME-SA/Ind2001 lineage. Vet Microbiol 178:181–189

41. Yoon SH, Lee KN, Park JH, Kim H (2011) Molecular epidemiology of foot-and-mouth disease virus serotypes A and O with emphasis on Korean isolates: temporal and spatial dynamics. Arch Virol 156:817–826

42. Madhanmohan M, Yuvaraj S, Nagendrakumar SB, Srinivasan VA, Gubbins S, Paton DJ, Parida S (2014) Transmission of foot-and-mouth disease virus from experimentally infected Indian buffalo (Bubalus bubalis) to in-contact naïve and vaccinated Indian buffalo and cattle. Vaccine 32:5125–5130

43. Gomes I, Ramalho AK, de Mello PA (1997) Infectivity assays of foot-and-mouth disease virus: contact transmission between cattle and buffalo (Bubalus bubalis) in the early stages of infection. Vet Rec 140:43–47

44. Alexandersen S, Mowat N (2005) Foot-and-mouth disease: host range and pathogenesis. Curr Top Microbiol Immunol 288:9–42

45. Domingo E, Sheldon J, Perales C (2012) Viral quasispecies evolution. Microbiol Mol Biol Rev 76:159–216

46. Kopliku L, Relmy A, Romey A, Gorna K, Zientara S, Bakkali-Kassimi L, Blaise-Boisseau S (2015) Establishment of persistent foot-and-mouth disease virus (FMDV) infection in MDBK cells. Arch Virol 160:2503–2516

47. Malirat V, De Mello PA, Tiraboschi B, Beck E, Gomes I, Bergmann IE (1994) Genetic variation of foot-and-mouth disease virus during persistent infection in cattle. Virus Res 34:31–48

# Permissions

The contributors of this book come from diverse backgrounds, making this book a truly international effort. This book will bring forth new frontiers with its revolutionizing research information and detailed analysis of the nascent developments around the world.

We would like to thank all the contributing authors for lending their expertise to make the book truly unique. They have played a crucial role in the development of this book. Without their invaluable contributions this book wouldn't have been possible. They have made vital efforts to compile up to date information on the varied aspects of this subject to make this book a valuable addition to the collection of many professionals and students.

This book was conceptualized with the vision of imparting up-to-date information and advanced data in this field. To ensure the same, a matchless editorial board was set up. Every individual on the board went through rigorous rounds of assessment to prove their worth. After which they invested a large part of their time researching and compiling the most relevant data for our readers.

The editorial board has been involved in producing this book since its inception. They have spent rigorous hours researching and exploring the diverse topics which have resulted in the successful publishing of this book. They have passed on their knowledge of decades through this book. To expedite this challenging task, the publisher supported the team at every step. A small team of assistant editors was also appointed to further simplify the editing procedure and attain best results for the readers.

Apart from the editorial board, the designing team has also invested a significant amount of their time in understanding the subject and creating the most relevant covers. They scrutinized every image to scout for the most suitable representation of the subject and create an appropriate cover for the book.

The publishing team has been an ardent support to the editorial, designing and production team. Their endless efforts to recruit the best for this project, has resulted in the accomplishment of this book. They are a veteran in the field of academics and their pool of knowledge is as vast as their experience in printing. Their expertise and guidance has proved useful at every step. Their uncompromising quality standards have made this book an exceptional effort. Their encouragement from time to time has been an inspiration for everyone.

The publisher and the editorial board hope that this book will prove to be a valuable piece of knowledge for researchers, students, practitioners and scholars across the globe.

# List of Contributors

**Yanqing Bao, Mingxing Tian, Peng Li, Jiameng Liu and Chan Ding**
Shanghai Veterinary Research Institute, Chinese Academy of Agricultural Sciences (CAAS), Shanghai, China

**Shengqing Yu**
Shanghai Veterinary Research Institute, Chinese Academy of Agricultural Sciences (CAAS), Shanghai, China
Jiangsu Co-innovation Center for Prevention and Control of Important Animal Infectious Diseases and Zoonoses, Yangzhou, China

**Liqian Zhu**
College of Veterinary Medicine, Yangzhou University, 48 Wenhui East Road, Yangzhou 225009, Jiangsu, China
Jiangsu Co-innovation Center for Prevention and Control of Important Animal Infectious Diseases and Zoonoses, 48 Wenhui East Road, Yangzhou 225009, Jiangsu, China
Department of Veterinary Pathobiology, Oklahoma State University, Center for Veterinary Health Sciences, Stillwater, OK 74078, USA

**Chen Yuan and Guoqiang Zhu**
College of Veterinary Medicine, Yangzhou University, 48 Wenhui East Road, Yangzhou 225009, Jiangsu, China
Jiangsu Co-innovation Center for Prevention and Control of Important Animal Infectious Diseases and Zoonoses, 48 Wenhui East Road, Yangzhou 225009, Jiangsu, China

**Xiuyan Ding**
College of Veterinary Medicine, Yangzhou University, 48 Wenhui East Road, Yangzhou 225009, Jiangsu, China
Jiangsu Co-innovation Center for Prevention and Control of Important Animal Infectious Diseases and Zoonoses, 48 Wenhui East Road, Yangzhou 225009, Jiangsu, China
Test Center, Yangzhou University, 48 Wenhui East Road, Yangzhou 225009, Jiangsu, China

**Clinton Jones**
Department of Veterinary Pathobiology, Oklahoma State University, Center for Veterinary Health Sciences, Stillwater, OK 74078, USA

**P. H. Phaswana, J. E. Crafford and H. van Heerden**
Department of Veterinary Tropical Diseases, University of Pretoria, Onderstepoort 0110, South Africa

**O. C. Ndumnego**
Department of Veterinary Tropical Diseases, University of Pretoria, Onderstepoort 0110, South Africa
Present Address: Africa Health Research Institute, K-RITH Tower Building, Umbilo Road, Durban 4013, South Africa

**S. M. Koehler**
Department of Livestock Infectiology and Environmental Hygiene, Institute of Animal Science, University of Hohenheim, Emil-Wolff-Strasse 14, 70599 Stuttgart, Germany
Present Address: Robert Koch Institute, Nordufer 20, 13353 Berlin, Germany

**W. Beyer**
Department of Livestock Infectiology and Environmental Hygiene, Institute of Animal Science, University of Hohenheim, Emil-Wolff-Strasse 14, 70599 Stuttgart, Germany

**Michael Muleme, Joanne M. Devlin, Alexander Cameron, Colin R. Wilks and Simon Firestone**
Asia–Pacific Centre for Animal Health, Faculty of Veterinary and Agricultural Sciences, The University of Melbourne, Parkville, VIC 3010, Australia

**Angus Campbell**
The Mackinnon Project, Faculty of Veterinary and Agricultural Sciences, The University of Melbourne, Werribee, VIC 3010, Australia

**John Stenos, Gemma Vincent and Stephen Graves**
Australian Rickettsial Reference Laboratory, Barwon Health, Geelong, VIC, Australia

**Hong Jo Lee, Kyung Youn Lee, Young Hyun Park and Hee Jung Choi**
Department of Agricultural Biotechnology, College of Agriculture and Life Sciences, and Research Institute of Agriculture and Life Sciences, Seoul National University, Seoul 08826, South Korea

**Yongxiu Yao and Venugopal Nair**
The Pirbright Institute, Woking, Pirbright, Surrey GU24 0NF, UK

**Jae Yong Han**
Department of Agricultural Biotechnology, College of Agriculture and Life Sciences, and Research Institute of Agriculture and Life Sciences, Seoul National University, Seoul 08826, South Korea
Institute for Biomedical Sciences, Shinshu University, Minamiminowa, Nagano 399-4598, Japan

**C. Fast, K. Tauscher and M. H. Groschup**
Friedrich-Loeffler-Institut, Institute of Novel and Emerging Infectious Diseases, Greifswald-Insel Riems, Germany.

**W. Goldmann and N. Hunter**
The Roslin Institute and Royal (Dick) School of Veterinary Studies, University of Edinburgh, Easter Bush, Midlothian, UK

**P. Berthon, I. Lantier, C. Rossignol and F. Lantier**
UMR 1282 ISP, Institut National de la Recherche Agronomique (INRA), University of Tours, 37380 Nouzilly, France

**O. Andréoletti**
INRA, UMR 1225, Interactions Hôtes Agents Pathogènes, Ecole Nationale Vétérinaire de Toulouse, Toulouse Cedex, France

**A. Bossers, J. G. Jacobs and J. P. M. Langeveld**
Wageningen BioVeterinary Research, Wageningen University & Research, Houtribweg 39, 8221RA Lelystad, The Netherlands

**Tian Liu**
Avian Disease Research Center, College of Veterinary Medicine, Sichuan Agricultural University, Wenjiang, Chengdu 611130, People's Republic of China
Institute of Preventive Veterinary Medicine, Sichuan Agricultural University, Wenjiang, Chengdu 611130, People's Republic of China

**Anchun Cheng, Mingshu Wang, Renyong Jia, Qiao Yang, Ying Wu, Kunfeng Sun, Shun Chen, Mafeng Liu and XinXin Zhao**
Avian Disease Research Center, College of Veterinary Medicine, Sichuan Agricultural University, Wenjiang, Chengdu 611130, People's Republic of China
Institute of Preventive Veterinary Medicine, Sichuan Agricultural University, Wenjiang, Chengdu 611130, People's Republic of China
Key Laboratory of Animal Disease and Human Health of Sichuan Province, Wenjiang, Chengdu 611130, People's Republic of China

**Dekang Zhu and Xiaoyue Chen**
Institute of Preventive Veterinary Medicine, Sichuan Agricultural University, Wenjiang, Chengdu 611130, People's Republic of China
Key Laboratory of Animal Disease and Human Health of Sichuan Province, Wenjiang, Chengdu 611130, People's Republic of China

**Hoang Trong Phan and Thuong Thi Ho**
Leibniz Institute of Plant Genetics and Crop Plant Research (IPK), Gatersleben, Germany
Institute of Biotechnology, Hanoi, Vietnam

**Ha Hoang Chu and Trang Huyen Vu**
Institute of Biotechnology, Hanoi, Vietnam

**Ulrike Gresch and Udo Conrad**
Leibniz Institute of Plant Genetics and Crop Plant Research (IPK), Gatersleben, Germany

**Gokhlesh Kumar and Mansour El-Matbouli**
Clinical Division of Fish Medicine, University of Veterinary Medicine, Veterinärplatz 1, 1210 Vienna, Austria

**Karin Hummel and Ebrahim Razzazi-Fazeli**
VetCore Facility for Research/Proteomics Unit, University of Veterinary Medicine, Vienna, Austria

**Timothy J. Welch**
National Center for Cool and Cold Water Aquaculture, Kearneysville, USA

**Maoda Pang, Lichang Sun, Tao He, Hongdu Bao, Lili Zhang, Yan Zhou, Hui Zhang, Ruicheng Wei and Ran Wang**
Key Laboratory of Control Technology and Standard for Agro-product Safety and Quality, Key Lab of Food Quality and Safety of Jiangsu Province-State Key Laboratory Breeding Base, Institute of Food Safety and Nutrition, Jiangsu

Academy of Agricultural Sciences, No. 50 Zhongling Street, Nanjing 210014, China

**Yongjie Liu**
College of Veterinary Medicine, Nanjing Agricultural University, No. 1 Weigang, Nanjing 210095, China

**Charlie Cador, Mathieu Andraud and Nicolas Rose**
Swine Epidemiology and Welfare Research Unit, French Agency for Food, Environmental and Occupational Health & Safety (ANSES), BP 53, 22440 Ploufragan, France
Université Bretagne Loire, Rennes, France

**Lander Willem**
Centre for Health Economics & Modeling Infectious Diseases, Vaccine and Infectious Disease Institute, University of Antwerp Research, Antwerp, Belgium

**Céline Ster, Valérie Lebeau, Julia Leclerc, Alexandre Fugère, Koui A. Veh and François Malouin**
Centre d'Étude et de Valorisation de la Diversité Microbienne (CEVDM), Département de Biologie, Faculté des Sciences, Université de Sherbrooke, Sherbrooke, QC J1K 2R1, Canada

**Jean-Philippe Roy**
Département de Sciences Cliniques, Faculté de Médecine Vétérinaire, Université de Montréal, C.P. 5000, St-Hyacinthe, QC J2S 7C6, Canada

**Min Sun, Jiale Ma, Zeyanqiu Yu, Zihao Pan, Chengping Lu and Huochun Yao**
College of Veterinary Medicine, Nanjing Agricultural University, Nanjing, Jiangsu, China

**Sarah Chuzeville, Jean-Philippe Auger, Audrey Dumesnil, David Roy, Sonia Lacouture and Marcelo Gottschalk**
Swine and Poultry Infectious Diseases Research Center (CRIPA), Saint-Hyacinthe, QC, Canada
Groupe de recherche sur les maladies infectieuses en production animale (GREMIP), Department of Pathology and Microbiology, Faculty of Veterinary Medicine, University of Montreal, 3200 Sicotte St., Saint-Hyacinthe, QC J2S 2M2, Canada

**Nahuel Fittipaldi**
Public Health Ontario Laboratory Toronto and Department of Laboratory Medicine and Pathobiology, University of Toronto, Toronto, ON, Canada

**Daniel Grenier**
Swine and Poultry Infectious Diseases Research Center (CRIPA), Saint-Hyacinthe, QC, Canada
Oral Ecology Research Group, Faculty of Dentistry, Laval University, Quebec City, QC, Canada

**José-Manuel Rojas and Noemí Sevilla**
Centro de Investigación en Sanidad Animal (CISA-INIA), Instituto Nacional de Investigación Agraria y Alimentaria, Ctra Algete a El Casar km 8, Valdeolmos, 28130 Madrid, Spain

**Teresa Rodríguez-Calvo**
Centro de Investigación en Sanidad Animal (CISA-INIA), Instituto Nacional de Investigación Agraria y Alimentaria, Ctra Algete a El Casar km 8, Valdeolmos, 28130 Madrid, Spain
Institute of Diabetes Research, Helmholtz Zentrum München, Deutsches Forschungszentrum für Gesundheit und Umwelt (GmbH), Neuherberg, Germany

**Nitin Machindra Kamble, Kim Je Hyoung and John Hwa Lee**
College of Veterinary Medicine, Chonbuk National University, Iksan Campus, Jeonju 570-752, Republic of Korea

**Barbara Brito, Carolina Stenfeldt and Helena C. de Carvalho Ferreira**
Foreign Animal Disease Research Unit, Plum Island Animal Disease Center, ARS, USDA, Orient Point, NY, USA
Oak Ridge Institute for Science and Education, PIADC Research Participation Program, Oak Ridge, TN, USA

**Steven J. Pauszek, Luis L. Rodriguez and Jonathan Arzt**
Foreign Animal Disease Research Unit, Plum Island Animal Disease Center, ARS, USDA, Orient Point, NY, USA

**Michael Eschbaumer**
Foreign Animal Disease Research Unit, Plum Island Animal Disease Center, ARS, USDA, Orient Point, NY, USA
Oak Ridge Institute for Science and Education, PIADC Research Participation Program, Oak Ridge, TN, USA
Friedrich-Loeffler-Institut, Federal Research Institute for Animal Health, Insel Riems, Germany

**Le T. Vu, Nguyen T. Phuong, Bui H. Hoang and Ngo T. Long**
Regional Animal Health Office No. 6, Department of Animal Health, Ministry of Agriculture and Rural Development, Ho Chi Minh City, Vietnam

**Nguyen D. Tho**
National Centre for Veterinary Diagnostics, Hanoi, Vietnam

**Pham V. Dong, Phan Q. Minh and Do H. Dung**
Department of Animal Health, Ministry of Agriculture and Rural Development, Hanoi, Vietnam

**Donald P. King and Nick J. Knowles**
The Pirbright Institute, Pirbright, UK

# Index

www.ingramcontent.com/pod-product-compliance
Lightning Source LLC
Chambersburg PA
CBHW082036190326
41458CB00010B/3383